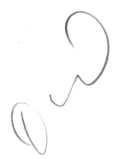

MW00344173

Comprehensive
Health Skills
for Middle School

Second Edition

by

Catherine A. Sanderson, PhD
Professor of Psychology
Amherst College
Amherst, Massachusetts

Mark Zelman, PhD
Professor of Biology
Aurora University
Aurora, Illinois

Pedagogy Developers

Lindsay Armbruster
Health Education Teacher
Burnt Hills, New York

Mary McCarley
National Health Education Specialist
National Board Certified Teacher in Health Education
Charlotte, North Carolina

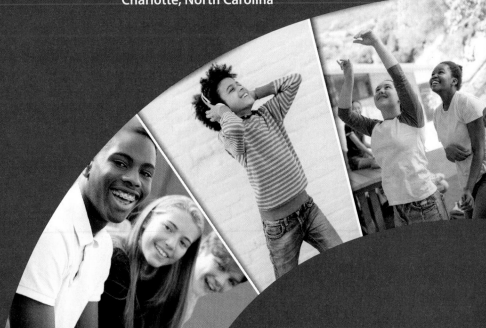

Publisher
The Goodheart-Willcox Company, Inc.
Tinley Park, Illinois
www.g-w.com

Introduction

We wrote this exciting textbook for middle school health and wellness classes based on our experiences as professors of psychology (Catherine Sanderson) and biology (Mark Zelman), and as the accomplished authors of high school and college-level textbooks. Our backgrounds give us a deep well of knowledge of the most current scientific theory and research to draw from.

Perhaps the most valuable experience we had in preparing us to write this book is our roles as parents to a combined total of seven children, ages 8 through 22. After all, in writing this book, we both reflected frequently on our experiences as parents and our goal of ensuring that our own children maintain excellent physical, mental and emotional, and social health.

This book includes all of the standard topics found in middle school health and wellness books—including self-talk, self-compassion, and self-care; body positivity, neutrality, and compassion; health effects of vaping; medication and drug abuse (including opioids); digital citizenship and personal digital footprint; affects of social media on physical, mental and emotional, and social health; and healthy relationships. We wanted our book to give middle school students the most current health information, presented in an engaging writing style so students would enjoy reading the book. Additionally, we included a focus on practical health skills that young people can use to develop and promote good health and wellness habits throughout their lives.

As the authors of high school and college-level textbooks, we felt confident in our research and writing abilities, but felt that the pedagogy was better left to health teachers. We would like to thank Lindsay Armbruster and Mary McCarley for developing the skills-based questions, activities, and features that are a vital part of this course. We are delighted with the final product, and wish all readers of this book a lifetime of good health.

About the Authors

Textbook Authors

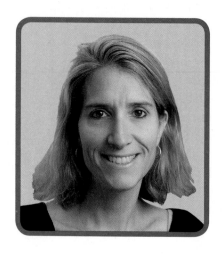

Catherine A. Sanderson is the Manwell Family Professor of Life Sciences (Psychology) at Amherst College. She received a bachelor's degree in psychology, with a specialization in Health and Development, from Stanford University, and received both master's and doctoral degrees in psychology from Princeton University. Professor Sanderson's research examines how personality and social variables influence health-related behaviors, such as safer sex and disordered eating. Her research also examines the development of persuasive messages and interventions to prevent unhealthy behavior and predictors of relationship satisfaction. This research has received grant funding from the National Science Foundation and the National Institutes of Health. Professor Sanderson has published more than 25 journal articles and book chapters; four college textbooks; high school and middle school health textbooks; and a trade book, *The Positive Shift*, which examines how mind-set influences happiness, health, and even how long people live. Her latest book, *Why We Act: Turning Bystanders into Moral Rebels*, examines why good people often stay silent or do nothing in the face of wrongdoing. In 2012, she was named one of the country's top 300 professors by the Princeton Review.

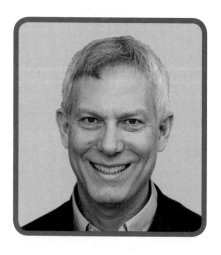

Mark Zelman is a Professor of Biology at Aurora University, Aurora, Illinois. He received a bachelor's degree in biology at Rockford College, with minors in chemistry and psychology. He received a PhD in microbiology and immunology at Loyola University of Chicago, where he studied the molecular and cellular mechanisms of autoimmune disease. During his postdoctoral research at the University of Chicago, he studied aspects of cell physiology pertaining to cell growth and cancer. Dr. Zelman supervises undergraduate research on streptococcal and staphylococcal infections, and mechanisms of antibiotic resistance. He teaches science education courses for high school teachers. He has published articles on microbiology, infectious disease, autoimmune disease, and biotechnology, and he has written two college texts on human diseases and infection control. Dr. Zelman works with the West Africa AIDS Foundation and other public health projects in the US and abroad. He is an officer of the Illinois State Academy of Sciences.

Pedagogy Developers

Lindsay Armbruster experiences, on a daily basis, the impact that positivity and happiness can have on a class, an individual, and on students' health behaviors. As a result, her teaching focuses on strengths and possibilities and is highly influenced by the theories of skills-based health education and positive psychology. Lindsay has been teaching Health Education since 2004, ranging all grade levels—kindergarten through twelfth grade as well as graduate school—with most of her experience occurring at the middle school level. Lindsay received her bachelor's degree in school and community health education from the State University of New York College at Brockport and her master degree in curriculum development and instructional technology from the University at Albany, while also completing coursework toward a master's degree in Public Health at the George Washington University. She is an award winner of the New York State Association for Health, Physical Education, Recreation and Dance (NYSAHPERD) Health Teacher of the Year award and the Society of Health & Physical Educators (SHAPE) America Eastern District Health Teacher of the Year award. Lindsay is a frequent presenter at local, state, and regional conferences.

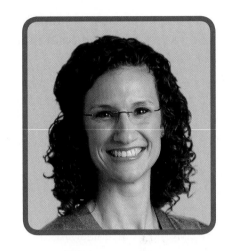

Mary McCarley is a National Health Education Specialist with 14 years of teaching experience in health education in Charlotte Mecklenburg Schools. She excels at creating an engaging student-centered environment with a focus on real-world learning. Mary graduated from UNC-Chapel Hill with an Exercise and Sports Science degree and East Carolina University with a Master of Arts in Education in Health Education. She is a National Board Certified Teacher in Health Education. In addition, Mary is the 2016 North Carolina High School Teacher of the Year for Health Education and the 2016 High School Southern District Teacher of the Year for the Advancement of Health Education. Mary presents at conferences and for school districts on various health education topics locally and nationally. She provides professional development and training for school districts to help teachers effectively implement skills-based health education curriculum.

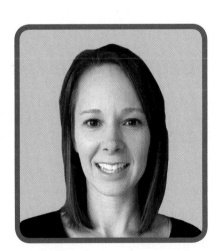

Reviewers

Professional Reviewers

Goodheart-Willcox Publisher would like to thank the following health professionals who reviewed selected chapters and contributed valuable input into the development of *Comprehensive Health Skills for Middle School*.

Jennifer Carroll, MSW
Resource Development
    Manager
National Eating Disorders
    Association
New York, New York

Michael Dorcas
Registered Pharmacist, Retired
Apple Valley, Minnesota

Pam Garramone, M.Ed.
Positive Psychology Keynote
    Speaker
pamgarramone.com
Quincy, Massachusetts

Shawn V. Giammattei, PhD
Psychologist
Quest Family Therapy
Santa Rosa, California

Courtney L. Hansen, PT, MPT, CMTPT
Physical Therapist/Owner
Fremont Therapy Group
Lander, Wyoming

Deb Kimberlin, PhD, RDN, LDN
Associate Professor
Olivet Nazarene University
Bourbonnais, Illinois

Linnea L. Mavrides, PsyD, CGP
Clinical Psychologist,
    Adjunct Professor
LIU-Post
Brookville, New York

Heather Noworatzky, MSED
School Counselor
Fond du Lac School District
Fond du Lac, Wisconsin

Rachael Woznick, RDN, CD
Renal Dietitian
Fresenius Medical Care
Milwaukee, Wisconsin

Teacher Reviewers

Goodheart-Willcox Publisher would like to thank the following teachers who reviewed selected chapters and contributed valuable input into the development of *Comprehensive Health Skills for Middle School*.

Gwyneth Aldridge
Randolph Middle School
Charlotte, North Carolina

Lynnea Allen
Wayzata East Middle School
Plymouth, Minnesota

Lindsay Armbruster
O'Rourke Middle School
Burnt Hills, New York

Kelsey Baker
Aliamanu Middle School
Honolulu, Hawaii

Heather Berlin
Harmon Middle School
Aurora, Ohio

Dawn Blevins
San Fernando Middle School
San Fernando, California

Scott Borowicz
Normandin Middle School
New Bedford, Massachusetts

Corbin Bray
Banks Trail Middle School
Fort Mill, South Carolina

Tammi Conn
Valley View School District
Romeoville, Illinois

Julie Connor
Wydown Middle School
Clayton, Missouri

Anita Dunham
Lexington Junior High School
Cypress, California

Cheryl Friske
Vernon Verona Sherrill
   Middle School
Verona, New York

Kim Gillick
Greenwich Middle School
Greenwich, Connecticut

Dwayne Hamlette
Amherst Middle School
Amherst, Virginia

Cathy Hawkins
Tri-North Middle School
Bloomington, Indiana

Emily Hill
Southern Hills Middle School
Boulder, Colorado

Diane Jones
Fairfield Middle School
Henrico, Virginia

Selene Kelley
Gahanna Middle School South
Gahanna, Ohio

Mike Kruse
Gilbert Middle School
Gilbert, Iowa

Dalis La
Stanford Middle School
Long Beach, California

Carleen Lawson
Hampton City School
Hampton, Virginia

Sheila Leamer
Chittenango Middle School
Chittenango, New York

Ben Leven
Twin Groves Middle School
Buffalo Grove, Illinois

Sarah Lewis
Rochester Community Schools
Rochester Hills, Michigan

Ashley Lubas
Ridley Middle School
Ridley Park, Pennsylvania

Charlie Means
Scott Middle School
Denison, Texas

Dawn Miller
Stewartville Middle School
Stewartville, Minnesota

Matthew Nichols
Lopez Middle School
San Antonio, Texas

Pam Nitsche
Madison Middle School
Trumbull, Connecticut

Judith R. Peters
School District of Philadelphia
Philadelphia, Pennsylvania

Marla Rickard
Suzanne Middle School
Walnut, California

Pam Riddle
Wayland Middle School
Wayland, Massachusetts

Misty Rodriguez
Jackson Middle School-NEISD
San Antonio, Texas

Jamie Rucci
Solon Middle School
Solon, Ohio

Tracey Rudnick
Bradley Middle School/NEISD
San Antonio, Texas

Susan Schoenrock
Stanley Middle School,
   Lafayette School District
Lafayette, California

Heidi Stan
Carmel Clay Schools
Carmel, Indiana

Shannon Todd
Lake Oswego Junior High
   School
Lake Oswego, Oregon

Craig Walter
Upper Moreland School District
Hatboro, Pennsylvania

Susie Woerner
Hinsdale Middle School
Hinsdale, Illinois

Brief Contents

Contents

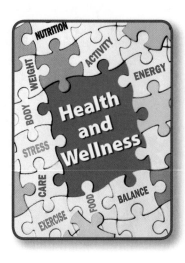

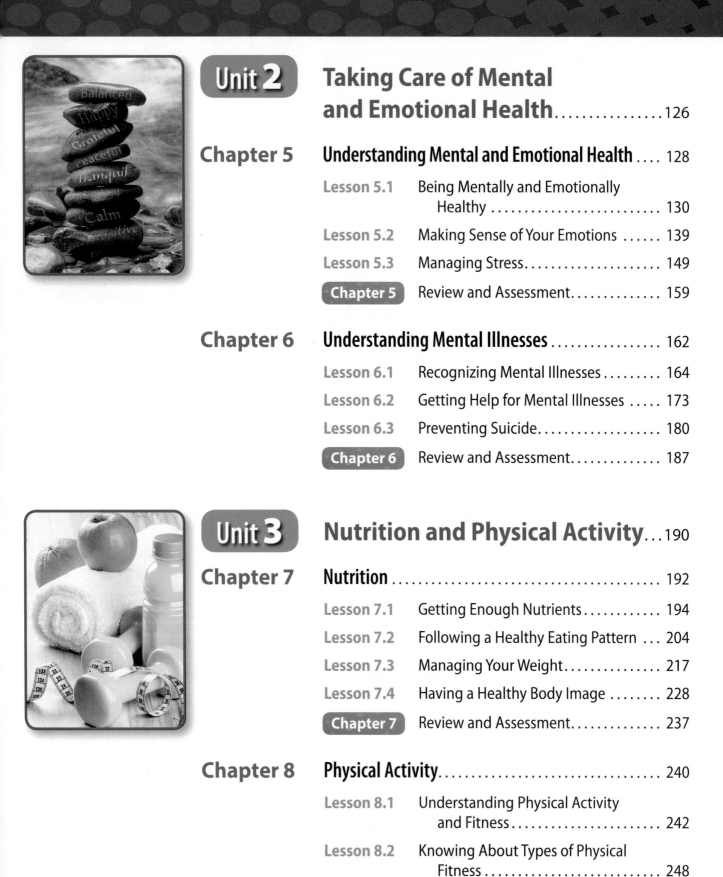

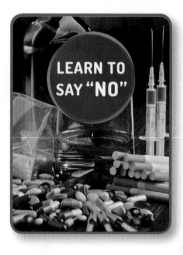
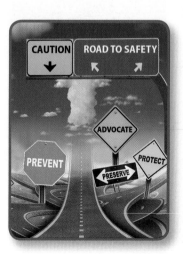

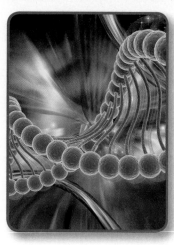

Infographics

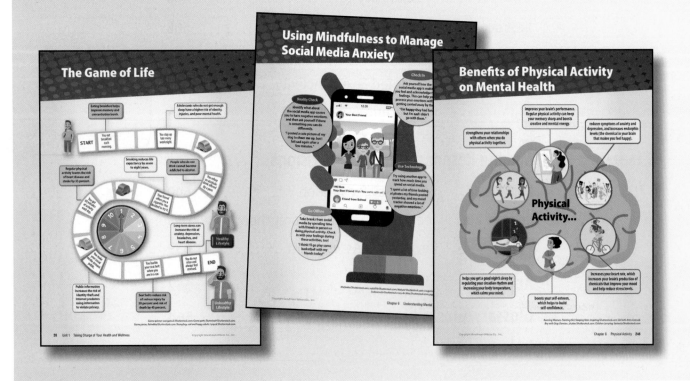

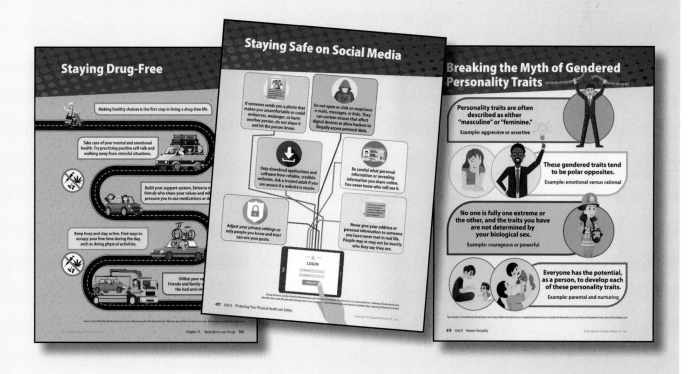

Features

To the Student

The best way to learn and develop your skills is not just to read, but to organize and apply the information you see. Getting ready to read and taking frequent breaks to complete activities can make reading seem less daunting. It can also help you remember information longer and understand it better. That is why this textbook does more than just *present* the information you need to know. It also contains features and activities to help you *understand* and *apply* what you learn. Knowing how to use these features will help you learn more quickly and effectively. To learn how best to use this textbook, join us on a walkthrough of a typical unit, chapter, and lesson.

Start with the Unit Opener

👁 1. Read the unit number and title.

👁 2. See what chapters are included in the unit. Think about what information you are excited to learn.

✏ 3. Complete the **Warm-Up Activity**. Some Warm-Up Activities ask you to come back to them after reading the chapters in the unit, so do not throw away your completed activity. Keep it so you can revisit it after reading the unit.

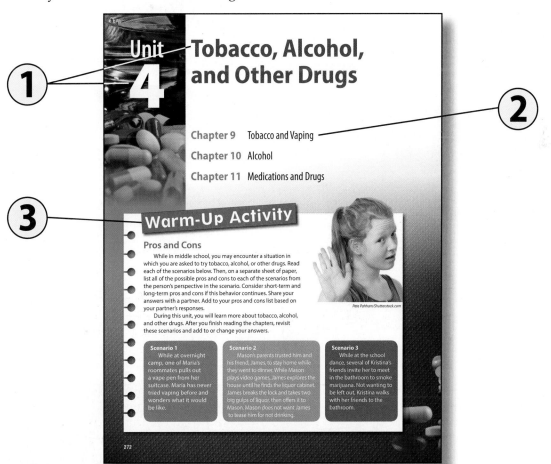

Read the Chapter Opener and Complete Chapter Opener Activities

1. Read the chapter number, title, and lessons included in the chapter. Think about questions you have that relate to each lesson.

2. Consider the **Essential Question**. You can discuss the question with your classmates and talk about related information you want to learn.

3. Complete the **Reading Activity**. The Reading Activity will help you understand and remember what you learn in the chapter.

4. Assess your own health habits using the **How Healthy Are You?** quiz. Answer "Yes" or "No" to each question and count your "Yes" or "No" answers. Use your answers to think about how you can improve your health.

5. Take a look at G-W Learning Companion Website feature. For each lesson, you can use flash cards and other vocabulary activities to remember key terms.

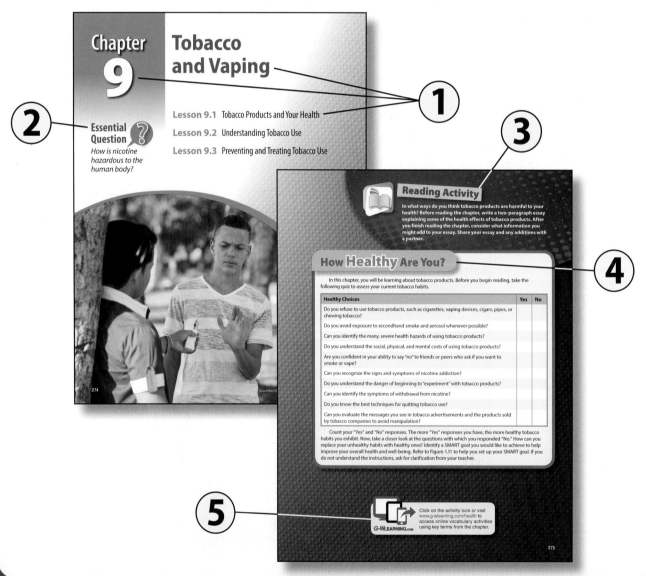

Chapter 9 — Tobacco and Vaping

Essential Question
How is nicotine hazardous to the human body?

Lesson 9.1 Tobacco Products and Your Health
Lesson 9.2 Understanding Tobacco Use
Lesson 9.3 Preventing and Treating Tobacco Use

Reading Activity

In what ways do you think tobacco products are harmful to your health? Before reading the chapter, write a two-paragraph essay explaining some of the health effects of tobacco products. After you finish reading the chapter, consider what information you might add to your essay. Share your essay and any additions with a partner.

How Healthy Are You?

In this chapter, you will be learning about tobacco products. Before you begin reading, take the following quiz to assess your current tobacco habits.

Healthy Choices	Yes	No
Do you refuse to use tobacco products, such as cigarettes, vaping devices, cigars, pipes, or chewing tobacco?		
Do you avoid exposure to secondhand smoke and aerosol whenever possible?		
Can you identify the many, severe health hazards of using tobacco products?		
Do you understand the social, physical, and mental costs of using tobacco products?		
Are you confident in your ability to say "no" to friends or peers who ask if you want to smoke or vape?		
Can you recognize the signs and symptoms of nicotine addiction?		
Do you understand the danger of beginning to "experiment" with tobacco products?		
Can you identify the symptoms of withdrawal from nicotine?		
Do you know the best techniques for quitting tobacco use?		
Can you evaluate the messages you see in tobacco advertisements and the products sold by tobacco companies to avoid manipulation?		

Count your "Yes" and "No" responses. The more "Yes" responses you have, the more healthy tobacco habits you exhibit. Now, take a closer look at the questions with which you responded "No." How can you replace your unhealthy habits with healthy ones? Identify a SMART goal you would like to achieve to help improve your overall health and well-being. Refer to Figure 1.11 to help you set up your SMART goal. If you do not understand the instructions, ask for clarification from your teacher.

Click on the activity icon or visit www.g-wlearning.com/health to access online vocabulary activities using key terms from the chapter.
G-WLEARNING.com

274

StevanMiles/S

275

Prepare to Read Each Lesson

1. Read the lesson number and title.
2. See what topics are covered in the lesson by reading the **Learning Outcomes**.
3. Look at the **Key Terms** in the lesson and read their definitions. You will learn more about these terms in the lesson. You will also see these definitions again in the **English and Spanish Glossary** in the back of the textbook.
4. Click on the activity icon or go to the G-W Learning Companion Website to use e-flash cards to review the terms.
5. Use the **Graphic Organizer** to take notes. You will need a separate piece of paper to create the organizer. Keep the organizer to help you study for the test.

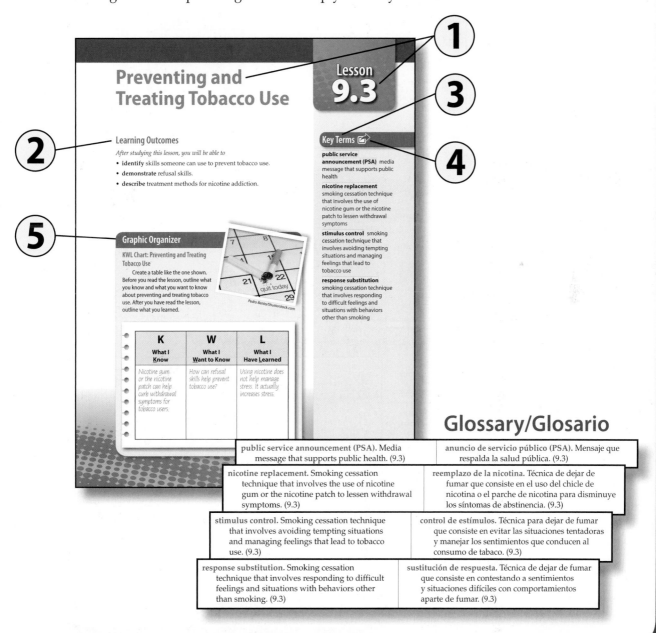

Preventing and Treating Tobacco Use

Lesson 9.3

Learning Outcomes

After studying this lesson, you will be able to

- **identify** skills someone can use to prevent tobacco use.
- **demonstrate** refusal skills.
- **describe** treatment methods for nicotine addiction.

Key Terms

public service announcement (PSA) media message that supports public health

nicotine replacement smoking cessation technique that involves the use of nicotine gum or the nicotine patch to lessen withdrawal symptoms

stimulus control smoking cessation technique that involves avoiding tempting situations and managing feelings that lead to tobacco use

response substitution smoking cessation technique that involves responding to difficult feelings and situations with behaviors other than smoking

Graphic Organizer

KWL Chart: Preventing and Treating Tobacco Use

Create a table like the one shown. Before you read the lesson, outline what you know and what you want to know about preventing and treating tobacco use. After you have read the lesson, outline what you learned.

Pedro Bento/Shutterstock.com

K	W	L
What I Know	What I Want to Know	What I Have Learned
Nicotine gum or the nicotine patch can help curb withdrawal symptoms for tobacco users.	How can refusal skills help prevent tobacco use?	Using nicotine does not help manage stress. It actually increases stress.

Glossary/Glosario

public service announcement (PSA). Media message that supports public health. (9.3)	anuncio de servicio público (PSA). Mensaje que respalda la salud pública. (9.3)
nicotine replacement. Smoking cessation technique that involves the use of nicotine gum or the nicotine patch to lessen withdrawal symptoms. (9.3)	reemplazo de la nicotina. Técnica de dejar de fumar que consiste en el uso del chicle de nicotina o el parche de nicotina para disminuye los síntomas de abstinencia. (9.3)
stimulus control. Smoking cessation technique that involves avoiding tempting situations and managing feelings that lead to tobacco use. (9.3)	control de estímulos. Técnica para dejar de fumar que consiste en evitar las situaciones tentadoras y manejar los sentimientos que conducen al consumo de tabaco. (9.3)
response substitution. Smoking cessation technique that involves responding to difficult feelings and situations with behaviors other than smoking. (9.3)	sustitución de respuesta. Técnica de dejar de fumar que consiste en contestando a sentimientos y situaciones difíciles con comportamientos aparte de fumar. (9.3)

Remember to Read the Captions and Features

1. As you are reading a lesson, do not forget to read the captions and features. Sometimes, captions have caption questions that you can answer to check your knowledge.

2. **Building Your Skills** features are activities that will help you act on the health skills you are learning.

3. **Case Study** features present lifelike scenarios in which young people have to make decisions about their health.

4. After reading each Case Study, complete the **Thinking Critically** questions. Discuss your answers with your classmates.

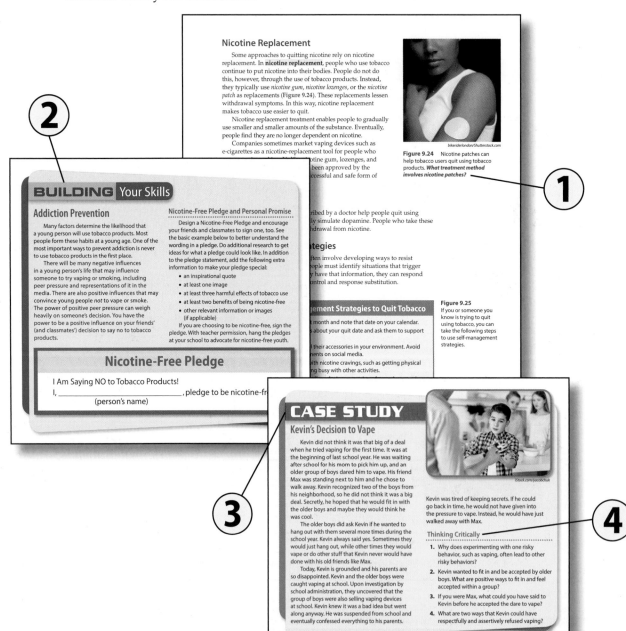

Nicotine Replacement

Some approaches to quitting nicotine rely on nicotine replacement. In **nicotine replacement**, people who use tobacco continue to put nicotine into their bodies. People do not do this, however, through the use of tobacco products. Instead, they typically use *nicotine gum, nicotine lozenges,* or the *nicotine patch* as replacements (Figure 9.24). These replacements lessen withdrawal symptoms. In this way, nicotine replacement makes tobacco use easier to quit.

Nicotine replacement treatment enables people to gradually use smaller and smaller amounts of the substance. Eventually, people find they are no longer dependent on nicotine.

Companies sometimes market vaping devices such as e-cigarettes as a nicotine-replacement tool for people who ... nicotine gum, lozenges, and ... been approved by the ... ccessful and safe form of ...

Figure 9.24 Nicotine patches can help tobacco users quit using tobacco products. *What treatment method involves nicotine patches?*

bikeriderlondon/Shutterstock.com

...ribed by a doctor help people quit using ...ly simulate dopamine. People who take these ...hdrawal from nicotine.

...tegies

...ften involve developing ways to resist ...ple must identify situations that trigger ...y have that information, they can respond ...ontrol and response substitution.

...ement Strategies to Quit Tobacco
...month and note that date on your calendar.
...s about your quit date and ask them to support

...l their accessories in your environment. Avoid ...ents on social media.
...with nicotine cravings, such as getting physical ...g busy with other activities.

Figure 9.25
If you or someone you know is trying to quit using tobacco, you can take the following steps to use self-management strategies.

BUILDING Your Skills

Addiction Prevention

Many factors determine the likelihood that a young person will use tobacco products. Most people form these habits at a young age. One of the most important ways to prevent addiction is never to use tobacco products in the first place.

There will be many negative influences in a young person's life that may influence someone to try vaping or smoking, including peer pressure and representations of it in the media. There are also positive influences that may convince young people *not* to vape or smoke. The power of positive peer pressure can weigh heavily on someone's decision. You have the power to be a positive influence on your friends' (and classmates') decision to say no to tobacco products.

Nicotine-Free Pledge and Personal Promise

Design a Nicotine-Free Pledge and encourage your friends and classmates to sign one, too. See the basic example below to better understand the wording in a pledge. Do additional research to get ideas for what a pledge could look like. In addition to the pledge statement, add the following extra information to make your pledge special:

- an inspirational quote
- at least one image
- at least three harmful effects of tobacco use
- at least two benefits of being nicotine-free
- other relevant information or images (if applicable)

If you are choosing to be nicotine-free, sign the pledge. With teacher permission, hang the pledges at your school to advocate for nicotine-free youth.

Nicotine-Free Pledge

I Am Saying NO to Tobacco Products!

I, _____, pledge to be nicotine-fr...
     (person's name)

CASE STUDY

Kevin's Decision to Vape

Kevin did not think it was that big of a deal when he tried vaping for the first time. It was at the beginning of last school year. He was waiting after school for his mom to pick him up, and an older group of boys dared him to vape. His friend Max was standing next to him and he chose to walk away. Kevin recognized two of the boys from his neighborhood, so he did not think it was a big deal. Secretly, he hoped that he would fit in with the older boys and maybe they would think he was cool.

The older boys did ask Kevin if he wanted to hang out with them several more times during the school year. Kevin always said yes. Sometimes they would just hang out, while other times they would vape or do other stuff that Kevin never would have done with his old friends like Max.

Today, Kevin is grounded and his parents are so disappointed. Kevin and the older boys were caught vaping at school. Upon investigation by school administration, they uncovered that the group of boys were also selling vaping devices at school. Kevin knew it was a bad idea but went along anyway. He was suspended from school and eventually confessed everything to his parents.

iStock.com/jacobchuk

Kevin was tired of keeping secrets. If he could go back in time, he would not have given into the pressure to vape. Instead, he would have just walked away with Max.

Thinking Critically

1. Why does experimenting with one risky behavior, such as vaping, often lead to other risky behaviors?

2. Kevin wanted to fit in and be accepted by older boys. What are positive ways to fit in and feel accepted within a group?

3. If you were Max, what could you have said to Kevin before he accepted the dare to vape?

4. What are two ways that Kevin could have respectfully and assertively refused vaping?

Answer Questions About Each Lesson

1. A **Lesson Review** follows each lesson. Read the Lesson Review number.

2. Answer the first four questions, which will test your knowledge of what you learned in the lesson.

3. The fifth **Critical thinking** question will have you think more deeply about what you learned. Take some time to consider and write an answer to this question. Discuss your answer with your classmates.

4. Complete the **Hands-On Activity**, which will ask you to put your learning into practice. Many Hands-On Activities ask you to work with your classmates.

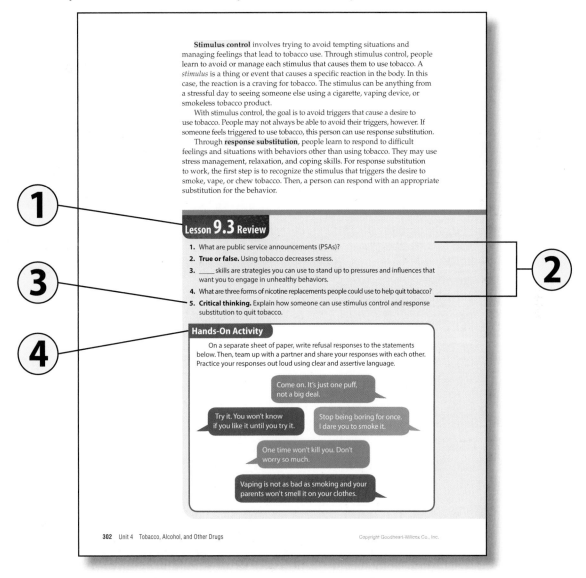

Stimulus control involves trying to avoid tempting situations and managing feelings that lead to tobacco use. Through stimulus control, people learn to avoid or manage each stimulus that causes them to use tobacco. A *stimulus* is a thing or event that causes a specific reaction in the body. In this case, the reaction is a craving for tobacco. The stimulus can be anything from a stressful day to seeing someone else using a cigarette, vaping device, or smokeless tobacco product.

With stimulus control, the goal is to avoid triggers that cause a desire to use tobacco. People may not always be able to avoid their triggers, however. If someone feels triggered to use tobacco, this person can use response substitution.

Through **response substitution**, people learn to respond to difficult feelings and situations with behaviors other than using tobacco. They may use stress management, relaxation, and coping skills. For response substitution to work, the first step is to recognize the stimulus that triggers the desire to smoke, vape, or chew tobacco. Then, a person can respond with an appropriate substitution for the behavior.

Lesson 9.3 Review

1. What are public service announcements (PSAs)?
2. **True or false.** Using tobacco decreases stress.
3. _____ skills are strategies you can use to stand up to pressures and influences that want you to engage in unhealthy behaviors.
4. What are three forms of nicotine replacements people could use to help quit tobacco?
5. **Critical thinking.** Explain how someone can use stimulus control and response substitution to quit tobacco.

Hands-On Activity

On a separate sheet of paper, write refusal responses to the statements below. Then, team up with a partner and share your responses with each other. Practice your responses out loud using clear and assertive language.

Come on. It's just one puff, not a big deal.

Try it. You won't know if you like it until you try it.

Stop being boring for once. I dare you to smoke it.

One time won't kill you. Don't worry so much.

Vaping is not as bad as smoking and your parents won't smell it on your clothes.

Recall What You Learned

1. Each chapter ends with a three-page chapter **Review and Assessment**. Start by reading the chapter number and heading.
2. Read each lesson number and title. Review the **Summary** for each lesson. While reading the bullets, look at your notes and add any information you missed.
3. Answer the **Check Your Knowledge** review questions.
4. Read the list of terms in the **Use Your Vocabulary** section.
5. Complete the vocabulary activities to review the meanings of the terms.
6. Click on the activity icon or go to the G-W Learning Companion Website to complete additional vocabulary activities online.

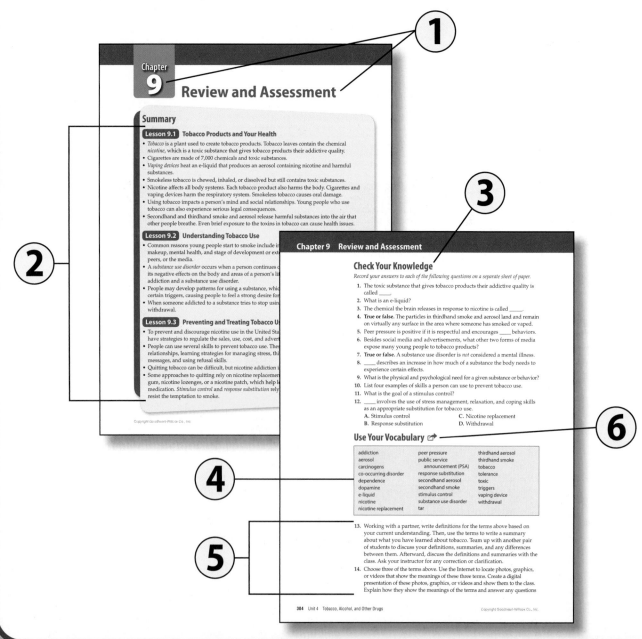

Act on What You Learned

1. The **Think Critically** questions ask you to think more deeply about what you learned in the chapter. Consider the questions and answer them. Some questions may need to be discussed with a partner or in small groups.

2. Complete the **Develop Your Skills** activities, which will help you improve your health and wellness skills. The type of skill the activity reinforces is bold and purple. Some activities involve working in groups and interacting with teachers and the community.

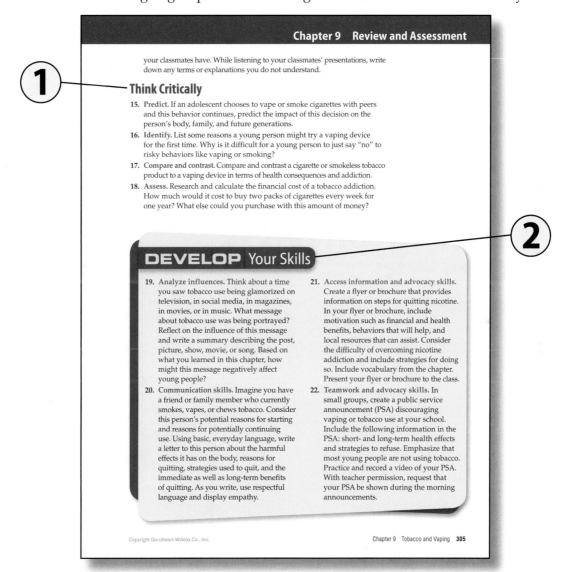

1

your classmates have. While listening to your classmates' presentations, write down any terms or explanations you do not understand.

Think Critically

15. **Predict.** If an adolescent chooses to vape or smoke cigarettes with peers and this behavior continues, predict the impact of this decision on the person's body, family, and future generations.

16. **Identify.** List some reasons a young person might try a vaping device for the first time. Why is it difficult for a young person to just say "no" to risky behaviors like vaping or smoking?

17. **Compare and contrast.** Compare and contrast a cigarette or smokeless tobacco product to a vaping device in terms of health consequences and addiction.

18. **Assess.** Research and calculate the financial cost of a tobacco addiction. How much would it cost to buy two packs of cigarettes every week for one year? What else could you purchase with this amount of money?

2

DEVELOP Your Skills

19. **Analyze influences.** Think about a time you saw tobacco use being glamorized on television, in social media, in magazines, in movies, or in music. What message about tobacco use was being portrayed? Reflect on the influence of this message and write a summary describing the post, picture, show, movie, or song. Based on what you learned in this chapter, how might this message negatively affect young people?

20. **Communication skills.** Imagine you have a friend or family member who currently smokes, vapes, or chews tobacco. Consider this person's potential reasons for starting and reasons for potentially continuing use. Using basic, everyday language, write a letter to this person about the harmful effects it has on the body, reasons for quitting, strategies used to quit, and the immediate as well as long-term benefits of quitting. As you write, use respectful language and display empathy.

21. **Access information and advocacy skills.** Create a flyer or brochure that provides information on steps for quitting nicotine. In your flyer or brochure, include motivation such as financial and health benefits, behaviors that will help, and local resources that can assist. Consider the difficulty of overcoming nicotine addiction and include strategies for doing so. Include vocabulary from the chapter. Present your flyer or brochure to the class.

22. **Teamwork and advocacy skills.** In small groups, create a public service announcement (PSA) discouraging vaping or tobacco use at your school. Include the following information in the PSA: short- and long-term health effects and strategies to refuse. Emphasize that most young people are not using tobacco. Practice and record a video of your PSA. With teacher permission, request that your PSA be shown during the morning announcements.

Now that you understand how to use this textbook, you are ready to begin your study of health and wellness skills. If you are ever not sure how to use a feature of the textbook, revisit this walkthrough. Remember to take advantage of the activities in this textbook. They will help you not only know information, but also apply it and use it in your life.

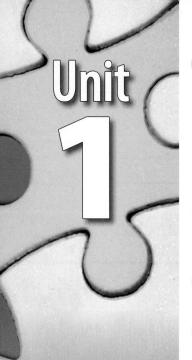

Unit 1

Taking Charge of Your Health and Wellness

Warm-Up Activity

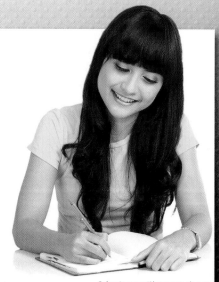

Odua Images/Shutterstock.com

Health Advice: Ask Avalon

Avalon is the regular advice columnist for your middle school newspaper. She has asked you to respond to the following letter she received from someone asking for advice:

Dear Avalon,

My dad has been in the hospital for the last two days. I overheard the doctor tell my mom that he would be okay, but needs to live a healthier life. While I'm only 13, I want to be healthy, too. I know it is important to take care of my health, but I'm not sure how to do it. Can you give me some advice on how to be healthy today and as I age?

Thanks,
Anonymous

When asked a difficult question, even an advice columnist will seek the help of a friend. Work with a partner to respond to Anonymous. Give at least four suggestions on how to be healthy. Include information on physical, mental and emotional, and social health. Give a detailed response and provide examples. Begin your response with "Dear Anonymous."

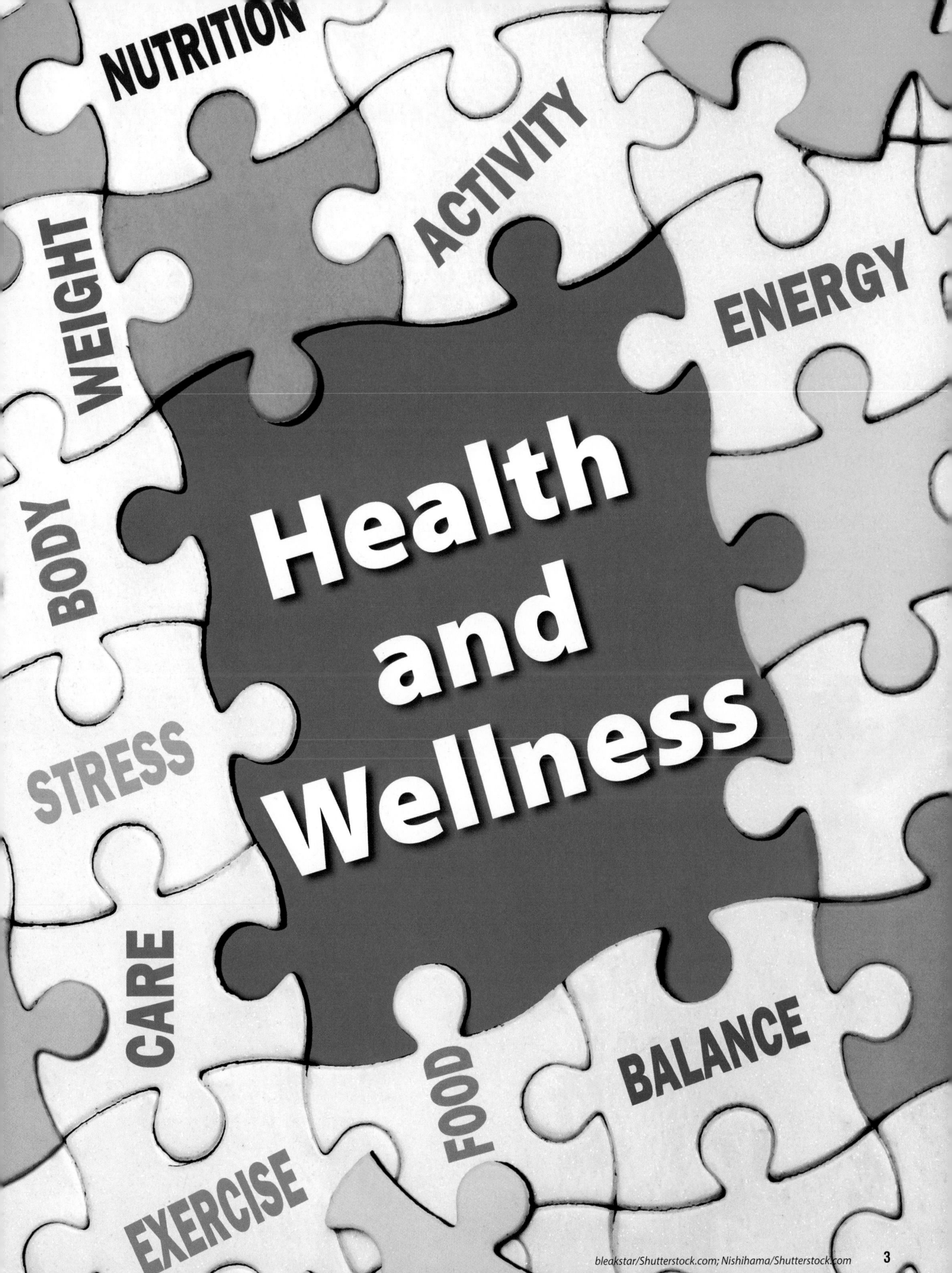

Health and Wellness

NUTRITION

ACTIVITY

WEIGHT

ENERGY

BODY

STRESS

CARE

FOOD

EXERCISE

BALANCE

Chapter 1

Understanding Your Health and Wellness

Essential Question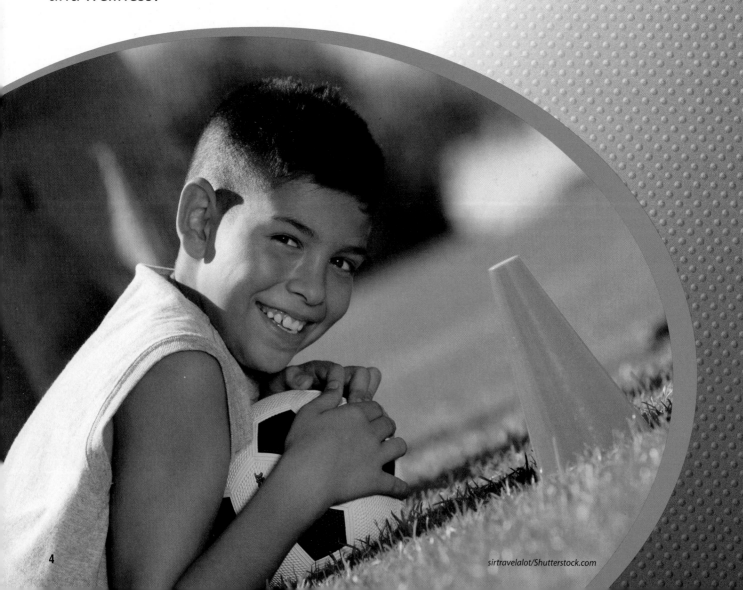

What is the difference between health and wellness?

Lesson 1.1 Learning About Health and Wellness

Lesson 1.2 Recognizing Factors That Affect Health and Wellness

Lesson 1.3 Building Skills for Health and Wellness

sirtravelalot/Shutterstock.com

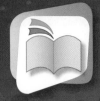

Reading Activity

List the headings in this chapter to create an outline for taking notes during reading and class discussion. Under each heading, list any key terms. Finally, write two questions you expect to have answered in class. After completing the chapter, ask your teacher any questions you still have about the concepts or terms you learned.

How Healthy Are You?

In this chapter, you will be learning about health and wellness. Before you begin reading, take the following quiz to assess your current health and wellness habits.

Healthy Choices	Yes	No
Do you regularly set short-term and long-term goals that are specific, measurable, achievable, relevant, and timely?		
Do you set a series of short-term goals to help you meet a long-term goal?		
Do you assume responsibility for your personal health behaviors?		
Do you avoid spending time with friends or family who engage in harmful behaviors such as smoking or bullying?		
Can you maintain mature relationships by respecting and valuing others and yourself?		
Do you cope well with stress?		
Can you identify reliable sources of health-related information?		
Do you clearly and honestly communicate your thoughts and feelings to others?		
Do you refuse to do things that go against your values and beliefs, regardless of what your friends and family do or say?		
Do you consider the impact of your decisions on others?		
Are you confident in your ability to learn and apply new knowledge, viewing learning as a chance to continually improve yourself?		

Count your "Yes" and "No" responses. The more "Yes" responses you have, the more habits you exhibit for promoting health and wellness. Now, take a closer look at the questions with which you responded "No." How can you make these healthy habits part of your daily life? Identify a SMART goal you would like to achieve to help improve your overall health and well-being. Refer to Figure 1.11 to help you set up your SMART goal. If you do not understand the instructions, ask for clarification from your teacher.

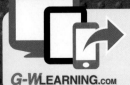

Click on the activity icon or visit www.g-wlearning.com/health to access online vocabulary activities using key terms from the chapter.

Learning About Health and Wellness

Key Terms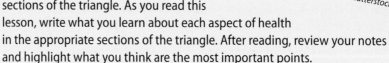

health state of complete physical, mental and emotional, and social well-being

well-being person's overall satisfaction that life's present conditions are good

wellness active process that involves becoming aware of and making choices toward improving aspects of health

physical health aspect of health that refers to how well a person's body functions

mental and emotional health aspect of health that has to do with a person's thoughts and feelings

social health aspect of health that involves interacting and getting along with others in positive, healthy ways

healthcare treatment and prevention of illnesses, injuries, or diseases to improve wellness

preventive healthcare going to the doctor when you are well to help you stay healthy; involves getting an annual physical exam, regular checkups, and screenings for conditions such as hearing or vision loss

Learning Outcomes

After studying this lesson, you will be able to

- **identify** the aspects of health and wellness.
- **describe** how the aspects of health are interrelated.
- **explain** how appropriate healthcare can promote personal health.

Graphic Organizer

The Health Triangle

Write *Health and Wellness* in the center of a triangle like the one shown. Then, add *physical*, *mental and emotional*, and *social* in the remaining sections of the triangle. As you read this lesson, write what you learn about each aspect of health in the appropriate sections of the triangle. After reading, review your notes and highlight what you think are the most important points.

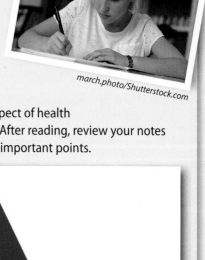

march.photo/Shutterstock.com

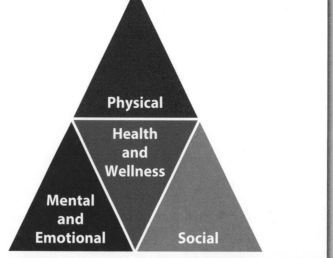

According to her doctor, 13-year-old Hannah passed her physical exam with flying colors and is the picture of health. At home, however, Hannah is often under stress and gets so anxious that she cannot sleep or focus on her schoolwork. She is frequently tired and eats on the go. She quit the soccer team and took up smoking with her boyfriend and his friends. Hannah avoids making decisions and planning for her future. Instead, she prefers to "go with the flow."

Aiden, also 13, was born with a breathing condition that makes running and playing most sports difficult. He manages his condition by following his doctor's orders. He takes his medicine, makes sure to eat well, and gets plenty of sleep. He also gets a moderate amount of physical activity. He does not smoke or drink. Aiden's positive attitude attracts other people to him, so he has many friends. He sets goals for his future, and is confident that he will succeed if he works hard.

So who do you think is healthier—Hannah or Aiden? Is Hannah healthier because her doctor said she is the picture of health? Is Aiden healthier because he seems to take better care of himself overall?

In this lesson, you will learn about the different aspects of health and wellness and overall well-being. You will also discover the connections between healthcare and wellness.

Aspects of Health and Wellness

The *World Health Organization (WHO)* is an international organization that promotes health across the world. The WHO defines **health** as not just the absence of disease, but as a state of complete physical, mental and emotional, and social well-being. **Well-being** refers to a person's overall satisfaction that life's present conditions are good. **Figure 1.1** shows common characteristics that describe people in a state of well-being.

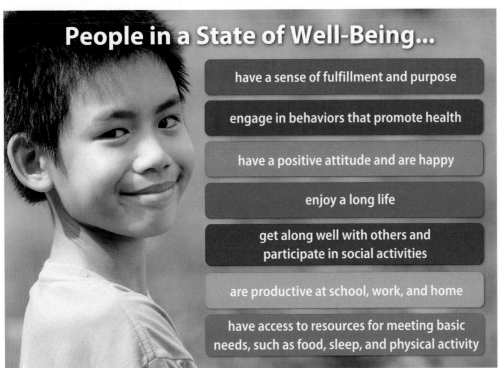

People in a State of Well-Being...

- have a sense of fulfillment and purpose
- engage in behaviors that promote health
- have a positive attitude and are happy
- enjoy a long life
- get along well with others and participate in social activities
- are productive at school, work, and home
- have access to resources for meeting basic needs, such as food, sleep, and physical activity

Sanmongkohl/Shutterstock.com

Figure 1.1
How you feel about yourself and your life affects your well-being. People who have a positive attitude and are happy often experience a higher level of well-being. *How would you describe your well-being? Are there steps you could take to improve your well-being?*

To achieve health, people practice wellness. *Wellness* is an active process that involves becoming aware of and making choices toward improving aspects of health. As you practice wellness, remember to consider all aspects of your health. This includes your physical health, mental and emotional health, and social health.

Physical Health

Physical health is the aspect of health that refers to how your body functions. If you have a physically healthy body, your body functions well. You are able to engage in the activities of daily life. You can also cope with the stresses of disease, injury, and aging and maintain an active lifestyle. In other words, being physically healthy enables you to do more than walk to school or lift a bag of books. You can recover from a sprained ankle, fight off the flu, and have the energy to cope with daily stresses.

Defining Mental and Emotional Health

Mental Health
- Describes how you observe and interpret information.
- Affects your ability to make decisions, solve problems, and examine situations.

Emotional Health
- Refers to how you express yourself and your thoughts and feelings.
- Your emotions, mood, feelings about yourself, and way of viewing the world are all parts of your emotional health.

Figure 1.2 While mental health and emotional health are related, they are not exactly the same.

Mental and Emotional Health

Your **mental and emotional health** has to do with your internal life—your thoughts and feelings (**Figure 1.2**). When you have good mental and emotional health, you can think clearly and critically. You can express your thoughts and feelings. You can cope well with stress. You can also realize your own skills and have a positive attitude and willingness to adapt, learn, and grow.

Sometimes people do not realize they are experiencing challenges with mental and emotional health. For example, ongoing feelings of sadness or worry are not healthy. These ongoing negative feelings can keep you from doing well in school or joining in your favorite activities. Ongoing negative feelings can also affect your sleep, diet, and activity level, and prevent you from forming healthy friendships. The good news is that treatment and skills for maintaining your mental and emotional health can help you feel better.

Social Health

Can you imagine your life with no human interaction? Living without contact from others is unhealthy. Humans are social animals who must interact and communicate with one another. **Social health** refers to how well you get along with other people.

Being socially healthy means having enjoyable and supportive relationships with others. In healthy relationships, you talk openly and honestly with family and friends. You trust others and others trust you. These are important parts of healthy relationships.

Unhealthy relationships are those that cause harm or make you feel bad about yourself. Social skills and healthy relationships give you the support you need to enjoy life and meet its challenges. Healthy relationships are among your most valuable resources.

Skills for Practicing Wellness

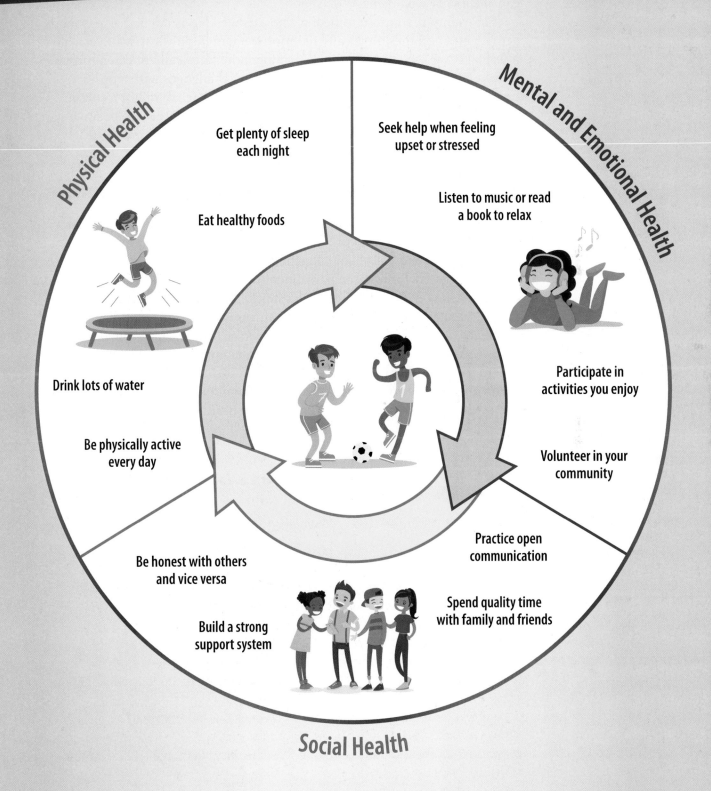

Physical Health

Get plenty of sleep each night

Eat healthy foods

Drink lots of water

Be physically active every day

Mental and Emotional Health

Seek help when feeling upset or stressed

Listen to music or read a book to relax

Participate in activities you enjoy

Volunteer in your community

Social Health

Be honest with others and vice versa

Build a strong support system

Practice open communication

Spend quality time with family and friends

Circular arrows: Arcady/Shutterstock.com; Center Photo and Trampoline: NotionPic/Shutterstock.com; Music and Group of Kids: Visual Generation/Shutterstock.com

How the Aspects of Health Are Interrelated

The aspects of your health are *interrelated*, meaning they all interact with and affect each other (**Figure 1.3**). Decline in one aspect of your health may lead to decline in another. Likewise, an improvement in one aspect of your health may lead to improvements in other aspects. Any changes in your health can affect your well-being.

For example, suppose someone who eats well but is not active gets more activity and becomes physically fit. Improvement in physical health can also affect all other aspects of health. Becoming more physically fit can improve how you feel about yourself and help you face challenges with a positive outlook (mental and emotional health). Being more active might result in participating in new activities with friends (social health). These positive changes can improve your overall health and well-being.

How Healthcare Promotes Personal Health

Healthcare directly relates to personal health and wellness. **Healthcare** involves the treatment and prevention of illnesses, injuries, or diseases to improve health and well-being. Practicing wellness means that you do not only go to the doctor to receive treatment when you are sick. You also go to the doctor when you are well to help you stay healthy (called *preventive healthcare*). **Preventive healthcare** involves getting an annual physical exam, regular checkups, and screenings for conditions such as hearing or vision loss.

In the United States, healthcare comes in many forms, takes place in different settings, and is delivered by many types of professionals. The following sections will introduce you to different types of healthcare services and settings, and explore how people pay for healthcare.

Figure 1.3
Only by paying attention to and practicing wellness in *each* aspect of health can people achieve good health and well-being. *What does the term* interrelated *mean?*

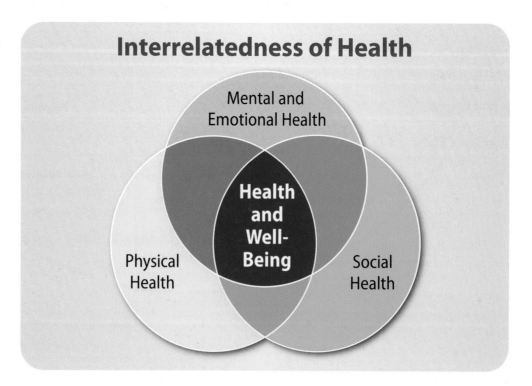

Interrelatedness of Health

Mental and Emotional Health

Health and Well-Being

Physical Health

Social Health

Healthcare Services

The healthcare field employs more people than any other type of business in the United States. The field is diverse and includes many types of professions and healthcare services. Some professions provide highly specialized services.

People usually see their *primary care physician* (regular doctor) to get routine checkups, diagnosis of conditions, and receive medical treatment. Physician assistants and nurse practitioners also provide primary care.

The *physician assistant* works under the supervision of physicians and usually provides the same types of healthcare services as a physician. A *nurse practitioner* has an advanced nursing education and can provide many of the same services as a doctor. Today, many people receive their primary care from physicians, physician assistants, and nurse practitioners.

Primary care physicians may also refer their patients to *specialists* who possess extra training and experience with certain types of diseases and disorders. **Figure 1.4** shows the common types of specialists and the care they provide.

CASE STUDY

A Day in the Life of Sarah

Next year, Sarah will be off to high school and almost old enough to get a job. Her mom works so hard, but there never seems to be enough money. As the oldest, it is Sarah's responsibility to take care of her younger siblings when her mom is at work. Sarah works so hard to take care of everyone else that she often does not take time to care for herself.

Sarah learned in school about the importance of eating healthy and being physically active to promote positive health. Sarah is always so busy, though. She finds it a lot easier to grab some fast food at the restaurant down the street or some snacks at the nearby gas station on her way home from school. Sarah recently noticed that she has gained some weight.

Due to her mom's work schedule, Sarah cannot remember the last time she visited a doctor for a yearly check, until today that is. Sarah had to see the doctor because she has been thirsty and tired all the time, and her vision is blurred. The doctor informed Sarah's mother that Sarah's blood work indicated that she has type 2 diabetes and she needs to eat better to improve her health. She also has to take medicine now and check the level of sugar in her blood every day.

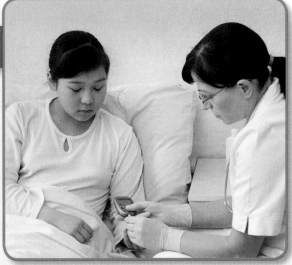

anetta/Shutterstock.com

Thinking Critically

1. How could preventive care have decreased the likelihood of Sarah's diagnosis of type 2 diabetes?

2. How might Sarah's life be different if Sarah and her mother received the guidance of a healthcare provider, such as a pediatrician?

3. If you were Sarah's doctor, what advice would you give Sarah and her mom to improve Sarah's health? Consider Sarah's obstacles to healthy eating and mental and physical activity.

4. How could Sarah's poor physical health affect her social and mental and emotional health?

Figure 1.4
Physician specialists
are expertly educated
and trained in their
particular fields.
*What type of specialist is
a dermatologist?*

Physician Specialists

Specialist	Treatment of...
Cardiologist	heart disease
Dermatologist	skin conditions
Gastroenterologist	diseases and disorders of the digestive system
Neurologist	diseases and disorders of the brain, nerves, and spinal cord
Oncologist	cancer
Orthopedist	bones, joints, and muscle conditions
Pediatrician	medical conditions of children from infancy through adolescence
Psychiatrist	mental illnesses and disorders
Pulmonologist	breathing issues and lung diseases
Rheumatologist	diseases of the joints, such as arthritis
Surgeon	surgical issues, such as gallbladder or appendix removal
Urologist	urination issues

Healthcare Settings

Healthcare workers work in inpatient and outpatient facilities. *Inpatient facilities* are hospitals where patients stay while they receive diagnosis, treatment, surgery, and therapy. *Outpatient facilities* treat patients who live in the community and who do not require a hospital. Most healthcare in the United States is delivered in outpatient settings. These settings include the following:

- doctors' offices and private healthcare clinics that provide checkups, physical therapy, outpatient surgery, counseling, addiction treatment, and eye and dental care
- hospital emergency rooms
- urgent care or walk-in clinics
- health clinics and counseling centers in high schools and colleges
- county public health clinics

Health Insurance

Healthcare is expensive, and most people cannot afford to pay the full cost of services. Instead, most people buy insurance to help pay for healthcare costs. Most people get insurance through their employer or purchase insurance from a health insurance marketplace. Other health insurance options, available through the United States government, include Medicare and Medicaid. *Medicare* is insurance available for people 65 years of age and older. *Medicaid* pays for healthcare costs of people living in poverty, pregnant people, older adults, and people with disabilities. Because of the *Patient Protection and Affordable Care Act (ACA)*, young people can get coverage through their parents' or guardians' insurance through age 26.

There are two main types of insurance plans available for people to buy to help pay for healthcare costs. These plans are the *health maintenance organization (HMO)* and the *preferred provider organization (PPO)*. **Figure 1.5** describes these two plans.

Main Types of Insurance Plans

HMO

- Pays for the costs of basic healthcare services and many other specialized services
- Users must use doctors, hospitals, clinics, and services that are members of the HMO network

PPO

- Pays for the costs of healthcare provided by doctors, healthcare providers, and hospitals
- Allows for more flexibility in choosing providers, but is more expensive

Figure 1.5
Understanding the differences between a PPO and an HMO can help people choose the best plan to meet their needs. *Which type of plan—a PPO or an HMO—is most likely to cost less?*

Although insurance can help some people afford healthcare services, other individuals still cannot access healthcare. Barriers to accessing healthcare may include the following:

- lack of availability
- high cost
- lack of insurance coverage

Without adequate healthcare, people cannot receive the care they need. As a result, they are more likely to have poor health status.

Lesson 1.1 Review

1. Describe the difference between health and wellness.
2. **True or false.** Focusing on wellness means that you go to the doctor to receive treatment only when you are sick.
3. The regular doctor patients see for routine checkups and medical treatment is a(n) _____.
4. What term involves getting an annual physical exam, regular checkups, and screenings for conditions such as hearing or vision loss?
5. How can healthcare help people promote personal health?
6. **Critical thinking.** Explain how a decline in mental and emotional health can affect the other aspects of health.

Hands-On Activity

Working in groups of three, create a digital or paper collage that includes at least five magazine pictures of healthy behaviors for one aspect of health: physical, mental and emotional, or social. Add captions to your photos as needed to clarify pictures. Show and discuss your collage in a group of four or five classmates. Are the other members of your group able to determine which aspect of health you tried to represent?

Recognizing Factors That Affect Health and Wellness

Key Terms 🖝

genes segments of DNA that determine the structure and function of a person's cells and affect individual development, personality, and health

risk factors aspects of people's lives that increase the chance of a disease, injury, or decline in health

environment circumstances, objects, or conditions that surround a person in everyday life

protective factors aspects of people's lives that reduce risk and increase the likelihood of optimal health

peers people who are similar in age to one another

culture beliefs, values, customs, and arts of a group of people

Learning Outcomes

After studying this lesson, you will be able to

- **identify** factors that can increase or reduce your level of health and wellness.
- **describe** actions you can take to help prevent genetically linked diseases and disorders.
- **give examples** of risk and protective factors within a person's physical, social, and economic environments.
- **evaluate** how the lifestyle choices you make now can affect your health and wellness in the future.

Graphic Organizer

Health and Wellness Risk Factors

While you are reading this lesson, think about the important facts you discover and areas you still question. After you finish reading, fill in a T-chart like the one shown.

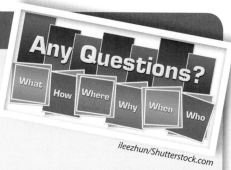

ileezhun/Shutterstock.com

Discoveries	Questions
There are factors that can increase or reduce my level of health and wellness. Some of these factors are within my control.	What factors can affect my health and wellness that are <u>not</u> within my control?

How would you describe your current health status? Are you in excellent health, or are you in poor health? Do you fall somewhere in between? If you have *optimal health*, you have the best health possible. You are in a state of excellent health and wellness in all areas of your life. This includes your physical, mental and emotional, and social health. A person's health status normally lies somewhere between the extremes of poor and excellent. This is because most people experience one or more factors that put their health status somewhere in the middle of the health and wellness spectrum.

Recall the examples of Hannah and Aiden from Lesson 1.1. Hannah passed her physical exam, but her health is far from excellent. Factors such as her stress, anxiety, and smoking habit negatively impact her health. On the other hand, Aiden has some physical health issues, but he does not smoke or drink, and he has a positive outlook on life. Hannah and Aiden each fall somewhere in the middle of the health and wellness spectrum.

As you can see in **Figure 1.6**, there are factors that can increase or reduce your level of health and wellness. Some factors, such as genetic factors, are not within your control. Many factors, however, are within your control. For example, a person who smokes can improve health and wellness by quitting smoking. The choices you make now largely determine your level of health and wellness, both today and in the future. By taking responsibility for the factors you *do* control and making healthy, informed decisions, you can improve all areas of your health.

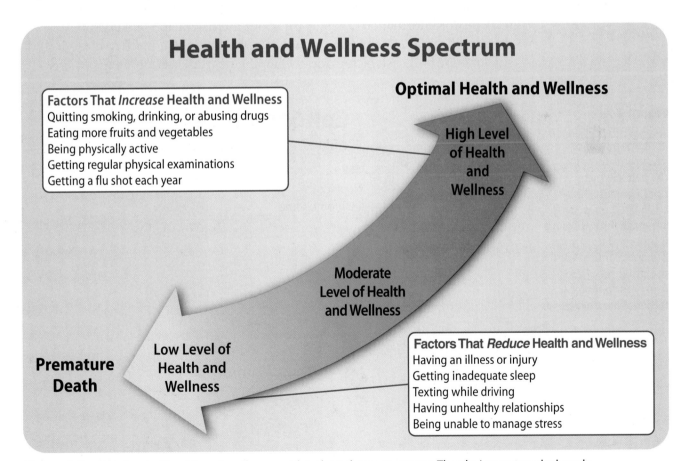

Health and Wellness Spectrum

Optimal Health and Wellness

Factors That *Increase* Health and Wellness
Quitting smoking, drinking, or abusing drugs
Eating more fruits and vegetables
Being physically active
Getting regular physical examinations
Getting a flu shot each year

High Level of Health and Wellness

Moderate Level of Health and Wellness

Premature Death

Low Level of Health and Wellness

Factors That *Reduce* Health and Wellness
Having an illness or injury
Getting inadequate sleep
Texting while driving
Having unhealthy relationships
Being unable to manage stress

Figure 1.6 Your level of health and wellness can be plotted on a spectrum. The choices you make largely determine where you are on the spectrum. *What kind of health do you have if you are at the top of the health and wellness spectrum?*

Genetic Factors

Genetic factors relate to your genes. Your **genes** are present in every cell in your body. They contain the blueprint for the structure and function of your cells. Genes direct how you grow and develop, influence your personality, and affect your health. Humans have 20,000 to 25,000 genes, which are composed of a chemical often referred to as *DNA*.

Located in a cell's nucleus, genes are bundled in packages called *chromosomes* (**Figure 1.7**). Humans inherit half of their chromosomes from each biological parent. The unique combination of genes from your parents determines many of your characteristics. For example, your nose might be shaped like one parent's nose. You and one parent may both have red, wavy hair. Perhaps you have blue eyes like your parents.

The genes you receive from your parents can affect your health and wellness by putting you at risk for developing certain diseases, such as heart disease. In this way, your family influences your health. To determine a person's genetic *risk factors* for developing a disease, doctors study a person's *family history*, the record of disease within a family. **Risk factors** are aspects of people's lives that increase the chance of a disease, injury, or decline in health. Although you cannot change the genes you receive, there are actions you can take to reduce the risk factors for developing genetically linked diseases and disorders.

The first step is to learn about your family's history of diseases. Do you have a family history of heart disease, cancer, or diabetes? Ask your biological relatives for information. Then, learn about the risk factors linked to the diseases that run in your family. For example, leading an inactive lifestyle and smoking are both risk factors for developing heart disease.

Figure 1.7
Each cell in your body contains a total of 46 chromosomes (23 pairs), which hold about 20,000 to 25,000 genes. One set of 23 chromosomes is inherited from your biological mother and the other set of 23 is from your biological father. *Where are genes located?*

Cell Structure

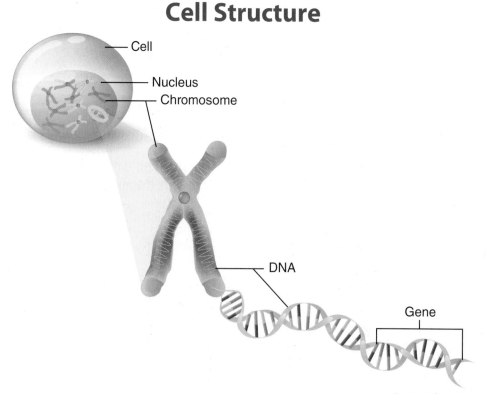

Cell

Nucleus

Chromosome

DNA

Gene

Designua/Shutterstock.com

Once you have this information, you can try to eliminate or reduce your risk factors for these diseases. Eliminating extra risk factors for a certain disease will lower your chances of getting that disease. Reducing these risk factors is just another way you can improve your health and wellness.

Environmental Factors

Environmental factors concern your environment. Your **environment** includes the circumstances, objects, or conditions that surround you. Every environment has risk factors that can affect health and wellness. The more you are exposed to risk factors within your environment, the more likely those factors are to reduce your level of health and wellness. Every environment also has protective factors. **Protective factors** are aspects of people's lives that reduce risk and increase the likelihood of good health. **Figure 1.8** shows examples of environmental protective and risk factors.

Physical Environment

Your *physical environment* consists of the places where you spend your time, such as your school, home, or community. Physical environment also consists of the region in which you live, the air you breathe, and the water you drink.

Risk factors within your physical environment differ from region to region, home to home, and school to school. Some hazards may include weather conditions, pollution, violence, unsafe drinking water, and other unsafe conditions. Certain hazards may depend on the policies at your school or in your community. To reduce the risk factors in your physical environment, you must first identify any hazards and unsafe conditions. Then, you can develop a plan of action to make your environment a safer place.

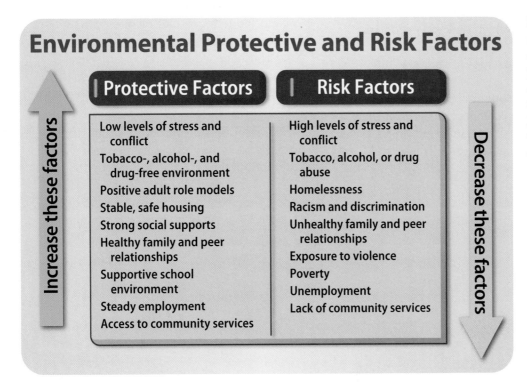

Environmental Protective and Risk Factors

Increase these factors →

Protective Factors	Risk Factors
Low levels of stress and conflict	High levels of stress and conflict
Tobacco-, alcohol-, and drug-free environment	Tobacco, alcohol, or drug abuse
Positive adult role models	Homelessness
Stable, safe housing	Racism and discrimination
Strong social supports	Unhealthy family and peer relationships
Healthy family and peer relationships	Exposure to violence
Supportive school environment	Poverty
Steady employment	Unemployment
Access to community services	Lack of community services

← Decrease these factors

Figure 1.8
Risk factors in your environment impact your health and wellness. *Reflect on what risk factors are present in your environment. What actions can you take to decrease these factors?*

Social Environment

The people around you make up your *social environment*. Your social environment may include family members, friends, **peers** (people similar in age to you), teachers, coaches, and neighbors. The people you interact with on social media sites are part of your social environment, too.

BUILDING Your Skills

The Power of Social Media to Inspire

How often do you spend time on social media sites? What kinds of messages do you receive in your online social community? Do the people within your social media network promote positive, healthy behaviors or negative, risky behaviors?

Social media can be a powerful tool to inspire healthy behaviors. It can also influence you to engage in risky behaviors, such as tobacco or alcohol usage or sexual activity. Just as peer pressure from your friends and classmates can impact the decisions you make regarding your health, so can the content you view on social media.

If the social network you see daily promotes negative, risky behaviors, you may feel pressured to engage in these behaviors too. For example, if your online friends are always posting mean comments to others or participating in hazardous viral or online challenges, you might think you need to do this too in order to fit in with the group.

Pay attention to how these posts impact the way you might think about risky behaviors. Carefully choose who you follow on social media based on how their messages could impact the way you view your own health and wellness. Surround yourself with a social network that cultivates a respectful, safe, and overall healthy lifestyle. In addition, inspire others to live this kind of lifestyle too, through the content you post on social media.

Inspire a Healthy Life

In this activity, you will create an inspiring digital representation of a social media post that encourages a healthy behavior. The materials you need depend on how you want to create your visual representation. You may choose to use a social media template or a paper representation using poster board or construction paper. To create your digital representation, complete the following steps:

1. Identify a healthy behavior that is meaningful and relevant to you, your classmates, or your friends. Topic examples may include green living, healthy eating, tobacco-free living, or physical activity. The healthy behavior you choose should positively affect a person's physical, mental and emotional, or social health.

2. Create a representation on the social media platform of your choice to raise awareness of this healthy behavior. Your digital representation may include infographics, pictures with captions to illustrate this behavior, famous quotes, and a hashtag or other link to a larger health community. Add other details as needed to make your representation inspiring, informative, creative, and visually appealing.

3. With permission, display these social media healthy posts around the classroom or throughout the school to inspire your peers. You may also want to post your message on a social media site, with permission, to get feedback from your online social community.

Astrovector/Shutterstock.com

Your **culture** (the beliefs, values, customs, and arts of a group of people) and community are also part of your social environment. The cultural practices and behaviors of your social group affect your health and wellness. Cultural practices that may affect your health and wellness are shown in **Figure 1.9**.

The risk factors in your social environment depend on the practices and behaviors of those in your group and their influences on you. If your parents practice healthy eating habits, you are more likely to practice them as well. If your friends smoke or drink and pressure you to do so, your risk of engaging in these harmful behaviors increases, too. Following are two ways to help reduce the risk factors within your social environment:

- maintain healthy relationships with others
- focus on engaging in healthy behaviors

Economic Environment

Your *economic environment* includes your family's and community's level of education, income, and resources. For example, education improves knowledge about the importance of nutrition and physical activity. Scientists have found that college graduates in the United States are less likely to experience overweight and obesity. Both of these conditions are related to nutrition and physical activity. The connection between education and health also relates to income. People with more education tend to earn more money. With more money, people are better able to pay for healthcare, activities, and resources that promote health.

Lifestyle Factors

The way you choose to live your life can greatly affect your health and wellness. For example, what you choose to eat and drink affects your health. How active or inactive you are makes a difference in your level of health, too. How much sleep

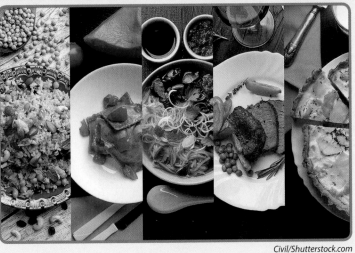

Cultural Practices That Affect Health and Wellness

- Food and taste preferences
- Eating patterns
- Religious or spiritual practices
- Activity preferences
- Medical treatment and customs

Civil/Shutterstock.com

Figure 1.9
The way your family and the wider culture you are part of eats, celebrates, gets physical activity, and treats illnesses affect your overall health and wellness.

The Game of Life

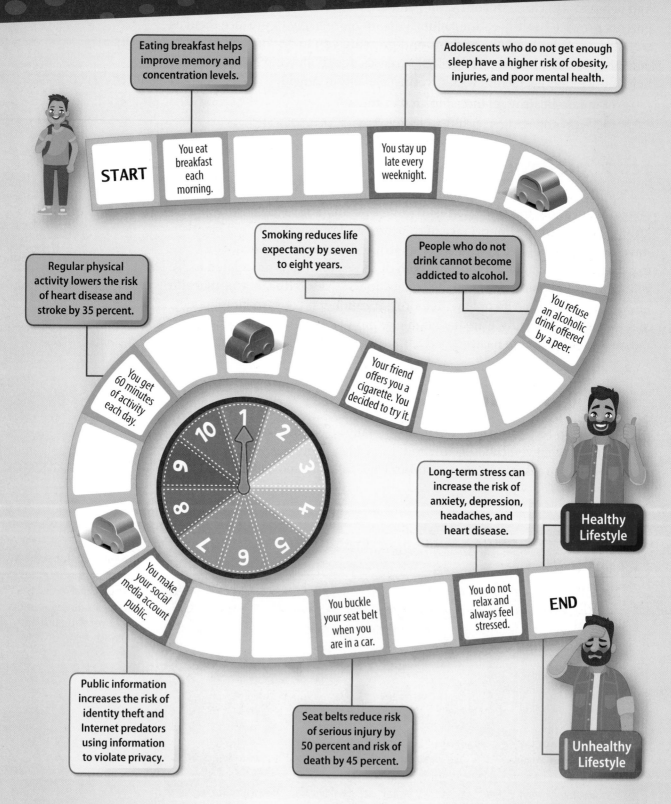

Eating breakfast helps improve memory and concentration levels.

Adolescents who do not get enough sleep have a higher risk of obesity, injuries, and poor mental health.

START

You eat breakfast each morning.

You stay up late every weeknight.

Smoking reduces life expectancy by seven to eight years.

People who do not drink cannot become addicted to alcohol.

Regular physical activity lowers the risk of heart disease and stroke by 35 percent.

You refuse an alcoholic drink offered by a peer.

You get 60 minutes of activity each day.

Your friend offers you a cigarette. You decided to try it.

Long-term stress can increase the risk of anxiety, depression, headaches, and heart disease.

Healthy Lifestyle

You make your social media account public.

You buckle your seat belt when you are in a car.

You do not relax and always feel stressed.

END

Public information increases the risk of identity theft and Internet predators using information to violate privacy.

Seat belts reduce risk of serious injury by 50 percent and risk of death by 45 percent.

Unhealthy Lifestyle

Game spinner: wongstock/Shutterstock.com; Game path: EkaterinaP/Shutterstock.com; Game pieces: Reinekke/Shutterstock.com; Young boy, sad and happy adults: tynyuk/Shutterstock.com you get each night can also have an impact on your health and wellness. Engaging in risky behaviors, such as drinking, smoking, or doing drugs, can reduce your level of health and wellness. Texting while driving is also an example of a risky behavior that can be a hazard to your health.

Some behaviors have an immediate impact on health and wellness. If you did not get enough sleep last night, you may lack energy and have trouble focusing. Other behaviors have both short-term and long-term effects. Sun exposure is just one example. Spending too much time in the sun can result in the short-term effect of sunburn. Regularly spending too much time in the sun without using sunscreen can increase your risk of developing skin cancer.

Many of the lifestyle choices you make and behaviors you develop begin in childhood and adolescence. Oftentimes, these behaviors continue into adulthood and can affect your health for years to come. If you have an inactive lifestyle as a child, you are more likely to become physically inactive as an adult. Inactive adults have a higher risk of developing high blood pressure and heart disease.

Parents and culture often influence lifestyle choices and behaviors that begin in childhood and adolescence. If your parents stay up late on a regular basis, you are more likely to stay up late as well. If your culture does not believe in taking medication, you will likely feel the same way. Your parents and culture may be a strong influence on you when you are young.

Making healthy lifestyle choices and practicing healthy behaviors promote your personal health and wellness today and in the future. Even if you do not make healthy lifestyle choices now, you have the power to change your behavior and take charge of your health and wellness.

Lesson 1.2 Review

1. The aspects of people's lives that reduce risk and increase the likelihood of good health are called _____factors.

2. Name the three types of environments that can affect a person's health and wellness.

3. **True or false.** Risk factors in your social environment depend on the practices and behaviors of those in your group and their influences on you.

4. Eating unhealthy foods, smoking, and not getting enough sleep are all examples of _____ _____ that can negatively impact your health and wellness.

5. **Critical thinking.** Give an example of a cultural practice that influences your family's health and wellness. Is this an example of a positive influence or a negative influence?

Hands-On Activity

In small groups, create a role play and script that shows the importance of making healthy lifestyle choices today to promote personal health and wellness in the future. Your role play may include your group's beliefs about preventive actions young people can take to avoid peer pressure to engage in unhealthy behaviors. It can also focus on your group's opinions about how to change an unhealthy behavior. Practice your role play and present it to the rest of the class.

Building Skills for Health and Wellness

Learning Outcomes

After studying this lesson, you will be able to

- **use** the decision-making process to solve problems and make healthy choices.
- **demonstrate** goal-setting skills by setting a SMART goal and developing an action plan to achieve it.
- **describe** how refusal skills help people avoid unhealthy behaviors.
- **identify** conflict management strategies.
- **demonstrate** how to access and evaluate health information.
- **explain** how to communicate about and advocate for health.

Graphic Organizer

Health and Wellness Skills

Each section of this organizer represents a set of skills necessary to achieve and maintain your health and wellness. As you read the lesson, record what you have learned by filling in the graphic organizer with techniques for mastering these skills.

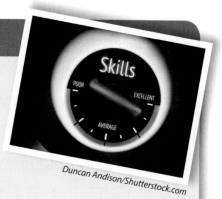

Duncan Andison/Shutterstock.com

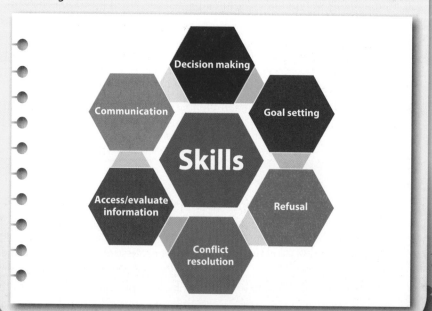

What is the best way to control asthma, muscle cramps, or acne? What can you do to manage the stress in your life? How can you help a friend who is going through a crisis? Do you know how you would find answers to these questions—good, reliable answers? You would not want answers based on rumors or unreliable sources of information.

Knowledge is power. Health knowledge gives you the power to prevent disease and promote your well-being. Consider Hannah and Aiden's situations, as described in the previous lessons. Hannah might improve her mental and emotional health if she researched counseling resources in her area. Aiden must be careful to get the best possible information about his breathing condition. With the right skills and resources, you can apply that knowledge and successfully take charge of your own health and wellness.

Making Healthy Decisions

As you grow up, you begin to make more of your own choices. Therefore, it is important to understand how the choices you make can affect your health and wellness. The best way to make healthy and informed decisions is to use a decision-making process. A **decision-making process** is a process of making choices by identifying the decision, brainstorming options, identifying possible outcomes, making a decision, and reflecting on the decision. **Figure 1.10** shows how to use the decision-making process.

Your personal needs, wants, values, and priorities are factors that will influence the decisions you make. Your *needs* are the things you must have to live, such as air, water, sleep, food, clothing, and housing. Your *wants* are the things you desire or would like to have. *Values* are the things that are important to you in life. Examples of values include family, peers, culture, health, and happiness. The things you value the most become your *priorities*.

How you approach making a decision is important. Sometimes you may make a decision on your own. Other times, you may *collaborate*, or

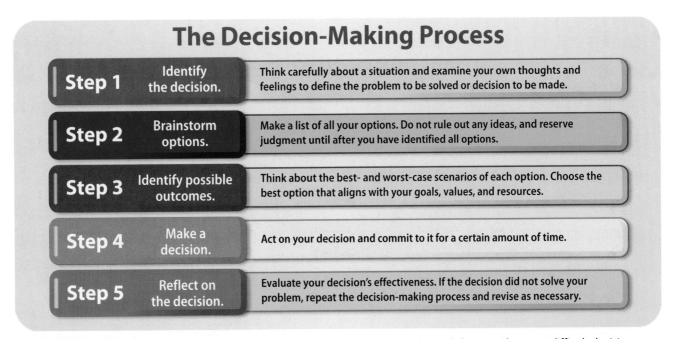

The Decision-Making Process

Step 1	Identify the decision.	Think carefully about a situation and examine your own thoughts and feelings to define the problem to be solved or decision to be made.
Step 2	Brainstorm options.	Make a list of all your options. Do not rule out any ideas, and reserve judgment until after you have identified all options.
Step 3	Identify possible outcomes.	Think about the best- and worst-case scenarios of each option. Choose the best option that aligns with your goals, values, and resources.
Step 4	Make a decision.	Act on your decision and commit to it for a certain amount of time.
Step 5	Reflect on the decision.	Evaluate your decision's effectiveness. If the decision did not solve your problem, repeat the decision-making process and revise as necessary.

Figure 1.10 Using the decision-making process can help you choose a healthy path for even the most difficult decisions.

work together, with others to make a group decision. Collaborating with others can give you options you may not have considered otherwise. Still other times, you may want to seek the advice of your family or friends. When you do ask others for their opinions, consider how their advice aligns with your values and priorities. In this way, you are more likely to make a good decision.

Setting and Achieving Goals

Goals are important for many aspects of life, including your health. Therefore, learning the skills you need to set and work toward goals is important. A **goal** is a desired result of something you plan to do. Goals motivate you and keep you focused on what you need to accomplish. Setting and working toward goals can help you change situations you do not like or help you get where you want to be. They can also give you a sense of satisfaction.

Goals can be short-term or long-term. A *short-term goal* is a goal you want to accomplish in the near future, within days or weeks. A *long-term goal* requires more time—months or years—to achieve. Reaching a long-term goal may involve achieving a series of short-term goals.

When setting goals, consider your values, or what is important to you, and assess your current situation. To make sure your goals are clearly stated and achievable, use the acronym **SMART** to guide your goal setting. SMART goals are specific, measurable, achievable, relevant, and timely (**Figure 1.11**). An example of a SMART goal is eating 2½ cups of vegetables every day for one month to improve healthy eating habits. This goal is more measurable, achievable, and timely than the goal of eating more vegetables.

To accomplish a goal you set, create an **action plan**, which is a detailed step-by-step method to reach a desired outcome. Your action plan should outline what you are going to do, how you are going to do it, and when it will be done. Be specific. Create short-term goals to outline what you need to do each day, week, or month to meet your long-term goal. Make sure that your

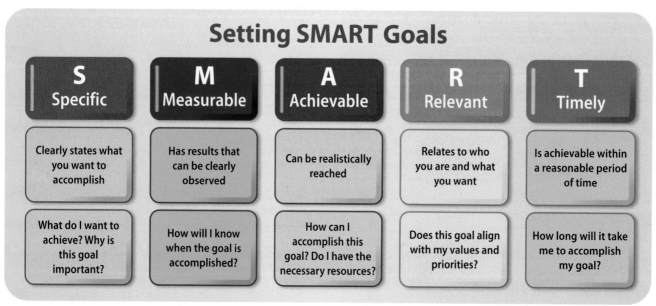

Figure 1.11 Use questions such as the ones in this figure to ensure you are setting SMART goals.

short-term goals are SMART goals with realistic deadlines. Identify any blocks that may prevent you from reaching your goal. Include in your plan what actions you can take to prevent these blocks from hurting your progress.

An action plan also includes how you plan to track your goal progress. You may want to use a goal planner or journal to monitor your progress. Free goal tracker apps are another way you can keep track of your goal progress.

Once you have completed your action plan, the next step is to follow it. As you track your progress, set time aside every month to evaluate whether your plan is working. You may need to adjust your plan along the way.

Sometimes, you may not achieve your goals. If this occurs, do not get discouraged. Consider the situation as a learning experience. Think about where things went wrong and what you could do differently. Then you can use this information as you set new goals. Mastering goal-setting skills will help you continually grow and improve yourself, your health, and your overall well-being.

Using Refusal Skills

Refusal skills are a set of skills designed to help someone avoid participating in unhealthy behaviors. These skills can help you respond to peer influences and behaviors without compromising your own goals, values, and health.

For example, you might be pressured to use drugs, tobacco, or alcohol. You could be pressured to engage in an activity that is illegal, inappropriate, or unhealthy. Your peers might pressure you into these activities, or you might see these behaviors modeled in television shows and movies you watch. You may think that this is what all young people are doing. These influences can make saying *no* difficult.

Using refusal skills helps you take responsibility for your health behaviors. By using refusal skills, you ensure that no one is responsible for your health but you. Practicing strong refusal skills will also help you avoid or reduce health risks. Behaviors such as smoking or drinking increase your risk of certain health issues. Refusing to engage in these behaviors helps you avoid the health risks associated with them.

Refusal skills help you make independent, informed decisions despite messages you may receive from peers, society, and the media. The tips in **Figure 1.12**, and information throughout this text, will help you learn and apply refusal skills to resist pressure.

Tips for Resisting Pressure

- Watch your body language—stand up straight and make eye contact.
- Say how you feel—use a firm voice to say *no*.
- Be honest and do not make excuses—your friends should accept your response when you say, "No, I don't want to." Remember, you have the right not to give a reason.
- Suggest something else to do—if your friends do not want to do another activity, find another friend who does.
- Stick up for yourself—be prepared to walk away to get out of the situation.

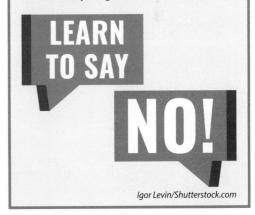

Igor Levin/Shutterstock.com

Figure 1.12 Pressure from others can be difficult to resist, but you have a right to say "no" and walk away from the situation.

Resolving Conflicts

As people interact with one another, *conflicts* (disagreements) are bound to arise. Conflicts can occur when people have different opinions or priorities. You may even have conflicts with your family or friends. Conflicts are a normal part of life. Some conflicts can be healthy, letting you see another person's point of view and even build relationships. Conflicts that are unhealthy cause stress and put strain on relationships.

Conflict resolution skills are strategies for resolving disagreements in a positive, respectful way to promote healthy relationships. Strategies in conflict resolution (also called *conflict management*) are shown in **Figure 1.13**.

In some cases, a conflict is too serious or too difficult for the people directly involved to manage by themselves. In this situation, an outside individual with a neutral perspective can help the people or groups find a good solution.

Mediation is a strategy for resolving difficult conflicts by involving a neutral third party, or *mediator*. During mediation, both parties in the conflict separately share their perspective of the conflict with the mediator. The mediator then brings the two parties together to share their views and tries to help them reach an agreement. You will learn more about conflict resolution later in this textbook.

Accessing and Evaluating Health Information and Services

As you learn about health-related terms, concepts, and facts, you will develop the ability to locate, evaluate, apply, and communicate information as it relates to your health. This is **health literacy**. Your health literacy builds on basic facts and concepts you learn at home and in school.

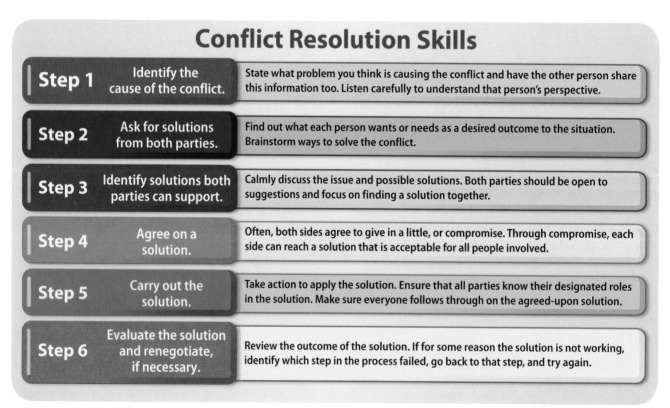

Conflict Resolution Skills

Step 1	Identify the cause of the conflict.	State what problem you think is causing the conflict and have the other person share this information too. Listen carefully to understand that person's perspective.
Step 2	Ask for solutions from both parties.	Find out what each person wants or needs as a desired outcome to the situation. Brainstorm ways to solve the conflict.
Step 3	Identify solutions both parties can support.	Calmly discuss the issue and possible solutions. Both parties should be open to suggestions and focus on finding a solution together.
Step 4	Agree on a solution.	Often, both sides agree to give in a little, or compromise. Through compromise, each side can reach a solution that is acceptable for all people involved.
Step 5	Carry out the solution.	Take action to apply the solution. Ensure that all parties know their designated roles in the solution. Make sure everyone follows through on the agreed-upon solution.
Step 6	Evaluate the solution and renegotiate, if necessary.	Review the outcome of the solution. If for some reason the solution is not working, identify which step in the process failed, go back to that step, and try again.

Figure 1.13 When you meet with the other person in the conflict, remember that each person is different. There is nothing wrong with someone having an opinion that is different from yours. Differences make people more interesting. *Why is it important to deal with arguments in a positive, respectful way?*

As you learn about health and wellness, you will discover that researchers are constantly finding out new information about the human body and its health. This means you will need to keep learning about health and wellness throughout your life.

Developing health literacy means you can also evaluate health-related products and services. Health literacy helps you analyze advertisements for products (**Figure 1.14**). With health literacy skills, you can find out whether various products actually promote health. Health literacy can help you determine which health services are right for you.

Technology can influence your health literacy. By using the Internet and a few key search words, you can find lots of health-related information. Just because health information is on the Internet, however, does not make it accurate or true. Developing health literacy can help you access valid health-related information on the Internet and evaluate health information.

Access Valid Information

Your health and wellness depend on your ability to access valid (accurate) information. You need to be able to tell information grounded in science from health claims based on rumors, opinions, and theories.

Science is a body of knowledge regarding the natural world, based on observation and experimentation. Science poses questions and proposes explanations about the natural world—including the human body, human health, and diseases. Scientists test these explanations repeatedly to prove or disprove them as factual. Therefore, science-based information is valid, unlike opinions and theories that have not been tested and verified as fact.

When using the Internet to answer questions about your health, you will see several websites. How do you decide which source you should trust? In general, you can access valid information from agencies or organizations whose main mission is education, research, or direct healthcare. Safe or reliable URL stems generally include *.gov*, *.edu*, and *.org*.

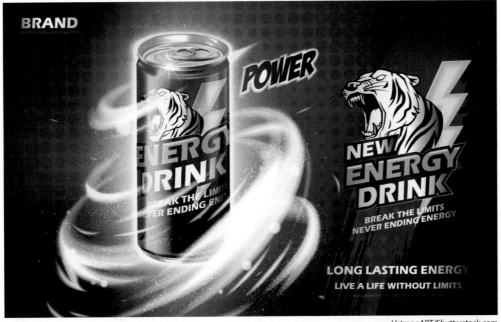

Figure 1.14
Health literacy helps you to analyze advertisements, such as this one. *What health claim is being made in this advertisement?*

Websites of businesses that earn profits or organizations promoting a particular cause are often not trustworthy. The main goal of a business is to make money by selling the product or service it provides. Information from a business may play up the benefits of the product or service and play down negative information. Organizations promoting a certain cause may only share information that supports its cause. Accessing valid information can help you locate reliable health-related products and services as well.

When searching for information, begin with a reliable, general source such as one of the agencies or websites in **Figure 1.15**. When in doubt, ask your school librarian or doctor about a reliable media source to find information about health and wellness. Librarians specialize in finding and evaluating sources, which means you can rely on their advice should questions arise.

Evaluating Health Information

"Get six-pack abs in two weeks!"
"You will catch a cold if you go outside with wet hair."
"The bumps on your skull reveal your character."
"Cell phones cause brain cancer."
"Caffeinated energy drinks will make you perform better on exams."

These are some examples of the thousands of health claims in magazines, on websites, in the media, and in advertisements. Claims such as these are not supported by science. If you act on these claims, you could waste money and time and harm your health. This is why carefully evaluating health-related information is so important.

Figure 1.15
These websites from reputable government and health agencies are a great place to start when looking for accurate health-related information. *What are three examples of safe or reliable URL stems?*

Health and Safety Information	
Sources of Information	**URLs**
Academy of Nutrition and Dietetics	www.eatright.org
American Academy of Pediatrics	www.aap.org
American Cancer Society	www.cancer.org
American Heart Association	www.heart.org
American Red Cross	www.redcross.org
Centers for Disease Control and Prevention (CDC)	www.cdc.gov
Mayo Clinic	www.mayoclinic.org
MedlinePlus® (U.S. National Library of Medicine, National Institutes of Health)	www.nlm.nih.gov/medlineplus/
National Highway Traffic Safety Administration	www.nhtsa.gov
National Institute of Mental Health	www.nimh.nih.gov
National Institute on Drug Abuse	www.drugabuse.gov
Office of the Surgeon General	www.surgeongeneral.gov
Tufts University Health & Nutrition Letter	www.nutritionletter.tufts.edu
United States Consumer Products Safety Commission	www.cpsc.gov
United States Department of Agriculture	www.choosemyplate.gov
United States Department of Health and Human Services	www.healthfinder.gov
United States Food and Drug Administration	www.fda.gov
World Health Organization	www.who.int

Refer to the information in **Figure 1.16** to learn more about evaluating health websites. When evaluating health information, including health claims about health products, ask yourself the following questions. Answering these questions can help you determine if the information is scientifically accurate:

- Is the source of the information reliable?
- Is the information current?
- Is the information relevant to my life stage and situation?
- Is the source making money or promoting a cause by publishing the story or article?
- Does the article refer to research published by medical scientists?
- Does the article give the names of the researchers and the journal that published the original research?
- Can you find other reliable sources with the same information?

Communicating Health Information

Once you have reliable health information, you can **advocate** for, or support, the health of your family and community by sharing it with others.

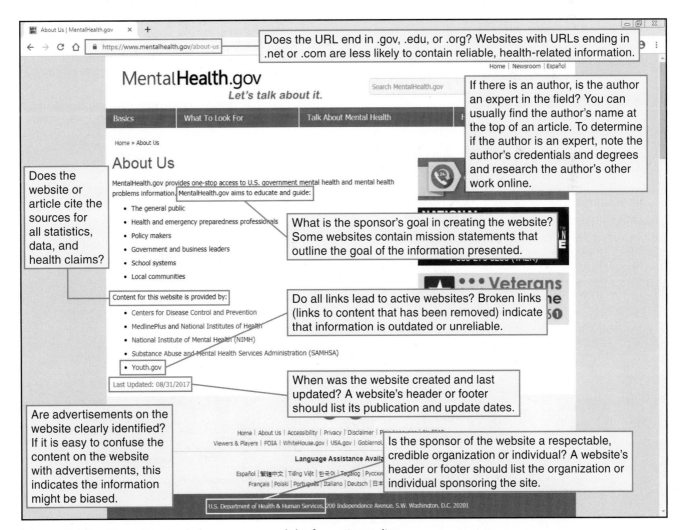

Figure 1.16 These tips can help you access valid information online.

This is called *health promotion*. For example, if your mother smokes, consider encouraging her to quit. Research the health risks of smoking and present the information to your mother. If your mother decides to quit smoking, support her effort.

Help your family access health information. For example, if your family members have questions about a health-related topic and do not understand English, help them by researching the topic on the Internet and translating the information you find.

If you are worried about a friend who is engaging in unhealthy behaviors, you can ask a school counselor how to help your friend. You might ask members of your community to help create health awareness posters. Collaborating with others can increase your personal ability to advocate for health.

BUILDING Your Skills

Your School Environment

Your school environment can have a positive or a negative influence on your health. Unhealthy food and beverage choices in the cafeteria can diminish student nutrition. School counseling services can help students who struggle with their mental and emotional health.

Your school environment can be influenced by initiatives and regulations on anything from banning weapons and alcohol to building speed bumps in the parking lot. Your voice or a collective group of voices has the power to change a school environment. Speaking up about your health needs and the needs of those around you is what can make you a health advocate in your community.

Be a Health Advocate at School

In this activity, you will create an inspiring school advocacy project for a new health initiative. To create your initiative, complete the following steps:

1. In small groups, discuss your school environment and what actions are being taken to encourage healthy students. Make a list of these positive actions.

2. Next, discuss which health needs are not currently being met at your school. Make another list of the actions not being taken to improve health and any actions that discourage healthy behavior.

3. Identify one school initiative or change that would improve the health of students.

4. Create a plan to gather student awareness and support to create this change.

5. Create a product to help raise awareness for your school advocacy project. Possible formats for this product include handmade posters, social media posts, and petitions.

6. Display your products around the classroom or school.

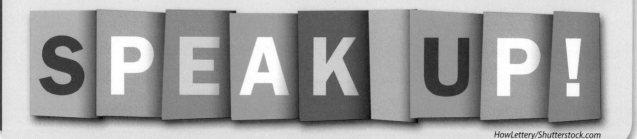

HowLettery/Shutterstock.com

You can also advocate for community health. *Community health* describes the overall health of a community. A *community* is a group of people who live in the same area and interact with one another (**Figure 1.17**). If a community is healthy, this means there are positive relationships among people and organizations. These organizations include health organizations and local, state, and national governments.

Suppose your state has a high rate of obesity. Begin by learning about existing public health services and write to your elected officials about supporting a healthy eating program. On a local level, start a fitness club at school. Attend community meetings and speak about health issues that concern you.

Community health depends on the actions of businesses, organizations, and each person in the community. This means you can promote the health of your community in the following ways:

- **Use community resources.** *Community resources* are organizations and programs that help the environment and people within a community (**Figure 1.18**).
- **Get involved in community service by volunteering.** *Community service* is work done without pay to help people in the community. Many organizations depend on volunteers. Some examples include nursing homes, food pantries, community gardens, shelters, or community outreach centers.

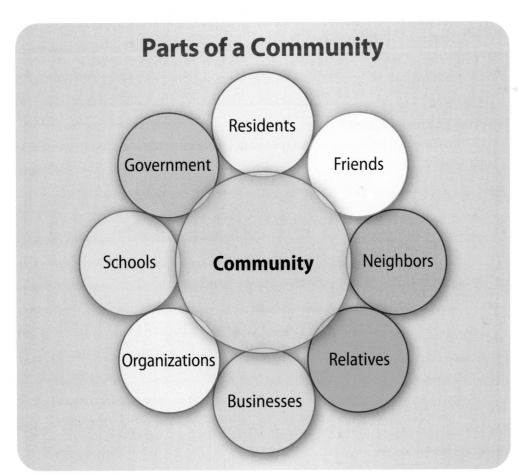

Parts of a Community

Residents
Government
Friends
Schools
Community
Neighbors
Organizations
Relatives
Businesses

Figure 1.17
Some communities are healthier than others, and communities can fall anywhere on the health spectrum.

Figure 1.18
Knowing how to find and use community resources can help you maintain your own health and advocate for the health of others. *What resources are available in your community?*

Examples of Community Resources	
City and county healthcare facilities	Hospitals
Community centers	Mental health centers
Crisis hotlines	Nursing homes
Department of human services	Public health departments
Financial assistance organizations	Rescue missions
Food pantries	Soup kitchens
Homeless shelters	Support groups

Lesson 1.3 Review

1. What are the five steps to making a good, healthy decision?
2. What are SMART goals?
3. To stand up to pressures and influences toward unhealthy behaviors, you can build _____ skills.
4. Health _____ is the ability to locate, interpret, apply, and communicate information as it relates to your health.
5. **Critical thinking.** Give an example of a long-term goal and the series of short-term goals involved in achieving it. Make sure that your goals are SMART.

Hands-On Activity

Imagine that the following text messages were sent to you during this school year:

My mom cooked. LOL Want to walk to McDonald's?

Nobody is home tonight. Want to come over and get drunk?

Hey, can we play video games today instead of going to the park?

On a separate sheet of paper, respond to the text messages using refusal skills and conflict resolution skills. With a partner, share how you responded to the text messages and discuss how refusing these offers would help maintain good health and wellness.

Review and Assessment

Summary

Lesson 1.1 Learning About Health and Wellness

- The term *health* refers to the state of complete physical, mental and emotional, and social well-being. *Wellness* is an active process that involves becoming aware of and making choices toward improving aspects of health.
- *Well-being* is a person's overall satisfaction that life's present conditions are good.
- Personal well-being depends on good physical, mental and emotional, and social health. These aspects of your health are *interrelated*, meaning they all interact with and affect each other.
- Focusing on wellness means that you not only go to the doctor to receive treatment when you are sick, you also go to the doctor when you are well to help you stay healthy.

Lesson 1.2 Recognizing Factors That Affect Health and Wellness

- *Risk factors* are aspects of people's lives that increase the chance of a disease, injury, or decline in health. Some risk factors, such as genetic factors, are not within your control. Many environmental and lifestyle risk factors, however, are within your control.
- *Protective factors* are aspects of people's lives that reduce risk and increase the likelihood of good health.
- Your *environment* includes the circumstances, objects, or conditions that surround you in everyday life and affect your health and wellness. This includes your physical, social, and economic environments.
- Your physical environment consists of the places where you spend your time, the region in which you live, the air you breathe, and the water you drink. Your social environment includes the people in your life and your culture (the beliefs, values, customs, and arts of a group of people). Your economic environment includes your level of education and income level.
- Making healthy lifestyle choices and practicing healthy behaviors promote your personal health and wellness today and in the future.

Lesson 1.3 Building Skills for Health and Wellness

- The *decision-making process* involves identifying a decision, brainstorming options, identifying possible outcomes, making a decision, and reflecting on the decision.
- Effective goals are *SMART goals*—specific, measurable, achievable, relevant, and timely.
- When peers or family members attempt to influence you to engage in unhealthy behaviors, refusal skills can help you respond without compromising your goals, values, or health.
- Conflict resolution skills, which involve negotiation and compromise, help you resolve arguments in a way that promotes healthy relationships.
- The ability to locate, interpret, apply, and communicate information as it relates to your health is called *health literacy*.
- Taking charge of your health and wellness involves playing an active role in your healthcare and advocating for your personal health.

Check Your Knowledge

Record your answers to each of the following questions on a separate sheet of paper.

1. **True or false.** To achieve health, people practice well-being.
2. Identify the aspects of your health. How are these aspects interrelated?
3. Which type of healthcare involves getting an annual physical exam, regular checkups, and screenings?
4. How do most people pay for the expensive cost of healthcare services?
5. The _____ you receive from your parents can affect your health and wellness by putting you at risk for developing certain diseases, such as heart disease.
6. Food and taste preferences and eating patterns are examples of _____ practices that may affect your social environment.
   A. peer
   B. physical
   C. cultural
   D. economic
7. **True or false.** Protective factors increase the chance of a disease, injury, or decline in health.
8. Identify three risky behaviors that can be a hazard to your health.
9. Using the _____ process can help you make good choices about health and wellness.
10. Which of the following URL stems is *not* generally a reliable source of health-related information?
    A. *.gov*
    B. *.org*
    C. *.edu*
    D. *.com*
11. What is at stake if you act on health claims that are *not* based in science?
12. Helping your grandfather research health information on the Internet is an example of _____ for family health.

Use Your Vocabulary ↱

action plan	goal	preventive healthcare
advocate	health	protective factors
conflict resolution skills	healthcare	refusal skills
culture	health literacy	risk factors
decision-making process	mental and emotional health	SMART
environment	peers	social health
genes	physical health	well-being
		wellness

13. Working in pairs, locate a small image online that visually describes or explains each of the terms above. Create flash cards by writing each term on a note card. Then paste the image that describes or explains the term on the opposite side.
14. With a partner, review each key term from this chapter and its definition. Then, write a short story about health and wellness in your life using at least 10 of the key terms. Share your short stories in class.

Think Critically

15. **Predict.** How can a change in a student's social health, such as experiencing violence or having close friends, also affect his or her physical and mental and emotional health?

16. **Identify.** What are three reasons young people may be tempted by risky behaviors? Explain why this group in particular is vulnerable.

17. **Draw conclusions.** How could you respond if you found that a claim about a health product was false? Whom would you tell about the false claim, and why?

18. **Determine.** In your opinion, does a young person have the power to change family health? Give a brief explanation to the class.

DEVELOP Your Skills

19. **Communication.** Imagine that you are in the following scenario: As a middle school student, life is pretty good. You have great friends, school is going well, and your family is a lot of fun. Last week, however, your grandma died and you are struggling to cope with the loss. You are sad, lack interest in everyday activities and friendships, and do not have much of an appetite. Write an essay reflecting on the following questions:
    - If you continue struggling with the loss of your grandma, how could it impact your physical and social health?
    - What would you do in this situation?
    - Who would you talk to, and how would you begin the conversation?
    - What self-help strategies could be helpful in coping?

20. **Goal setting.** Reflect on the parts of your health that you think could use more development. What improvements would you like to see in your health and wellness? Establish three or more long-term personal health goals. For each long-term goal, create three or more short-term goals. Your short-term goals should act as stepping stones for each of your long-term goals. Make sure to follow the SMART goal guidelines to make the most effective goals for you. Make a creative product that will serve as a reminder of your goals.

21. **Analyze influences.** Analyze a social media post, online article, or website that could potentially have a negative influence on a young person's physical, mental and emotional, or social health. Write a short paragraph about how this post, article, or website could negatively affect a teenager's behavior or health. Share your reflection with the class. Include the post, article, or website for the class to view during your presentation.

22. **Advocacy.** Imagine that your family has a history of a health condition, such as diabetes, heart disease, cancer, or obesity. Despite this, your family continues to make poor lifestyle decisions and you are worried about their health across the life span. Write a letter to your family talking about their current lifestyle choices and offer a plan to improve family health. This plan should include the big and small lifestyle changes that you would want to make with your family. It should also include a way to hold each other accountable for achieving these goals, such as a rewards system.

Chapter 2

Knowing How Your Body Works

Essential Question

What are the body systems and what are their main functions?

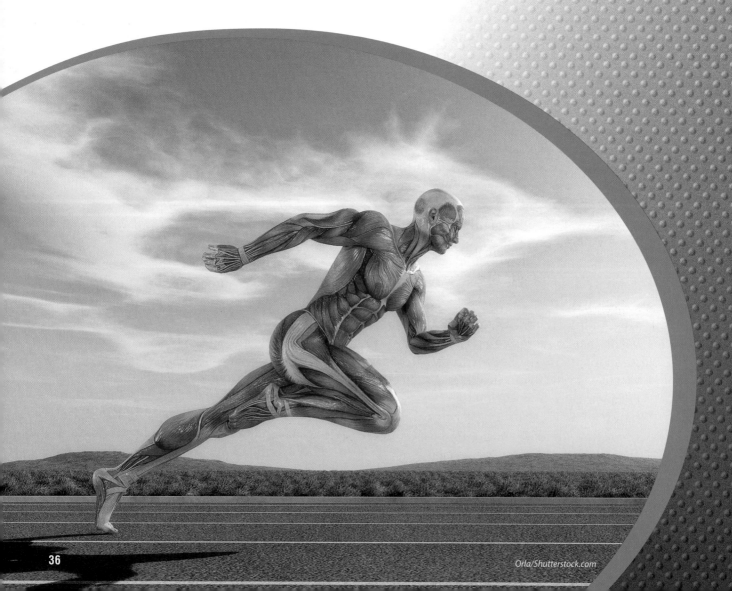

Reading Activity

In this chapter, you will read about body systems. Specific terminology will help you understand these systems and their functions. Prior to reading, list any key terms for each lesson with which you are not familiar. Look up these terms in a dictionary and write the definitions in your own words. As you listen to your teacher present the chapter, revise your definitions as needed. Ask your teacher questions if terms are still unclear to you.

How Healthy Are You?

In this chapter, you will be learning about the human body and its systems. Before you begin reading, take the following quiz to assess your current understanding of the human body systems and how each system affects your health and wellness.

Health Concepts to Understand	Yes	No
Do you know what is the basic unit of life?		
Can you name the body system that includes the skin, hair, and nails?		
Do you know which body system is made of 206 bones that provide structure, shape, and protection to the body?		
Can you name the three types of muscle tissue in the muscular system?		
Do you know which body system moves blood throughout the body to provide oxygen, nutrients, and energy?		
Do you know which body system exchanges oxygen and carbon dioxide through inhaling and exhaling?		
Can you name the body system that brings food into the body and breaks it down?		
Do you understand which organs are involved in the removal of liquid waste from the body in the urinary system?		
Do you know which body system removes foreign substances from the body?		
Can you name the body system that involves the brain, spinal cord, and nerves?		
Do you understand how the endocrine system uses hormones to control the body?		

Count your "Yes" and "No" responses. The more "Yes" responses you have, the more you understand human body systems. Now, take a closer look at the questions with which you responded "No." Develop your health literacy skills by accessing valid information about each of the concepts you do not understand. Evaluate any health websites you find using the information in Figure 1.16 of this text. If you do not understand the instructions, ask for clarification from your teacher.

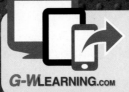

Click on the activity icon or visit www.g-wlearning.com/health to access online vocabulary activities using key terms from the chapter.

Supporting and Moving the Body

body system collection of organs that work together

integumentary system body system that covers and protects the entire body

epidermis outermost layer of the skin

dermis middle layer of the skin, which contains hair follicles

hypodermis innermost layer of the skin, which contains fat, blood vessels, and nerve endings; attaches to underlying bone and muscle

skeletal system body system made up of 206 bones that provides structure, shape, and protection to the body

joint location in the body where two or more bones meet and are held together

ligaments strong bands of tissue that hold together bones at joints to allow movement

muscular system body system that helps the body move and aids other body systems

tendons structures made of tough tissue that connect muscle to bone

Learning Outcomes

After studying this lesson, you will be able to

- **explain** how different elements of the human body work together.
- **describe** how the integumentary system protects the body.
- **summarize** the importance of a strong skeletal system.
- **describe** how the muscular system enables movement and prevents injury.

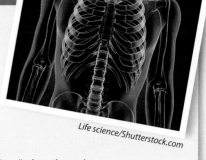

Life science/Shutterstock.com

Graphic Organizer

Support and Movement

As you read through this lesson, use a graphic organizer like the one shown to take notes on each system of the body that helps with the support and movement functions of humans. Make sure to note the structures, body parts, and organs involved in each body system. For each system, answer the question "what does this system allow my body to do?"

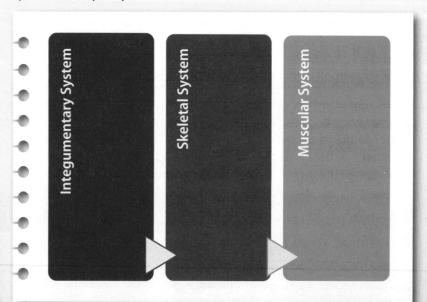

Integumentary System

Skeletal System

Muscular System

Have you ever wondered why you sweat when you play sports, or why your skin gets darker after being in the sun? Do you know what parts of your body allow you to sit, stand upright, walk, or run? These are just a few examples of tasks your body accomplishes every day. Each task requires the cooperation of cells, tissues, and systems throughout your body.

In this lesson, you will learn about the body systems that provide support and movement for the body. These systems include the following:

- integumentary system
- skeletal system
- muscular system

Organization of the Body

The body is organized into cells, tissues, organs, and body systems (**Figure 2.1**). *Cells* are the basic unit of life. All living things, including the human body, are made of cells.

In the body, cells are organized as tissues. A *tissue* is a collection of similar cells that do a certain job for the body. For example, muscle tissue is made of muscle cells. Muscle tissue can contract and shorten, enabling muscles to move.

Some tissues form glands. A *gland* is a group of cells that produce and release substances into the body. For example, the salivary glands in the mouth release saliva. This liquid breaks down food so that it can be swallowed.

Tissues work together to form organs. An *organ* is a collection of tissues that perform a specific job. For example, the stomach is an organ. Its job is to store and digest food. The stomach is made of several kinds of tissue, which include the following:

- muscle
- connective tissue
- nerve tissue

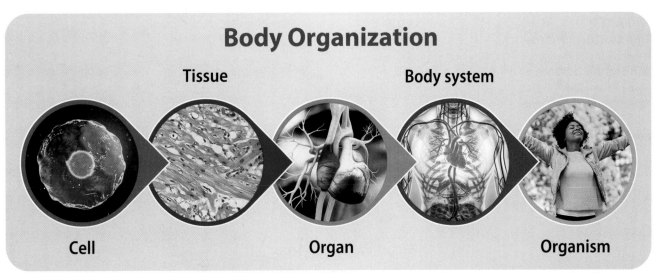

Body Organization

Tissue   Body system

Cell   Organ   Organism

Left to right: 3Dstock/Shutterstock.com; steeehc/Shutterstock.com; Liya Graphics/Shutterstock.com; yodiyim/Shutterstock.com; Syda Productions/Shutterstock.com

Figure 2.1 At the cellular level, different cells perform functions in the body. These cells form tissues, and different tissues form organs, which carry out specific jobs. Organs make up body systems, and body systems combine to make the human organism. *What is the basic unit of life that makes up everything in the human body?*

Organs work with other organs. A collection of organs that works together is a **body system**. This chapter reviews most of the major body systems. You will learn about the male and female reproductive systems in Chapter 17.

Each body system performs a set of important functions and makes up the human organism. Like the dimensions of health, body systems work very closely together. For example, the skeletal and muscular systems work together so you can walk and run and move your arms. The respiratory and circulatory systems work closely together to bring air into the body and move it through the blood. Taking care of each system enables the others to work effectively.

Integumentary System

The **integumentary system** is one of three systems that support and move the body. The integumentary system includes the skin, hair, and nails. It covers and protects the entire body and may be the most familiar body system. You see the integumentary system as you look at another person and when you look in the mirror. It is the only body system completely exposed to the world outside the body.

Skin

The *skin* is the largest organ in the human body (**Figure 2.2**). If spread flat, the skin would cover 17 to 20 square feet, about the size of a bedsheet. Skin protects the body and does a surprising number of important jobs. Taking care of the skin ensures it can do these jobs. Some of the tasks the skin performs include the following:

- keep out germs that could infect the body
- remove some waste and make vitamin D to build strong bones
- house nerve endings that allow people to sense pain, touch, and pressure

Figure 2.2
This diagram shows the three distinct layers of skin and the locations of your nerves, hair follicles, sweat glands, pores, and arteries and veins. *What are the three layers of skin called?*

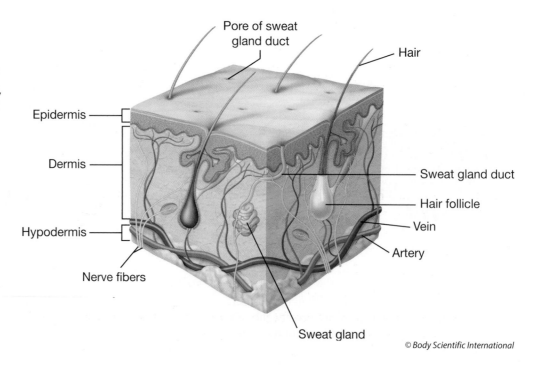

Pore of sweat gland duct

Hair

Epidermis

Dermis

Sweat gland duct

Hair follicle

Vein

Hypodermis

Artery

Nerve fibers

Sweat gland

© Body Scientific International

The skin houses various nerves, pores, arteries, veins, and hair follicles. These items are housed within the three main layers of the skin: the epidermis, the dermis, and the hypodermis, as you saw in Figure 2.2.

The outermost layer of the skin is the **epidermis**. The epidermis, which consists of five layers of its own, is the thinnest layer of the skin. The main function of the epidermis is to protect the body from infection by stopping foreign substances from entering into the body.

The middle layer of the skin is the **dermis**. This layer contains two proteins, *collagen* and *elastin*. These proteins provide support to the skin and give skin the ability to stretch and return to its normal shape. With age, the body creates less of these proteins, which leads to the appearance of wrinkles and sagging skin.

The innermost layer of the skin is the **hypodermis**. This layer consists of fat, blood vessels, and nerve endings. It also connects the skin to the bone and muscle underneath. Additional functions of each layer of skin are listed in Figure 2.3

Hair and Nails

Hair and nails are made by cells in the skin. Both hair and nails are made of the protein *keratin*. Hair grows on all skin surfaces except the palms, soles, lips, nipples, and some areas of the genitals. Each hair grows from a specialized cell called a *hair follicle*. Hair, like the skin, helps protect the body. For example, eyelashes and eyebrows shield the eyes. Nose hair prevents dust and particles from entering the airways. Head hair helps regulate temperature and protects the head from sunlight.

Nails protect the ends of fingers and toes. They grow on the upper sides of fingers and toes near the ends. As they grow, the older cells are pushed out, making the nails longer.

Skeletal System

The **skeletal system** is the body system made up of 206 bones that provides structure, shape, and protection to the body (**Figure 2.4**). For example, you can stand upright because of your sturdy and flexible backbone.

Layers of the Skin	
Layers	**Functions**
Epidermis	• Continually sheds and replaces the outer layer of skin cells. • Contains *keratin*, which protects the skin from drying out and from minor cuts and scratches. • Contains *melanin*, which gives the skin pigment.
Dermis	• Contains nerve endings that sense heat, cold, pain, and pressure. • Contains hair follicles, oil glands, and sweat glands.
Hypodermis	• Contains cells that store fat and help the body keep a steady temperature. • Connects the skin to underlying bone and muscle.

Figure 2.3
The three layers of skin contain keratin, melanin, nerve endings, collagen, elastin, and fat cells. Together, they form the largest organ in the human body. *Which layer of skin is the outermost layer?*

Figure 2.4
The individual bones that make up the human skeleton come in many different sizes and shapes, each uniquely designed to serve a specific function. *How many bones are in the skeletal system?*

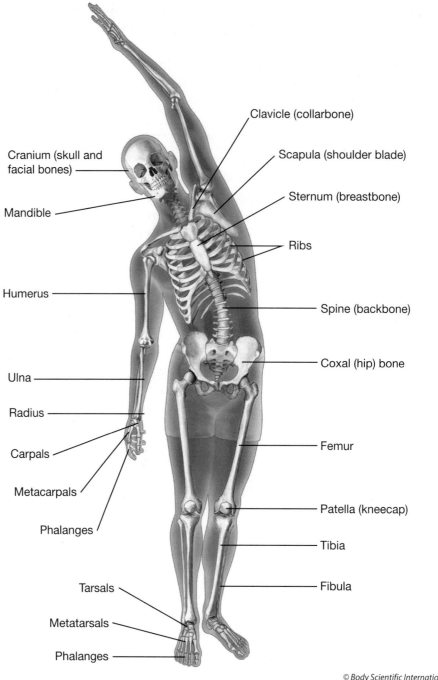

Clavicle (collarbone)

Scapula (shoulder blade)

Sternum (breastbone)

Cranium (skull and facial bones)

Mandible

Ribs

Humerus

Spine (backbone)

Coxal (hip) bone

Ulna

Radius

Carpals

Femur

Metacarpals

Patella (kneecap)

Phalanges

Tibia

Fibula

Tarsals

Metatarsals

Phalanges

© Body Scientific International

You can walk because your leg bones are strong and movable. The ribs protect the heart, lungs, and other internal organs. The skull and backbone protect the brain and spinal cord. Bones also make movement possible when they are attached to muscles.

Bone Tissue

Bones develop, grow, and change throughout life. They are made of minerals, proteins, and living cells. Bone hardness comes from the minerals *calcium* and *phosphate*. Bone flexibility comes from the protein *collagen*. To envision bone tissue, think of a gelatin dessert with marbles in it. The marbles represent the hard minerals. The firm, flexible gelatin represents collagen. Together, the gelatin and marbles have hardness and flexibility, like bones.

Bones can grow and change because they contain living bone cells. Some bone cells can make more bones. Other cells dissolve bones. Weight-bearing physical activities, such as running and lifting weights, put stress on bones. That stress pushes bone-making cells to make more bone tissue.

Bone Structure

Bones come in many shapes and sizes (**Figure 2.5**). For example, bones of the arms and legs are long. Bones of the skull, hip, and backbone are flat or have an irregular shape. Most bones have a dense outer tissue. Inside that dense tissue is a softer, spongy bone tissue. This spongy tissue contains cells that can make blood cells. The long bones of the arms and legs also have a hollow space filled with fat.

The ends of some bones are covered with *cartilage*, which is not as hard as bone. The cartilage slowly turns into bone tissue until it is all used up, causing growth. This growth stops at different ages in different people. Some people stop growing in their mid-teens. Others continue growing into their mid-twenties.

Joints

The skeletal system can move because of joints. A **joint** is a location where two or more bones meet. Some joints, such as those in the shoulder, move a great deal. Other joints, such as those in the skull, do not allow bones to move.

In joints that allow movement, bones are held together by strong bands of tissue called **ligaments**. For example, the tibia, or lower leg bone, and the femur, or large thighbone, meet at the knee joint. Ligaments hold the femur and tibia together.

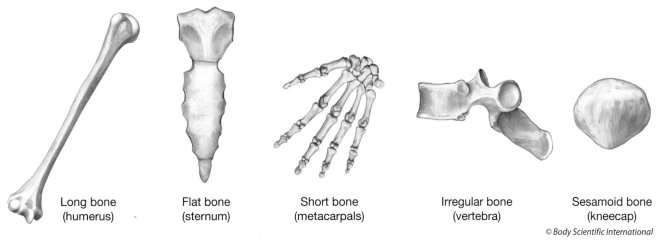

Long bone (humerus)   Flat bone (sternum)   Short bone (metacarpals)   Irregular bone (vertebra)   Sesamoid bone (kneecap)

© Body Scientific International

Figure 2.5   Bones found in the body include long bones, flat bones, short bones, irregular bones, and sesamoid bones. *Which shape are the bones of the arms and legs?*

The knee joint and other moving joints are kept moist by a special fluid. This fluid reduces the amount of friction between moving bones. It also cushions the bones that meet in the joint. In a joint that moves, cartilage covers the bones' surfaces. This tissue absorbs shock in the joint and protects the ends of the bones.

Muscular System

The **muscular system** helps the body move and plays important parts in other body systems (**Figure 2.6**). For example, the skeletal and muscular systems work together to move the body. A healthy muscular system can help you achieve tasks and prevent injury.

Muscles are made of specialized tissue that can shorten and stretch. Muscle that is attached to a bone can make the bone move.

Muscles are connected to bones by **tendons** made of tough tissues. Like muscles, tendons can shorten or lengthen. Muscles, bones, and tendons work closely together.

Figure 2.6
Muscles in the human body make it possible to walk, run, and lift objects. Muscles also control the beating of your heart and the movement of food through the digestive system.

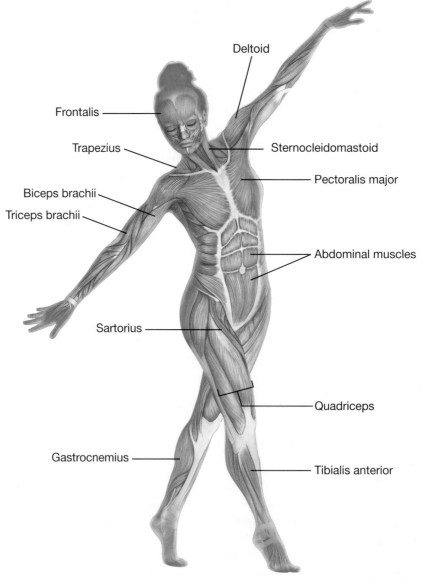

Deltoid

Frontalis

Trapezius

Sternocleidomastoid

Pectoralis major

Biceps brachii

Triceps brachii

Abdominal muscles

Sartorius

Quadriceps

Gastrocnemius

Tibialis anterior

© Body Scientific International

Muscle Tissue

Muscles are built from bundles of muscle cells. Different muscle cell arrangements create different types of muscle. Following are the three types of muscle tissue:

- *Skeletal muscles* are attached to bones and can be controlled. For example, you can choose to move your legs to walk or move them faster to run.
- *Smooth muscles* cannot be controlled. These muscles do very important work without you realizing it. For example, the smooth muscles in your intestines digest food.
- *Cardiac muscle* is found in the heart. This muscle pumps blood through the body.

Muscle Pairs

Muscles can contract (become shorter and tighter) and relax. Most skeletal muscles contract to move the bones of the body. When muscles relax, body parts return to an original state. Throughout the body, most skeletal muscles work in pairs to move certain body parts. Some examples of muscle pairs include the following:

- The biceps muscle contracts to bend the arm at the elbow. The triceps muscle contracts to straighten the arm at the elbow (**Figure 2.7**).
- The hamstring muscle contracts to bend the leg at the knee. The quadricep muscle contracts to extend the leg at the knee.
- The gluteus medius muscle contracts to bend the leg at the hip. The gluteus maximus muscle contracts to extend the leg at the hip.

Tension in biceps

Triceps relaxed

© Body Scientific International

Figure 2.7 When muscles contract, they can move bones. For example, when the biceps on the front of your arm contracts, it pulls your lower arm toward your upper arm. *What is the name of the tough tissue that connects muscles to bones?*

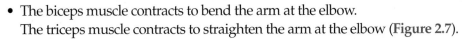

Lesson **2.1** Review

1. A body system is a collection of _____ that work together to perform a set of important functions.
2. **True or false.** The integumentary system includes the skin, hair, and nails.
3. What is a joint?
4. Which type of muscle can be controlled?
5. **Critical thinking.** Explain how the skeletal and muscular systems work together to cause movement.

Hands-On Activity

In small groups, outline one group member's entire body on large paper. Add drawings to "your body" of the organs and structures from this lesson. On your drawing, start a list of behaviors that will keep these structures and organs healthy. Choose one of these behaviors that you do not already do and add it into your life this week. Save this drawing for use in the other lessons.

Lesson 2.2

Moving and Exchanging Substances

Key Terms 👉

circulatory system body system formed by all the structures that move blood through the body; also called the *cardiovascular system*

heart hollow, muscular organ located in the center of the chest; pumps blood into the circulatory system

arteries blood vessels that carry oxygen-rich blood

capillaries small arteries that deliver oxygen and nutrients to cells and pick up cells' waste

veins blood vessels that carry oxygen-poor blood

plasma liquid part of blood

respiratory system body system of organs that obtain vitally important oxygen from the outside world

bronchi two air passages, each of which connects the trachea to a lung

respiration exchange of oxygen and carbon dioxide between the body and the air around it

diaphragm sheet of muscle beneath the lungs and above the abdomen that contracts and relaxes to help the chest expand so a person can inhale or shrink so a person can exhale

Learning Outcomes

After studying this lesson, you will be able to

- **describe** the importance of a healthy circulatory system.
- **identify** the role of the respiratory system in supporting health.

Graphic Organizer

Movement and Exchange of Substances

Before you read this lesson, create a table similar to the one shown. Write down three predictions about the circulatory and respiratory systems. Base these predictions on your prior knowledge of the human body. As you read the lesson, make any corrections necessary to the predictions you made and include as many notes as needed to help you better understand the information.

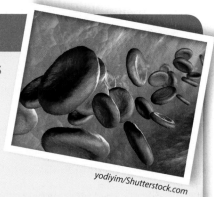

yodiyim/Shutterstock.com

Body Systems	Predictions	Notes
Circulatory system	1. 2. 3.	• • •
Respiratory system	1. 2. 3.	• • •

Two body systems do the work of exchanging substances with the outside world and moving them through the body. The circulatory system moves substances through the blood. The respiratory system brings air into and out of the body. These two body systems will be explained in this lesson.

Circulatory System

The **circulatory system** (also called the *cardiovascular system*) is formed by all the structures that move blood through the body (**Figure 2.8**). The circulatory system consists of the heart, blood vessels, and blood. The heart pumps the blood that the blood vessels transport to every cell in the human body. Functions of the circulatory system include the following:

- transporting oxygen and other nutrients to cells in the body
- removing carbon dioxide and other waste products
- regulating body temperature
- assisting with immune function

Caring for the circulatory system through healthy eating and physical activity supports these functions. In the next sections, you will learn more about the heart and how blood circulates in the heart. You will also learn more about blood vessels and blood.

Heart

The **heart** is a hollow, muscular organ located in the center of the chest. The heart is a steadily working muscle. It beats around 30 million times per year and pumps about 4,000 gallons of blood each day.

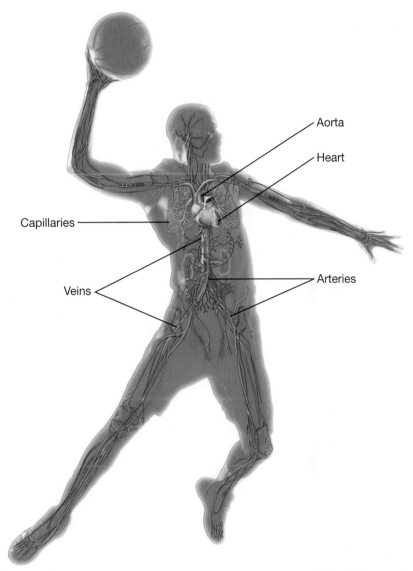

© Body Scientific International

Figure 2.8 The human body must have a continual supply of oxygen and other nutrients. The structures of the circulatory system work together to move the blood that contains these substances throughout the body. *Which organ pumps blood through the circulatory system?*

The heart contains four hollow spaces called *chambers*. The top two chambers are called *atria*. The bottom two chambers are called *ventricles*. Valves control the direction of blood flow in the heart. Like doors that open only one way, the valves make sure blood flows in the right direction. For example, one valve makes sure that blood flows from an atrium to a ventricle. It will not let blood flow from a ventricle to an atrium. Other valves make sure that blood leaving a ventricle does not flow backward into the ventricle.

The heartbeat you feel and hear is caused by the contraction of the heart chambers and closing of valves. The first heart sound is the atria squeezing blood into the ventricles. The second sound is the ventricles pumping blood out of the heart.

Blood Circulation

Blood circulation follows a path that provides the body with a continual supply of oxygen-rich blood. You can trace this path in **Figure 2.9**.

Oxygen-poor blood flows from around the body into the right atrium, which passes this blood into the right ventricle. The right ventricle pumps oxygen-poor blood out of the heart to the lungs, where this blood obtains oxygen.

Then oxygen-rich blood is returned from the lungs into the left atrium of the heart, which passes blood into the left ventricle. Finally, the left ventricle pumps oxygen-rich blood into the aorta. The oxygen-rich blood is then pumped around the body. After oxygen is used up, the oxygen-rich blood becomes oxygen-poor blood and flows back into the right atrium. The process then begins again.

Figure 2.9
The oxygen-poor blood (shown in blue) enters the heart where it is sent to the lungs and returns as oxygen-rich blood (shown in red) to the heart. From there, the blood is sent to the rest of the body. *What is responsible for controlling the direction of blood flow in the heart?*

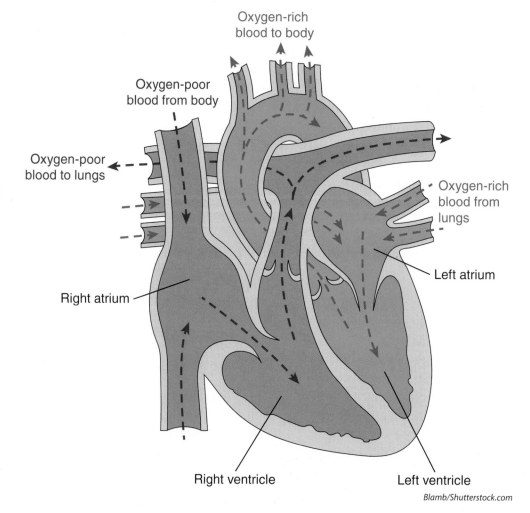

Oxygen-rich blood to body

Oxygen-poor blood from body

Oxygen-poor blood to lungs

Oxygen-rich blood from lungs

Left atrium

Right atrium

Right ventricle

Left ventricle

Blamb/Shutterstock.com

Blood Vessels

Blood vessels are an extensive network of pipes that carry blood throughout the entire body (**Figure 2.10**). There are three types of blood vessels. These vessels are the arteries, capillaries, and veins.

Arteries carry oxygen-rich blood. The largest artery is the *aorta*, which carries blood from the left ventricle of the heart to other arteries. Most arteries carry blood from the heart to the rest of the body. These arteries have muscular walls that can handle the pressure created by the heart's pumping. Arteries branch into smaller blood vessels, and these branch into even smaller ones.

The smallest arteries are the **capillaries**. Capillaries have very thin walls with no muscle. They deliver oxygen and nutrients to body cells and pick up cells' waste. Capillaries lead into tiny veins, which lead into larger veins.

Veins carry oxygen-poor blood. Two large veins, called the *vena cavae*, carry blood into the right atrium of the heart. One vena cava brings blood from the head and upper body. The other brings blood from the lower body.

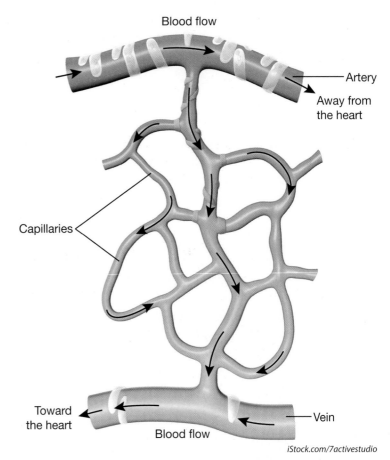

Blood flow

Artery

Away from the heart

Capillaries

Toward the heart

Vein

Blood flow

iStock.com/7activestudio

Figure 2.10 Arteries deliver oxygen-rich blood to capillaries. Blood flows through capillaries to deliver oxygen to body tissues. Once oxygen has been taken out of the blood, the blood returns to the heart through veins. *Arteries, capillaries, and veins are three types of what body part?*

Blood

Blood plays an important role in maintaining a person's health and sustaining life. As you already learned, blood carries oxygen and nutrients through the body, while also removing carbon dioxide and waste. Blood regulates a person's body temperature, similar to how a thermostat regulates the temperature in a room. Blood also protects the body against infection.

Because of blood's vital role in the human body, many people donate blood to organizations such as the American Red Cross. In fact, one pint of donated blood can save up to three lives. For this reason, people who donate blood are actually giving the gift of life.

Blood is made up of both liquid and solid parts (**Figure 2.11**). The liquid part of blood is called **plasma**. Plasma makes up at least half of blood's content. It is responsible for carrying all parts of blood throughout the body.

The solid parts of blood consist of red blood cells, white blood cells, and platelets.

- *Red blood cells* make up one-half the blood's volume. Red blood cells contain a red substance called *hemoglobin*, which can carry and release oxygen. As a result, red blood cells transport oxygen throughout the body.

Blood Donation

According to the American Red Cross, every two seconds someone in the United States needs blood. Some people may need blood due to a serious injury. Others may need blood for cancer treatments and chronic illnesses. Patients who are having surgery also require blood. These people need a blood transfusion to keep their bodies healthy.

A blood *transfusion* is the process of moving the blood from one person into the bloodstream of another person. People who need a blood transfusion receive donated blood of the same or a compatible blood type. A person who volunteers to donate blood is a *blood donor*. Blood donors with Type O blood are known as *universal donors* because this blood type can be used for people with any blood type. (See chart below.)

Once blood is donated, the blood is processed and tested to determine that it is safe to use. Blood that is safe to use is stored in a *blood bank*, such as the one that the American Red Cross maintains, until it is shipped to hospitals.

There is a high demand for blood donations, but only about 10 percent of the population donates blood annually. A person in a serious car accident may need as many as 100 pints of blood.

Some diseases require people to receive blood transfusions throughout their lives. Donating blood can save up to three lives for each pint of blood donated.

Becoming a Blood Donor

How much do you know about being a blood donor? What questions do you have about blood donation? Write them down and use a valid and reliable source of information, such as the American Red Cross Blood Services, to find the answers. Questions can include the following:

- Who can donate blood? What are the requirements?
- How does someone become a donor?
- How often can someone donate blood?
- What types of blood donations are available?
- Why does the United States need blood donors?
- Who can receive different types of blood?

Based on the information you learned, create a letter, poster, voicemail, text message, or graphic that will encourage people who are able to donate blood to sign up to be a donor. Use accurate information to show people the importance of donation. Provide simple, clear directions on how to become a blood donor. Share your information with the class.

Blood Type Donations

Type A	can donate to	Type A Type AB
Type B	can donate to	Type B Type AB
Type AB	can donate to	Type AB
Type O	can donate to	Type O Type A Type B Type AB

Parts of Blood

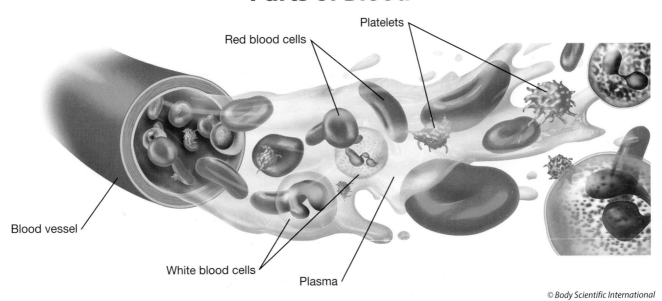

© Body Scientific International

Figure 2.11 The basic parts of blood include plasma, which is the liquid part, and red blood cells, white blood cells, and platelets, which are all solid in form. *Which part of the blood is reponsible for transporting oxygen throughout the body?*

- *White blood cells* move through the blood and live in various organs of the body. They help defend the body against infections.
- *Platelets* are responsible for blood clotting. Clotting stops blood from flowing outside the wall of a blood vessel. This action helps prevent blood loss when blood vessels are injured.

Respiratory System

The circulatory system cannot deliver oxygen to the body's cells without the help of the respiratory system. The **respiratory system** includes organs that obtain vitally important oxygen from the outside world (**Figure 2.12**). This body system draws oxygen into the lungs and delivers it to blood vessels. It also takes carbon dioxide—another gas—out of the blood and sends it outside the body. Since the body's cells require oxygen, a healthy respiratory system enables all other body functions. Respiratory organs can be divided into the upper and lower respiratory systems.

Upper Respiratory System

The upper respiratory system allows air containing oxygen to enter the body. Air enters the nose and mouth and passes down through the throat to the *larynx* and then through the *trachea* to the lungs. You can feel the larynx as a bump in the front of your throat. It vibrates when you speak, as air passes across the vocal cords. A small structure covers the larynx when you swallow and prevents food from entering the trachea.

The walls of the respiratory passages make a sticky substance called *mucus*. This mucus traps bacteria and dust particles so they cannot enter the lungs.

Figure 2.12
The main function of the respiratory system is to make sure a constant supply of fresh oxygen is always available to the body.

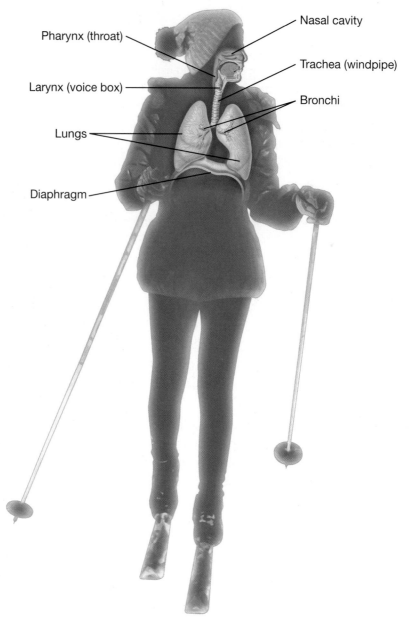

Pharynx (throat)
Nasal cavity
Larynx (voice box)
Trachea (windpipe)
Bronchi
Lungs
Diaphragm

© Body Scientific International

Extra mucus is made when someone has an infection or an allergic reaction. The passage behind the nose is also lined with mucus and with blood vessels that warm and moisten air. You see evidence of this on cold days when you exhale. The warm, exhaled air forms water vapor as it contacts the cold outside air.

Lower Respiratory System

The trachea branches into two **bronchi**, which are air passages that lead to each lung. The bronchi branch into smaller passages called *bronchioles* inside the lungs. These smaller airways end as sacks called *alveoli*. When you inhale, air fills the alveoli. The alveoli are important for oxygen exchange in the lungs. If they fill with fluid, as in pneumonia, air and oxygen cannot enter them. This can disrupt the vital process of respiration.

Respiration

Respiration is the exchange of oxygen and carbon dioxide in the respiratory system. It includes two steps: inhaling and exhaling. When you inhale, you take in air, which reaches the lungs. Air fills the alveoli, and oxygen moves into the blood in tiny capillaries. These capillaries then deliver oxygen-rich blood to the heart.

At the same time, carbon dioxide moves from the blood into the alveoli. This air travels back into the respiratory passages. When you exhale, you push the air with carbon dioxide out of the body (**Figure 2.13**).

Muscles help the lungs take in and push out air. During inhalation, muscles enlarge the chest. This draws air in through the mouth and nose. The chief muscle doing this work is the **diaphragm**. The diaphragm is a sheet of muscle beneath the lungs and above the abdomen. As the diaphragm moves down, the chest expands. Other muscles of the chest, especially those between the ribs, also help the chest expand. Exhalation happens when these muscles relax. The chest collapses and squeezes air out the mouth and nose.

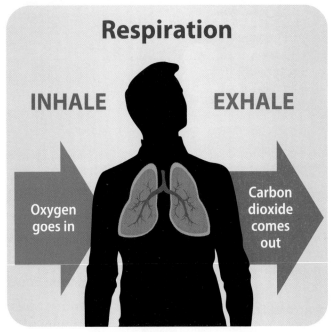

Silhouette: Chipmunk131/Shutterstock.com; Lungs: Inspiring/Shutterstock.com

Figure 2.13 In respiration, the body inhales air from the environment. Oxygen leaves the air and enters the blood. Carbon dioxide leaves the blood and enters the air. Air is then exhaled outside the body. *Which type of vessel delivers oxygen-rich blood to the heart?*

Lesson 2.2 Review

1. Name two functions of the circulatory system.
2. Which heart chamber pumps oxygen-rich blood out to the rest of the body?
3. **True or false.** Veins carry oxygen-poor blood to the heart.
4. What is the name of the blood cell responsible for blood clotting?
5. Explain what happens during respiration.
6. **Critical thinking.** What kind of blood vessels obtain oxygen from air in the lungs?

Hands-On Activity

Pull out your drawing from the first lesson. Add drawings to "your body" of the organs and structures from this lesson. Add to your list of behaviors that will keep these structures and organs healthy. What medical specialists help care for these body systems? Are these specialists available in your community? Locate the website of a national organization associated with one or more of these body systems. Find out how you can help get their message out in your community.

Lesson 2.3

Digesting and Removing Substances

Key Terms 📖

digestive system body system that breaks down food to provide nutrients and energy; also removes solid waste from the body

pancreas fish-shaped organ behind the stomach that makes many kinds of enzymes needed for digestion

liver large brown organ to the right of the stomach that has many jobs, including making bile

gallbladder organ in which bile is stored until needed to digest food

appendix finger-shaped organ attached to the large intestine; made of lymphatic tissue

urinary system body system that removes liquid waste from the body

kidneys two bean-shaped organs that filter blood and make urine

bladder organ that stores urine until it can be pushed out of the body

lymphatic system body system of organs and tissues that help fight infections

spleen organ filled with white blood cells; filters blood

Learning Outcomes

After studying this lesson, you will be able to

- **explain** how the structures of the digestive system digest food and promote health.
- **describe** how the urinary system ensures health.
- **identify** ways the lymphatic and immune systems prevent communicable diseases.

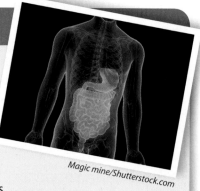

Magic mine/Shutterstock.com

Graphic Organizer

Digest and Remove

On a separate sheet of paper, create a graphic organizer like the one shown. As you read this lesson, fill in the organizer with the bodily processes involved in bringing substances into the body, digesting them, and removing them from the body. Make sure to note body parts and organs involved in the digestive, urinary, lymphatic, and immune systems.

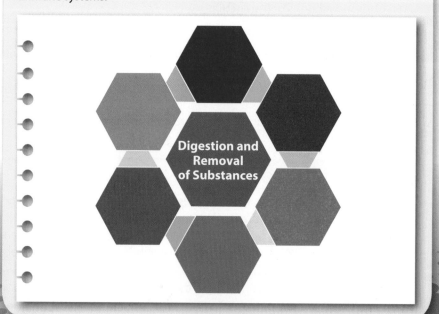

Digestion and Removal of Substances

Three body systems help digest and remove substances. The digestive system brings food into the body. It also breaks down food to provide nutrients the body needs and removes waste. The urinary system takes liquid waste out of the body. The lymphatic and immune systems help the body fight disease. In this lesson, you will learn about the digestive, urinary, and lymphatic and immune systems.

Digestive System

The **digestive system** brings food into the body and breaks it down to provide nutrients and energy the body needs. It also removes solid waste from the body. The digestive system begins at the mouth and continues through the throat, esophagus, and stomach. It also includes the small and large intestines, liver, gallbladder, pancreas, appendix, rectum, and anus (**Figure 2.14**).

Mouth and Teeth

Digestion, or the process of breaking down food, begins in the mouth. Here, teeth break down food into a soft mass that can be swallowed.

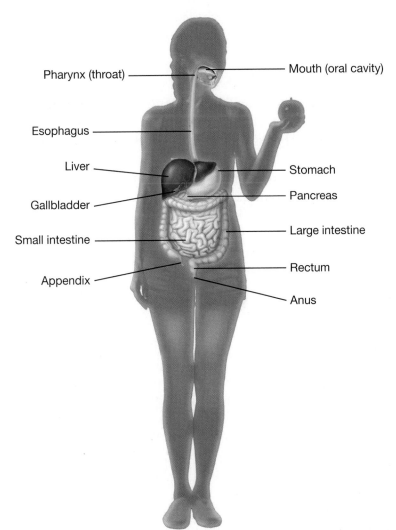

Pharynx (throat)

Esophagus

Liver

Gallbladder

Small intestine

Appendix

Mouth (oral cavity)

Stomach

Pancreas

Large intestine

Rectum

Anus

Figure 2.14
Food travels through the digestive system from the mouth all the way to the anus. *What is the name of the process that occurs in this system and what does it do?*

© Body Scientific International

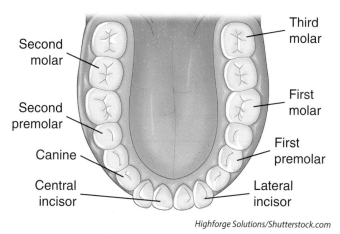

Second molar

Second premolar

Canine

Central incisor

Third molar

First molar

First premolar

Lateral incisor

Highforge Solutions/Shutterstock.com

Figure 2.15 The incisors and canines (front teeth) have sharp surfaces for tearing food. Premolars and molars (back teeth) have a flat surface for crushing and chewing food.

Teeth have different shapes to do different jobs. The teeth in the front, which are more pointed, tear food. The flatter, larger teeth toward the back crush food. Teeth play an important role in digestion, so their health is important (**Figure 2.15**).

Salivary glands are found in and around the mouth. These glands produce a liquid called *saliva*, which moistens food. Saliva also contains substances called *enzymes* that help digest food. Enzymes use chemical reactions to break down food into nutrients and energy.

The tongue is also part of the digestive system. It pushes chewed food into the throat. Food passes from the throat into the esophagus.

Esophagus

The *esophagus* is a muscular tube that connects the throat to the stomach. Chewed food moves down the esophagus during digestion. A small, donut-shaped muscle called a *sphincter* joins the esophagus to the stomach and opens to let food pass into the stomach. The sphincter closes after food enters the stomach to prevent backflow into the esophagus.

Stomach and Small Intestine

The *stomach* is a muscular bag that is slightly to the left of the center of the body and below the ribcage. The stomach makes a mixture of enzymes and a powerful acid. Muscles of the stomach wall mix digesting food with chemicals to break it down further.

Food passes from the stomach into the *small intestine*. Another sphincter controls the flow of food from the stomach into the small intestine. Once food is in the small intestine, muscles in the walls of the small intestine contract rhythmically. These movements push the food along the small intestine. In the small intestine, nutrients are also absorbed into the blood.

The walls of the small intestine make enzymes needed to digest food. Most digestion happens in the first part of the small intestine. The pancreas and liver release substances to help this process.

Pancreas and Liver

The **pancreas** is a fish-shaped organ behind the stomach. It connects to the small intestine and makes many kinds of enzymes needed for digestion. These enzymes pass into the small intestine through a thin tube.

The **liver** is a large brown organ to the right of the stomach that has many jobs in the body. It helps digestion by making bile. *Bile* breaks down large fat droplets into very small fat particles that can be digested and transported through the body.

Bile is stored in the **gallbladder**. The gallbladder is a small, pear-shaped bag under the liver. It squeezes bile through a tube into the small intestine.

Large Intestine

Nutrients and materials that are not absorbed into the blood pass into the *large intestine*. This part of the digestive system prepares solid food waste for removal from the body.

Some water and minerals from food are absorbed into the blood from the large intestine. The remaining material is eliminated as *feces*. It takes about six to eight hours for food to move from the stomach to the large intestine. Undigested food spends 24 to 48 hours in the large intestine. The exact time depends on the kind of food eaten. Protein meals, such as meat and fish, take longer to digest. Time in the digestive system also varies from person to person.

Feces are stored in a part of the large intestine called the *rectum*. They are eliminated from the body when large intestine muscles push them out through an opening called the *anus* (**Figure 2.16**).

The Digestion Process

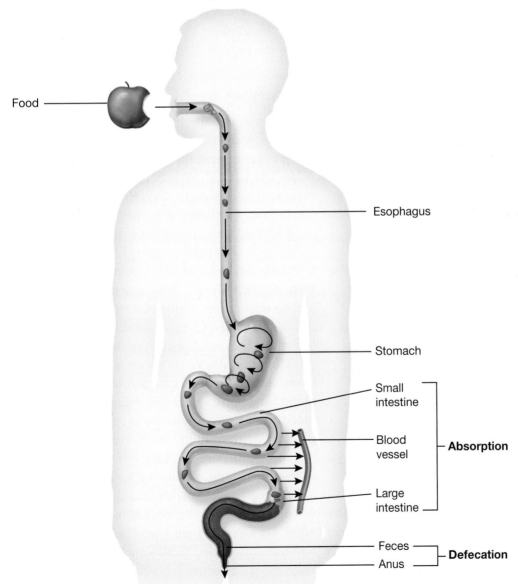

Food

Esophagus

Stomach

Small
intestine

Blood
vessel

Absorption

Large
intestine

Feces

Defecation

Anus

Figure 2.16
Review the steps of digestion using this illustration. Food enters the mouth and travels down the esophagus to the stomach. In the small intestine and large intestine, nutrients, water, and minerals are absorbed into the blood. Material that is not absorbed becomes feces in the large intestine and is removed through the anus.

© Body Scientific International

The **appendix** is attached to the large intestine, but it does not play a role in digesting food. The appendix is a finger-shaped organ made of lymphatic tissue, which you will learn about later in this lesson. The job of the appendix is unclear, but it might help protect the digestive tract from infections.

Sometimes the appendix gets infected by bacteria in the colon. Such an infection—a condition called *appendicitis*—is dangerous. An infected appendix swells as it fills with bacteria and pus. If it swells and bursts, bacteria will infect the body cavity and circulatory system. An infected appendix must be removed by surgery.

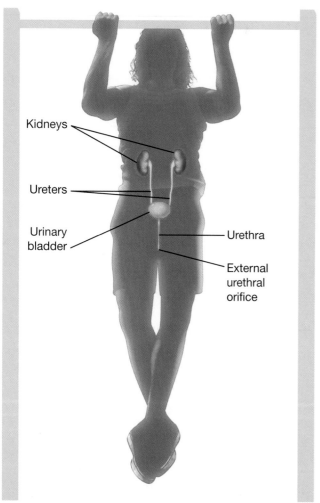

Kidneys

Ureters

Urinary bladder

Urethra

External urethral orifice

© Body Scientific International

Figure 2.17 The primary function of the urinary system is to take liquid waste out of the body. *Which organs have the most important role to play in the functioning of the urinary system?*

Urinary System

The **urinary system** removes liquid waste from the body (**Figure 2.17**). The kidneys play an important role in this system. The urinary system includes the following:

- two kidneys and ureters
- the bladder
- the urethra

Kidneys

Two bean-shaped **kidneys** begin the process of urine production by filtering blood. Both kidneys lie against the lower back wall of the body. The left kidney is behind the spleen. The right kidney is smaller than the left kidney and lies behind and below the liver.

Kidneys remove waste from the blood. Kidneys also control the amount of water, minerals, and acid in blood. As blood moves through the kidneys, the waste that is filtered out becomes *urine*. Urine exits the kidney through a ureter. Cleansed and filtered blood returns to the circulatory system.

Though kidneys are smaller than the stomach, they receive an enormous amount of blood. The body sends up to 25 percent of its blood to the kidneys. Kidneys must continually filter waste from blood and form urine.

You would not live long if your kidneys stopped working. Waste and toxins would build up in blood quickly and soon poison every organ, including the brain. This is why making decisions that promote a healthy urinary system is important. One way to help keep the urinary system healthy is to drink more water and less caffeinated drinks such as soda.

Ureters, Bladder, and Urethra

A *ureter* is a tube that carries urine from a kidney to the bladder. The urinary system includes two ureters. Each ureter enters the top of the bladder.

The **bladder** is a muscular bag that sits at the level of the pubic area above the genitals. The bladder stores urine. When the bladder is full, the bladder muscle squeezes urine into the urethra. Two sphincters join the urethra to the bladder (**Figure 2.18**). The outermost sphincter, also called the *external urethral sphincter*, gives you some control over urination. During toilet training, small children learn how to control this sphincter.

The *urethra* is a small tube that transports urine out of the body. The urethra exits males at the tip of the penis. The urethra is shorter in females. It exits females above the vagina.

Lymphatic and Immune Systems

The **lymphatic system** is responsible for removing foreign substances from the body. This body system includes the *immune system* and has organs and tissues that help fight infections. Communicable diseases can develop often if this system is not healthy. The main organs of the lymphatic and immune systems include the following:

- lymphatic vessels
- lymph nodes
- tonsils
- the spleen
- the thymus
- white blood cells

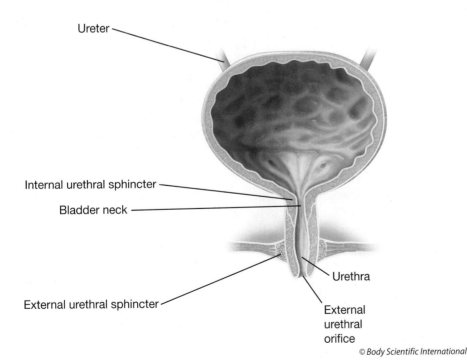

Ureter

Internal urethral sphincter

Bladder neck

External urethral sphincter

Urethra

External urethral orifice

© Body Scientific International

Figure 2.18
The internal and external urethral sphincters control the flow of urine out of the body. The internal urethral sphincter is involuntary. The external urethral sphincter is voluntary. ***Which sphincter gives some control over urination?***

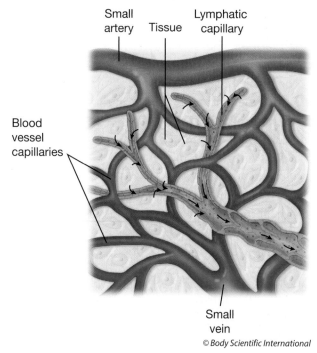

Small artery   Tissue   Lymphatic capillary

Blood vessel capillaries

Small vein

© Body Scientific International

Figure 2.19 Lymphatic capillaries (green) collect lymph from the fluid pushed out of blood vessel capillaries. Lymph travels through lymphatic vessels in the body. *While blood vessels carry blood, what do lymphatic vessels carry?*

Lymphatic Vessels and Lymph Nodes

The *lymphatic vessels* are similar to blood vessels, but they do not carry blood. Instead, they carry fluid that builds up in tissues of the body. This fluid comes from the body's millions of tiny capillaries. Each time the heart beats, it creates blood pressure in capillaries. This pressure pushes fluid out of the capillaries and into tissues. The fluid becomes *lymph* when it enters the lymphatic capillaries and flows into other lymphatic vessels (**Figure 2.19**). Lymphatic vessels collect and transport lymph to the chest. There, lymph rejoins the blood.

Lymph is filtered by *lymph nodes* before it reenters the blood. Inside the lymph nodes, lymph contacts white blood cells. These cells remove bacteria and viruses from the fluid. They can also grow and reproduce to fight infections. In some infections, lymph nodes become swollen because of the buildup of extra white blood cells. For this reason, swollen lymph nodes are a sign that the body is fighting an infection.

CASE STUDY

Fighting Off Infections: Brian Gets a Cold

Brian is 12 years old, and last month he had a fever and a terrible sore throat that lasted for a few days. His parents took him to the doctor, who said that Brian's lymph nodes and tonsils in his throat were both swollen from infection, which is why it hurt.

His parents never seem to get colds, but Brian gets one at least once a year. His three-year-old sister gets sick even more often. Brian asked his dad about it, and he told Brian that bodies can fight off infections better as they develop. Children get sick less often as they grow up and their body systems mature.

Brian does not want to get sick anymore. It is not fun and he does not like missing baseball practice. At his next regular checkup with his doctor, he asks her what he can do to keep from getting sick. She tells Brian that he should minimize stress, be physically

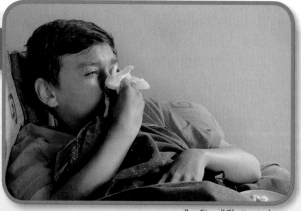

Ben Gingell/Shutterstock.com

active, sleep well, and eat nutritious foods. According to her, Brian can also avoid getting sick with respiratory etiquette, such as washing his hands.

Thinking Critically

1. Which body system, when weak or underdeveloped, is the cause of infections?

2. Why are the recommendations of Brian's doctor helpful for not getting sick?

Tonsils are lymphatic tissues that guard the throat from infection. They are located on the sides and top of the back of the throat. The tonsils also contain white blood cells. When the throat is infected, tonsils enlarge and become red. Swollen tonsils are a sign that your body is fighting a throat infection.

Spleen and Thymus

The **spleen** is an organ that is filled with white blood cells and filters blood. The spleen is located to the left of the stomach and is shaped like a flattened bean. The spleen also removes dead red blood cells.

The *thymus* is a lymphatic organ located over the large blood vessels in the upper chest. In the thymus, certain kinds of white blood cells learn how to recognize and attack bacteria and viruses.

White Blood Cells

A variety of white blood cells are part of the lymphatic system. Some take in and destroy bacteria (**Figure 2.20**). Others specialize in controlling viruses. Some white blood cells make antibodies. *Antibodies* are proteins that stick to bacteria and viruses and help destroy these invaders. All these white blood cells are a vital part of the body's immune system.

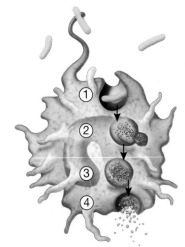

① White blood cell engulfs enemy cell (bacteria, dead cells)

② Enzymes start to destroy enemy cell

③ Enemy cell breaks down into small fragments

④ Indigestible fragments are discharged

© *Body Scientific International*

Figure 2.20 White blood cells can engulf and destroy enemy cells such as bacteria. *What are the proteins made by white blood cells that help protect against viruses and bacteria?*

Lesson 2.3 Review

1. Which of the following connects the throat to the stomach?
   A. Esophagus.
   B. Small intestine.
   C. Salivary glands.
   D. Large intestine.

2. **True or false.** In the small intestine, nutrients are absorbed into the blood.

3. Which organ removes waste from the blood and produces urine?

4. Lymphatic organs that filter lymph before it reenters the blood are called _____ _____.

5. **Critical thinking.** What would happen if your kidneys stopped working?

Hands-On Activity

Pull out your body systems drawing from the previous lessons. Add drawings to "your body" of the organs and structures from this lesson. Add to your list of behaviors that will keep these structures and organs healthy. Create a flyer or poster for younger students encouraging them to do one of these behaviors. With your teacher's permission, hang it around the school.

Controlling and Regulating the Body

nervous system body system that allows people to think, use the senses, move, and maintain important body processes

neuron cell that is specialized to receive and send signals

cerebrum largest part of the brain, which interprets information from the sensory organs; controls muscle actions and is responsible for intelligence, memory, and personality

cerebellum part of the brain that controls coordinated, smooth muscle activity

brain stem part of the brain that controls the heartbeat and breathing rate

spinal cord part of the nervous system that carries nerve signals between the brain and the body

endocrine system body system that produces chemical messengers called *hormones*, which regulate body processes

pituitary gland master gland of the body, which releases hormones to control other endocrine organs

thyroid hormone substance produced in the thyroid that increases the rate at which the body uses energy

Learning Outcomes

After studying this lesson, you will be able to

- **explain** why the nervous system plays an essential role in overall health.
- **list** the sensory organs and their impact on health.
- **identify** how a healthy endocrine system helps the body work effectively.

Graphic Organizer

Nervous and Endocrine Systems

The body systems involved in the control and regulation of the body contain many different structures and organs. On a separate sheet of paper, create a graphic organizer like the one shown. As you read this lesson, fill in the organizer with notes on each body system, the body parts involved, and what each system does. Examples are provided for you.

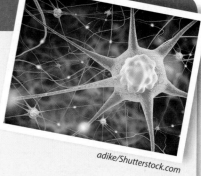
adike/Shutterstock.com

Nervous system
- The nervous system allows a person to think, use the senses, send signals to the body to move, and control important body processes.
-
-

Endocrine system
- The endocrine system controls the body using hormones.
-
-

The nervous system, sensory organs, and endocrine system help regulate the body's function internally and with the outside world. They allow the body to function smoothly and efficiently and do many complicated things. For example, the nervous system helps the body remember and perform complex tasks such as playing the piano. The nervous and endocrine systems both guide the female body through labor and the birth of a baby. In this final lesson, you will learn about the nervous system, sensory organs, and endocrine system.

Nervous System

The **nervous system** is organized into two parts. The first is the *central nervous system (CNS)*, which includes the brain and the spinal cord. The second is the *peripheral nervous system (PNS)*, which includes the nerves and sensory organs. A healthy nervous system allows people to think, perform tasks, and maintain important body processes (**Figure 2.21**).

Neurons

Neurons are the building blocks of the nervous system. A **neuron** is a cell specialized to receive and send signals. Neurons make up the brain, spinal cord, and nerves. In addition to neurons, the nervous system has millions of other cells that protect and support them.

There are three types of neurons. Some neurons carry signals from the body to the CNS. These are *sensory neurons*. In contrast, *motor neurons* carry information from the CNS to the body. Motor neurons control the body's glands and tell muscles to contract or relax. A third type of neuron is the *interneuron*. Interneurons carry signals between neurons.

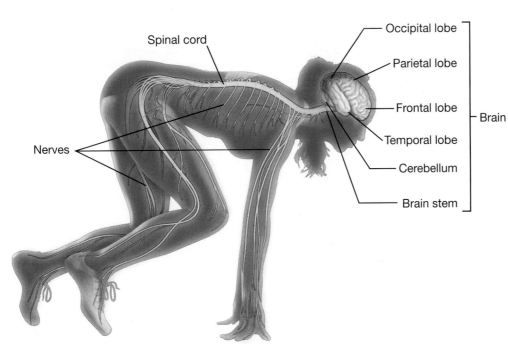

Spinal cord

Occipital lobe

Parietal lobe

Frontal lobe

Temporal lobe

Cerebellum

Brain stem

Brain

Nerves

Figure 2.21
The nervous system is amazing in its ability to direct many different functions at one time. *Which part of the nervous system includes the brain and spinal cord?*

© Body Scientific International

Brain

The brain controls nearly all body functions. For example, to bend the knee, the brain tells muscles on the back of the thigh to contract. At the same time, the brain tells muscles on the front of the thigh to relax. The brain also stores information and makes sense of signals coming from the sensory organs.

The brain is protected by the bones of the skull. Under the skull, layers of tissues cover and also protect the brain. A fluid flows over the brain and cushions it.

The largest part of the brain is the **cerebrum**. The cerebrum performs important functions. It interprets information coming to the brain from the sensory organs as well as controls muscle actions. The cerebrum also is responsible for intelligence, memory, and personality.

The cerebrum is divided into two nearly equal halves—the left and right hemispheres. The halves are connected by nerves that allow them to communicate. The inner region of the cerebrum is called *white matter*. The outer, wrinkled region of the cerebrum is the *cerebral cortex*, or *gray matter*. The cerebral cortex is divided into lobes and each lobe has a different function (**Figure 2.22**).

Figure 2.22
The different lobes of the brain have different functions. *Which lobe of the brain is responsible for controlling personality, judgment, and memory?*

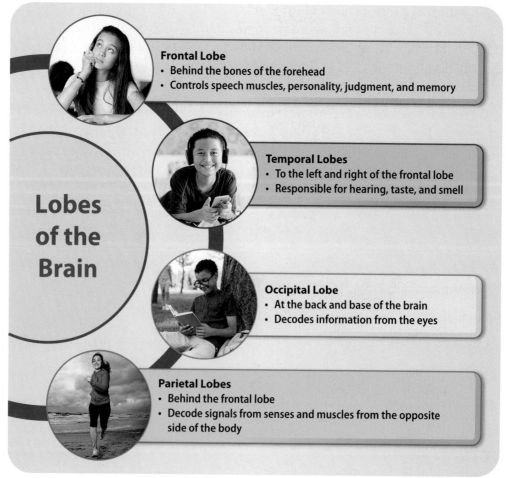

Lobes of the Brain

Frontal Lobe
- Behind the bones of the forehead
- Controls speech muscles, personality, judgment, and memory

Temporal Lobes
- To the left and right of the frontal lobe
- Responsible for hearing, taste, and smell

Occipital Lobe
- At the back and base of the brain
- Decodes information from the eyes

Parietal Lobes
- Behind the frontal lobe
- Decode signals from senses and muscles from the opposite side of the body

Girl thinking: Tyler Olson/Shutterstock.com; Boy with headphones: Creativa Images/Shutterstock.com; Boy reading: LightField Studios/Shutterstock.com; Girl running: Jacek Chabraszewski/Shutterstock.com

Brain Powers: The Different Abilities of the Left and Right Brain

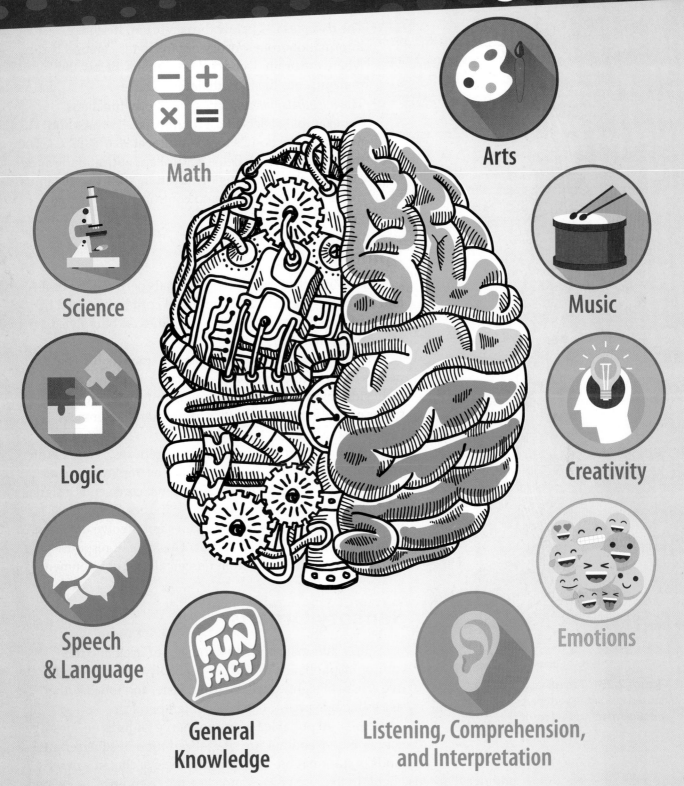

Math

Arts

Science

Music

Logic

Creativity

Speech & Language

Emotions

General Knowledge

Listening, Comprehension, and Interpretation

Brain: Macrovector/Shutterstock.com; Left icons, top to bottom: Creative Stall/Shutterstock.com; Alekseeva Yulia/Shutterstock.com; Anna_leni/Shutterstock.com; LuckyDesigner/Shutterstock.com; Alex Gorka/Shutterstock.com; Right icons, top to bottom: 3DDock/Shutterstock.com; Olha Zinovatna/Shutterstock.com; Bloomicon/Shutterstock.com; Andre Luiz Gollo/Shutterstock.com; Panda Vector/Shutterstock.com

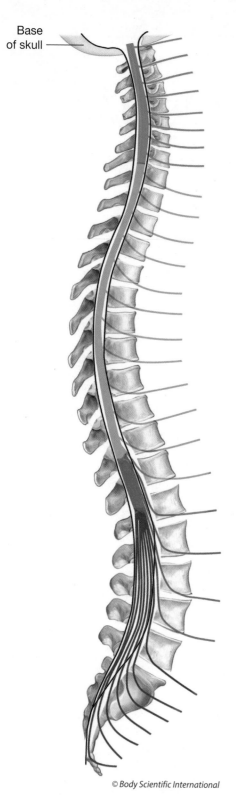

Base
of skull

© Body Scientific International

Figure 2.23 The spinal cord is housed inside the vertebrae. *What is the function of the spinal cord?*

The base of the brain includes the cerebellum and the brain stem. The **cerebellum** lies below the occipital lobe, which controls coordinated, smooth muscle activity. The **brain stem** connects the brain to the spinal cord. It controls heartbeat and breathing rate.

The brain also includes the following structures:

- The *thalamus* lies below the cerebrum. It sends information from sensory organs to the cerebral cortex, where the brain decodes these signals. Below the thalamus lies the hypothalamus.
- The *hypothalamus* regulates vital body functions. For example, it acts like a thermostat. It senses and maintains the body's temperature, at 98.6°F (37°C). The hypothalamus also helps control appetite and the cycle of waking and sleeping. In addition, the hypothalamus makes some hormones and controls the endocrine system.

Spinal Cord

The **spinal cord** carries nerve signals between the brain and the body (**Figure 2.23**). The spinal cord is protected by bones of the spine called *vertebrae*. Tissues and fluid also cover the spinal cord.

Many nerves run up and down the spinal cord. The nerves branch from the spinal cord and run to the left and right sides of the body. Some nerves control the muscles. Other nerves carry sense information from the sensory organs to the brain.

The spinal cord also controls some reflexes. A *reflex* is an automatic response to a sensation. For example, if extreme heat is sensed at the fingertips, the spinal cord sends a signal to arm muscles to contract and move the arm away from the source of heat. This response does not involve the brain. That is why a reflex can be so fast. This type of response helps keep the body safe from dangers in the environment.

Sensory Organs

Senses allow the body to know about itself and the environment outside it. You are probably familiar with the five senses of sight, smell, hearing, taste, and touch. Other senses include pressure, pain, and temperature.

Senses are possible because of nerve endings on sensory nerves. Nerve endings are specialized for detecting certain kinds of information. For example, the eye contains nerve endings that sense light. In the case of eyes and ears, nerve endings are helped by numerous other structures. The eyes and ears are sensory organs. Caring for these structures promotes health.

Eye

The eyes and brain work together to make vision possible. The eyes detect light with nerve endings. Nerves then carry this information to the occipital lobe of the brain, which forms images from the information it receives. Numerous structures help the eye capture light and send signals to the brain.

The inner, back layer of the eyeball is the *retina* (**Figure 2.24**). The retina is made of nerve endings that are very receptive to light. These nerve endings allow the brain to see color, black and white, and shades of gray. In the center of the retina is an area rich in nerve endings. This area is responsible for forming sharp images.

The front of the eyeball's surface is covered by the *cornea*. Light enters the cornea and passes through a *lens*. The lens focuses light on the retina. The *iris*, the colored part of the eye, lies in front of the lens, under the cornea. The iris appears round and has a black, circular opening called the *pupil*. The pupil allows light into the eyeball. The iris can change the pupil's size. In bright light, the iris shrinks the pupil to let in a small amount of light. In darkness, the iris widens the pupil to let in more light.

The eyeball is protected by the bones of the skull. A strong tissue gives the eye its spherical shape. A firm gel fills the inside of the eye to help keep the eyeball's shape.

In front of the eyeball are *eyelids*, skin-covered flaps that can close and protect the eye. Tear glands are located above each eye. The tears lubricate and clean the eye's outer surface.

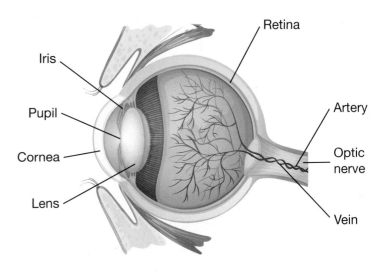

BlueRingMedia/Shutterstock.com

Figure 2.24 The cornea, iris, pupil, lens, and retina work together in the eye to give you vision. *How do the eyes detect light?*

Ear

The ear has three main parts, and each serves a different, but important, role (**Figure 2.25**). The outer ear, called the *pinna*, is the large part of the ear that people can see. The main job of the pinna is to help bring sounds into the ear. Sounds then enter the *auditory canal*, the part of the ear that extends inward. Earwax is also produced in the auditory canal. This part of the ear also *amplifies* (increases the volume of) sounds so they can be clearly heard and interpreted.

After sound is gathered by the outer ear and sent through the auditory canal, it reaches the middle ear. The middle ear includes the *eardrum*, which vibrates when sounds reach it. This part of the ear also includes the following three small bones:

- hammer (malleus)
- anvil (incus)
- stirrup (stapes)

Anatomy of the Ear

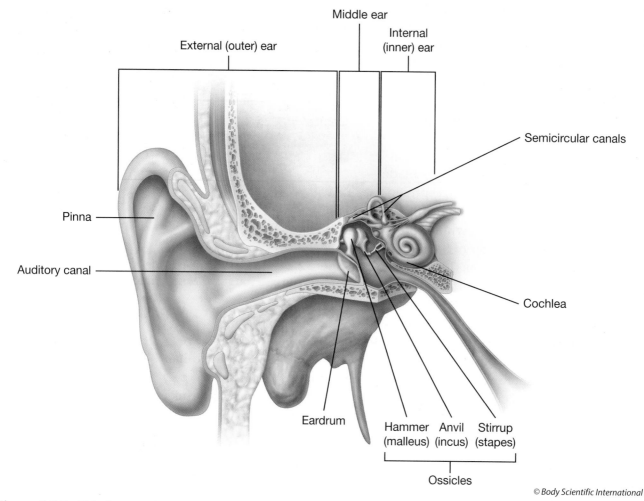

Figure 2.25 This diagram shows the anatomy of the ear. *Where in the ear is earwax produced?*

© Body Scientific International

The inner ear converts sound vibrations produced in the middle ear into neural impulses that the brain recognizes as sound. This part of the ear includes the *cochlea*, which is a spiral tube. The cochlea is covered with nerve cells, which pick up different vibrations. These vibrations are then sent to the brain through the auditory nerve. The inner ear also includes the *semicircular canals*, which are attached to the cochlea. These canals are filled with fluids that move when you move, helping you to keep your balance.

Endocrine System

The **endocrine system** produces chemical messengers called *hormones*, which regulate body processes. The organs that produce these hormones are part of the endocrine system (**Figure 2.26**). These organs release hormones into the blood, which carries them all over the body. Certain organs respond to certain hormones. They respond by growing or developing or by making other hormones and products.

Pituitary Gland

The **pituitary gland** is called the *master gland* of the endocrine system and is located beneath the hypothalamus in the brain. The pituitary gland uses hormones to control other endocrine organs. For example, the pituitary gland makes hormones that control growth, birth, puberty, and other activities. The pituitary gland itself is controlled by the brain's hypothalamus.

Thyroid

The *thyroid* is a gland located on the front of the neck, just below the larynx. It makes thyroid hormone. **Thyroid hormone** increases the rate at which the body uses energy. This also controls the body's temperature.

Parathyroid Glands

The *parathyroid glands* are four tiny glands located on the back of the thyroid gland. These glands make *parathyroid hormone (PTH)*. The parathyroid glands raise the blood levels of calcium and phosphate. Calcium and phosphate are minerals important for bone growth and the growth of all the body's cells.

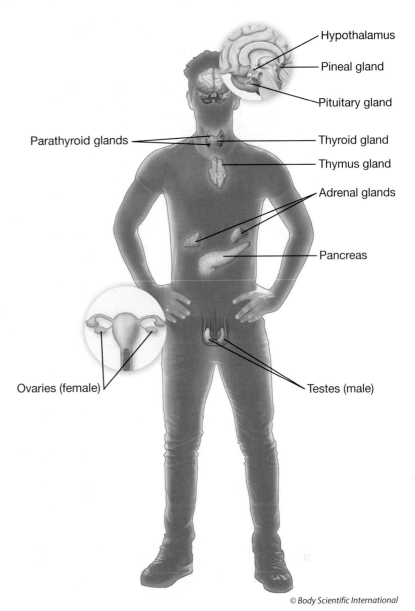

© *Body Scientific International*

Figure 2.26   The pituitary gland, which hangs beneath the hypothalamus, is controlled by the hypothalamus and regulates all other endocrine glands.

Adrenal Glands

The *adrenal glands* are located on top of each kidney. These glands produce several hormones that control the blood levels of minerals and salts. Adrenal hormones also control how the body uses energy sources such as carbohydrates.

During stress, the adrenal glands make adrenaline. *Adrenaline* prepares the body to cope with stress by increasing the heart rate and breathing rate. Adrenaline also increases blood flow to the muscles, heart, lungs, and brain. The adrenal glands also make *cortisol*, which prepares the body to deal with stress.

Pancreas

The *pancreas* is an endocrine organ as well as part of the digestive system. As part of the endocrine system, the pancreas makes the hormones insulin and glucagon. Insulin and glucagon have opposite effects on blood sugar.

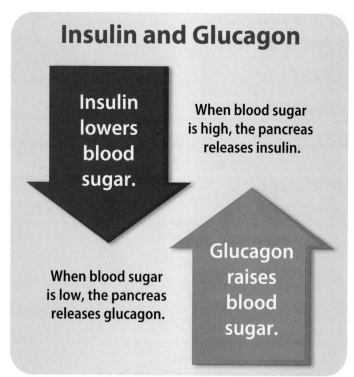

Insulin and Glucagon

Insulin lowers blood sugar.

When blood sugar is high, the pancreas releases insulin.

When blood sugar is low, the pancreas releases glucagon.

Glucagon raises blood sugar.

Figure 2.27 Together, insulin and glucagon keep blood sugar steady. The pancreas releases them when blood sugar becomes too high or too low. *Which disease can develop if insulin and glucagon do not work properly in the body?*

Insulin lowers blood sugar, and *glucagon* elevates blood sugar. Together, these hormones keep blood sugar at a healthy level (**Figure 2.27**). If they do not work properly, a person can develop the disease *diabetes*. Diabetes results in abnormally high blood sugar. Untreated diabetes leads to kidney and eye damage. Diabetes can also cause heart disease.

Ovaries and Testes

The *ovaries* and *testes* are part of the endocrine system as well as part of the reproductive system. As you will read in Chapter 17, the ovaries produce the hormones estrogen and progestin. These hormones regulate the sexual development of females, female sex characteristics, and the female reproductive cycle.

The testes produce testosterone. This hormone controls the sexual development of males and male sex characteristics.

Lesson 2.4 Review

1. Which type of neuron carries information from the CNS to the body?

2. The _____ lobe of the brain decodes information from the eyes.
   - **A.** temporal
   - **B.** parietal
   - **C.** occipital
   - **D.** frontal

3. **True or false.** The pituitary gland is the master gland of the endocrine system.

4. Which endocrine gland produces adrenaline and cortisol?

5. **Critical thinking.** Are the neurons that carry information from the eyes and ears to the CNS motor or sensory neurons? Explain.

Hands-On Activity

Pull out your body systems drawing from the previous lessons. Add drawings to "your body" of the organs and structures from this lesson (brain, spinal cord, sense organs, glands, etc.). Reflect on your behaviors to keep these structures and organs healthy. Set a goal to follow that identifies how you will keep the structures healthy.

Summary

Lesson 2.1 Supporting and Moving the Body

- Cells are the basic unit of life. A tissue is a collection of similar cells that do a certain job. An organ is a collection of tissues that perform a specific job.
- The integumentary system includes the skin, hair, and nails. It covers and protects the body, keeps out germs, makes vitamin D, and houses nerve endings.
- The skeletal system is made of 206 bones that provide structure, shape, and protection. At joints, bones are held together by ligaments.
- The muscular system helps the body move as muscle tissue contracts. There are three types of muscle tissue: skeletal muscles, smooth muscles, and cardiac muscle.

Lesson 2.2 Moving and Exchanging Substances

- The circulatory system, also called the cardiovascular system, is responsible for the flow of blood and substances through the body. Arteries carry oxygen-rich blood while veins carry oxygen-poor blood. Capillaries deliver oxygen and nutrients to body cells and pick up cell waste.
- Blood carries oxygen and nutrients through the body, removes carbon dioxide and waste, regulates a person's body temperature, and protects the body against infection.
- The respiratory system delivers oxygen to blood vessels, then sends carbon dioxide out of the body. This exchange is called *respiration*.

Lesson 2.3 Digesting and Removing Substances

- The digestive system breaks down food to provide nutrients and energy for the body. It also removes waste from the body.
- Undigested food passes into the large intestine, where it is removed from the body as feces. The urinary system removes liquid waste from the body using the kidneys, ureters, bladder, and urethra.
- The lymphatic system, including the immune system, is responsible for removing foreign substances from the body. The main organs of this system are the lymphatic vessels, lymph nodes, tonsils, spleen, thymus, and white blood cells.

Lesson 2.4 Controlling and Regulating the Body

- The nervous system contains the brain, spinal cord, nerves, and sensory organs. The brain controls body functions, stores information, and makes sense of signals coming from sensory organs. The spinal cord carries nerve signals between the brain and the body.
- Senses allow the body to know about itself and the surrounding environment.
- The endocrine system uses hormones to control the body. This system uses the pituitary gland, thyroid, parathyroid glands, and adrenal glands to produce various hormones. The pancreas, ovaries, and testes also produce hormones for the endocrine system.

Check Your Knowledge

Record your answers to each of the following questions on a separate sheet of paper.

1. **True or false.** A tissue is a collection of organs that works together.
2. Which of the following is a function of the skin?
   A. Keep out germs.
   B. Provide structure and shape.
   C. Enable movement.
   D. Circulate blood.
3. Which muscle contracts to bend the arm at the elbow?
4. Which body system is formed by all the structures that move blood through the body?
5. **True or false.** Arteries carry oxygen-rich blood, and veins carry oxygen-poor blood.
6. What is the name of the watery portion of blood?
7. The _____ is the site of oxygen and carbon dioxide exchange in the lungs.
8. Which organ of the digestive system makes bile?
9. **True or false.** Ureters carry urine from the bladder out of the body.
10. Why do the lymph nodes swell when the body is fighting infections?
11. **True or false.** In a reflex, the spinal cord signals the body to move without involving the brain.
12. Explain the major role of each main part of the ear.
13. Which of the following hormones lowers blood sugar?
    A. Glucagon.
    B. Thyroid hormone.
    C. Parathyroid hormone.
    D. Insulin.

Use Your Vocabulary ⤤

appendix	endocrine system	neuron
arteries	epidermis	pancreas
bladder	gallbladder	pituitary gland
body system	heart	plasma
brain stem	hypodermis	respiration
bronchi	integumentary system	respiratory system
capillaries	joint	skeletal system
cerebellum	kidneys	spinal cord
cerebrum	ligaments	spleen
circulatory system	liver	tendons
dermis	lymphatic system	thyroid hormone
diaphragm	muscular system	urinary system
digestive system	nervous system	veins

14. The spelling of English words often follows set rules or patterns. Applying these rules will result in words being spelled correctly. Write a paragraph about one of the body systems discussed in this chapter. Use the correct terms related to that system. Make an effort to spell each word correctly.

15. Work with a partner to write the definitions of the terms based on your current understanding. Then, team up with another pair to discuss your definitions and any discrepancies. Finally, discuss the definitions with the class.

Think Critically

16. **Make inferences.** Each body system performs essential functions. Choose one body system and summarize why it is important to keep its organs in good working order.

17. **Compare and contrast.** List the body systems discussed in this chapter and their major functions. Then, compare and contrast the functions. Note any functions that body systems have in common.

18. **Identify.** Healthy behaviors can affect the health and functionality of all body systems. Identify five physical, mental, or social health behaviors that would improve health. Explain how the behaviors would help each body system.

19. **Predict.** Choose one body system and predict how its failure would affect the body.

DEVELOP Your Skills

20. **Teamwork and communication skills.** Working in a small group, discuss what you know about the body and its systems using basic, everyday language. Review the chapter and your notes and create a digital presentation with visuals summarizing the most important information. In your presentation, use new terms you have learned to describe the body systems. Then, reteach the chapter to your peers using the presentation and at least two activities. Take a few minutes after the presentation to answer any questions

21. **Accessing information and literacy skills.** Visit a library and find a children's book about the human body. Read the children's book and compare the information in the book to the information in this chapter. How accurate is the children's book? To which age group would the children's book appeal? What would you change about the book to make it more accurate or engaging?

22. **Accessing information and communication skills.** Talk with a trusted adult about your most recent physical examination at the doctor. Review what happened during the examination and identify all the body systems and organs that the doctor evaluated. Did the doctor focus on one system more than the others? Why do you think the doctor did this? Discuss any questions or comments you have about the physical examination with the trusted adult.

23. **Access information.** Choose one body system and research ways to keep it healthy. Use only reliable websites and resources. Keep track of your sources and why they are good ones. Take notes about the information you find. Then, identify 10 things you can do today to keep the body system healthy, including at least one situation that would require professional help and one high-quality product that people can buy to promote health. Share these 10 things with the class.

Chapter 3

Developing Good Personal Hygiene

Essential Question ❓

Which aspects of good hygiene are important to your health?

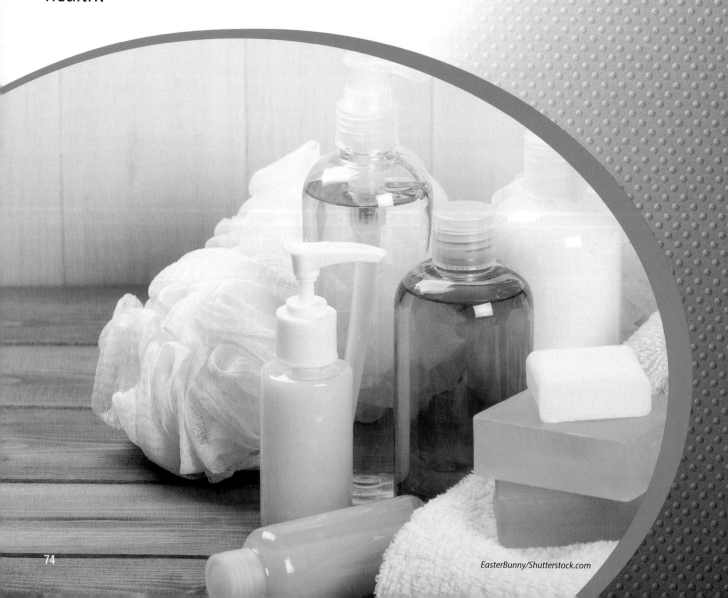

EasterBunny/Shutterstock.com

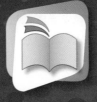

Reading Activity

Write a short dialogue that narrates a discussion between friends about personal hygiene concerns. As you read the chapter, note any concerns your dialogue did not address. Write a paragraph detailing what might happen if the friends addressed only the concerns you originally noted.

How Healthy Are You?

In this chapter, you will be learning about personal hygiene. Before you begin reading, take the following quiz to assess your current personal hygiene habits.

Healthy Choices	Yes	No
Do you wear deodorant and regularly wash your face, body, and hair?		
Do you drink plenty of water to keep your skin hydrated?		
Do you wash your face (and rinse well) twice a day to prevent acne?		
Do you avoid tanning beds, tanning booths, and sunlamps?		
Do you follow the cleanliness guidelines for any piercings you may have?		
Do you use sunscreen every time you go out in the sun?		
Do you avoid listening to music at a high volume, especially when using headphones?		
Do you wear a mouth guard during activities that can result in broken teeth, such as basketball or ice hockey?		
Do you floss after meals and brush your teeth at least twice a day?		
When spending time outdoors, do you wear sunglasses that block at least 99 percent UVB and UVA rays, or provide UV 400 protection?		
Do you keep your nails dry and clean and regularly trim your fingernails?		
Do you avoid exposure to very high levels of noise, such as construction sites or rock concerts?		

Count your "Yes" and "No" responses. The more "Yes" responses you have, the more healthy personal hygiene habits you exhibit. Now, take a closer look at the questions with which you responded "No." How can you make these healthy habits part of your daily life? Identify a SMART goal you would like to achieve to help improve your overall health and well-being. Refer to Figure 1.11 to help you set up your SMART goal. If you do not understand the instructions, ask for clarification from your teacher.

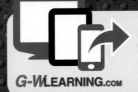

G-WLEARNING.com

Click on the activity icon or visit www.g-wlearning.com/health to access online vocabulary activities using key terms from the chapter.

Caring for Your Skin, Hair, and Nails

Key Terms 👉

deodorant product designed to cover up body odor

antiperspirant product designed to stop or dry up sweat

acne skin condition in which inflamed, clogged hair follicles cause pimples

dermatologist skin specialist who diagnoses and treats skin conditions

eczema chronic condition that causes swollen, red, dry, and itchy patches of skin on one or more parts of the body

body art permanent decorations that are applied to the body; examples include tattoos and piercings

dandruff dead skin that flakes off the scalp due to dryness, infrequent shampooing, or irritation

lice tiny insects that attach to hair and feed on human blood

Learning Outcomes

After studying this lesson, you will be able to

- **demonstrate** ways to care for the skin.
- **give examples** of conditions that affect the skin and how to treat them.
- **identify** strategies to keep hair healthy and looking good.
- **recognize** common hair conditions and how to treat them.
- **practice** effective nail care.

Graphic Organizer

Grooming Routines

Grooming tasks are a normal part of people's daily routines. Create a chart like the one shown and write "Grooming Tasks" in the center. As you read this lesson, list grooming routines that involve taking care of your skin, hair, and nails. In addition, include how often you should perform each routine.

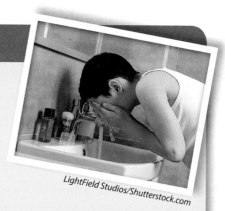
LightField Studios/Shutterstock.com

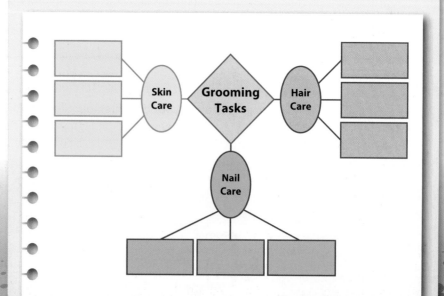

Twelve-year-old Gabriela spends much more time on her grooming than ever before. On days when she has basketball practice, she showers and applies deodorant twice a day. Her face seems to get oily all the time, so she washes it every morning and night. Gabriela knows this grooming routine is necessary to keep her skin healthy.

Levi is 11 years old and likes to hang out with his friends outside. They enjoy playing soccer, riding their bikes around the neighborhood, and swimming in Levi's backyard pool. To avoid sunburns, Levi applies sunscreen every few hours and reminds his friends to do the same.

Taking care of your personal hygiene is hard work, but Gabriela and Levi know that caring for their bodies by keeping them clean will keep them healthy. In this lesson, you will learn some basic steps to ensure that your body is healthy and clean and that you present your best self to the world. The good personal hygiene skills you develop now can help to promote your health and wellness throughout your life.

Skin

The skin, which is the largest organ of the human body, is the outer covering of the entire body. Your skin plays a very important role in keeping you healthy. First, the skin protects everything inside the body. This includes muscles, bones, and other organs, such as the brain, heart, and liver. The skin serves as a barrier for keeping bacteria and viruses from entering your body. Your skin also plays an important role in regulating your body temperature. In this section, you will learn techniques to care for your skin. You will also learn about common types of skin conditions and how to prevent and treat these conditions.

Caring for Your Skin

Keeping your skin healthy requires care. Take a bath or shower every day to remove sweat and bacteria, which cause body odor. When bathing or showering, use a mild soap and warm water to rid your skin of dirt and oil. After bathing, applying a lotion or moisturizer can keep skin from becoming too dry. Also, apply a deodorant or antiperspirant to help prevent body odor (**Figure 3.1**). A **deodorant** covers up the odor of sweat, while an **antiperspirant** actually stops or dries up sweat.

In addition to these basic skin care steps, caring for your skin also involves making healthy lifestyle choices. Eating healthy foods, such as fruits and vegetables, and drinking lots of water can help keep your skin looking its best. Getting enough sleep each night, managing your stress, and avoiding tobacco products are all choices that can also keep your skin looking healthy.

Deodorant Versus Antiperspirant

Deodorant covers up the odor of sweat

ODOR

Antiperspirant stops or dries up sweat

SWEAT

Girl in mirror: wavebreakmedia/Shutterstock.com;
Deodorant & antiperspirant vectors: Rvector/Shutterstock.com

Figure 3.1 Many people think deodorant and antiperspirant are the same, but they are not. Knowing the difference will help you understand which product is best for you.

Spending too much time in the sun can damage your skin. Therefore, applying sun protection whenever you go outside is very important. A sunscreen protects the skin by absorbing, reflecting, or scattering ultraviolet (UV) light. *Ultraviolet (UV) light* is an invisible kind of radiation that comes from the sun, tanning beds, and sunlamps. UV light can seriously harm your skin.

Common Skin Conditions

People may experience several common types of skin conditions. Examples of conditions that affect the skin include acne, eczema, and sunburn. Body decorations, such as tattoos and body piercings, may also cause skin conditions.

In the following sections, you will learn about these skin conditions. You will also learn how to prevent or treat them.

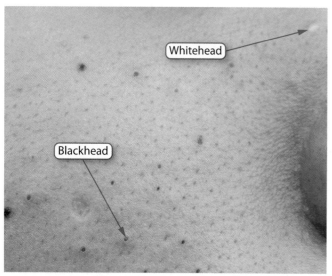

ThamKC/Shutterstock.com

Figure 3.2 Pimples are common among adolescents and can be treated and prevented. ***What are pores?***

Acne

Acne, a skin condition characterized by pimples, commonly develops during adolescence. Acne occurs when the oil glands produce too much oil and clog the pores.

Pores are hair follicles under the skin. The excess oil mixes with dead skin cells and creates a blockage in the pore. Over time, oil and bacteria leak into the skin surrounding this pore. This causes infection and inflammation, including redness, swelling, and pus.

A pimple called a *whitehead* gets its name from the whitish pus inside a clogged pore that has only a tiny opening to the skin's surface. In contrast, a *blackhead* is a yellow or blackish bump inside a clogged pore that is more open to the air. When air gets inside the follicle, it causes the oil inside the follicle to become darker (**Figure 3.2**).

Fortunately, there are steps you can take to prevent and treat acne breakouts. The following strategies can help:

- Wash your face gently with soap or face scrub twice a day. After washing your face, rinse well so that the soap does not stay on your skin.
- Do not squeeze pimples. Doing so can lead to permanent acne scars.
- Avoid touching your face with your fingers. This can spread bacteria and cause inflammation and irritation to other parts of your face or body.
- Make sure anything that touches your face is clean, including glasses, headbands, and hats. Keep your hair clean and pulled away from your face.
- Protect your skin from sunburn, which can make acne appear even worse.
- Wash any makeup off your skin before going to sleep. Throw away old makeup as it can contain bacteria.
- Shave your face lightly, and not too frequently, to avoid accidentally cutting a skin blemish.

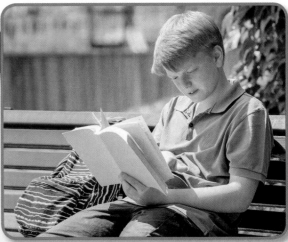
- Use over-the-counter acne medication to clear and prevent acne. For serious cases of acne, consult a **dermatologist** (doctor who is a skin specialist). A dermatologist can give you useful information about caring for your skin type, and prescribe medication, if necessary.

Eczema

Eczema, or *dermatitis*, is a condition that causes swollen, red, dry, and itchy patches of skin on one or more parts of the body (**Figure 3.3**). Eczema is a chronic disease, which means it typically reoccurs over time. Colds or other minor illnesses, irritating substances, and stress may all trigger eczema flare-ups. Eczema is not contagious, meaning you cannot catch it from someone else.

You can often treat symptoms of eczema using over-the-counter products. To relieve the dryness and itching of eczema, apply a lotion or cream when

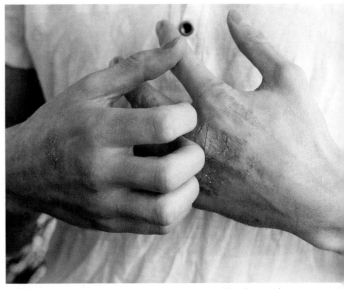

Ternavskaia Olga Alibec/Shutterstock.com

Figure 3.3 Eczema patches can occur anywhere on the body, but are commonly found on the hands, feet, face, and creases of the elbows and knees. *Is eczema contagious?*

Health in the Media

Mass media messages aim to directly affect people's health behaviors. Some media messages, such as those that focus on tobacco-free living and heart disease prevention, are positive and encourage healthy behaviors. Other media messages focus on behaviors that can have harmful effects on people's health, such as drinking alcohol or eating foods that are high in fat and low in nutrients. Additionally, only some media messages tell the truth. False advertising is common in health products—from "no sugar added" foods to "anti-aging" skin creams.

Browsing skin care or hair care products can be daunting. The options seem endless, and the products all look the same. Most advertisements say the same things. How do you know which products are scams? What will work best for you?

You must be able to analyze how messages from media and labels on products may influence your purchases. You also need to be able to evaluate which products will improve your health and which ones will not.

Evaluating Skin and Hair Care Products

The best way to fight against false advertising for health claims on skin care and hair care products is to do your research. Evaluate the scientific studies done on that brand, product, and any ingredients used.

Working in groups of four, choose two skin care products and two hair care products to evaluate. For each product, research and record your answers to the following questions. Then, write a review of each product. Rate the products on a scale of one to five, with one being poor and five being excellent. Share your reviews with the rest of the class.

1. Was this product tested on human subjects? Tests conducted on animals or tissue samples can have different effects.

2. What are the ingredients in the product? Can any of these ingredients be harmful to your skin or hair? Can they cause any side effects?

3. Are any health claims of this product backed by scientific research? All true health claims will have scientific data in multiple studies to back them up.

4. Do the products contain added colors, preservatives, or fragrances? Large amounts of these may irritate sensitive skin.

Yana Lesnik/Shutterstock.com

the skin is damp, such as after bathing or washing your hands. This locks in moisture and can help reduce itching. Avoid scratching any patches of eczema. Doing so may cause an infection.

Suntans, Sunburns, and Skin Cancer

Spending too much time in the sun's UV rays can damage your skin. Suntans and sunburns are both indicators of damage to the skin because of too much time in the sun. Scientific evidence suggests that overexposure to UV rays and damage to the skin can lead to skin cancer. There are three main types of skin cancer (**Figure 3.4**).

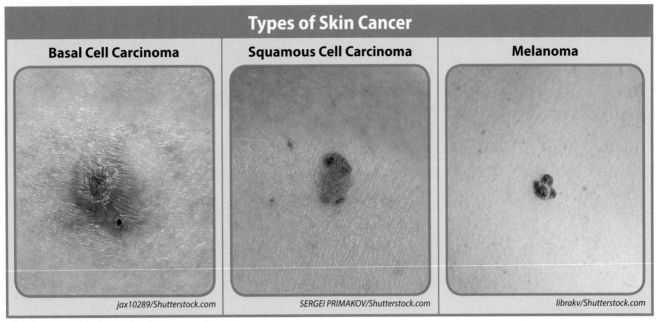

Types of Skin Cancer

| Basal Cell Carcinoma | Squamous Cell Carcinoma | Melanoma |

jax10289/Shutterstock.com   *SERGEI PRIMAKOV/Shutterstock.com*   *librakv/Shutterstock.com*

Figure 3.4 Preventing skin cancer and detecting signs of it early are important to protect your health. *What is the most dangerous type of skin cancer?*

Two types of skin cancer are common and curable. These two types are *basal cell carcinoma* and *squamous cell carcinoma*. *Melanoma* is the most dangerous type of skin cancer because it spreads rapidly throughout the body, sometimes before the initial skin cancer is recognized.

To protect your skin and prevent skin damage, which can lead to skin cancer, reduce intentional UV exposure and increase sun protection. Other ways to protect your skin are shown in **Figure 3.5**. Sometimes you might feel pressure from friends to spend time in the sun without protection. You can resist this influence by encouraging others to be safe too.

Figure 3.5 Sun safety tips such as these can help you protect your skin from harmful UV rays.

Sun Safety Tips

- Avoid outdoor activities during the midday hours when the sun's rays are the strongest.
- Wear a hat with a large brim to protect your face, head, ears, and neck.
- Stay in the shade whenever possible.
- Apply sunscreen to all exposed areas of skin. The higher the *sun protection factor (SPF)* of a sunscreen, the greater the protection it provides from UV rays. For the best protection against UV rays, use sunscreen with a SPF of at least 15.
- Keep sun protection handy and reapply sunscreen at least every two hours, or more often if you sweat or swim.
- Wear tightly woven clothing that protects any skin exposed to the sun's UV rays. Certain fabrics have built-in SPF protection.
- Avoid tanning beds, tanning booths, and sunlamps. The UV rays these machines produce are just as dangerous as the sun's UV rays, and are just as likely to cause skin cancer. Monitor your skin for any new or unusual spots. Consult a doctor if any new or unusual spots are found.

Tips for Choosing Care Products

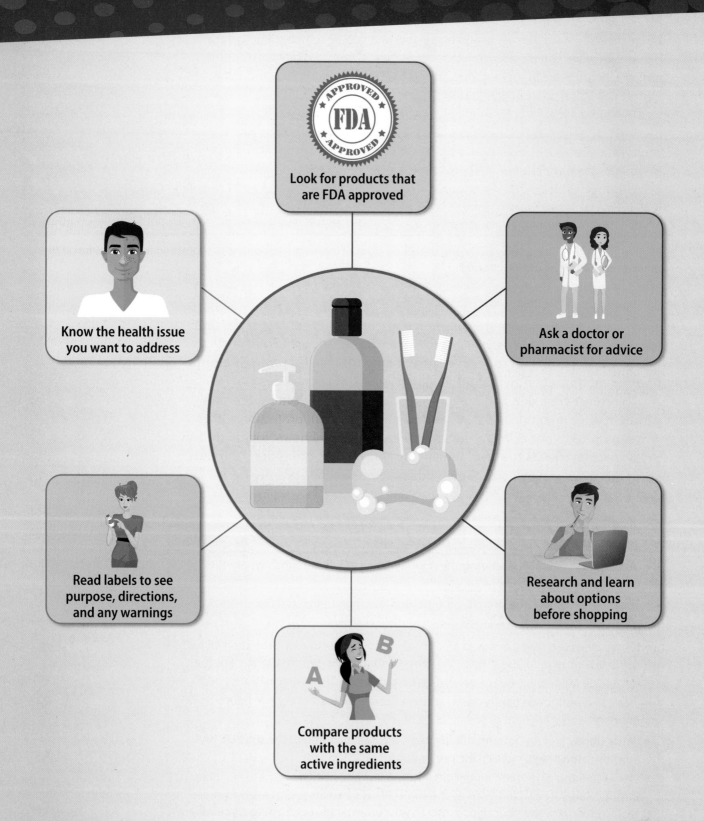

Look for products that are FDA approved

Ask a doctor or pharmacist for advice

Research and learn about options before shopping

Compare products with the same active ingredients

Read labels to see purpose, directions, and any warnings

Know the health issue you want to address

Center image: Focus_Vector/Shutterstock.com; Outside images, clockwise from the top: carmen2011/Shutterstock.com; Inspiring/Shutterstock.com; subarashii21/Shutterstock.com; pikepicture/Shutterstock.com; Lorelyn Medina/Shutterstock.com; Fedorenko Kateryna/Shutterstock.com

Tattoos and Piercings

Since ancient times, people have chosen to decorate their bodies in permanent ways. Two of the most common types of body decoration, or **body art**, are tattoos and piercings. These types of body decorations can potentially impact health.

Tattoos are designs on the skin made by using a needle to insert colored ink under the skin. *Body piercing* involves the use of a needle to make a hole in the skin to insert jewelry. The most common body piercing is to the earlobe. Other pierced body parts often include ear cartilage, the belly button, the nose, and the tongue.

In most states, people are required to be at least 18 years of age or have written permission by a legal guardian to get a tattoo or body piercing. To reduce the risk of complications from tattoos or piercings, people should have them done at clean, safe, and well-regarded facilities by licensed professionals. In addition, following the care instructions closely can help decrease the possibility of infection.

Although getting a tattoo or a body piercing may seem harmless, it is a big decision—and a permanent one. People should think carefully about the risks involved with these procedures before making a decision (**Figure 3.6**).

Hair

Although you have more than 100,000 hairs on your head, you lose about 50 to 100 hairs every day through normal activities such as washing, brushing, or combing your hair. These hairs are replaced by new hairs, which grow from the same follicles. Practicing good hair care will help you keep your hair looking clean and healthy. Maintaining the health of your hair can also be easy when you understand common hair conditions and know how to prevent and treat them.

Caring for Your Hair

Keeping your hair healthy requires routine care. One simple hair care technique is to regularly wash and condition your hair and scalp. This helps

---

Risks of Body Art

- Any needles not sterilized or properly cleaned before use can cause serious infections to the body.
- Some people can have allergic reactions to either the tattoo ink or the jewelry worn in the pierced area.
- Tearing of the skin or excessive bleeding could occur since the skin is being broken.
- Some businesses do not allow their employees to have visible tattoos or piercings. Employees with a piercing or tattoo may be asked to remove it or cover it up.
- Tattoos can be removed, but removing a tattoo is a painful, expensive, and time-intensive process. It can also leave scarring.

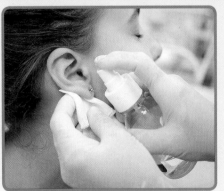

Pavel L Photo and Video/Shutterstock.com

Figure 3.6
Consider the risks of body art before making the decision to get a piercing or tattoo.

keep hair clean and prevents it from becoming too dry. When washing your hair, get it really wet. Use only a small amount of shampoo and gently massage it into your scalp. Then, rinse really well to remove all the shampoo from your hair.

After showering, gently dry your hair with a towel. Let your hair air dry when possible. Using a blow dryer too often can dry out your hair and increase the chance of breakage. In addition, comb your hair carefully. Do not tug on it to decrease the chances of breaking or pulling the hair out.

In addition to washing your hair regularly, following are some other techniques that can help keep your hair healthy:

- Eat a healthful diet (**Figure 3.7**). Some hair conditions are caused in part by a lack of certain vitamins and fats.
- Avoid sharing items that have touched your hair with other people, such as combs or hats.
- Wash your hair after swimming, especially after swimming in a chlorinated pool.
- Get a haircut regularly, such as every six to eight weeks, to remove split ends.

Common Hair Conditions

A common hair condition many people experience is having oily hair. This is especially true for adolescents who are going through puberty. Every hair follicle is attached to a gland that produces oil. When these glands produce too much oil, such as during puberty, a person's hair may look greasy.

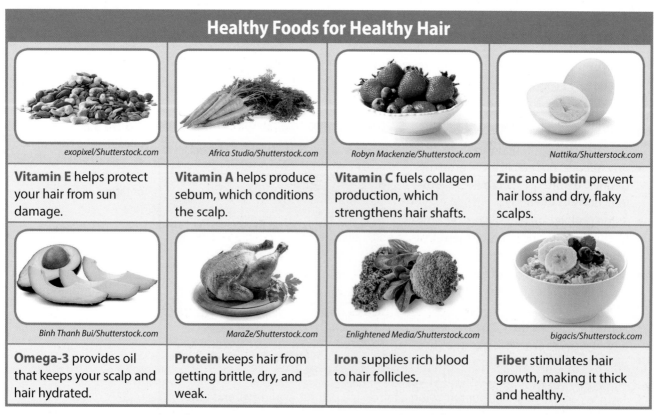

Healthy Foods for Healthy Hair

exopixel/Shutterstock.com	Africa Studio/Shutterstock.com	Robyn Mackenzie/Shutterstock.com	Nattika/Shutterstock.com
Vitamin E helps protect your hair from sun damage.	**Vitamin A** helps produce sebum, which conditions the scalp.	**Vitamin C** fuels collagen production, which strengthens hair shafts.	**Zinc** and **biotin** prevent hair loss and dry, flaky scalps.
Binh Thanh Bui/Shutterstock.com	MaraZe/Shutterstock.com	Enlightened Media/Shutterstock.com	bigacis/Shutterstock.com
Omega-3 provides oil that keeps your scalp and hair hydrated.	**Protein** keeps hair from getting brittle, dry, and weak.	**Iron** supplies rich blood to hair follicles.	**Fiber** stimulates hair growth, making it thick and healthy.

Figure 3.7 Hair is made up of protein and is kept long, full, healthy, and strong by the nutrients we eat.

Oily hair can be treated by washing hair regularly. People can also use shampoos designed to help treat oily hair.

Another common hair condition people may experience is **dandruff**, which is the flaking of dead skin cells from the scalp. A common cause of dandruff is having dry skin. People who have dandruff because of dry skin often notice white flakes of dead skin in their hair and on their shoulders (**Figure 3.8**). Dandruff is usually worse in the fall and winter, when indoor heating can dry out skin. Infrequent shampooing, which allows oils and skin cells from the scalp to build up, is another common cause of dandruff. Shampooing too often or using too many hair care products may irritate the scalp and lead to dandruff, too. If you have dandruff, try using a medicated shampoo that can be purchased at stores. If the dandruff continues, see your doctor or dermatologist for treatment options.

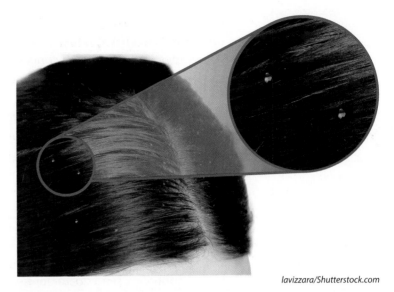

lavizzara/Shutterstock.com

Figure 3.8 White flakes of dead skin cells on the scalp are the result of a common hair condition called *dandruff*. *What is one possible cause of dandruff?*

A highly contagious hair condition some people may contract is lice. **Lice** are tiny insects that attach to the hair and feed on human blood. Lice can transmit easily from one person to another through direct head-to-head contact or if people share combs, brushes, or hats. Although lice do not cause any major health conditions, they are very itchy and uncomfortable. If you become infected with lice, use a medicated shampoo to kill the lice and their eggs (or *nits*). You also need to wash all bedding, towels, and other items that have touched your hair in hot water.

Nails

Fingernails and toenails are made up of layers of a hard protein called *keratin*. This hard substance protects the sensitive tissues on the tips of your fingers and toes. Nails grow out from the area at the base of the nail. As new cells continuously grow, older cells are pushed out.

It is relatively easy to keep your nails strong and healthy. Keep your nails dry and clean to prevent bacteria and other organisms from growing under them. If you must soak your hands, such as while washing dishes, or if you must use harsh chemicals, wear gloves. Be sure to trim your fingernails regularly using clippers, manicure scissors, or a nail file.

In addition, moisturize your hands regularly, including your fingernails and cuticles. Do not bite your fingernails, pick at your cuticles, or pull off your hangnails. Doing so can cause infections.

Before using the services of a salon for nail care, make sure the salon and the nail technician are licensed. All tools should be properly sterilized between customers to avoid spreading infections.

Healthy fingernails and toenails are smooth, free of spots or discoloration, and consistent in color. Some irregularities in the nails, such as white spots or vertical ridges, are normal. Other conditions, however, such as nail discoloration, curled nails, or redness and swelling around the nail, can sometimes indicate health concerns (**Figure 3.9**). Some common nail conditions can be treated at home while some may need to be treated by a professional.

Common Nail Conditions

Condition	Treatment	Prevention
Hangnail: tiny piece of torn skin next to a fingernail.	Wash hands, clip loose piece of skin with clean nail clipper, and apply ointment if area is inflamed.	Use hand lotion or cream to keep hands moisturized and prevent dryness.
Ingrown toenail: toenail pushes too far into the skin along the side of the toe.	For home remedies, soak your feet, insert cotton under your toenail, apply antibiotic cream, and bandage. If swelling and pain continues, see a doctor for treatment.	Trim toenails straight across and do not wear shoes that are too tight.
Nail infection (fungal): infection that causes nail to become discolored, thick, crack, and break.	Use a prescription antifungal pill prescribed by a doctor. In severe cases, the nail may have to be removed completely.	Keep your hands and feet clean and dry, do not walk barefoot in public areas, and do not share nail clippers.
Split nail: also called *nail separation*, the nail becomes loose and separates from nail bed.	Trim away the damaged area, if possible. Cover the split with over-the-counter products. If splitting worsens, see a doctor for treatment.	Keep nails dry, neatly trimmed, and do not bite your fingernails or cuticles. Avoid harsh nail care products.

Figure 3.9 It is important to recognize signs of unhealthy nails and how to treat and prevent them.

Lesson 3.1 Review

1. What is the difference between a deodorant and an antiperspirant?

2. **True or false.** Your diet, sleeping patterns, and water intake have a big impact on how healthy your skin looks.

3. Swollen, red, dry, and itchy patches of skin on one or more parts of the body describes a skin condition called _____.

4. Name the characteristics of healthy nails.

5. **Critical thinking.** Name three different hair conditions and explain different ways to prevent and treat them.

Hands-On Activity

In small groups, create an advertisement about how to take care of the skin, hair, or nails. Include the following information in your advertisement:

- conditions due to poor hygiene
- products needed for good personal hygiene
- tips for taking care of this region of the body

Possible formats for your advertisement include posters, videos, and social media posts. Present your advertisement to the class and answer any questions your classmates may have about words or concepts they do not understand.

Keeping Your Mouth, Eyes, and Ears Healthy

Learning Outcomes

After studying this lesson, you will be able to

- **demonstrate** ways to take care of the mouth and teeth.
- **summarize** common mouth and teeth conditions people may experience.
- **identify** ways to protect the eyes.
- **list** common vision conditions and how they can be treated.
- **explain** how people can protect their ears.
- **describe** common hearing conditions.

Graphic Organizer

Mouth, Ear, and Eye Health

Create a KWL chart like the one shown. Before reading this lesson, write what you know and what you want to know about mouth, eye, and ear health in the appropriate columns. After studying the lesson, write what you have learned.

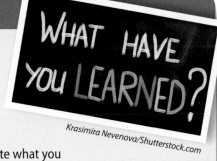

Krasimira Nevenova/Shutterstock.com

K What I <u>K</u>now	W What I <u>W</u>ant to Know	L What I <u>H</u>ave Learned
I should brush and floss my teeth at least twice a day.	What are different events that can cause ear damage?	Decrease screen time to reduce eyestrain.

Key Terms

plaque sticky, colorless film that coats the teeth and dissolves their protective enamel surface

cavities holes in the teeth that occur when plaque eats into a tooth's enamel

gingivitis inflammation of the gums

periodontitis infection caused by bacteria getting under the gum tissue and destroying the gums and bone

orthodontist dental specialist who prevents and corrects teeth misalignments

optometrist eye care specialist who examines and treats eyes for vision conditions

nearsightedness condition in which objects close to the eye appear clear, while objects farther away appear blurry

farsightedness condition in which distant objects are seen more clearly than nearby objects

astigmatism condition in which the eye does not focus light evenly onto the retina; objects appear blurry and stretched out

tinnitus pain or ringing in the ears after exposure to excessively loud sounds

The mouth, teeth, ears, and eyes are important parts of the body that help people live their lives to the fullest. In this lesson, you will learn ways to care for your mouth, teeth, eyes, and ears. You will also read about some common health conditions relating to these parts of your body and how you can treat and prevent them.

Mouth and Teeth

Having good oral health is important to your overall health (**Figure 3.10**). *Oral health* refers to your mouth, teeth, and gums. In order for your mouth and teeth to help with digestion, you need to take care of them. In addition, it is important to recognize common mouth and teeth conditions so proper treatment and prevention can occur.

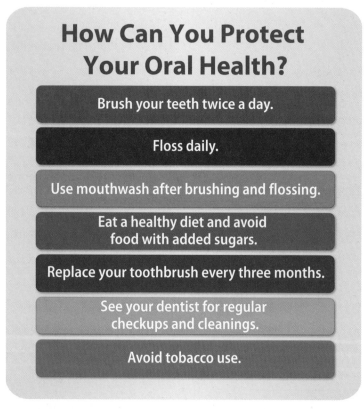

How Can You Protect Your Oral Health?

Brush your teeth twice a day.

Floss daily.

Use mouthwash after brushing and flossing.

Eat a healthy diet and avoid food with added sugars.

Replace your toothbrush every three months.

See your dentist for regular checkups and cleanings.

Avoid tobacco use.

Figure 3.10 It is important to protect your oral health by using healthy practices such as flossing daily and seeing your dentist for regular cleanings.

Caring for the Mouth and Teeth

Taking care of your mouth and teeth requires regular attention. To start, brush your teeth, including your tongue, at least twice a day with a soft-bristle brush and toothpaste that contains fluoride (**Figure 3.11**). *Fluoride* is a chemical that helps prevent tooth decay. Brushing your teeth daily cleans your mouth and teeth and prevents the buildup of plaque. Replace your toothbrush about every three months or sooner if the bristles are worn. Flossing is also important to do every day. Flossing gets rid of any food particles stuck between your teeth and removes plaque from between the teeth and under the gums.

It is also important to visit the dentist twice a year. The dentist will check and clean your teeth to help prevent tooth decay and gum disease. The dentist can also detect teeth conditions, such as cavities, early on when they can be more easily treated.

There are additional healthy lifestyle choices that you can do to keep your mouth and teeth healthy. Choose to eat healthful foods, such as fruits and vegetables, instead of sticky foods that are high in sugar and starch, such as candy and soda. If you choose to eat food high in sugar, brush your teeth as soon as possible to prevent oral conditions. When playing sports such as football or ice hockey, wear a mouth guard. This will protect your teeth from being broken. Avoid using any type of tobacco product, which can stain your teeth. You will learn more about the physical effects of tobacco products in Chapter 9.

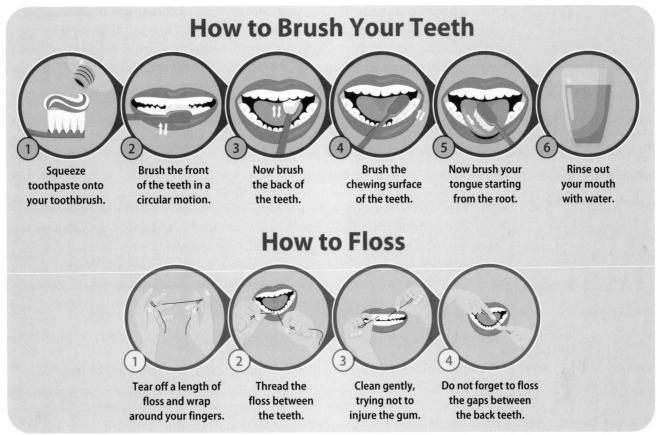

How to Brush Your Teeth

1 Squeeze toothpaste onto your toothbrush.

2 Brush the front of the teeth in a circular motion.

3 Now brush the back of the teeth.

4 Brush the chewing surface of the teeth.

5 Now brush your tongue starting from the root.

6 Rinse out your mouth with water.

How to Floss

1 Tear off a length of floss and wrap around your fingers.

2 Thread the floss between the teeth.

3 Clean gently, trying not to injure the gum.

4 Do not forget to floss the gaps between the back teeth.

Brushing: Inspiring/Shutterstock.com; Water: runLenarun/Shutterstock.com; Flossing: Inspiring/Shutterstock.com

Figure 3.11 Brushing your teeth cleans your mouth and teeth and prevents buildup of plaque and tooth decay. *How many times a day should you brush your teeth?*

Common Mouth and Teeth Conditions

Many people experience mouth and teeth conditions at some point. These conditions can interfere with important daily life functions such as chewing, swallowing, and even talking. Some of the common mouth conditions people may experience include tooth decay, gum disease, teeth misalignment, impacted wisdom teeth, cold sores, bad breath, and teeth grinding.

Tooth Decay

When you eat or drink something, a substance in your saliva breaks down the food particles and sugars for digestion. This process turns everything you eat or drink into a type of acid. When this acid combines with the bacteria in your mouth, as well as saliva and small food particles, it forms plaque. **Plaque** is a sticky, colorless film that coats the teeth and dissolves their protective enamel surface. If plaque is not removed, it mixes with minerals to become tartar, a harder substance. Tartar removal requires professional cleaning.

If you do not brush and floss your teeth daily, food particles remain in your mouth and promote bacterial growth (**Figure 3.12**). This results in tooth decay. Over time, tooth decay causes **cavities**, or holes in the teeth that occur when plaque eats into a tooth's enamel. Cavities are also known as *dental caries*.

Sergii Kuchugurnyi/Shutterstock.com

Figure 3.12 Cavities occur when plaque eats into a tooth's enamel. *What is another name for cavities?*

As the decay continues, the hole gets deeper and eventually reaches the nerve layer under the enamel known as the *dentin*. This causes painful nerve damage. The *death of the tooth* occurs when the decay reaches the deepest layer of the tooth (the *pulp cavity*).

Gum Disease

Your *gums* consist of the pinkish tissue that surrounds your teeth. The gums lie on top of the bones of the jaw, and cover the entire root of each tooth. The gums help keep your teeth in place.

Gum disease occurs when plaque and tartar build up on the teeth (**Figure 3.13**). The bacteria in plaque cause toxins to form in the mouth, which irritates the gums. Over time, this irritation can lead to **gingivitis**, an inflammation of the gums. It can also lead to periodontitis. **Periodontitis**, or *periodontal disease*, is an infection caused by bacteria getting under the gum tissue and destroying the gums and bone. Early signs of gum disease include swelling and bleeding of the gums. If gum disease goes untreated, it can damage the gums and jawbone.

Teeth Misalignment and Impacted Wisdom Teeth

Sometimes teeth do not always come in straight. Teeth may be crooked, overcrowded in the mouth, have too much space in between, or are misaligned. A misalignment (incorrect position) of the upper teeth and the lower teeth may result in an overbite or underbite. An *overbite* is a condition in which the upper teeth extend significantly over the lower teeth. An *underbite* is a condition in which the lower teeth extend significantly past the upper teeth. An orthodontist may apply braces to fix crooked or misaligned teeth. An **orthodontist** is a dental specialist who prevents and corrects teeth misalignments (**Figure 3.14**).

Wisdom teeth may become stuck under the gum tissue, or may only be able to partially come through the gums. This can be caused by lack of room in the jaw. When this occurs, the condition is called *impacted wisdom teeth*. In this case, the teeth may need to be removed by an oral surgeon because the wisdom teeth can become infected or displace other teeth.

Figure 3.13
Brushing your teeth can help remove plaque, but it can also be removed professionally at the dentist. *If you do not remove plaque buildup on your teeth, what conditions can occur?*

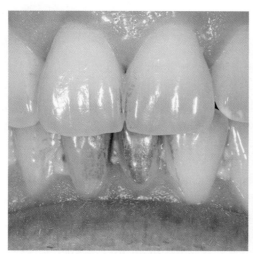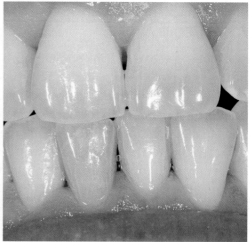

Lighthunter/Shutterstock.com

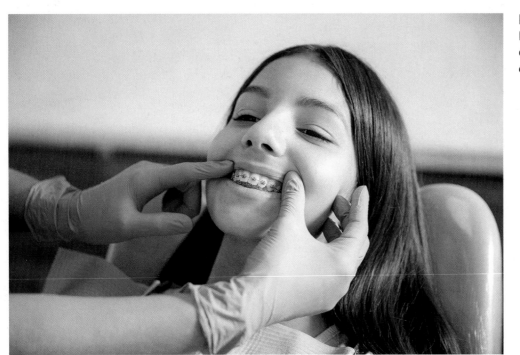

Figure 3.14
Braces are applied by dental specialists called *orthodontists*.

antoniodiaz/Shutterstock.com

Cold Sores

Cold sores, or *fever blisters*, are small blisters that appear on the lips and inside the mouth (**Figure 3.15**). These blisters are red, swollen, and painful, especially when touched. Cold sores are caused by a virus spread from person to person through passing saliva in some way, such as sharing a utensil. Cold sores typically last several days, but can last as long as two weeks. Cold sores generally clear up without treatment. Cold sores that are painful can be treated with a skin cream or ointment to speed up the healing and help ease the pain.

Bad Breath and Teeth Grinding

Bad breath, or *halitosis*, can be caused by poor oral hygiene. Bad breath is also caused by gum disease, cavities, trapped food particles, and certain medical conditions. For example, respiratory tract infections, diabetes, and chronic bronchitis can all cause bad breath.

Ways people can help prevent bad breath include the following:

- practicing good oral hygiene
- seeing the dentist every six months for checkups
- using an antiseptic mouth-rinse to reduce the bacteria that causes bad breath

Teeth grinding involves repeatedly clenching and grinding one's teeth. This condition may be caused by stress or anxiety, having an abnormal bite, or missing or crooked teeth. Many people who grind their teeth are unaware they do it because it often occurs during sleep. They may learn from other people that they grind their teeth.

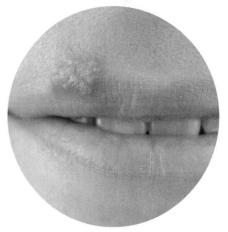

Levent Konuk/Shutterstock.com

Figure 3.15
Painful blisters, called *cold sores*, are contagious through saliva, such as through sharing a beverage or a utensil. *How long do cold sores last?*

Take Charge of Your Personal Hygiene

Are you taking charge of your personal hygiene to treat current health issues or prevent future conditions? Practicing good personal hygiene can boost self-confidence and help you stay healthy. Examples of good personal hygiene tasks include the following:

- bathing or showering regularly
- washing your face daily
- applying lotion to your skin
- using deodorant or antiperspirant
- brushing and flossing your teeth
- keeping your nails dry, clean, and trim
- eating healthy foods
- drinking plenty of water
- getting enough sleep
- managing stress
- wearing sunglasses outside
- avoiding loud noises

Setting Personal Hygiene Goals

If you are currently skipping any healthy personal hygiene habits, you may want to set some personal hygiene goals. Remember to write SMART (specific, measurable, achievable, relevant, and timely) goals. After developing your goals, create a *Personal Hygiene Goal Chart* like the one shown to monitor daily and weekly progress. If you are successful in meeting your goal for the day, add a smiley face, a star, or a checkmark in your chart.

Based on your results, what changes, if any, should you make to your goals? Continue to adjust your goals each week as needed until these healthy habits are part of your lifestyle.

Personal Hygiene Goal Chart

Goals	Monday	Tuesday	Wednesday	Thursday	Friday	Saturday	Sunday
Floss							
Turn my music down							
Sleep for 9 hours							
Wash my face							

Although teeth grinding is usually harmless, persistent teeth grinding can lead to tooth damage, a sore jaw, headaches, and even hearing loss. A dentist can determine whether you are grinding your teeth. If you do grind your teeth, the dentist may suggest that you wear a mouth guard during sleep to protect your teeth.

Eyes

Most people rely on their sense of vision more than their other senses. You need good vision for many activities in your daily life, from kicking a soccer ball to taking a photograph to riding a bicycle. Keeping your eyes healthy is important. In the following sections, you will learn some good strategies for keeping your eyes healthy. You will also learn about common vision conditions that can affect the eyes.

Protecting Your Eyes

Following are simple strategies to help you keep your eyes as healthy as possible throughout your lifetime:

- Wear protective eyewear when playing contact sports or doing activities that can create flying debris that could hit the eyes.
- When spending time outdoors, wear sunglasses to block harmful UV rays.
- Avoid sharing eye makeup and eye care products as germs can easily spread.
- If something gets in your eye, flush it out with either clean water or eye drops.

It is also important to reduce eyestrain. *Eyestrain* occurs when your eyes grow tired from intense use, such as staring at a digital device for an extensive time or reading in dim light. There are several methods to help reduce eyestrain (**Figure 3.16**). One simple way to reduce eyestrain is to reduce the amount of time spent looking at a screen.

Tips to Reduce Eyestrain

Take Breaks
- Rest your eyes by looking away from the screen.
- Try the 20-20-20 rule: every 20 minutes, look at something 20 feet away for at least 20 seconds.

Adjust Screen Settings
- Make text larger so it is easier to read.
- Adjust screen brightness and contrast to a comfortable level.

Blink Often
- Make a habit of blinking more often when looking at a screen.
- Blinking produces tears that refresh your eyes.

Adjust the Lighting
- Avoid light shining directly into your eyes.
- Try using a shaded light or dimming room lights to a comfortable level.

Figure 3.16 Making adjustments in your daily routine, such as looking at a digital device, can help reduce eyestrain. *When does eyestrain occur?*

Perhaps the simplest step you can take to protect your eyes is to get regular eye exams. An **optometrist** is an eye care specialist who examines eyes for vision conditions and prescribes corrective lenses. They also may conduct tests for eye diseases. It is recommended to get an eye exam at least once a year.

Common Vision Conditions

For many people, especially young people, vision works well. Other people, however, experience vision conditions. For example, in some people, the shape of the eyeball is such that light does not focus where it needs to focus—on the retina. People whose parents have vision conditions are also more likely to have vision conditions themselves. Vision conditions are more common in older people because aging can cause changes in parts of the eye.

The following are the most common vision conditions:

- **Nearsightedness** (or *myopia*) is a condition in which objects close to the eye appear clear, while objects farther away appear blurry. In the eye of someone who is nearsighted, light focuses in front of the retina instead of on the retina.
- **Farsightedness** (or *hyperopia*) is a condition in which distant objects are seen more clearly than nearby objects. In the eye of someone who is farsighted, light focuses behind the retina instead of on the retina.
- **Astigmatism** is a condition in which the eye does not focus light evenly onto the retina. As a result, objects appear blurry and stretched out.

Fortunately, these conditions can usually be corrected with glasses or contact lenses (**Figure 3.17**). Surgery can also correct, or improve, some vision conditions. LASIK (or *laser in-situ keratomileusis*) is a surgery that reshapes the cornea. This allows light to reach the retina, and helps improve vision.

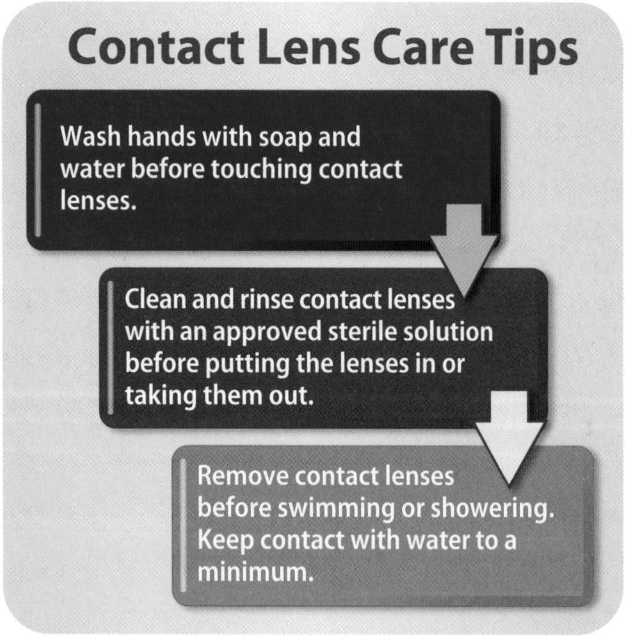

Some people may experience slight differences in the way they see colors. People who see colors very differently from the way others see colors have color blindness. People with *color blindness* are not aware of differences among colors.

The most common form of color blindness is an inability to distinguish red from green (**Figure 3.18**). Another form is blue-yellow color blindness. A complete lack of color vision is *total color blindness*, which is very rare.

Unlike nearsightedness or farsightedness which can be corrected with lenses, there are no treatments for most types of color blindness. People with color blindness have an option to wear a colored filter over their glasses or a colored contact lens that may enhance the perception of contrasts between colors. These lenses, however, will not improve the ability to see all colors.

Contact Lens Care Tips

Wash hands with soap and water before touching contact lenses.

Clean and rinse contact lenses with an approved sterile solution before putting the lenses in or taking them out.

Remove contact lenses before swimming or showering. Keep contact with water to a minimum.

Figure 3.17 Proper care of contact lenses is essential to eye health.

Ears

What do the following activities have in common: target shooting, woodworking, playing in a band, attending rock concerts, and using a leaf blower? All of these activities can contribute to hearing loss. Many teens

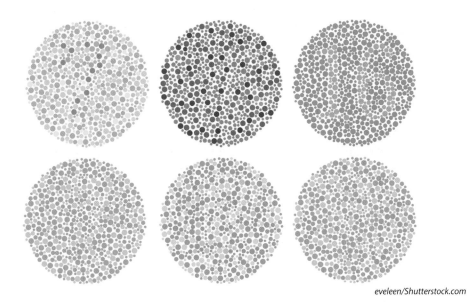

Figure 3.18
A common test to check for red-green color blindness is shown here. *What are the two most common forms of color blindness?*

regularly expose themselves to loud noises, often through headphones. The sense of hearing allows you to listen to music you enjoy, talk with friends, and be alerted to approaching cars and other dangers. Your ears also play a role in helping you keep your balance. In the following sections, you will learn about strategies for maintaining your hearing and common hearing conditions.

Protecting Your Ears

One of the best methods to protect your ears is to protect your hearing. There are several simple ways to protect your hearing.

In addition to protecting your hearing, there are healthy practices you can follow to help keep ears healthy (**Figure 3.19**).

Figure 3.19
Using healthy practices to protect your ears and keep them healthy can help maintain your hearing and prevent common hearing conditions.

Protecting and Keeping Ears Healthy

Protecting Your Ears

- Avoid exposure to very high levels of noise, such as at rock concerts, dances, or construction sites, whenever possible.
- If you are around loud noises for a long period of time, wear earplugs or noise cancelling headphones to decrease the sound.
- When wearing headphones, avoid listening to music at high volume levels.
- If people around you can hear your music through the headphones, turn the volume down.

Keeping Your Ears Healthy

- Clean your ears regularly by wiping the outside of the ear with a damp towel. This will remove excess dirt or earwax on the outside of the ear.
- Avoid using cotton swabs in your ears.
- If water gets stuck in your ear, use special ear drops to dry out the water.
- Wear a hat, earmuffs, or a hood when the weather is cold.

Common Ear Conditions

The most serious health condition associated with the ears is permanent loss of hearing. Hearing loss is typically caused by damage to the inner ear. This damage is often the result of repeated exposure to excessively loud sounds. This may mean exposure to loud music through headphones (**Figure 3.20**).

Sound *intensity*, or loudness, is measured in units called *decibels*. You can experience hearing loss by listening to sounds at or above 85 decibels over an extended period of time. The louder the sound, the less time it takes for hearing damage to occur.

Hearing loss can also be caused more suddenly by a ruptured eardrum. This may occur as a result of loud blasts of noise, sudden changes in pressure, insertion of an object into the ear, or an infection. In fact, just one exposure to a very loud sound, blast, or impulse (at or above 120 decibels) can cause hearing loss.

Unfortunately, many people do not notice that they are losing their hearing because damage from noise exposure is usually gradual. By the time they notice, they have substantial symptoms of permanent hearing loss. Early signs of hearing damage include the following:

- difficulty hearing relatively soft sounds, such as doorbells
- difficulty understanding speech during telephone conversations or in noisy environments
- pain or ringing in the ears, or **tinnitus**, after exposure to excessively loud sounds

If you suddenly lose your hearing, seek immediate medical attention. If you notice hearing gradually decreasing over time, talk to your doctor about symptoms. In addition, schedule regular hearing exams to ensure that your hearing is working properly.

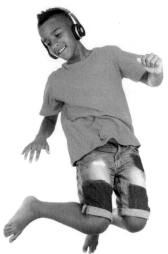

Samuel Borges Photography/ Shutterstock.com

Figure 3.20
One recent study found that 12.5 percent of children and teens (6 to 19 years of age) experience hearing loss caused by using headphones or earbuds at too high a volume. *What level of sound intensity can cause hearing damage?*

Lesson 3.2 Review

1. Name two common mouth and teeth conditions people may experience.
2. You should brush and floss your teeth at least _____ a day.
3. A(n) _____ is a specialist who examines eyes.
4. **Critical thinking.** Describe three ways to protect your hearing.

Hands-On Activity

In small groups, create a life-size guide to personal hygiene. To begin, have a group member lie down to allow the others to trace the person's body on paper. Outside the outline, draw arrows from various body parts to the following information: personal hygiene tips to care for this area, hygiene products to care for it, and the benefits to using the product.

Summary

Lesson 3.1   Caring for Your Skin, Hair, and Nails

- *Personal hygiene* is the act of caring for and cleaning your body. Taking a bath or shower and applying deodorant or antiperspirant every day will help prevent body odor.
- Eating healthy foods, drinking lots of water, and getting enough sleep can help your skin look and stay healthy.
- Spending too much time in the sun, or in tanning beds, can damage skin and possibly lead to skin cancer. Take precautions such as applying sunscreen with a minimum of 15 SPF to protect yourself when outdoors.
- *Acne* is a skin condition commonly developed during adolescence. It occurs when glands produce too much oil and clog pores. Washing your face gently twice a day can help treat and prevent acne.
- A condition that causes swollen, red, dry, and itchy patches of skin on one or more parts of the body is *eczema*, or dermatitis. Eczema is not contagious and is often treatable with over-the-counter products.
- Getting a tattoo or a body piercing is a permanent decision. People should think carefully about the risks involved with these procedures before making a decision.
- Having oily hair or dandruff are common conditions during puberty. Regularly washing your hair and eating a diet of healthy foods will help keep your hair healthy.
- To care for your nails, keep them dry, clean, and trimmed. Wear gloves when using harsh chemicals.

Lesson 3.2   Keeping Your Mouth, Eyes, and Ears Healthy

- *Oral health* refers to your mouth, teeth, and gums. If you have poor oral hygiene, bacteria can cause infections or disease.
- You should brush and floss your teeth at least twice a day to prevent cavities and plaque from forming. Plaque can harm the enamel surface of your teeth and lead to gingivitis in the gums.
- Poor oral hygiene, gum disease, cavities, trapped food particles, and certain medical conditions can cause bad breath.
- Certain mouth and teeth conditions can be treated at home while others need to be treated by a dentist or orthodontist.
- Common vision conditions can be corrected with glasses, contact lenses, or surgery (like LASIK). Protect your eyes with eyewear during contact sports or in construction areas and with sunglasses when outdoors.
- Exposure to loud sound through headphones can damage the inner ear and cause hearing loss. The louder the sound, the less time it takes to inflict hearing damage. Hearing loss can also be caused by a ruptured eardrum from changes in pressure, insertion of an object into the ear, or an infection.
- Get regular vision and hearing exams to treat any conditions before they get worse.

Check Your Knowledge

Record your answers to each of the following questions on a separate sheet of paper.

1. **True or false.** You can damage your skin with exposure to UV light from the sun, tanning beds, and sunlamps.

2. Which of the following strategies will help prevent and treat acne breakouts?
   A. Cover up existing acne with makeup.
   B. Pop pimples on your skin.
   C. Avoid touching dirty glasses, headbands, and hats to your face.
   D. Cover pimples with your hair.

3. A doctor who specializes in skin conditions is called a(n) _____.

4. The higher the _____, the more a sunscreen will protect skin from UV rays.

5. What are the two most common types of body art?

6. Which hair condition can be the result of either dry or irritated skin or infrequent shampooing?

7. **True or false.** Irregularities in toenails and fingernails, such as redness and swelling, discoloration, or curled nails, are normal.

8. **True or false.** Plaque helps protect teeth and gums from diseases caused by small food particles or bacteria in the mouth.

9. What are two potential causes of bad breath?

10. Which of the following types of specialists helps prevent and correct teeth misalignments?
    A. Dentist.
    B. Dermatologist.
    C. Orthodontist.
    D. Cardiologist.

11. **True or false.** You should brush your teeth at least twice a day, and especially after eating foods that are sticky or high in starch and sugar.

12. What are the three most common vision conditions?

13. An eye care specialist who examines eyes for vision conditions and prescribes corrective lenses is called a(n) _____.

14. What is an early sign of hearing damage?

Use Your Vocabulary ↗

acne	dermatologist	nearsightedness
antiperspirant	deodorant	optometrist
astigmatism	eczema	orthodontist
body art	farsightedness	periodontitis
cavities	gingivitis	plaque
dandruff	lice	tinnitus

15. Prepare a presentation about two of the terms from the list above. In your presentation, explain each term as it might apply to your own life. Then, provide a more scientific explanation of the term. Answer any questions your classmates may have after your presentation.

16. Review the terms list above. If there are any terms you do not know how to pronounce, research their pronunciations online. Make flash cards with the phonetic spellings for these terms to help you remember.

Think Critically

17. **Analyze.** Are there differences in the rules and expectations of personal hygiene between different races and cultures? Give a detailed answer.

18. **Determine.** How can a child's environment and family impact his or her desire to get a tattoo or body piercing?

19. **Identify.** What are some reasons someone would not take care of his or her personal hygiene?

20. **Cause and effect.** How can personal hygiene affect how someone feels about himself or herself and his or her relationships with others?

DEVELOP Your Skills

21. **Advocacy and teamwork skills.** In small groups, create three flyers to raise awareness of personal hygiene issues that affect the students at your school. Choose three personal hygiene issues in this chapter to research. For each issue, create one flyer that provides important health information about the topic. The flyers should provide accurate information and be colorful and creative. With permission, hang these flyers in the school bathrooms to help raise awareness about these issues among people your age.

22. **Access information and technology skills.** Choose a personal hygiene issue commonly affecting middle school students. Search reliable health resources online to learn more about some of the hygiene products suggested for people in your age group to treat or prevent this issue. Evaluate two different products and each product's information. Were the products scientifically tested? Are they safe and effective? Compare and contrast these products. Is one product more expensive, healthy, or useful than the other? Which one would you recommend to your peers? Create a presentation highlighting the information learned. Present your findings to the class.

23. **Technology and communication skills.** Imagine your best friend confesses her insecurities about her personal hygiene in the following text message. Write a response with respectful, encouraging words and honest feedback. What advice can you share? Should your friend speak to a trusted adult about Devon?

> PE was horrible today. We had to run three miles! My armpits were so sweaty and Devon made fun of me. I smelled horrible and now I have two pimples on my nose.

24. **Decision-making skills.** Imagine your family has to cut back on basic hygiene products such as deodorant, soap, floss, toothpaste, and hair and skin products due to financial problems. In addition, you have less access to water to bathe and wash your clothes. As a result, your clothes are not being washed regularly and you shower less often. Recently, you have begun to notice an increase in body odor. Lastly, your teeth have a film and yellow stain on them. Write a short essay about how you would respond to a situation like this. What would you do? What resources are available to you? Who would you go to for guidance? What would you say to begin the conversation?

Chapter 4

Getting the Sleep You Need

Essential Question ?

What health benefits accompany getting enough sleep?

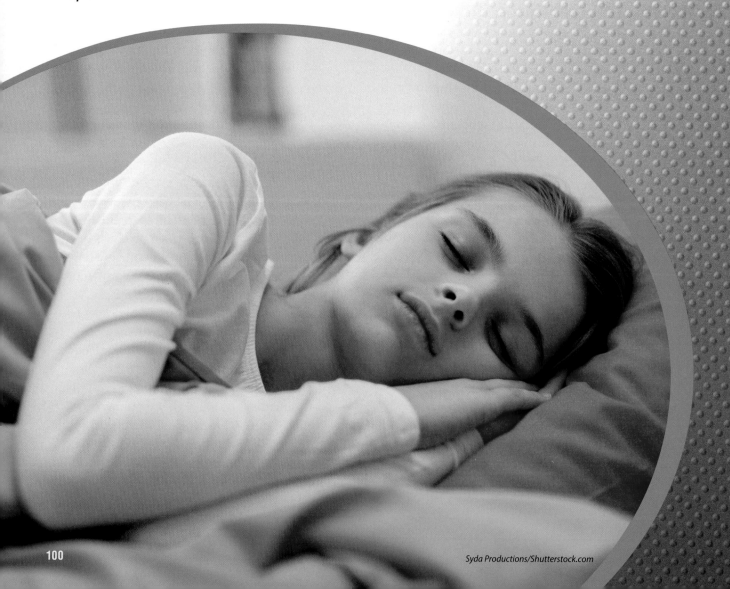

Syda Productions/Shutterstock.com

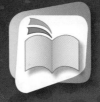

Reading Activity

Using reliable online resources, find an article discussing strategies for getting quality sleep. Take detailed notes as you read the article and then this chapter. Compare your notes on the article and the chapter and assess how the article is similar to or different from this chapter. Write a summary of the main ideas from your notes.

How Healthy Are You?

In this chapter, you will be learning about sleep. Before you begin reading, take the following quiz to assess your current sleep habits.

Healthy Choices	Yes	No
Do you get 8½ to 9½ hours of sleep every night?		
If you suffer from a sleep disorder, such as sleep apnea or nightmares, have you sought forms of treatment?		
Do you go to bed at approximately the same time each night and get up at approximately the same time each morning?		
Do you follow the same sleeping pattern on weekends as throughout the week?		
Are you physically active for 20 to 30 minutes a day?		
Do you avoid caffeine in food or drinks in the hours leading up to your bedtime?		
Do you practice relaxation techniques, such as reading a book or taking a warm shower, to wind down before bed?		
Have you created a cool, dark, and quiet environment in which you can sleep?		
Do you minimize the time you spend in front of a television, computer, or phone screen near the end of the day?		
Do you avoid napping for too long or too close to your bedtime, so you do not disrupt your normal sleep cycle?		

Count your "Yes" and "No" responses. The more "Yes" responses you have, the more healthy sleep habits you exhibit. Now, take a closer look at the questions with which you responded "No." How can you make these healthy habits part of your daily life? Think about how implementing these ideas can help improve your overall health. Identify a SMART goal you would like to achieve to help improve your overall health and well-being. Refer to Figure 1.11 to help you set up your SMART goal. If you do not understand the instructions, ask for clarification from your teacher.

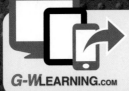

G-WLEARNING.com

Click on the activity icon or visit www.g-wlearning.com/health to access online vocabulary activities using key terms from the chapter.

Understanding Sleep

Key Terms ☞

sleep deprived term used to describe a person who gets inadequate amounts of sleep

short sleepers people who can function well on less sleep than other people

sleep deficit condition that occurs when people frequently get less sleep than they should

circadian rhythms naturally occurring physical, behavioral, and mental changes in the body that typically follow the 24-hour cycle of the sun

sleep-wake cycle pattern of sleeping in a 24-hour period

melatonin hormone that increases feelings of relaxation and sleepiness and signals that it is time to go to sleep

jet lag fatigue that people feel after changing time zones when they travel

blue light type of light from many digital devices, such as phones, tablets, televisions, and computers, that produces large amounts of energy

REM sleep active stage of sleep during which your breathing changes, your heart rate and blood pressure rise, and your eyes dart around rapidly

Learning Outcomes

After studying this lesson, you will be able to

- **understand** why sleep is important.
- **describe** the sleep needs of each age group.
- **explain** the science of sleep, the stages of sleep, and dreams.

Graphic Organizer

The Importance of Sleep

In a graphic organizer similar to the one shown, write five to six statements describing what you already know about the importance of sleep to your health. As you read the content in this lesson, add any health benefits of sleep that you did not previously know.

TO-DO LIST:
1.
2. SLEEP
3.

iQoncept/Shutterstock.com

I need to sleep because...

it enhances productivity

Sanjay is 12 years old and rarely gets 10 to 11 hours of sleep, the recommended amount for his age group. He has to wake up at 5:30 a.m. to get to school on time. He also likes to stay up late at night because this is when his favorite TV shows air. When he tries to go to bed, it takes him a long time to fall asleep. Sanjay knows he is sleep deprived. He has a hard time paying attention in class and maintaining his energy during football practice. He has been getting sick more often, too.

Sleep is an important process that his body needs each night. Without sleep, Sanjay's body is unable to heal or rest after performing daily activities. This can pose serious risks to his health and lifestyle.

In this lesson, you will learn why sleep is so important to your overall health and wellness, and how much sleep you need based on your age. You will also learn about the processes in your body that influence sleep. Finally, you will learn about the effects of not getting enough sleep.

The Importance of Sleep

How did you feel when you woke up this morning? Did you spring out of bed to face the new day, feeling completely refreshed and rested? Did you hit the snooze button a few times before crawling out of bed, dragging yourself to school, and nearly nodding off in class? How much sleep you get can affect your overall health and wellness (**Figure 4.1**).

If you felt completely refreshed, you likely got an *adequate* amount of sleep. This means that you got enough sleep to function properly throughout the day. If you find yourself falling asleep in class, however, you likely got an *inadequate* amount of sleep. This means you did not get enough sleep to function. *Insufficient* is another term for inadequate. A person who is **sleep deprived** gets inadequate amounts of sleep.

Getting enough sleep is just as important to good health as eating well or being physically active. If you do not get enough sleep during the week, you cannot make up for it by sleeping in on the weekend. Getting insufficient

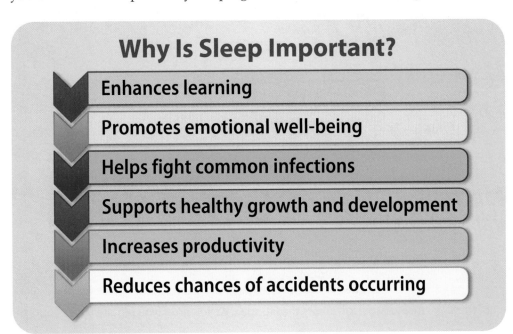

Why Is Sleep Important?

- Enhances learning
- Promotes emotional well-being
- Helps fight common infections
- Supports healthy growth and development
- Increases productivity
- Reduces chances of accidents occurring

Figure 4.1
Regularly getting enough sleep can benefit your health and wellness in many ways. *What is the term for a person who gets inadequate amounts of sleep?*

sleep on a regular basis can lead to health conditions, accidents, and poor performance in both school and athletics. For example, people who do not get enough sleep are more likely to get colds and other types of infections. People who drive while drowsy are just as likely to have an accident as those who drive while drunk. Students who do not get enough sleep often have trouble paying attention in class.

Getting an adequate amount of sleep helps the body heal, rest, and *rejuvenate* itself. The term *rejuvenate* means to refresh and feel more energetic. Getting an inadequate amount of sleep can result in feeling cranky, being unable to think clearly, and getting into arguments more easily.

You are likely to notice the benefits of a good night's sleep. After getting an adequate amount of sleep, you likely feel refreshed and ready to tackle a new day. If you go without sleep, you may not feel like yourself. It is important to get an adequate amount of sleep each night so your body and brain can function properly each day.

Sleep Needs and Age

The amount of sleep that a person needs depends on the individual's age (**Figure 4.2**). Infants, children, and teens need considerably more sleep than adults need. Young people need more sleep because their bodies and brains are still developing. Sleep encourages the development process and helps young people grow.

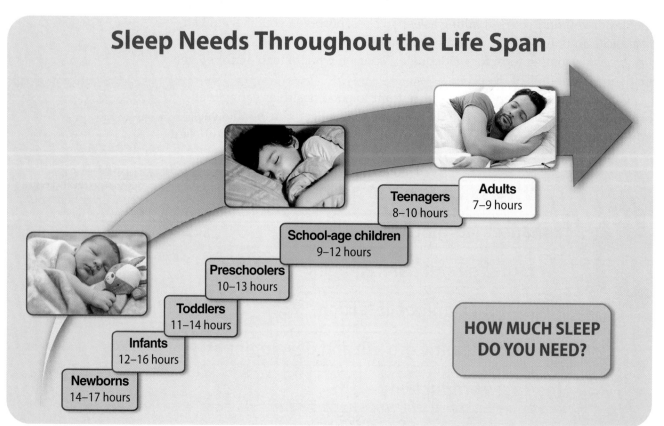

Sleep Needs Throughout the Life Span

Adults
7–9 hours

Teenagers
8–10 hours

School-age children
9–12 hours

Preschoolers
10–13 hours

Toddlers
11–14 hours

Infants
12–16 hours

Newborns
14–17 hours

HOW MUCH SLEEP DO YOU NEED?

Baby: Brandon Blake/Shutterstock.com; Child: Zurijeta/Shutterstock.com; Adult: Rido/Shutterstock.com

Figure 4.2 Sleep needs are not the same for every person across the life span. As you grow, you require fewer hours of sleep each night.

Some people may need more or less sleep than others. For example, some people are **short sleepers**, meaning they can function well on less sleep. These people often feel fully awake after sleeping for only 4 to 6 hours. Other people may need more than 9 hours of sleep to feel fully rested.

Think about how much sleep you usually get each night. Do you get enough sleep according to the amounts identified in Figure 4.2? Not meeting these sleep requirements causes people to experience a **sleep deficit**. This means that they frequently get less sleep than they should. People might experience a sleep deficit for a variety of reasons. They may go to sleep too late based on when they have to wake up in the morning. Over time, a sleep deficit can result in health concerns.

The Science of Sleep

The body and brain are very active during sleep, and this activity is essential to staying healthy. This healing activity cannot occur unless you sleep. Systems in your body help you get this necessary rest. Certain *mechanisms*, or processes, in the body control when you feel tired and when you feel awake. These mechanisms include circadian rhythms and the release of hormones such as melatonin.

Circadian rhythms are naturally occurring physical, behavioral, and mental changes in the body that typically follow the 24-hour cycle of the sun (**Figure 4.3**). For example, the body's temperature drops during the night and rises during the day. Most circadian rhythms are controlled by the body's master biological "clock." This "clock" controls circadian rhythms such as the following:

- sleep-wake cycle
- hormone levels
- brain wave activity

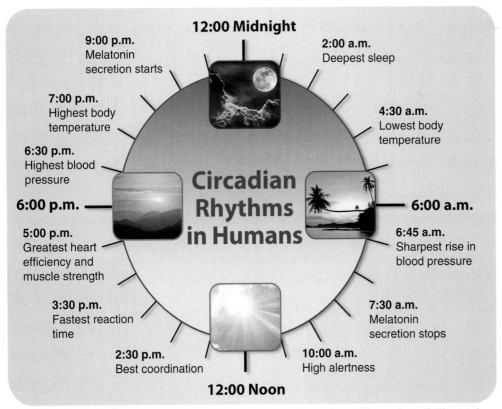

12:00 Midnight

9:00 p.m.
Melatonin secretion starts

2:00 a.m.
Deepest sleep

7:00 p.m.
Highest body temperature

4:30 a.m.
Lowest body temperature

6:30 p.m.
Highest blood pressure

Circadian Rhythms in Humans

6:00 p.m.

6:00 a.m.

5:00 p.m.
Greatest heart efficiency and muscle strength

6:45 a.m.
Sharpest rise in blood pressure

3:30 p.m.
Fastest reaction time

7:30 a.m.
Melatonin secretion stops

2:30 p.m.
Best coordination

10:00 a.m.
High alertness

12:00 Noon

Figure 4.3
The body automatically adjusts to specific times, providing better coordination and alertness during the day and deepest sleep at night. *When does the body start secreting melatonin to help encourage sleep?*

Clockwise from top: kdshutterman/Shutterstock.com; Sanit Fuangnakhon/Shutterstock.com; estherpoon/Shutterstock.com; sihy/Shutterstock.com

The **sleep-wake cycle** is a person's pattern of sleeping in a 24-hour period. The biological clock regulates the sleep-wake cycle in two ways. First, it monitors the amount of light in the environment. If it senses light, the biological clock sends signals in the body that result in activity. If there is less light, the biological clock can send signals to make the body less active. The biological clock also causes a gland located in the brain to release the hormone **melatonin** when it gets dark. Melatonin increases feelings of relaxation and sleepiness and signals that it is time to go to sleep.

When the natural circadian rhythm is disrupted, the body's biological clock takes a while to readjust. This explains **jet lag**, which is a fatigue that people feel after changing time zones when they travel. When people travel by plane from California to New York, their bodies feel like they "lost" three hours. When their alarms ring the next morning at 7 a.m. in New York, they are tired because it is only 4 a.m. in California according to their biological clocks. Working night shifts, adjusting the clock for daylight savings, or simply being exposed to **blue light** (light that produces large amounts of energy) at night can trick your body into an unnatural circadian rhythm (**Figure 4.4**).

Stages of Sleep

Each night, you usually pass through four distinct stages of sleep (**Figure 4.5**). These four stages include non-REM and REM sleep. A complete sleep cycle lasts about 90 to 110 minutes. Over the course of a night, you go through this sleep cycle about four to five times, depending on how long you sleep. The amount of time you spend in each stage of sleep, however, changes as the night progresses.

When a person first falls asleep, they are in non-REM (*non-rapid eye movement*) sleep. Non-REM sleep is broken out into the first three stages of sleep as follows:

- **Stage N1** occurs when a person gets drowsy and makes the transition from being awake to falling asleep.
- **Stage N2** is a period of light sleep. In this stage, eye movement stops, heart rate slows, and the body begins to relax.
- **Stage N3** is referred to as *deep sleep*. This stage is needed for a person to feel rested for the next day.

After the final stage of non-REM, a person enters the REM (*rapid eye movement*) sleep stage. The first period of REM sleep usually occurs about 70 to 90 minutes after you fall asleep. **REM sleep** is an active stage of sleep during which a person's breathing changes and becomes irregular, shallow, and more rapid. Heart rate and blood pressure also rise. A person's eyes dart about rapidly from side to side under the eyelids, and muscles are temporarily paralyzed.

The first sleep cycles of the night contain relatively short REM periods and long periods of deep sleep (Stage N3). The periods of REM sleep get longer with each sleep cycle, while the deep sleep periods get shorter.

There are smartphone apps available that track users' sleep cycle patterns (**Figure 4.6**). These apps can identify if the user is getting enough good quality

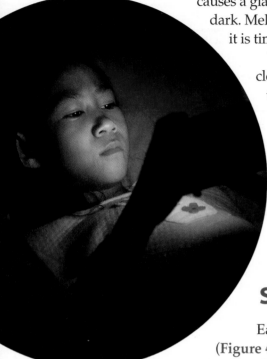

My Life Graphic/Shutterstock.com

Figure 4.4 Looking at digital screens, such as phones, tablets, televisions, and computers, before bed interrupts sleep. Researchers have found that people exposed to blue light before sleep showed lower levels of melatonin. *What is the body's physical reaction to the hormone melatonin?*

Sleep Stages

Non-REM Sleep (Stages 1–3)	
N1 (Stage 1)	You are making the transition from being awake to falling asleep. Heart and breathing rates start to slow, body temperature lowers, and muscles begin to relax.
N2 (Stage 2)	You enter a period of light sleep. Eye movement stops, heart rate slows, and muscles relax further.
N3 (Stage 3)	You fall into deep sleep. Heart and breathing rates are at their lowest point, body temperature lowers further, blood pressure lowers, and muscles slow. This is the stage when sleepwalking or sleep talking may occur.
REM Sleep (Stage 4)	You enter REM sleep after going through all 3 stages of non-REM sleep. Eyes move rapidly, heart rate and blood pressure rise slightly, and body temperature is at its lowest point. This is the stage when dreaming occurs.

One cycle: 90–110 minutes

Figure 4.5 You should cycle through all four stages of sleep multiple times each night, experiencing noticeable changes in the body's temperature, movement, and systems. *During which stage of sleep does your blood pressure lower?*

sleep. They also offer techniques and tools for falling and staying asleep. They can even wake the user at the ideal time, while entering the first stage of sleep. It is important to note, however, that many sleep experts do not believe that a sleep app can provide reliable, accurate data regarding a person's quality of sleep.

Dreaming

Even though you may not remember your dreams, you do dream every night. On most nights, people spend more than two hours dreaming. Many of these dreams will last between 5 and 20 minutes. What a person dreams about, however, may change a lot from night to night. Sometimes dreams may closely relate to what is going on in someone's daily life. At other times, dreams may appear bizarre and unreal.

Although most dreams occur during REM sleep, they can also occur during other sleep stages (**Figure 4.7**). Dreams that occur during REM sleep—when the brain is particularly active—are very vivid. People who wake up at the end of a REM sleep period are more likely to remember their dreams.

How dreams influence a person's psychological (mental) and physical well-being is unclear because it is difficult to study dreams. This difficulty is because people often

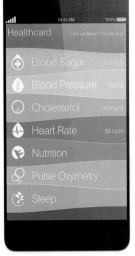
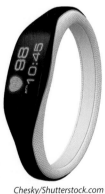

Chesky/Shutterstock.com

Figure 4.6 Smartphone apps can connect to devices, such as smart watches, which will record heart rate, blood pressure, and more to track the sleep patterns of the user.

Figure 4.7

These fun facts about dreaming explore this body function that people do not fully understand. *During which stage of sleep does dreaming typically occur?*

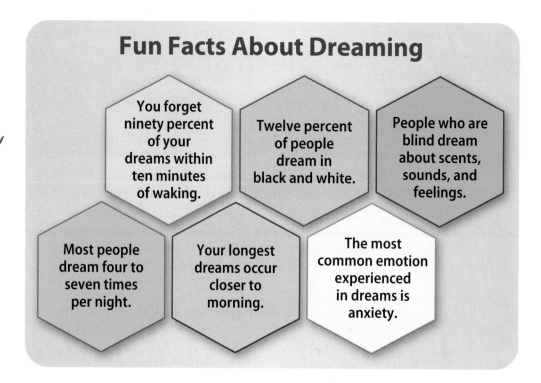

Fun Facts About Dreaming

You forget ninety percent of your dreams within ten minutes of waking.

Twelve percent of people dream in black and white.

People who are blind dream about scents, sounds, and feelings.

Most people dream four to seven times per night.

Your longest dreams occur closer to morning.

The most common emotion experienced in dreams is anxiety.

forget most of their dreams. Some sleep researchers believe that dreams play a valuable role in daily life. Dreams may provide important information about a person's deepest feelings, thoughts, and motives. Researchers believe dreams help people do the following:

- remember information
- resolve conflicts
- regulate their moods

Lesson 4.1 Review

1. How much sleep do school-age children and teens need each night?
2. The naturally occurring physical, behavioral, and mental changes in the body that typically follow the 24-hour cycle of the sun are known as _____ _____.
3. The body releases the hormone _____ in the late evening to encourage sleep.
4. **True or false.** People typically go through the sleep cycle once over the course of a night.
5. **Critical thinking.** List three possible consequences of not getting enough sleep.

Hands-On Activity

Explore starting and ending times of middle schools in and surrounding your community. What impact do start and end times have on students' sleep and performance in school and activities? If needed, recommend an appropriate adjustment to your school's schedule and support your recommendation with information about sleep needs of people your age.

Recognizing Sleep Disorders

Learning Outcomes

After studying this lesson, you will be able to

- **explain** symptoms of delayed sleep phase syndrome and insomnia.
- **describe** common types of parasomnia.
- **understand** the symptoms of and treatment for sleep apnea.
- **explain** the symptoms of narcolepsy.

Graphic Organizer

Sleep Disorders

As you read this lesson, use a table like the one shown to list the sleep disorders and possible causes of each one. If multiple disorders have possible causes in common, highlight each repeated cause in a different color.

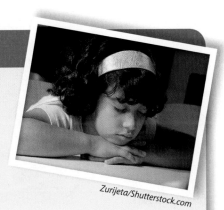

Zurijeta/Shutterstock.com

Sleep Disorders	Possible Causes

Key Terms

delayed sleep phase syndrome (DSPS) condition that results from a delay in the sleep-wake cycle that affects a person's daily activities

insomnia trouble falling or staying asleep

parasomnia term for sleep disorders that occur when people are partially, but not completely, awoken from sleep

sleep apnea potentially serious disorder in which a person stops breathing for short periods of time during sleep

narcolepsy disorder that affects the brain's ability to control the sleep-wake cycle

Have you ever spent an hour or more trying and failing to fall asleep? Have you had nightmares or experienced sleepwalking? Remember the example from Lesson 4.1. Sanjay stays up late watching TV at night and has a hard time falling asleep, which is causing him not to get enough sleep. His sleep deficit is causing him to get sick more often and to struggle to pay attention and work hard in class and at football practice.

Common sleep disorders such as these may cause you to lose sleep, but they are usually not serious. Long-term sleep disorders, however, can cause issues at school and in your life. Most importantly, sleep disorders have health consequences. Fortunately, most sleep disorders can be treated once the person recognizes the condition and seeks help. In this lesson, you will learn about some common sleep disorders, as well as available treatments.

Delayed Sleep Phase Syndrome

A common sleep disorder that affects a person's sleep-wake cycle is **delayed sleep phase syndrome (DSPS)**, also called *"night owl" syndrome*. DSPS is a disorder that results in a person being unable to fall asleep until very late at night and naturally not waking up until much later in the morning.

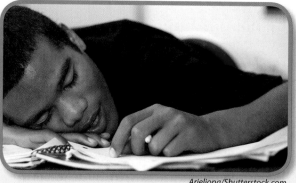

Arieliona/Shutterstock.com

CASE STUDY

Time to Wake Up, Beckett!

Beckett lies in his bed, unable to fall asleep. He keeps rolling over to check the time—10:30 p.m., 11 p.m., 11:30 p.m., 12 a.m., 12:30 a.m. Beckett is starting to worry because he isn't falling asleep and he knows that he needs to get up early in the morning to catch his school bus.

Beckett's alarm goes off at 6:30 a.m., but he hits the snooze button. He knows he has to wake up, but he can't keep his eyes open. He just feels so tired. Maybe if he gets five more minutes of sleep.

The next thing Beckett hears is his dad yelling from the kitchen for him to get up. *Oh man, that must mean it's after 7 a.m.* His dad gets so angry every time he has to wake up Beckett on school days. Beckett realizes his dad just thinks he is being lazy or is sleeping in on purpose or something. He is running late now and will not have time to eat breakfast. Beckett barely has time to get dressed and brush his teeth before the bus arrives.

The extra 30 minutes of sleep Beckett got this morning does not seem to help at all. He still falls asleep during math, which is his first subject of the

day. Beckett's teacher gently shakes him awake and Beckett can tell that his teacher is annoyed. Mad at himself, Beckett promises himself that tonight he *will* go to sleep at 10:00 p.m. No matter what!

Thinking Critically

1. Consider what you know about sleep among adolescents. Is Beckett's experience common? Why or why not?

2. What sleep disorder may explain Beckett's inability to fall asleep and wake up early?

3. If this happens to Beckett again, what strategies could help him fall asleep?

4. What could Beckett adjust in his life to prevent this from happening again?

DSPS can affect anyone, but is most common during adolescence. This is because teens' bodies are going through many changes as part of the normal growth process. One of these changes is the body's release of melatonin later in the night. This means teens are unable to fall asleep earlier in the evening. As a result, teens often do not get enough sleep because they go to bed late, but must still get up early to go to school.

The most common treatment method for DSPS is slowly changing the time a person goes to bed. People with DSPS can try to go to sleep a few minutes earlier each night until they reach the desired bedtime. Once they reach the desired time, the next step is to stick to that new time. If a person stays up late just one night, even on the weekend, the sleep-wake cycle can reset.

Oleg Golovnev/Shutterstock.com

Figure 4.8
People who have insomnia do not get adequate amounts of sleep. This often affects their ability to function the next day at work or school. *Why is long-term use of sleeping pills to combat insomnia discouraged?*

Insomnia

Almost everyone experiences **insomnia**, which is trouble falling asleep or staying asleep. Some people with insomnia lay awake for hours at night without being able to fall asleep. Others wake up several hours early and are unable to go back to sleep. Having insomnia can negatively affect all aspects of a person's health and well-being (**Figure 4.8**).

Insomnia may be a short-term, temporary condition that is a result of changes in a person's normal routine. For example, if you are going on a family vacation tomorrow, you may not be able to fall asleep on time the night before you leave. Insomnia like this usually goes away on its own.

Long-term insomnia is more serious than short-term insomnia. Long-term insomnia lasts a month or longer. It is often a symptom or side effect of another issue, such as a medical condition, substance abuse, or a sleep disorder. People with long-term insomnia can get help from a doctor, therapist, or counselor.

The most common cause of insomnia is stress. This stress may be a result of issues in a person's life. The stress could even be about the insomnia. Worrying about being unable to fall asleep or about being tired the next day can make insomnia worse.

Insomnia may be treated in many ways. Treatment can include sleeping pills, which are a type of medication that helps people sleep. Long-term use of sleeping pills is discouraged, however, because using them can interfere with good sleeping habits. It is important to talk to a doctor before using sleep medications or other sleep aids.

Parasomnia

Parasomnia is a term for sleep disorders that occur when people are partially, but not completely, aroused from sleep. Parasomnia occurs more commonly in young people because their brains are still developing. These disorders can occur when people first fall asleep, between sleep stages, or aroused from sleep. There are five common types of parasomnia. These types include bed-wetting, nightmares, sleepwalking, restless leg syndrome (RLS), and teeth grinding. **Figure 4.9** describes the five common types of parasomnia.

Types of Parasomnia

Bed-Wetting

- Disorder that occurs when a person unintentionally urinates (pees) at night during sleep.
- Very common in children younger than five years of age.
- May occur in young children because they have small bladders or do not have full bladder control.
- Reduce or avoid instances of bed-wetting by drinking more liquid during the day and less at night and by going to the bathroom immediately before bedtime.
- Other treatments include bed-wetting alarms, bladder training, and some medications.

Nightmares

- Scary dreams associated with negative feelings, such as anxiety, fear, and sadness.
- May cause people to wake up and have difficulty falling back asleep, or develop a fear of going to sleep.
- Usually occur during the last hours of sleep.
- May be caused by stress; trauma; illness; reading books, watching television, and eating before bed; lack of sleep; or alcohol, illegal drugs, and some types of medications.

Sleepwalking

- Sleep disorder in which people get out of bed and walk around while in a state of deep sleep.
- May occur when a person is sick, has a fever, is not getting enough sleep, or is experiencing stress.
- While sleepwalking, a person's eyes are typically open. The person will not respond to questions or remember sleepwalking, however.
- Sleepwalking is not usually a serious condition.

Restless Leg Syndrome (RLS)

- Disorder in which people experience sensations such as tingling, itching, cramping, or burning, as well as aches and pains in their legs.
- One of the most common sleep disorders among older adults.
- Possible causes may include another disease or health condition, such as anemia, pregnancy, or some medications.
- Substances such as caffeine, alcohol, and tobacco can worsen symptoms.
- Treatment includes lifestyle changes such as regular sleep habits, relaxation techniques, and moderate physical activity during the day. Certain medications may also help lessen the symptoms.

Teeth Grinding

- Disorder that involves grinding and clenching the teeth. Also known as *bruxism*.
- May be caused by stress or anxiety, having an abnormal bite, or missing or crooked teeth.
- Behavior is usually harmless, although long-term teeth grinding can lead to tooth damage, a sore jaw, headaches, and hearing loss.
- Treatment may include wearing a mouth guard, also called a *night guard*; relaxing the jaw and teeth; reducing stress; staying hydrated; and taking a prescription medication.

Sleep Apnea

Sleep apnea is a potentially serious disorder in which a person stops breathing for short periods of time during sleep. This disorder is usually associated with loud snoring, but not everyone who snores has this disorder. Many people have sleep apnea, but do not know it, or have not been diagnosed. Sleep apnea is most common among older people, and it is more common in males than in females. There are two types of sleep apnea (**Figure 4.10**).

People with sleep apnea can suffer numerous side effects due to inadequate sleep and a lack of oxygen in their blood. These side effects include the following:

- excessive daytime sleepiness
- irritability or depression
- morning headaches
- decline in mental functioning
- high blood pressure
- irregular heartbeats
- increased risk of heart attack and stroke
- accidents, including car accidents

Once a doctor diagnoses someone with sleep apnea, the doctor will suggest possible treatments. One common treatment for sleep apnea is continuous positive airway pressure (CPAP) therapy. CPAP therapy consists of a special machine that increases air pressure in the throat and keeps the airway open to help a person breathe. Someone with sleep apnea may wear a CPAP machine while sleeping (**Figure 4.11**).

Types of Sleep Apnea

Obstructive Sleep Apnea

- Occurs when a person's airway is *obstructed*, or blocked.
- Follows a cycle that may repeat hundreds of times a night.

Central Sleep Apnea

- Occurs when the brain fails to send the right signals to the muscles that control breathing.
- Is less common than obstructive sleep apnea.

Figure 4.10 The two types of sleep apnea, obstructive and central, are caused by different factors. *What is the most common treatment for sleep apnea?*

Between the 2016 and 2017 seasons, minor league pitcher Josh James experienced heavy snoring, decreased performance, increased fatigue, and weight gain.

He was diagnosed with sleep apnea, which meant he was not getting the sleep he needed to perform well. James began CPAP therapy for his sleep apnea. Once he was getting the sleep he needed, he regained the energy to perform well on the field.

With his sleep apnea in check, Josh James was even called up to the major league with the Houston Astros. He now pitches faster than ever, exceeding 100 mph.

Figure 4.11 Sleep apnea, like all sleep disorders, prevents people from getting the sleep they need. This can cause many disruptions in daily life, including athletic performance.

poylock19/Shutterstock.com

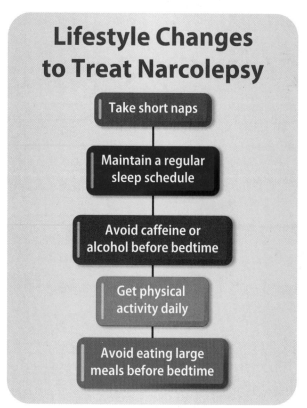

Lifestyle Changes to Treat Narcolepsy

Take short naps

Maintain a regular sleep schedule

Avoid caffeine or alcohol before bedtime

Get physical activity daily

Avoid eating large meals before bedtime

Figure 4.12 Certain lifestyle changes can help treat the symptoms of narcolepsy. *When might a narcolepsy sleep attack be dangerous?*

Narcolepsy

Narcolepsy is a disorder that affects the brain's ability to control the sleep-wake cycle. People with narcolepsy have frequent *sleep attacks* at various times of the day, even if they have had a normal amount of nighttime sleep.

During a sleep attack, a person falls asleep suddenly for several seconds or even more than 30 minutes. Strong emotions, such as fear, stress, or excitement, may trigger sleep attacks. These sleep attacks can be embarrassing and dangerous. They may occur when people are walking, driving, or performing other forms of physical activity.

Symptoms of narcolepsy typically appear between the ages of 10 and 25, but diagnosis may not occur right away. The causes of narcolepsy are still unclear. This disorder tends to run in families. People whose parents have narcolepsy are more likely to develop it themselves. Narcolepsy may also be caused by brain damage resulting from a head injury or brain-related disease.

Narcolepsy can be treated with medications that help control the symptoms. People with narcolepsy can also make lifestyle changes to treat their symptoms (**Figure 4.12**).

Lesson 4.2 Review

1. What age group is most commonly affected by "night owl" syndrome?
2. **True or false.** Parasomnia occurs when people are partially, but not completely, aroused from sleep.
3. What are the two types of sleep apnea?
4. Which sleep disorder involves having sleep attacks at various times of the day?
   A. Delayed sleep phase syndrome.
   B. Insomnia.
   C. Sleep apnea.
   D. Narcolepsy.
5. **Critical thinking.** Name three types of parasomnia and what might cause them.

Hands-On Activity

Make a list of resources (print, online, and personal) that could help someone who is dealing with difficult or abnormal sleep. Rank the list in order from easiest to most difficult to access. Which resources would you be most comfortable accessing? Which resources do you think are the best? Is there a difference? Why or why not?

Developing Strategies for Getting Enough Sleep

Learning Outcomes

After studying this lesson, you will be able to

- **create** a sleep schedule based on your needs.
- **explain** the best way to take naps.
- **demonstrate** how physical activity can help you sleep better.
- **describe** which substances interfere with sleep.
- **understand** how relaxing before bedtime can help you sleep.
- **demonstrate** how to create a comfortable sleep environment.
- **explain** how to control exposure to light before bedtime.

Key Terms

sleep-wake schedule routine for going to bed at about the same time each night and getting up at about the same time each morning

caffeine substance that increases energy, alertness, and attention, making it difficult to sleep

tryptophan amino acid that can help boost serotonin levels, which aid in sleep

night-light small lamp, often attached directly to an electrical outlet, that provides dim light during the night

Graphic Organizer

Sleep Tips

Write the phrase *Improving Sleep* in the middle of a graphic organizer like the one shown. As you read this lesson, brainstorm and write what you learn about techniques for improving sleep in the surrounding circles.

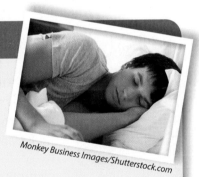

Monkey Business Images/Shutterstock.com

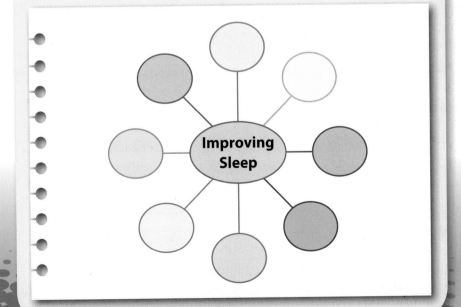

Improving Sleep

Getting enough sleep is an essential part of staying healthy. You need plenty of sleep to help protect your physical, social, and mental and emotional health and well-being. While you are sleeping, your brain is gearing up for the next day. Your body is getting the rest it needs to function well and be productive throughout the day.

Sanjay, the boy from the previous lessons, rarely gets enough sleep. It negatively affects his health and well-being, hurting his abilities in school and sports and making him more vulnerable to getting sick. What strategies can Sanjay use to improve his sleep habits?

Keep in mind that different sleep strategies work best for different people. The strategies that work best for Sanjay may be different from the strategies that work best for his parents, siblings, or friends. They may also be different from the strategies that work best for you. In this lesson, you will learn some sleep strategies that may help you get the sleep you need.

Apps and Devices to Improve Sleep

Drown Out Distracting Noise

- Especially benefit light sleepers
- Nature sounds, white noise, music, etc.
- Blocks other apps from making sounds

Calm Down and Prepare to Sleep

- Step-by-step instructions for relaxation
- Relaxing music
- Reduces alertness and slows thoughts

Monitor and Track Sleep

- Sleep duration (how long you sleep)
- Sleep quality (tossing and turning)
- Sleep stages and sleep patterns

Figure 4.13 The predictable pattern of a sleep-wake schedule makes it easier for the body to fall asleep and wake up. *What is a common reason it is difficult to wake up on Monday morning?*

Set and Follow a Schedule

Setting and following a sleep-wake schedule is one of the best ways to make sure you get enough sleep. When you follow a **sleep-wake schedule**, you go to bed at about the same time each night and get up at about the same time each morning. Maintaining this schedule creates a sleep-wake pattern for your body to follow (**Figure 4.13**).

Use the same schedule every day of the week—not just Monday through Friday. Many people get too little sleep during the week and then try to "catch up" on the weekend. Sleeping in for two or three extra hours on Saturday and Sunday disrupts your body clock. This makes it more difficult to get up early again on Monday morning.

There may be times when you want to change your sleep schedule. For example, you may be able to sleep later than usual during your summer vacation. You can help your body adjust to a new sleep schedule by changing the time you go to bed and the time you wake up by a few minutes each day. Going to bed and waking up just 15 or 20 minutes later each day helps you reset your biological clock to the new time and get better sleep.

Take Naps

Taking short naps is a better way of catching up on sleep than sleeping in late on the weekends. Taking naps during the day can help you get some extra sleep without disrupting your regular sleep schedule.

BUILDING Your Skills

Create Your Own Sleep-Wake Schedule

Busy lives can make it difficult to fall asleep on time. After you get home from sports practice or another after-school program, you may still need to finish your homework. After you finish your homework and relax for a few minutes, you may be falling asleep late. The next night, you may not have any after-school programs and not much homework, meaning that you get to sleep earlier. Having an irregular sleep-wake schedule like this can mean that you are not getting enough sleep.

As with any health behavior change, getting enough sleep starts with understanding where you are right now. Start the process of getting enough sleep by tracking your sleep habits for the next week using a chart similar to the one shown.

After a week, look at your log to review your sleep-wake cycle. Are you going to bed and waking up at consistent times each day? Are you getting 8–10 hours of sleep each night? If not, it is time to set a sleep-wake schedule. Remember, the sleep-wake schedule you set has to work for you, and this option may be different from what works for a friend.

If you discover that you need to fall asleep earlier, start by adjusting your bedtime to five minutes earlier than usual. After you are comfortable with this new bedtime, set it another five minutes earlier. Once you are comfortable with this new bedtime, set it yet another five minutes earlier. Do this as many times as needed to get to your goal bedtime. Another way to increase your total sleep is by gradually setting your morning alarm clock five minutes later each week. Five minutes may not seem like a huge deal, but over time it adds up.

Writing down your sleep-wake schedule and discussing it with someone who can help you follow it is likely to make you more successful. Review your progress regularly in following your sleep-wake schedule and make adjustments to your schedule as needed.

Sleep-Wake Schedule							
	Day 1	Day 2	Day 3	Day 4	Day 5	Day 6	Day 7
Last night, I went to bed at:							
Last night, I fell asleep around:							
This morning, I woke up at:							
Total number hours slept:							
Notes about the day: (include mood, activity level, naps, etc.)							

Naps have other benefits as well. People who take even a short nap—for 20 to 30 minutes—feel more alert, find it easier to learn new skills, and are better able to use their memory. They are also more creative. If you choose to take naps during the day, remember the strategies in **Figure 4.14**.

Be Physically Active

Have you noticed you feel more tired on nights after sports practice or time outside with friends? This is because your body uses up energy during physical activity and has to rest to get that energy back. Engaging in physical activity has many benefits, such as helping you get enough sleep.

Generally, young people should try to get at least 60 minutes of physical activity each day. Being physically active for even 20 to 30 minutes a day, however, can help you fall and stay asleep. To sleep better, find ways to add at least this much physical activity to your routine. Remember, you do not need to do the 20 to 30 minutes of physical activity all at once. Sometimes it can be easier to find smaller periods of time for physical activity. Even being active for five to 10 minutes several times during the day will help you sleep at night.

Try to be physically active at least five or six hours before you plan to go to sleep. Physical activity in the evening can make it difficult to fall asleep. It is best to get physical activity in the morning or afternoon if you can.

Understand Substances That Affect Sleep

Avoiding substances that make it harder to sleep can help you fall asleep more quickly and sleep more deeply. One example of a substance that interferes with sleep is caffeine. **Caffeine** is a substance that increases energy, alertness, and attention. This temporary increase makes it difficult to sleep. Avoiding drinks, foods, and medications that contain caffeine can help you

Figure 4.14
If you use the napping strategies listed at the right, you can get a small amount of extra sleep without disrupting your regular sleep-wake cycle.

Napping Strategies

- **Set an alarm.** Naps that are longer than 30 minutes can prevent you from getting adequate sleep at night. Short naps are best because they refresh you during the day while allowing you to get a full night's sleep.
- **Nap in the early afternoon.** Your body's biological clock tells your body it is time to rest in the early afternoon. Listening to your biological clock can help you get the most out of naps.
- **Do not nap after dinner.** This can disrupt your regular sleep schedule. If you are drowsy after dinner, do something active to avoid falling asleep.

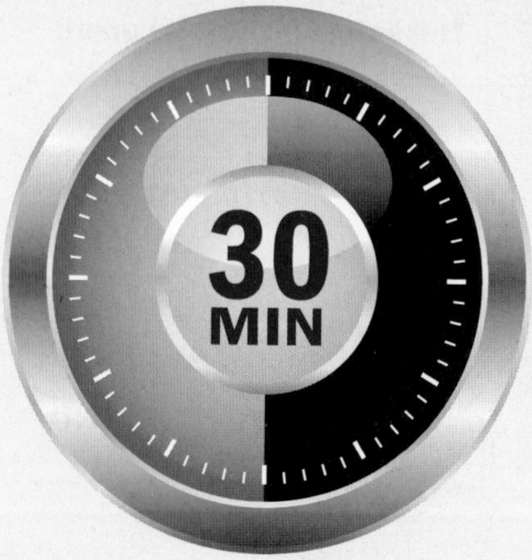

30 MIN

Arcady/Shutterstock.com

sleep better. Some products that contain caffeine include coffee, chocolate, energy drinks, soft drinks, nonherbal teas, and diet pills.

Consuming certain substances can also calm the body and help you sleep better. For example, **tryptophan** is an amino acid that can help boost serotonin levels, which aid in sleep. Bedtime snacks that contain tryptophan include a turkey sandwich, glass of milk, or banana. **Figure 4.15** lists other foods and drinks that may help people sleep. Avoid eating large meals or snacks shortly before bedtime.

Sleep medications and sleep supplements, such as melatonin, can also help a person sleep. A person should talk with a doctor before taking these medications and supplements, however. Sleep medications and supplements can have side effects such as dizziness, nausea, and headaches. They can also lead to dependence and long-term sleep issues.

Relax Before Bedtime

At the end of the day, people may focus on stressful experiences or worry about upcoming events. For example, you may feel worried about a test in one of your classes. You may feel stressed about a big assignment that is due, or feel angry about an argument you had with a friend. Thinking about these things at the end of a busy day is natural, but worries can cause you not to get enough sleep.

Fortunately, there are ways to clear your mind of stressful thoughts. One of the easiest and most effective ways is to create a bedtime routine. A peaceful bedtime routine sends a powerful signal to your brain that it is time to relax and let go of the day's stresses. Practicing relaxation techniques before bed is also a great way to wind down, calm the mind, and prepare for sleep (**Figure 4.16**).

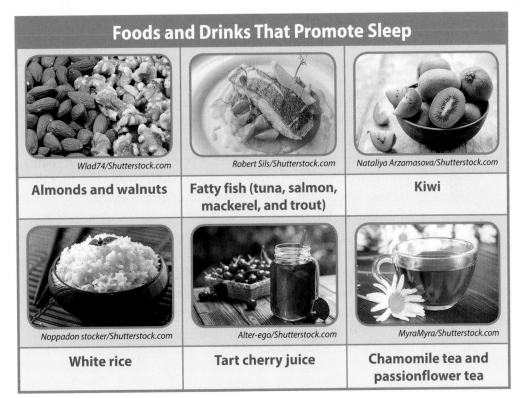

Foods and Drinks That Promote Sleep

Wlad74/Shutterstock.com	Robert Sils/Shutterstock.com	Nataliya Arzamasova/Shutterstock.com
Almonds and walnuts	**Fatty fish (tuna, salmon, mackerel, and trout)**	**Kiwi**
Noppadon stocker/Shutterstock.com	Alter-ego/Shutterstock.com	MyraMyra/Shutterstock.com
White rice	**Tart cherry juice**	**Chamomile tea and passionflower tea**

Figure 4.15
You could experiment with eating different types of foods or drinks to see whether they help you get to sleep.

Relaxation Techniques

- Take slow, deep breaths.
- Relax all of the muscles in your body, starting at your toes and working up to your head.
- Think about being in a peaceful, calm place, such as a warm beach or a lush forest.
- Read a book or magazine or listen to an audiobook.
- Write in a journal to help your mind stop thinking about the day.
- Take a warm bath or shower.
- Listen to quiet music.
- Have a warm drink, such as a cup of herbal tea.
- Perform gentle stretches to relax your body and mind.
- Avoid lying in bed if you are wide awake. Get up for 10 minutes and try to do something relaxing.

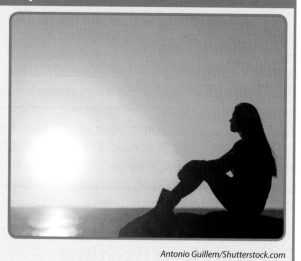

Antonio Guillem/Shutterstock.com

Figure 4.16 Creating a relaxed and peaceful bedtime routine through various relaxation techniques helps prepare your brain and body for sleep. *What should you do if you cannot sleep?*

If you cannot sleep, or if you wake up in the middle of the night and are unable to get back to sleep, get out of bed and do something relaxing. Feeling anxious about not sleeping makes it even harder to get to sleep. Read a book or listen to soft music until you feel tired. Avoid watching television or checking your phone or computer. These activities will keep your mind active.

Create a Comfortable Sleep Environment

It is easier to sleep in an environment you find comfortable. Even if you share a bedroom with a sibling, you can take certain actions to improve the sleep environment. The following techniques can help you create a comfortable environment for sleeping:

- **Reduce the room's temperature.** Most people sleep best in a slightly cool room with a temperature around 65°F.
- **Keep the bedroom dark.** If light comes through a window, install a room-darkening shade. If you share a bedroom with a sibling, consider wearing an eye mask to create a feeling of darkness or decide on a lights-out time (**Figure 4.17**).
- **Maintain quiet.** If you cannot eliminate noise, consider wearing earplugs or sleeping with a fan or a white noise machine to mask sounds.
- **Make your bed as comfortable as possible.** Try to have enough room in your bed to stretch and turn comfortably. If your mattress is uncomfortable, you might need a new one. Speak with your parent or guardian about it. Adding a foam mattress cover may solve the issue. A new pillow can also help.

pedrolieb/Shutterstock.com

Figure 4.17 Wearing a sleep mask can help you sleep when it is not dark enough in your environment.

Ways to Get a Good Night's Sleep

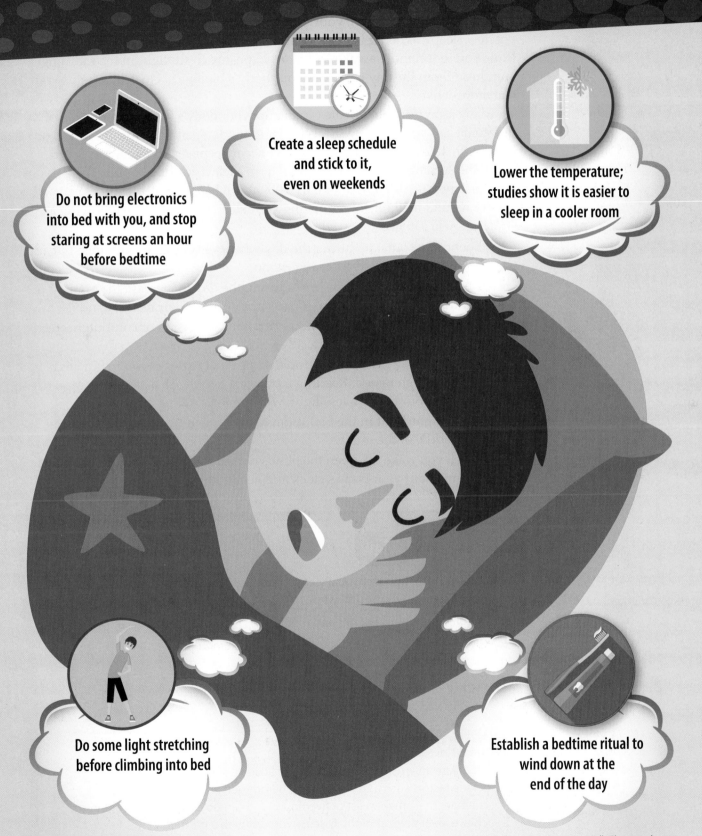

Do not bring electronics into bed with you, and stop staring at screens an hour before bedtime

Create a sleep schedule and stick to it, even on weekends

Lower the temperature; studies show it is easier to sleep in a cooler room

Do some light stretching before climbing into bed

Establish a bedtime ritual to wind down at the end of the day

Middle: Rimma Z/Shutterstock.com; Thought Bubbles: Kotenko Oleksandr/Shutterstock.com; Clockwise from top left: ten_thriller/Shutterstock.com; Jane Kelly/Shutterstock.com; KYY26871/Shutterstock.com; LesyaD/Shutterstock.com; gmast3r/iStock.com

Control Exposure to Light

As you have learned, melatonin is a naturally occurring hormone that helps regulate the sleep-wake cycle. Light affects the body's production of melatonin. When it is dark, your body produces more melatonin, which makes you feel sleepy. When it is light, your body produces less melatonin, which leads you to feel more awake and alert. Exposure to sunlight in the morning and throughout the day regulates your body's biological clock and helps you feel more active.

Many aspects of modern life can disrupt your body's natural production of melatonin and your sleep-wake cycle. For example, spending time in a school or home with little natural light can make you feel sleepier during the day. If you spend the evening exposed to blue light from a television or computer screen, your body may produce less melatonin, which makes it harder to feel sleepy.

Try natural methods of regulating your sleep schedule. The following are strategies you can use:

- Spend time outside during the day whenever possible. Eat lunch outside or go for a walk in the late afternoon.
- Keep curtains and blinds open during the day to increase the amount of natural light in your room. Move your desk or chair near a window.
- Minimize the time you spend in front of a television or computer screen at the end of the day.
- Avoid reading from an electronic device that exposes you to blue light before you go to bed. Reading a physical book with a bedside lamp exposes your body to less light, which makes falling asleep easier.
- Use a **night-light** in the bathroom to avoid turning on a bright light in the middle of the night.
- When you wake up, open the blinds or curtains and turn on bright lights to jump-start your body's clock and help you feel more awake and alert.

Lesson 4.3 Review

1. **True or false.** Being physically active for 20–30 minutes late in the evening can help you fall asleep and stay asleep.
2. People should avoid drinks and foods with _____ near bedtime.
3. Give two examples of strategies you can use to relax before bedtime.
4. When does the body produce more melatonin?
5. **Critical thinking.** How can you change your body's sleep-wake schedule in a healthy way (for example, over school breaks)?

Hands-On Activity

Create an artistic representation of an ideal sleeping situation for you. Include factors such as environment, before-bed behaviors, and sleep schedule. Then, make a list of five things you can do each day or evening to achieve ideal sleep at night. Discuss your list with a partner.

Chapter 4

Review and Assessment

Summary

Lesson 4.1 **Understanding Sleep**

- People who get insufficient sleep are sleep deprived, which prevents their bodies from rejuvenating, healing, and resting. Those who do not get enough sleep experience a sleep deficit.
- Naturally occurring physical, behavioral, and mental changes in the body that follow the 24-hour cycle of the sun are called *circadian rhythms*. The body monitors light in the environment and releases melatonin at night. Disruptions to the circadian rhythm, such as being exposed to blue light at night, can take a while to overcome.
- *Melatonin* is a hormone that increases feelings of relaxation and sleepiness and signals that it is time to go to sleep. *Blue light* is a type of light from many digital devices, such as phones, tablets, televisions, and computers, that produces large amounts of energy.
- Throughout one evening, you cycle through four distinct stages of sleep multiple times.

Lesson 4.2 **Recognizing Sleep Disorders**

- Delayed sleep phase syndrome (DSPS) or "night owl" syndrome is a disorder that results in a person being unable to fall asleep until very late at night and naturally not waking up until much later in the morning. DSPS is common during adolescence.
- Trouble falling or staying asleep is called *insomnia*. This affects a person's ability to get enough sleep.
- The most common forms of parasomnia are bed-wetting, nightmares, sleepwalking, restless legs syndrome (RLS), and teeth grinding.
- Sleep apnea is a potentially serious disorder in which a person stops breathing for short periods of time during sleep. This can be due to an obstruction in the person's airway (obstructive sleep apnea), or the brain failing to send the right signals to the muscles that control breathing (central sleep apnea).
- Narcolepsy affects the brain's ability to control the sleep-wake cycle, which can cause people to suddenly fall asleep for seconds or minutes at a time.

Lesson 4.3 **Developing Strategies for Getting Enough Sleep**

- Setting and following a sleep-wake schedule every day of the week is one of the best ways to avoid an irregular sleeping pattern. Naps can be helpful for getting some extra sleep throughout the day as long as they are no longer than 30 minutes or are not too close to bedtime.
- Being physically active at least 20–30 minutes every day can help people fall asleep and stay asleep.
- Even if they do not struggle with sleep disorders, people should avoid drinks and foods with caffeine near bedtime.
- Practicing relaxation techniques before bed can help prepare the body for sleep. A comfortable sleep environment is also important for getting the best sleep possible. Most people sleep best in a cool, dark, and quiet room.
- Spending time in places with little natural light and being exposed to blue light from digital devices can disrupt the body's production of melatonin and the sleep-wake cycle.

Check Your Knowledge

Record your answers to each of the following questions on a separate sheet of paper.

1. A person who gets an inadequate amount of sleep is _____ _____.
2. The fatigue people feel after traveling across time zones, called _____ _____, is a disruption to the body's natural circadian rhythm.
3. During which stage of sleep do most dreams occur?
4. **True or false.** Lack of sleep can lead to health conditions, accidents, and poor performance in school and athletics.
5. What is the most common cause of insomnia?
6. Nightmares, teeth grinding, bed-wetting, and sleepwalking are all examples of _____.
7. **True or false.** Obstructive sleep apnea occurs when the brain fails to send the right signals to the muscles that control breathing.
8. List three lifestyle changes that can help treat the symptoms of narcolepsy.
9. One of the best ways to make sure you get enough sleep is to set and follow a(n) _____ _____.
10. Which of the following nap strategies can disrupt your sleep-wake schedule?
    A. Set an alarm for no more than 30 minutes.
    B. Nap in your bed.
    C. Nap in the early afternoon.
    D. Nap after dinner.
11. Why does exposure to blue light from a digital screen make it difficult to fall asleep?
12. **True or false.** Spending time outside during the day can help you fall asleep better at night.

Use Your Vocabulary ↗

blue light	melatonin	sleep apnea
caffeine	narcolepsy	sleep deficit
circadian rhythms	night-light	sleep deprived
delayed sleep phase syndrome (DSPS)	parasomnia	sleep-wake cycle
insomnia	REM sleep	sleep-wake schedule
jet lag	short sleepers	tryptophan

13. For each of the terms above, identify a word or group of words describing a quality of the term—an *attribute*. Team together with a classmate and discuss your list of attributes. Then, discuss your list with the whole class to increase understanding.
14. Before reading, work with a partner to write the definitions of each term above based on your current understanding of them. After reading the chapter, discuss any differences between your definitions and those of another pair of partners. Finally, discuss the definitions as a class and ask your instructor for any necessary correction or clarification.

Think Critically

15. **Determine.** Why do people, especially teens, need sufficient sleep? What is a good bedtime for teens in your community?

16. **Cause and effect.** Explain the sleep cycle and how someone might feel if that person wakes up before the end of the sleep cycle. How do naps fit into this cycle?

17. **Analyze.** What is the connection between sleep and digital screen time in the hours before bedtime?

18. **Draw conclusions.** Using reliable sources (print, online, and in person), find information, tips, and suggestions about getting better sleep. Draw conclusions from the information and share your thoughts with the class. Be sure to cite your sources.

19. **Evaluate.** Is it healthy to sleep less on weekdays and "catch up" on weekends by sleeping more? Explain.

DEVELOP Your Skills

20. **Technology and advocacy skills.** Middle school and high school students struggle to get enough sleep on a regular basis. Research the health information in this chapter on sleep, including how much sleep your age group needs and strategies for getting enough sleep. Plan an app that helps students get the sleep they need. Consider appearance as well as function. This app should represent at least one way to utilize technology to benefit the health of you and your peers.

21. **Communication skills.** Imagine you have a friend who has been having trouble sleeping. He tosses and turns almost every night for a few hours. You know this is probably because after dinner he drinks a caffeinated soda and plays video games until bedtime. Write a dialogue using appropriate, informal language between you and your friend about his sleeping habits. Have him explain the health impacts he experiences from lack of sleep. What warning signs and tips for improvement would you share with him?

22. **Refusal and decision-making skills.** Imagine you have a friend who frequently invites you to come over to her house to watch movies on weeknights. You enjoy watching movies with your friend, but you stay up so late. Then, you always feel exhausted and sluggish the next day. How would you respond to your friend's next offer? Write a few possible responses.

23. **Communication and conflict resolution skills.** Imagine you are having a disagreement with your parents or guardians about your bedtime. What are the likely details of this disagreement? Role-play this situation with a classmate. Express your thoughts and feelings, as well as what you believe your parents' or guardians' thoughts and feelings would be. Consider the information you learned in this chapter. How would you resolve the conflict so everyone agrees?

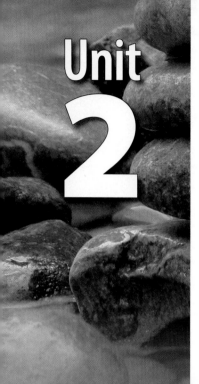

Unit 2

Taking Care of Mental and Emotional Health

Warm-Up Activity

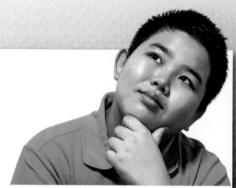

Pair Srinrat/Shutterstock.com

Prove or Disprove

Recreate the chart shown at the right on a separate sheet of paper. Before reading the chapters in this unit, fill in your thoughts for each quadrant of the chart.

When you finish reading the chapters, look at what you wrote in your chart. If what you wrote corresponds with information from the chapters, indicate that by noting the page number next to your statement. If what you wrote is disproved by your readings, cross out the statement and indicate on which page your thought was disproved.

In a different color, add additional information that you learned from the chapters. Be sure to indicate the page number on which you found the information. Then, think about the way your thoughts have been validated and changed as a result of your learning.

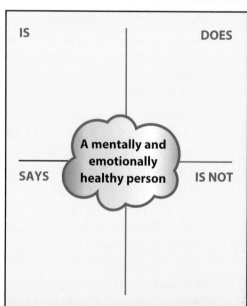

IS — DOES

SAYS — IS NOT

A mentally and emotionally healthy person

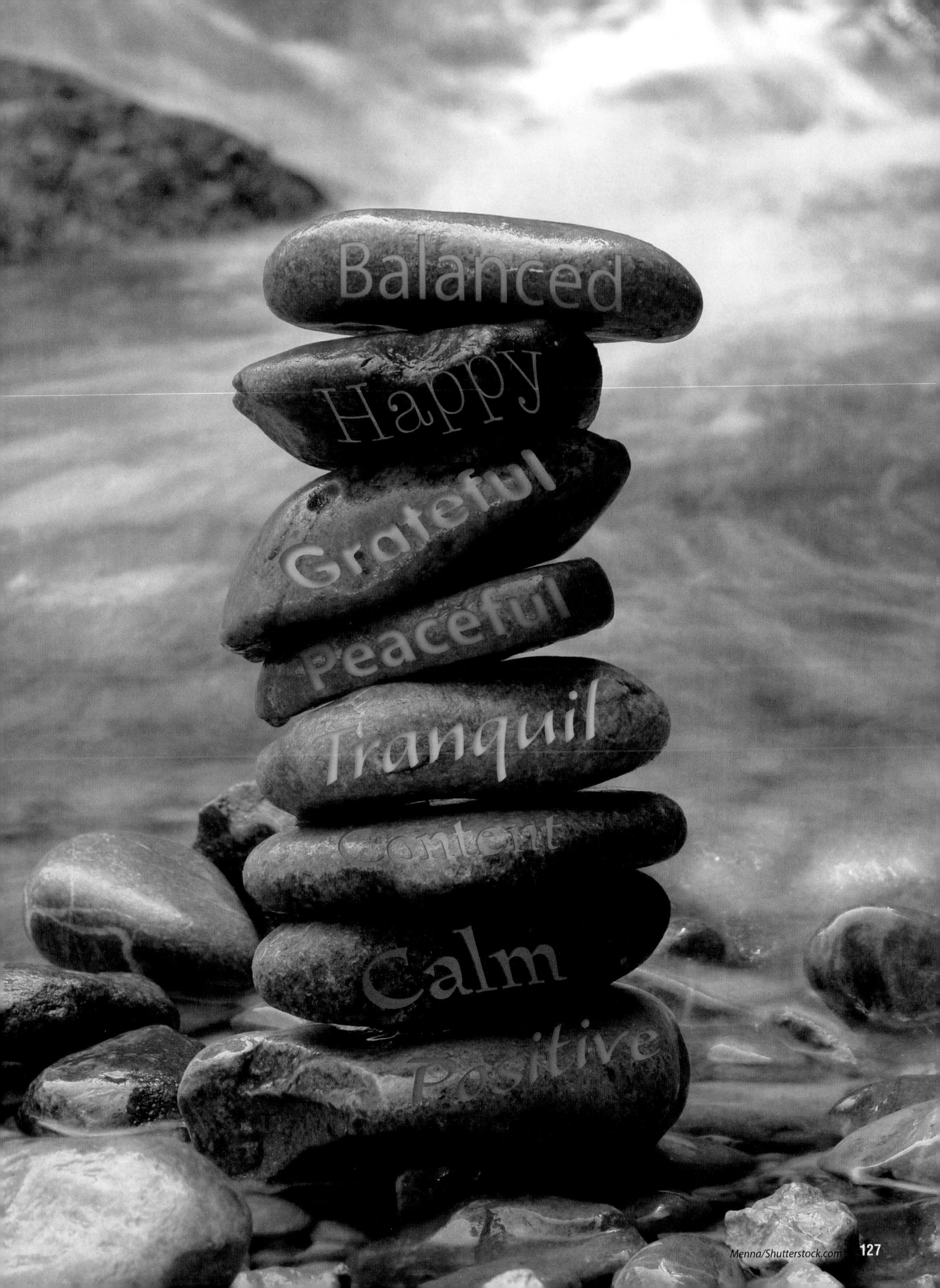

Balanced
Happy
Grateful
Peaceful
Tranquil
Content
Calm
Positive

Menna/Shutterstock.com

Chapter 5

Understanding Mental and Emotional Health

Essential Question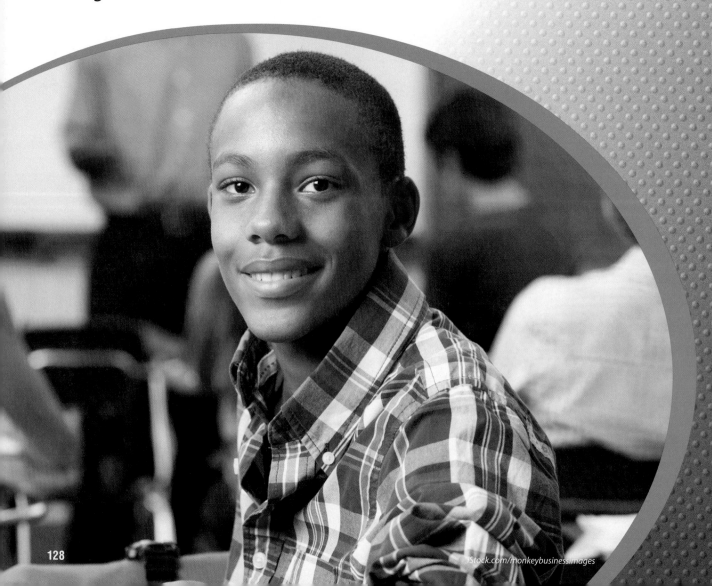

Can you make sense of your own thoughts and feelings?

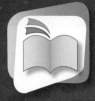

Reading Activity

As you read this chapter, take notes about skills for maintaining mental and emotional health. Make a list of what each skill might teach you about your mental and emotional health. After reading, pick three skills from your list and write a few paragraphs about how these skills can help you understand yourself. Use proper grammar and spelling in your paragraphs.

How Healthy Are You?

In this chapter, you will be learning about mental and emotional health. Before you begin reading, take the following quiz to assess your current mental and emotional health habits.

Healthy Choices	Yes	No
Can you keep a positive outlook in stressful situations and focus on the good aspects of these situations?		
Are you tolerant and accepting of other people's beliefs, values, and feelings?		
Do you accept your strengths and weaknesses as different parts of who you are?		
Are you honest and fair in your interactions with others?		
Can you recognize your emotions and feelings and understand why you experience them?		
Can you enjoy spending time with other people, as well as spending time alone?		
Instead of bottling up your emotions, do you express them clearly to others?		
Do you help people in need and thank those who help you?		
Do you trust your own judgment and feel confident that you can make the right decision, even in difficult situations?		
Can you understand others' wants, needs, and points of view?		
Do you practice relaxation techniques, like deep breathing or mindfulness, to manage how your body responds to stress?		

Count your "Yes" and "No" responses. The more "Yes" responses you have, the more healthy mental and emotional health habits you exhibit. Now, take a closer look at the questions with which you responded "No." How can you make these healthy habits part of your daily life? Identify a SMART goal you would like to achieve to help improve your overall health and well-being. Refer to Figure 1.11 to help you set up your SMART goal. If you do not understand the instructions, ask for clarification from your teacher.

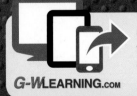

Click on the activity icon or visit www.g-wlearning.com/health to access online vocabulary activities using key terms from the chapter.

G-WLEARNING.com

Being Mentally and Emotionally Healthy

Key Terms ↪

mental health conditions patterns of thoughts and feelings that decrease mental and emotional health

mental distress mental and emotional state in which negative thoughts interfere with daily function for a short amount of time

identity who you are, which includes your physical traits, social connections, and internal thoughts and feelings

beliefs ideas or thoughts a person knows to be true, based on real experiences, scientific facts, or what a person has learned from others

attitudes set ways a person thinks or feels about someone or something

self-image your mental picture of yourself, which includes how you look, how you act, your skills and abilities, and your weaknesses; also called *self-concept*

self-esteem how you feel about yourself

self-talk thoughts and feelings about oneself

Learning Outcomes

After studying this lesson, you will be able to

- **summarize** the meaning of mental and emotional health.
- **describe** the different parts of a person's identity.
- **identify** personal values, beliefs, and attitudes.
- **differentiate between** self-image and self-esteem.
- **identify** factors that can affect a person's self-esteem.
- **explain** the difference between healthy self-esteem and low self-esteem.
- **practice** methods to assess mental and emotional health.

Graphic Organizer

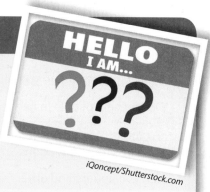

iQoncept/Shutterstock.com

Who Am I?

As you read this lesson, complete a chart like the one shown below for the physical, social, and psychological parts of your identity. For each box, identify specific examples of traits that would fall under each main topic.

Who Am I?		
Physical	**Social**	**Psychological**

As you read this lesson, you will learn ways to understand yourself through self-discovery. Understanding yourself relates to your overall mental and emotional health. By discovering who you are, how you see yourself, and how you feel about yourself, you can get to know yourself a little better. You will figure out how you feel about this person you are becoming.

If you discover that you are not happy with what you find, you can follow strategies to improve the way you feel about yourself. You will also learn about methods to assess your mental and emotional health. It is important to identify sources you can turn to for help when looking to improve your overall mental and emotional health.

Understanding Mental and Emotional Health

As you previously learned in Chapter 1, *mental and emotional health* has to do with your internal life—your thoughts and feelings. *Mental health* describes how you observe and understand information. It affects how you make decisions, solve problems, and examine situations in your daily life. *Emotional health* refers to how you express yourself and your thoughts and feelings. It includes your emotions, mood, feelings about yourself, and way of viewing the world. People with positive mental and emotional health share similar traits and characteristics (**Figure 5.1**).

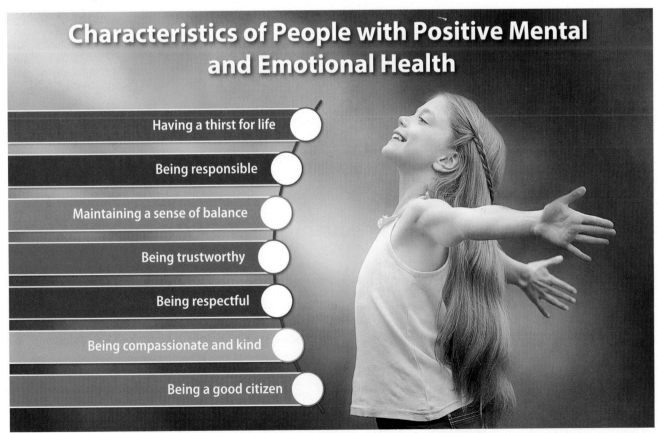

Characteristics of People with Positive Mental and Emotional Health

- Having a thirst for life
- Being responsible
- Maintaining a sense of balance
- Being trustworthy
- Being respectful
- Being compassionate and kind
- Being a good citizen

MANDY GODBEHEAR/Shutterstock.com

Figure 5.1 The characteristics shown here are good indicators of someone who has positive mental and emotional health. *Which characteristics on this list do you possess?*

Positive mental and emotional health have many benefits. They help people make meaningful contributions to their family, school, and community. This means people benefit from feeling good about themselves. It also means people benefit when other people in the community feel positively. In addition, people with positive mental and emotional health are better able to

- work productively in school and activities
- feel successful and content
- cope with minor and major stresses
- work through difficult situations
- know when to ask for help from family, friends, or other trusted adults

Having positive mental and emotional health does not mean feeling good all the time. It is normal to have ups and downs. Sometimes people feel happy, have a positive outlook, and feel they can take on any challenge. Other times, people feel sad or tired or have negative thoughts and feelings during stressful events.

Some people have **mental health conditions** (thoughts and feelings that decrease mental and emotional health). When mental health conditions interfere with daily function for a short amount of time, they are known as **mental distress**. For example, you might feel very sad or angry after a fight with a sibling. Your feelings might interrupt your life for a brief time. Eventually, these feelings of sadness and anger will pass. When a mental health condition becomes long-term and interferes with daily function, it is a mental illness. You will learn about mental illnesses in Chapter 6.

Discovering Your Identity

How would you answer the question "Who are you?" Your answer will probably depend on which part of your **identity** (who you are) is your current focus. Your focus may be on your physical, social, or psychological identities (**Figure 5.2**).

People often focus on different parts of their identities at different ages. During early childhood, children typically define themselves by their physical identities. This includes children's physical characteristics and abilities.

Figure 5.2
All three different aspects of your identity combine to make up who you are. *Which part of your identity is your current focus?*

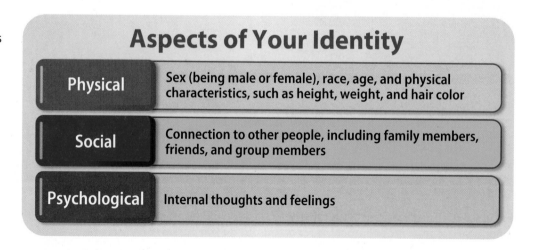

Aspects of Your Identity

Physical	Sex (being male or female), race, age, and physical characteristics, such as height, weight, and hair color
Social	Connection to other people, including family members, friends, and group members
Psychological	Internal thoughts and feelings

For example, a four- or five-year-old boy may describe himself as a tall boy with black hair and green eyes who runs fast.

As children enter middle childhood, around six years of age, their focus often shifts to their social identities. Social identity is a person's connection to other people, including family and friends. It is also a person's relationship with cultural, ethnic, political, national, and religious groups in a community. Children may define their social identities by focusing on these connections. As children age, their interests expand, and they get involved in new activities. They begin to interact more with friends, family, and community members. Children want to be a part of social groups with people who share similar interests.

During the teen years, teens tend to focus on their unique personal qualities and psychological identities. They define themselves in terms of their personal values, beliefs, and attitudes. *Values* are the things a person considers to be the most important in life. Personal **beliefs** are ideas or thoughts a person knows to be true, based on real experiences, scientific facts, or what a person has learned from others. **Attitudes** are set ways a person thinks or feels about someone or something. A person's psychological identity can be a combination of many values, beliefs, and attitudes, which often change throughout life.

Exploring Your Self-Image

Now that you have identified who you are, consider how you see yourself. Do you generally like the way you look? Do you think of yourself as a good person? Are you happy with the personality traits you possess (**Figure 5.3**)?

Personality Traits			
Adaptable	Dependable	Insecure	Planner
Adventurous	Detailed	Kind	Pleasant
Ambitious	Diplomatic	Leader	Productive
Analytical	Efficient	Listener	Reserved
Assertive	Emotional	Logical	Resourceful
Athletic	Empathetic	Loyal	Respectful
Bashful	Enthusiastic	Mediator	Self-reliant
Bold	Expressive	Musical	Sensitive
Calm	Faithful	Optimistic	Shy
Careful	Flexible	Orderly	Sociable
Cheerful	Forgiving	Outspoken	Spontaneous
Competitive	Friendly	Patient	Stubborn
Confident	Funny	Peaceful	Sympathetic
Considerate	Helpful	Perfectionist	Talkative
Consistent	Imaginative	Persistent	Thoughtful
Cooperative	Impulsive	Persuasive	Tolerant
Creative	Independent	Pessimistic	Understanding

Figure 5.3
This table offers some examples of the many personality traits that can describe who you are. These traits can also help you reflect on whether you are happy with yourself as a person. *Which five personality traits best describe you?*

Do you accept your strengths and weaknesses? Answering questions such as these can give you a sense of your self-image.

Your **self-image**, also called *self-concept*, is your mental picture of yourself. Your self-image is how you view your appearance, personality, skills and abilities, and weaknesses. People with positive mental and emotional health accept themselves for who they are. They accept the way they look—even though they may not like all of their physical features. They have confidence in their skills and abilities and work toward improving their weaknesses.

You are not born with a self-image. It forms gradually over time, starting in childhood. Your life experiences and interactions with others influence your self-image. As you experience different events and interact with different people, your self-image may change.

The view you have of yourself is likely different from how others see you. This is because your unique personal values, beliefs, and attitudes shape your opinion of yourself. The way you see yourself affects how you relate to others. If you view yourself in a positive way, people will probably respond positively to you. If the view you have of yourself is negative, others may view you in this way, too.

Determining Your Level of Self-Esteem

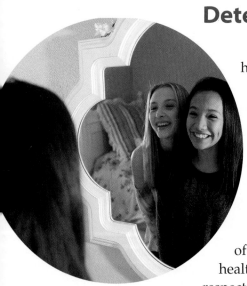

How you feel about yourself, or your **self-esteem**, closely relates to how you see yourself. How you feel about yourself has a major impact on many different aspects of your life (**Figure 5.4**). Self-esteem varies from person to person, and many factors can affect how you feel about yourself. Some people have healthy self-esteem, while other people have low self-esteem. Self-esteem also changes with life experiences and new understanding.

Factors That Affect Self-Esteem

Many different factors can affect self-esteem. Other people are one of the biggest factors that can affect how you see yourself. For example, healthy relationships with family and friends who accept and treat you with respect can help you develop a sense of pride in who you are. On the other hand, if you receive constant criticism and rejection from others, you may develop low self-esteem. Your personal relationships with others, whether positive or negative, can have a lasting effect on how you feel about yourself.

Another big factor is how you view yourself. Your thoughts about yourself, called **self-talk**, affect your self-esteem. Positive self-talk is encouraging and supportive and improves self-esteem. An example is thinking about how well you prepared for a test. Negative self-talk constantly criticizes and finds faults. This type of self-talk can make you feel worse and lead to low self-esteem. Other factors that can affect self-esteem are shown in **Figure 5.5**.

Healthy Self-Esteem

People who have a realistic view of and value themselves have *healthy self-esteem*. If you have healthy self-esteem, you feel good about yourself—

Mat Hayward/Shutterstock.com

Figure 5.4
How you feel about yourself affects your relationships with others, how well you do in school, and how you manage disappointments and frustrations. *What is the term for how you feel about yourself?*

Factors Affecting Self-Esteem

- Self-image
- Social interactions with family members, friends, and others
- Home, school, community, and cultural environments
- Life events and personal experiences
- Media, such as television, movies, and social networking sites

including your skills and abilities—and you have a positive self-image. If you have healthy self-esteem, you also feel good about your relationships with other people. You feel loved, appreciated, and accepted by your friends and family members.

Having healthy self-esteem does not mean that you only experience good situations and never face problems or have days when you feel a little down. It just means that you cope well with unpleasant situations and disappointments.

BUILDING Your Skills

How You Can Build Your Self-Esteem

Building self-esteem is not easy, but it can happen as you learn to work through issues and accept who you are. As you gain experience, you will see how you can take charge and have a positive outcome.

If you do not see yourself in a positive way, choose one of the following strategies to help build your self-esteem. Set a reasonable goal to improve your self-care:

- Take good care of yourself. Eat healthy foods, get plenty of sleep, and be physically active.
- Make a list of activities you really enjoy doing. Then, pick something from the list to do every day. Keep adding to your list as you discover new activities you enjoy.
- Spend time with people who make you feel good about yourself. Also, be someone who makes others feel good, too. Do something nice for someone else. Say a few kind words to someone. Hold the door open for someone the next time you are at a public place, such as a restaurant or store.

- Make a list of your skills and abilities. If you cannot think of anything on your own, ask friends or relatives what they think your skills and abilities are. The next time you feel down about yourself, look at the list and remember your strengths.
- Focus on your strengths. Look at your positive qualities and concentrate on those. Acknowledge your weaknesses and figure out what you can do to try to improve them.

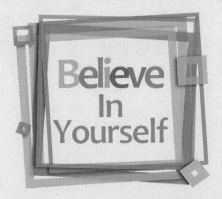

ileezhun/Shutterstock.com

Questions to Help Assess Mental and Emotional Health

How often and intensely do you worry about situations?

Do you feel in control of your emotions and actions?

How happy or sad have you been feeling?

Has anyone mentioned changes in your behavior?

Do you enjoy the activities that you are doing?

Have you been confident or critical of your abilities?

How healthy are your relationships with friends and family?

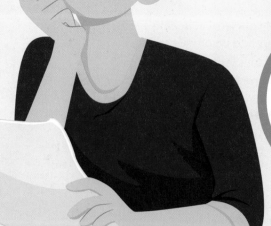

Male: Lorelyn Medina/Shutterstock.com; Question Marks: Blan-k/Shutterstock.com

People with healthy self-esteem view negative events and failures as learning experiences, not as proof of their weaknesses. Moreover, when they run into obstacles, people with healthy self-esteem can accept reality or criticism and make a new plan. They are also more comfortable asking other people for help and support in times of need.

People who have healthy self-esteem have great decision-making skills. They trust their own judgment and follow their own values. They are confident that they can make the right decision, even in difficult situations. When they feel pressure to go along with the crowd, people with healthy self-esteem have the courage to make the choice they believe is right or take responsibility for a poor choice.

Low Self-Esteem

People who have *low self-esteem* doubt their own self-worth and may engage in negative self-talk about their traits, skills, and abilities (**Figure 5.6**). If you have low self-esteem, you may wish you could change your looks, intelligence, or skills. You may feel left out of social groups and disconnected from other people. You may also question whether other people like or respect you, in part, because you do not really like or respect yourself.

People with low self-esteem often worry about what other people think of them. They may try to show off because they want to convince other people of their worth. Being concerned about the opinions of others makes people with low self-esteem vulnerable to pressure. People with low self-esteem may feel unable to resist pressure to engage in unhealthy behaviors. Unfortunately, these behaviors can have long-term health consequences.

Most people experience periods of low self-esteem from time to time. This is a normal part of life. As young people try to figure out who they are, they can feel uncertain about themselves, lost, or think they do not measure up

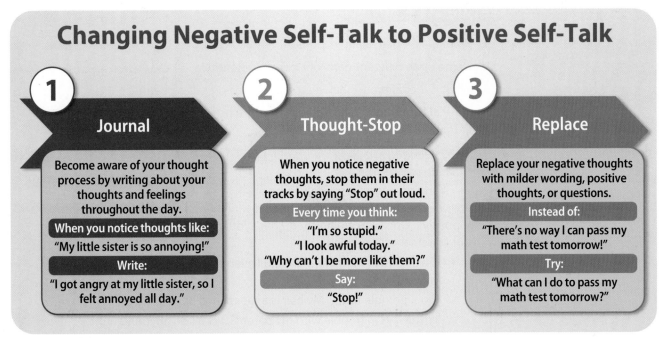

Figure 5.6 Learning to recognize and replace negative self-talk with positive self-talk can help improve your self-esteem.

to others. This does not have to last forever. Young people can learn to work through these issues and accept who they are. They can improve their self-esteem by caring for themselves, avoiding perfectionism, and celebrating their strengths and successes.

Assessing Your Mental and Emotional Health

Everyone experiences times when they feel good and times when they feel worse. These changes in mood are a normal part of life. Sometimes, however, mental health conditions and negative thoughts can make it difficult to perform daily tasks, maintain relationships, and reach goals. Regularly assessing the health of your thoughts and feelings can help you improve or maintain your mental and emotional health.

Assessing your mental and emotional health involves considering the thoughts and feelings you experience throughout the day. First, identify what events, if any, trigger certain feelings. Then examine the pattern of your thoughts and feelings. Think about whether most of your feelings are positive or negative and about whether your thoughts are encouraging or criticizing. You can work to improve these areas of your mental and emotional health. For example, if you notice you have negative self-talk, you can make an effort to notice what you are doing well and focus on positive self-talk.

Assessing your mental and emotional health can also determine if you need to seek help from others. It can be helpful to talk with someone about your thoughts and feelings. Seeking help can offer a new point of view to a situation. Seeking help can be as simple as talking to a trusted adult or friend. It can also involve meeting with a therapist. Serious mental health conditions and mental illnesses require professional treatment to manage symptoms.

Lesson 5.1 Review

1. What is a mental health condition?
2. Name three different parts of a person's identity.
3. What is the difference between self-image and self-esteem?
4. **Critical thinking.** What strategies can you use to assess your mental and emotional health?

Hands-On Activity

Changing negative self-talk to be positive self-talk takes practice. On a separate sheet of paper, rewrite the following negative self-talk statements to be positive. Once you are finished, share your answers with a partner. Revise your statements as needed.

- "I'm so bad in math. Why should I even try? I'll get an F on the next test anyway."
- "I look terrible today. My hair is a mess and I have pimples on my face."
- "I'm always in trouble with my parents. I can't do anything right."

Making Sense of Your Emotions

Learning Outcomes

After studying this lesson, you will be able to

- **identify** pleasant and unpleasant emotions.
- **explain** what it means to have emotional awareness.
- **describe** how identifying and accepting your feelings can help you control your emotions.
- **demonstrate** how to express your emotions in a healthy way.
- **identify** characteristics of people with high emotional intelligence.

Graphic Organizer

My Emotions

Write "Making Sense of My Emotions" at the top of a graphic organizer like the one shown. Then, write the three main (green) headings of the lesson underneath. As you read the lesson, fill in the main concepts from each section. How does this information help you understand your emotions?

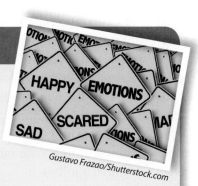

Gustavo Frazao/Shutterstock.com

Making Sense of My Emotions

Understanding Your Emotions	Controlling Your Emotions	Developing Emotional Intelligence
	Identifying What You Are Feeling First step: Think about events or factors that might trigger an emotion	

Key Terms

emotions moods or feelings you experience

emotional awareness skill of knowing which emotions you feel and why

self-compassion treating oneself with kindness and understanding, even when experiencing setbacks and disappointments

emotional intelligence (EI) skill of understanding, controlling, and expressing your emotions and sensing the emotions of others

optimism ability to keep a positive outlook and focus on the good aspects of stressful situations

empathy ability to put yourself in someone else's shoes, and to understand someone else's wants, needs, and viewpoints

gratitude emotion that means being thankful or grateful

resilience ability to bounce back from traumatic or stressful events

Making sense of your feelings can be challenging at times, especially when you feel like you are on an emotional roller coaster. Many people go through emotional ups and downs, which are a normal part of experiencing life. Understanding these feelings can help you learn about yourself and others.

In the previous lesson, you explored who you are and how you feel about yourself. You also learned how to assess your mental and emotional health. In this lesson, you will explore how you feel about and react to people and situations around you.

How you react to your feelings—what you think, say, and do—can have positive or negative effects on your mental and emotional health. People who are mentally and emotionally healthy understand their moods and feelings. They know how to control and express those feelings to others in positive ways.

Understanding Your Emotions

People experience many different emotions. Your **emotions** are the moods or feelings you experience. They reveal to you how you feel about certain events and situations. They can also help you understand yourself and make healthy decisions that relate to your values and beliefs. Emotions, which are a normal part of life, can be pleasant or unpleasant (**Figure 5.7**). Pleasant emotions represent positive feelings that make you feel good. Unpleasant emotions represent negative feelings that often make you feel bad.

As you experience life, you may feel pleasant and unpleasant emotions at the same time. For example, when the school year ends, you may feel happy because you will not have to do homework. You might also feel sad because you will not see some of your friends every day.

Sometimes, understanding your emotions can be challenging because one emotion masks or hides another emotion. If you try out for and do not make the sports team, you might feel angry with the coach for not selecting you.

Figure 5.7
Everyone experiences many different pleasant and unpleasant emotions throughout life, often at the same time. *How does emotional awareness help you control your emotions?*

How Are You Feeling Today?

Alhovik/Shutterstock.com

Alhovik/Shutterstock.com

Pleasant Emotions			Unpleasant Emotions		
Happy	Grateful	Proud	Angry	Jealous	Guilty
Loved	Excited	Hopeful	Scared	Helpless	Rejected
Kind	Cheerful	Joyful	Disgusted	Lonely	Sad

This feeling of anger may only be a result of sadness, however, because you really wanted to be part of the team.

Understanding your emotions involves knowing which emotions you feel and why. When you are aware of your emotions, you have **emotional awareness**. You are not just reacting to your emotions. Instead, you use emotional awareness to control them.

Controlling Your Emotions

Controlling your emotions is not easy. As a young child, you probably reacted to what you felt without thinking. As you grow up, however, you can learn to control your emotions by following the steps in **Figure 5.8**.

In the following sections, you will learn about the process for controlling your emotions. You will read about the feelings Jennifer is experiencing and how she responds to the situation. As you are reading, think about how you would react if you were in Jennifer's shoes. What would you do? Reflect on how identifying, accepting, and expressing your feelings in healthy, positive ways can help you control your emotions.

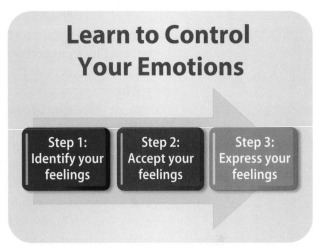

Learn to Control Your Emotions

| Step 1: Identify your feelings | Step 2: Accept your feelings | Step 3: Express your feelings |

Figure 5.8 Learning how to control your emotions can have a positive effect on your mind and body.

Identifying What You Are Feeling

The first step in controlling your emotions is to identify what emotion or emotions you are feeling. This is not always an easy task. Sometimes, identifying feelings of sadness and fear or other emotions can be confusing. To help you determine the actual emotion you are experiencing, and why, think about events or factors that might have triggered the emotion (**Figure 5.9**).

Consider Jennifer's situation. Jennifer started the day in a bad mood. She argued with her sister when her sister said it was Jennifer's turn to take the dog for a walk. On the way to school, she yelled at her brother for not keeping up with her. At lunch, Jennifer snapped at her best friend, Alia, for no reason. Alia asked Jennifer why she was in such a bad mood.

As it turns out, Jennifer was reacting negatively to a conversation she had with her mother the night before. Jennifer's mother had mentioned that she was applying for a new job in another city. If her mother gets the job, Jennifer will probably have to move, which she does not want to do. Rather than telling her mother that she did not want to move, Jennifer took out her frustrations on those around her, which is unhealthy.

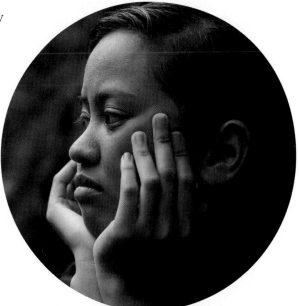

Francis Wong Chee Yen/Shutterstock.com

Figure 5.9
Spending time thinking about how you feel, and why, can help you identify your emotions.

Jennifer apologized to Alia for snapping at her and then they talked about Jennifer's situation. Jennifer identified that she was angry, but as they talked about it, Jennifer also identified that she was anxious and afraid. She was anxious about the thought of leaving her friends. She was afraid that others would not accept her at a new school. By identifying and sorting out her feelings, Jennifer took the first step toward accepting her feelings.

Accepting Your Feelings

Now that Jennifer knows her anger is a result of being anxious and afraid, she must learn to accept her feelings. Accepting your feelings does not mean that those feelings will just go away. It simply means that you allow yourself to experience your emotions. When you experience your emotions, you can work through what you are feeling so you can let it go.

Sometimes you may want to cover up or deny your emotions and hope they just simply go away. Try to avoid judging or changing your emotions. Instead, accept your emotions as they are by showing self-compassion. **Self-compassion** means treating yourself with kindness and understanding, even when you experience setbacks and disappointments. Your emotions belong to you, and you are not wrong for feeling them. Denying or burying your emotions deep inside can have a negative effect on you both physically and mentally. Realize that your emotions cannot hurt you as long as you accept them and manage them in healthy ways.

Healthy, positive ways to accept and express your emotions may include sharing your feelings with friends, family members, or a trusted adult. Writing about what you are feeling in a journal is another positive way to work through your feelings. You can also work through your emotions by crying if you feel sad or running if you feel angry. **Figure 5.10** shows other healthy ways to accept and express your feelings.

Jennifer began to accept her emotions when she admitted that her anger was a result of being anxious and afraid about moving. Talking with Alia was a healthy, positive way for Jennifer to begin to work through her emotions. Once Jennifer acknowledged her feelings and calmed down, she felt that she was ready to express her feelings to her mother.

Healthy, Positive Ways to Accept and Express Emotions

- Sharing with friends, family, or a trusted adult
- Writing in a journal
- Crying
- Taking a walk or run
- Reducing stress
- Doing an activity you enjoy
- Taking a long bath or shower
- Finding a reason to laugh
- Documenting a positive moment

Figure 5.10 People who allow themselves to express their emotions are better able to release them and move past them. *Why should you not deny or bury your emotions?*

Expressing Your Feelings to Others

Controlling your emotions involves expressing your feelings clearly to others. When you are telling others how you feel, it is important to stay calm and keep your emotions under control. If you are negative and lash out or try to hurt someone, then you are expressing your emotions in an unhealthy way.

What to Do If You Feel...

Happy

Write down what made you happy that day so you can reflect on it the next time you feel down.

Express gratitude to those who helped you feel that way.

Spread the good mood to friends and family through kind words and actions.

Sad

Confide in a friend, loved one, or a trusted adult about how you are feeling.

Exercise or do something else that is physically active.

Do activities that you enjoy.

Stressed

Close your eyes and focus on your breathing for a few minutes.

Visualize a place that makes you feel happy and relaxed.

Distract yourself. Go for a walk or focus on something else for a while.

Nervous

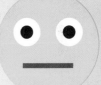

Close your eyes and take a few deep breaths. Focus on your breathing until you feel calm.

Talk to a friend, family member, or trusted adult about what you are feeling.

Think of five things that make you feel happy and focus on those positive thoughts.

Angry

Take a mental step back before you react. Do not take action until you no longer feel angry.

Take some time alone. Get some space to clear your mind and calm down. Try taking a walk.

Once you calm down, work toward solutions. Discuss what angered you once you can keep your cool.

Lonely

Make plans to do something with friends.

Join a team, club, or activity with others who share your interests.

Spend time with family.

Play with a pet.

Faces: flower travelin' man/Shutterstock.com

You may cause serious harm to the relationship. Instead, be positive and think about the effect your words may have on the other person. Explain how you feel without being hurtful or negative (**Figure 5.11**). In healthy relationships, people are not afraid to express their emotions. Your friends or family members will want to hear about how you feel and may be able to help by offering support.

Sometimes, you can make a situation worse if you try to confront the person who caused you to feel a certain way while you are still angry. Instead, wait until you cool off before talking about your feelings. By waiting, you can control your emotions and express them in a more positive, healthy way. You are allowing yourself time to work through and get relief from your feelings of anger. This will help you keep your emotions under control.

When Jennifer talked with her mother, she had already worked through her anger and was able to remain calm and explain her feelings about the potential move. By talking with her mom, Jennifer began to have a more positive outlook about the situation.

Developing Emotional Intelligence

Do you know people who always seem to remain positive, calm, and in control of their emotions in stressful situations? Do you know people who sense that you are feeling down, even before you say anything to them?

People who are skilled at understanding, controlling, and expressing their emotions and sensing the emotions of others have high **emotional intelligence (EI)**. Having EI is necessary to develop close personal relationships with others.

People with high EI share similar abilities and characteristics (**Figure 5.12**). In the following sections, you will learn more about these abilities and characteristics. In the process, you will discover ways to develop your emotional intelligence and enhance personal relationships.

Figure 5.11
When expressing your feelings to others, be careful to avoid aggressive messages that lay blame on someone else. Instead, focus on your own actions, feelings, and needs. *Why might it be a good idea to wait a bit before talking to someone who made you angry?*

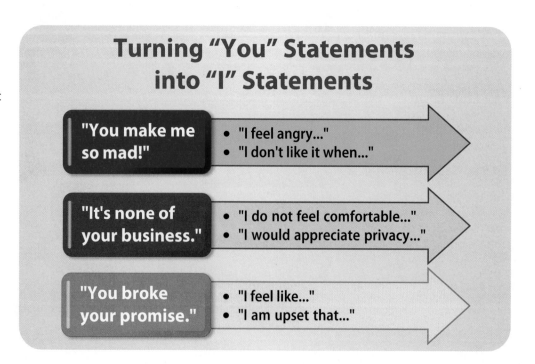

Turning "You" Statements into "I" Statements

"You make me so mad!"
- "I feel angry..."
- "I don't like it when..."

"It's none of your business."
- "I do not feel comfortable..."
- "I would appreciate privacy..."

"You broke your promise."
- "I feel like..."
- "I am upset that..."

Control Negative Emotions

People with high EI are able to control or reduce their negative emotions. The negative emotions you experience, such as anger, jealousy, or fear, can easily become overwhelming and cloud your judgment. Controlling or reducing these emotions can help you live a happier, more fulfilling life.

One way to control your negative emotions is to change the way you think about a situation. Instead of thinking negatively about the issue, try to view it in different, more positive ways. For example, if your friend does not respond to your messages, try not to think that your friend is ignoring or rejecting you. Look at other possible explanations. Perhaps your friend is very busy. Maybe your friend's cell phone is off or has a low battery.

Your friend's actions are probably more a result of your friend than a result of you. Try not to take your friend's lack of response personally and avoid jumping to conclusions. Instead, have optimism. **Optimism** is the ability to keep a positive outlook and focus on the good aspects of situations (**Figure 5.13**). People who have optimism are better able to cope with stressful situations because they realize situations are temporary. They know that circumstances will eventually improve. If you respond with optimism, you understand that your friend will eventually message you back.

Emotional Intelligence Abilities and Characteristics

- Control negative emotions
- Show resilience
- Have empathy
- Show gratitude

Figure 5.12 You probably have high EI if you have the ability to control your negative emotions, be optimistic, have empathy, and show gratitude. *What skills do people with high emotional intelligence have?*

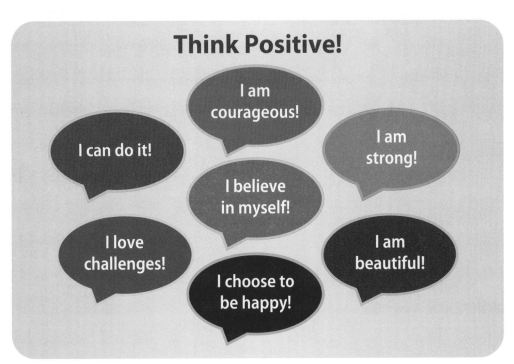

Think Positive!

- I am courageous!
- I can do it!
- I am strong!
- I believe in myself!
- I love challenges!
- I choose to be happy!
- I am beautiful!

Figure 5.13 Responding to positive or negative situations with optimism can help you control negative emotions. *How would you rate yourself on being optimistic? Can you be more positive?*

Have Empathy

Having high emotional intelligence involves having empathy. People who have **empathy** are able to put themselves in someone else's shoes. They understand other people's wants, needs, and viewpoints. They treat others as they would expect to be treated. As a result, people who have empathy are better able to support their friends and family members who are in need.

Can you remember a time when someone showed you empathy? How did this make you feel? Perhaps you felt valued and respected, which means you are more likely to feel good about yourself. In turn, when you show empathy to others, you are more likely to make them feel good about themselves. Having empathy helps you sense the emotions of others and respond in open, positive ways.

Developing empathy involves keeping an open mind and listening carefully to what others have to say (**Figure 5.14**). People have differing opinions, and you must be able to listen to understand what people are feeling and what they need. You do not necessarily have to agree with someone else's opinion, but you can see why they feel the way they do.

Show Gratitude

The ability to have gratitude has many benefits on your personal health and wellness. **Gratitude** is an emotion that means being thankful or grateful. People with high emotional intelligence have the ability to appreciate what is good and meaningful in their lives. This enables people to be happier, which, in turn, often results in the ability to be nicer to others and show them gratitude.

Figure 5.14
If you can recognize and understand someone else's feelings, you can better respond to their emotional needs. *What is the term for the ability to understand other people's perspectives?*

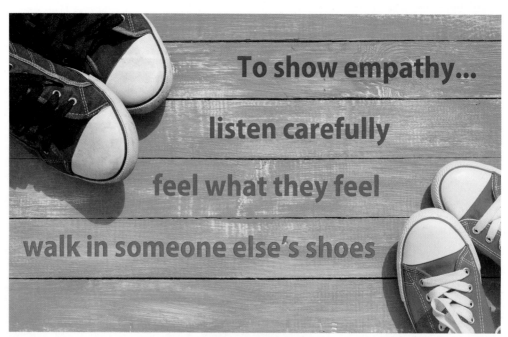

To show empathy...

listen carefully

feel what they feel

walk in someone else's shoes

Natalya Danko/Shutterstock.com

People who can openly show gratitude to others, including friends, family members, and even strangers, demonstrate that they appreciate others and recognize what these people have done for them. As a result, their relationships with others improve and grow stronger.

BUILDING Your Skills

Being Thankful Makes You Healthier

> **Gratitude:** the quality of being thankful; readiness to show appreciation for and to return kindness.

Perhaps *gratitude* is not a new word to you. Do you realize the power of affirming the good things and people in your life? Expressing gratitude can have an immense and positive impact on your mental health, which can then translate into positive outcomes for your social and physical health. All of this from the simple act of purposefully being thankful.

Most obviously, expressing gratitude is one of the most reliable methods for improving happiness. Expressing gratitude can also reduce symptoms of depression and anxiety and help people be more resilient. There's more, too! Affirming the good in your life helps your body to work and feel better and encourages you to take better care of yourself. Social lives also improve with expressions of gratitude. People who regularly express gratitude have stronger relationships, are better able to forgive, are more connected with their communities, and are more helpful and compassionate.

Expressing Thanks

With all those reasons understood, it is time to put thankfulness into practice. Think of a person for whom you are thankful. It could be a family member, a teacher, a friend, a coach…anyone! Now write a letter and say why you are thankful for this person. What has this person done for and with you? How has this person made you feel? What is so wonderful about this person?

When you are done, choose one of the following options:

- **Option 1.** Do nothing with the letter. Just by writing the letter, you expressed gratitude and improved your health.
- **Option 2.** Give the letter to the person you wrote it to. This will boost your mental health and the other person's mental health a bit more than the first choice.
- **Option 3.** Read the letter aloud to the person you wrote it to. This will boost your mental health the most and the person you wrote it to will appreciate hearing those words in your voice.

Regardless of which option you choose, you expressed gratitude and boosted your mental health. If you continue to be thankful for someone or something each day, you will notice the biggest impact on your health.

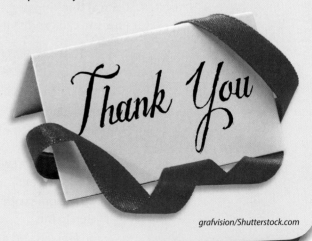

grafvision/Shutterstock.com

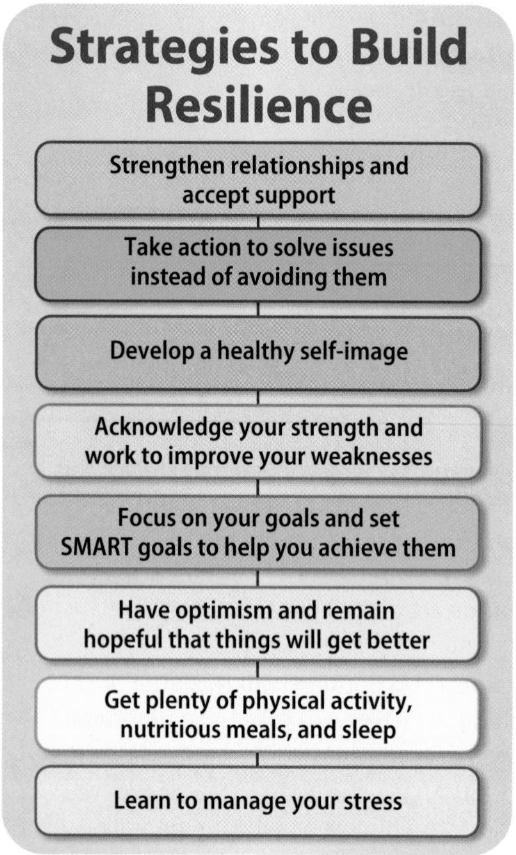

Strategies to Build Resilience

Strengthen relationships and accept support

Take action to solve issues instead of avoiding them

Develop a healthy self-image

Acknowledge your strength and work to improve your weaknesses

Focus on your goals and set SMART goals to help you achieve them

Have optimism and remain hopeful that things will get better

Get plenty of physical activity, nutritious meals, and sleep

Learn to manage your stress

Figure 5.15 People utilize different strategies to build resilience. *Which strategy would you use to build resilience and why?*

Show Resilience

People respond to challenges differently, and many demonstrate resilience. People who show **resilience** are able to bounce back from traumatic and stressful events, such as an act of violence, a serious health condition, or a family crisis. They are flexible and adapt, change, and grow as they encounter difficult experiences. When facing a life-changing situation, they think about the best way to respond to the situation and figure out what they can learn from the experience.

Having resilience requires strength, which means you need to engage in a healthy lifestyle. When you take care of yourself, you have more energy to handle challenges and respond to issues.

The care and support of others often helps people show resilience. Relationships that are positive, loving, and trusting help build a person's resilience. When experiencing emotional pain and sadness, it helps to have a strong support system of people who can offer encouragement.

Because people react to traumatic and stressful events differently, they tend to use various strategies for building resilience. The strategies that work for one person may not work for another. **Figure 5.15** identifies different strategies a person could use to help build resilience.

Lesson 5.2 Review

1. Knowing which emotions you feel and why is called _____ _____.
2. **True or false.** Covering up or denying your feelings will make what you feel go away.
3. What are the characteristics of having high emotional intelligence?
4. **Critical thinking.** List two positive emotions and two negative emotions. Explain how you can express these emotions in a healthy way.

Hands-On Activity

With a partner, change the following You-Statements to I-Statements. Reference Figure 5.11 to help. Then, identify healthy and positive methods someone can use to accept and express emotions in these situations. See Figure 5.10 for ideas.

- You are arguing with your sibling and say, "You always think you are better than me."
- You disagree with your parent and say, "You are so unfair. You don't even listen to me."
- You feel sad and a friend tries to comfort you. You say, "You don't know how I feel. You are always happy."

Managing Stress

Learning Outcomes

After studying this lesson, you will be able to

- **differentiate between** acute stressors and chronic stressors.
- **describe** different types of stress.
- **explain** how the body responds to stress.
- **give examples** of strategies you can use to manage the stress in your life.
- **recognize** when you should seek professional help for stress.

Graphic Organizer

What to Do About Stress

Prior to reading the lesson, identify the top stressors you are experiencing right now. Record your stressors in a graphic organizer like the one shown. As you read the lesson, list healthy ways to manage each stressor. A sample is done for you.

Olivier Le Moal/Shutterstock.com

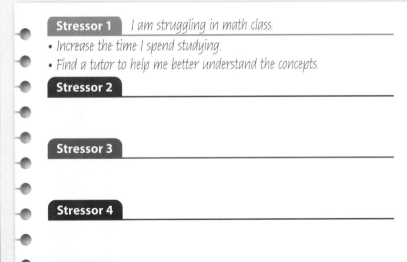

Stressor 1   *I am struggling in math class.*
- *Increase the time I spend studying.*
- *Find a tutor to help me better understand the concepts.*

Stressor 2

Stressor 3

Stressor 4

Stressor 5

Key Terms

stress physical, mental, and emotional reactions of your body to the challenges you face

stressor any factor that causes stress

eustress positive stress that encourages growth and motivation

distress stress that causes negative feelings and harmful health effects

trauma extreme stress due to deeply disturbing events, such as disasters, sexual assault, or violence

toxic stress stress caused by repeated, long-lasting exposure to severe stressors, such as neglect and abuse, violence, or loss of a loved one

fight-or-flight response body's impulse to either fight off or flee from threatening situations

relaxation response reaction in which the body returns to its resting state after a stressful event

stress management process of using strategies to reduce the impact of the stress response and handle threatening situations in positive ways

self-care practice of taking an active role in protecting your own health; involves eating healthy and getting plenty of sleep and physical activity

Y ou explored how you feel about and react to people and situations around you in the previous lesson. You also learned about the importance of developing emotional intelligence. One of the abilities of people who have high emotional intelligence is the ability to manage stress.

In this lesson, you will learn about different sources and types of stress and how stress can impact your health. You will also learn some effective strategies that can help you manage the stress in your life to promote positive mental and emotional health.

Sources of Stress

The physical, mental, and emotional reactions of your body to the challenges you face is **stress**. Stress is unavoidable. Some common sources of stress are shown in **Figure 5.16**.

Everyone experiences stress at times. For example, a student may experience stress when starting a new school year or preparing for a test. An argument between family members can be a source of stress for both family members, as well as for other family members who are aware of the disagreement. An adult may experience stress when starting a new job or giving a presentation in front of coworkers. All of these situations contain **stressors**, or factors that lead to stress.

Figure 5.16
Learning how to avoid or manage common sources of stress can have a positive effect on your health and well-being.

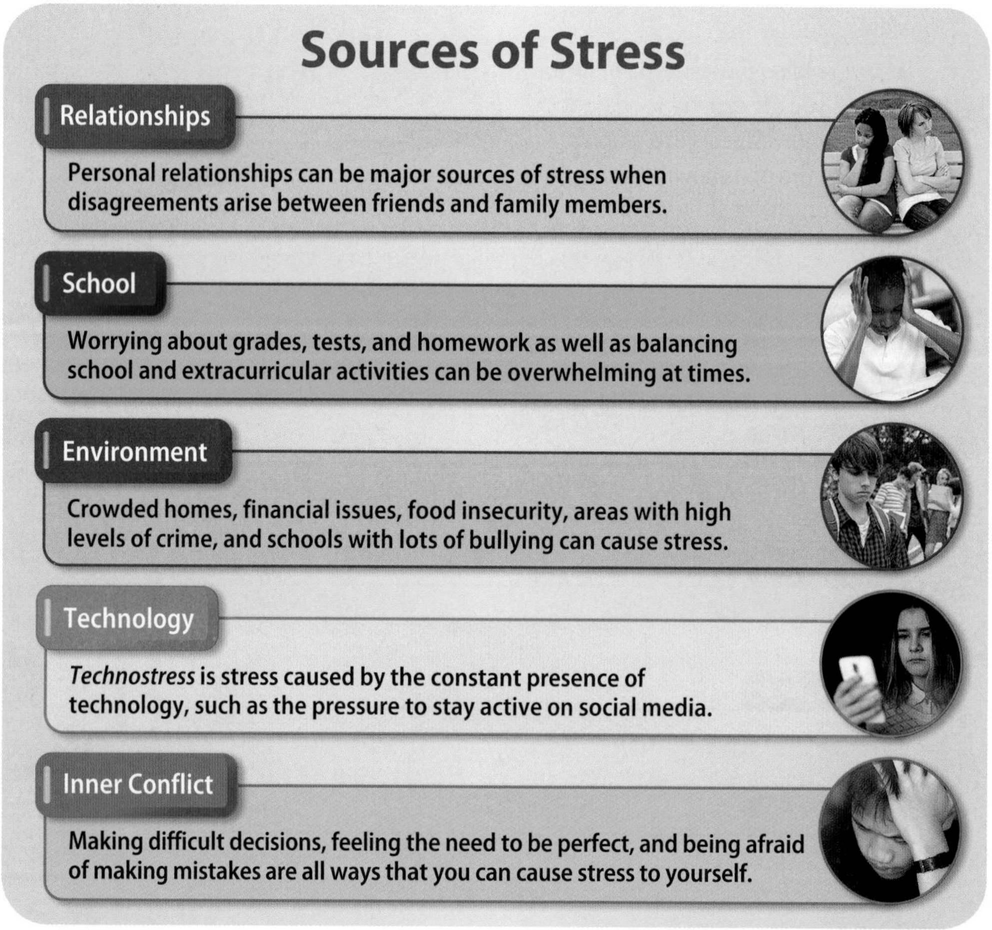

Sources of Stress

Relationships
Personal relationships can be major sources of stress when disagreements arise between friends and family members.

School
Worrying about grades, tests, and homework as well as balancing school and extracurricular activities can be overwhelming at times.

Environment
Crowded homes, financial issues, food insecurity, areas with high levels of crime, and schools with lots of bullying can cause stress.

Technology
Technostress is stress caused by the constant presence of technology, such as the pressure to stay active on social media.

Inner Conflict
Making difficult decisions, feeling the need to be perfect, and being afraid of making mistakes are all ways that you can cause stress to yourself.

Girls on bench: Elena Elisseeva/Shutterstock.com; Boy studying: Monkey Business Images/Shutterstock.com; Sad boy: Daisy Daisy/Shutterstock.com; Girl with phone: Burdun Iliya/Shutterstock.com; Stressed boy: smolaw/Shutterstock.com

Stressors may be major, life-event stressors, such as moving to a new school, losing a loved one, or experiencing an illness or health condition, or minor, daily stressors. Examples of minor, daily stressors include losing a favorite pair of jeans, arriving late for class, or arguing with a sibling. Many young people face similar stressors in their lives and share experiences of coping with stress.

Types of Stress

People of all ages experience many types of stress. Some stress is positive. This type of positive stress, which encourages growth and motivation, is called **eustress**. Positive stress is healthy for you because it creates feelings of excitement, can be motivating, and can help you improve your performance (**Figure 5.17**). Stress that causes negative feelings and harmful health effects is called **distress**. Major events such as losing a loved one, experiencing bullying, or dealing with a conflict with family or friends, are examples of distress. Extreme stress due to deeply disturbing events, such as disasters, sexual assault, and violence, is called **trauma**.

Stress can be short-lived or long-lasting. One type of stress, called *acute stress*, is sudden and does not last long. Acute stressors come from the normal pressures of daily life experiences such as getting to school on time or taking a final exam. People can also experience *chronic stress*, which continues over long periods of time. Chronic stress seems to have no clear end in sight. Examples include feeling unsafe in your neighborhood or worrying about a loved one who has a health condition.

Repeated exposure to severe, chronic stressors can lead to **toxic stress**. Some examples of severe, chronic stressors include exposure to neglect and abuse, family rejection, intimate partner violence, death of a loved one, extreme poverty, substance abuse, a loved one going to jail, or community violence. Toxic stress can lead to negative short- and long-term physical and mental and emotional health consequences. If you or someone you know is experiencing toxic stress, it is important to talk to a trusted adult and get professional help.

The Body's Response to Stress

Sometimes stress feels unpleasant—a knot in the stomach before a big test, for example. Stress can also produce excitement, such as the surge of energy before a championship game. Your body reacts in specific ways when you encounter situations that seem threatening (for example, standing up to someone who is picking on you). All types of stress can trigger the same bodily responses.

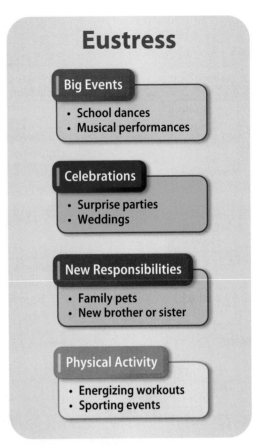

Eustress

Big Events
- School dances
- Musical performances

Celebrations
- Surprise parties
- Weddings

New Responsibilities
- Family pets
- New brother or sister

Physical Activity
- Energizing workouts
- Sporting events

Figure 5.17 Eustress is a positive type of stress that is good for you because it can make you feel confident and excited by the challenges you experience.

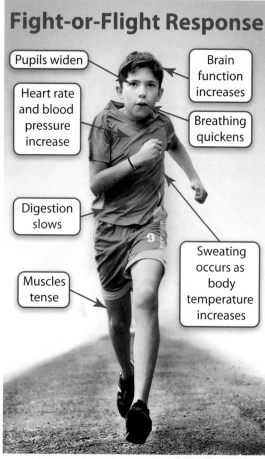

Fight-or-Flight Response

- Pupils widen
- Brain function increases
- Heart rate and blood pressure increase
- Breathing quickens
- Digestion slows
- Sweating occurs as body temperature increases
- Muscles tense

Lapina/Shutterstock.com

Figure 5.18 In the alarm stage of your body's response to stress, your body mobilizes resources to either attack or get away from a threat. *What is the second stage of your body's response to stress?*

This type of reaction to a stressful experience is called the **fight-or-flight response**, or *stress response*. When a person experiences some type of threat, the body's immediate response is to mobilize resources for fighting off or escaping from the threat. In the fight-or-flight response, a person may not react by literally fighting or escaping. Fighting might take the form of studying hard for a test or confronting a conflict. Flight might take the form of avoiding a task or freezing.

Generally, the body's response to stress progresses through the following three stages:

1. **Alarm stage.** When faced with a stressful event, your body mobilizes all of its resources to fight off or escape from a perceived threat. To prepare for fighting or escaping, your body undergoes several changes (**Figure 5.18**).

2. **Resistance stage.** Your body continues to devote energy to maintaining its stress response. Heart rate, blood pressure, and breathing are still rapid, which helps deliver oxygen and energy quickly to various parts of your body.

3. **Exhaustion stage.** If the threat persists, the body may stay in a state of high alert for a long time. In this case, the body will use up its resources and exhaustion will occur.

The **relaxation response** occurs after a stressful event is over. This is the opposite of the fight-or-flight response. The body gradually returns to its resting state. Blood pressure and heart rate return to normal and muscles relax. If the stressful event does not end, or if the body maintains the stress response for a long time, however, negative health effects can occur.

Strategies for Managing Stress

Learning how to manage stress is an important part of staying healthy. **Stress management** is the process of using strategies to reduce stress and handle stressful situations in positive ways. Not everyone will find the same stress-management strategies useful. Trying several strategies can help you learn about yourself and identify effective methods of stress management (**Figure 5.19**). Some strategies work better in certain situations than in others.

Express Your Feelings

Talking with people you trust about issues is a good way to manage or reduce your stress. The people you confide in may have useful advice for how to handle situations. They might be able to provide helpful insight and suggestions. They might also help you think about the issue in a new way.

Stress Management Strategies

Express Your Feelings	Maintain a Positive Attitude	Take Care of Yourself
• Talk through an issue with a person you trust • Ask for advice from someone who was in a similar situation • Write about your stress in a journal	• Shift your focus to something positive that has happened • See mistakes as opportunities to learn and grow • Look for the positive aspect of a negative situation	• Get enough nutrients and energy • Get plenty of sleep • Get physical activity • Spend time with your friends or family
Manage Your Time	**Distract Yourself**	**Use Relaxation Techniques**
• Break down your big tasks into smaller, more manageable ones • Create a reasonable schedule and stick to it • Say "no" to new commitments when you are already too busy	• Go for a walk • Read a good book • Find something to laugh at—a movie, TV show, videos, etc. • Work on a jigsaw or crossword puzzle	• Take slow, deep breaths • Visualize your "happy place" • Engage in muscle relaxation • Be present in the moment and pay attention to your feelings

Figure 5.19 There are many healthy ways to manage stress and become more resilient. Some ideas are shown above.

CASE STUDY

Sameera Is in a Slump

Sameera, an eighth grader, has always enjoyed school. She likes the challenge of learning new things and the constant social interaction that comes with being in school with her friends. Math and science come pretty easily for her and she enjoys them, which makes her willing to work hard to understand the concepts. Social studies is not as interesting, but this year Sameera has a really dynamic teacher who is more like a storyteller than a teacher. This year has been great so far, until recently.

For the past few weeks, Sameera is not as excited to go to school as she used to be. Even knowing that she will see her friends in school does not motivate her to get going in the morning. She dreads waking up in the morning more than she did just a few months ago. She does not really feel like trying in any of her classes, not even math and science.

Overall, Sameera does not really feel like herself. Her friends and parents have mentioned similar thoughts to her. She is trying really hard to get back to her normal self, but she just can't.

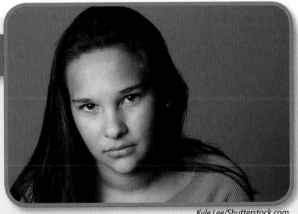

Kyle Lee/Shutterstock.com

Thinking Critically

1. What may be going on with Sameera's mental health?

2. If you were Sameera's friend and noticed these changes in her, what would you do? Explain the importance of friends advocating for friends' health during the school years.

3. Who could Sameera reach out to for help dealing with her situation? What could she say to start a conversation with these trusted people?

4. If you found yourself experiencing a dramatic change from your "normal," what would you do? Who would you reach out to for help?

Even if you do not find a solution, simply talking about an issue can be effective for reducing stress.

If you do not feel like talking with someone, you can always express your feelings by writing them down in a journal. Sharing your thoughts and feelings—instead of keeping them bottled up inside you—can reduce the amount of stress you feel.

Maintain a Positive Attitude

Focusing on negative events can trigger anxiety. It is healthier to focus on the good events in your life. When negative thoughts enter your mind, shift your focus to something positive that has happened. Try to see mistakes or disappointments as opportunities to learn and grow, and not as major crises.

You can reduce stress by thinking about certain situations in a new and positive way (**Figure 5.20**). For example, if a family member picks you up late after school you may feel frustrated and anxious. Instead of focusing on your family member being late, you could come up with productive ways of using the time. For example, you could read a book or start a homework assignment while you wait.

You can also look for positive aspects of stress-causing events—even negative events. Suppose you tried out for a role in a play or for a spot on the basketball team and you were not chosen. Not being chosen means you will have more time for homework, to do other activities you enjoy, or to hang out with friends and family.

Figure 5.20
Having a positive attitude is a healthy way to reduce stress, and can be achieved by seizing opportunities to gain new experiences and being grateful for the life you have.

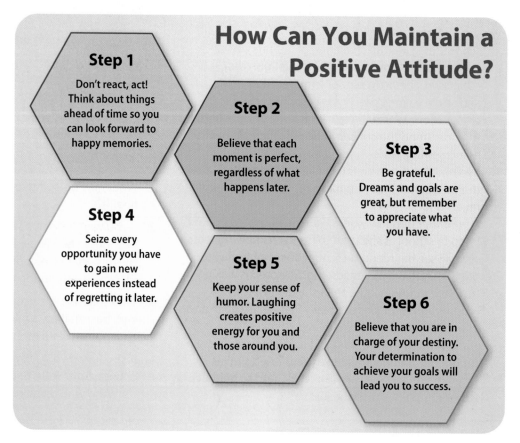

How Can You Maintain a Positive Attitude?

Step 1
Don't react, act! Think about things ahead of time so you can look forward to happy memories.

Step 2
Believe that each moment is perfect, regardless of what happens later.

Step 3
Be grateful. Dreams and goals are great, but remember to appreciate what you have.

Step 4
Seize every opportunity you have to gain new experiences instead of regretting it later.

Step 5
Keep your sense of humor. Laughing creates positive energy for you and those around you.

Step 6
Believe that you are in charge of your destiny. Your determination to achieve your goals will lead you to success.

Take Care of Yourself

During times of stress, many people neglect their physical needs. Failing to take care of yourself increases your risk for illness, which can further contribute to stress. During these times, it is important to practice self-care. When you practice **self-care**, you take an active role in protecting your own health. You eat healthy foods to provide your body with the energy and nutrients it needs. You also get plenty of sleep and physical activity. Physical activity reduces the effect of stress on heart rate and blood pressure. Physical activity also helps to relax the muscles.

Manage Your Time

You can avoid many stressors—such as the feeling of having too much to do at once—with careful planning, or *time management*. **Figure 5.21** shows some strategies you can use to manage your time well.

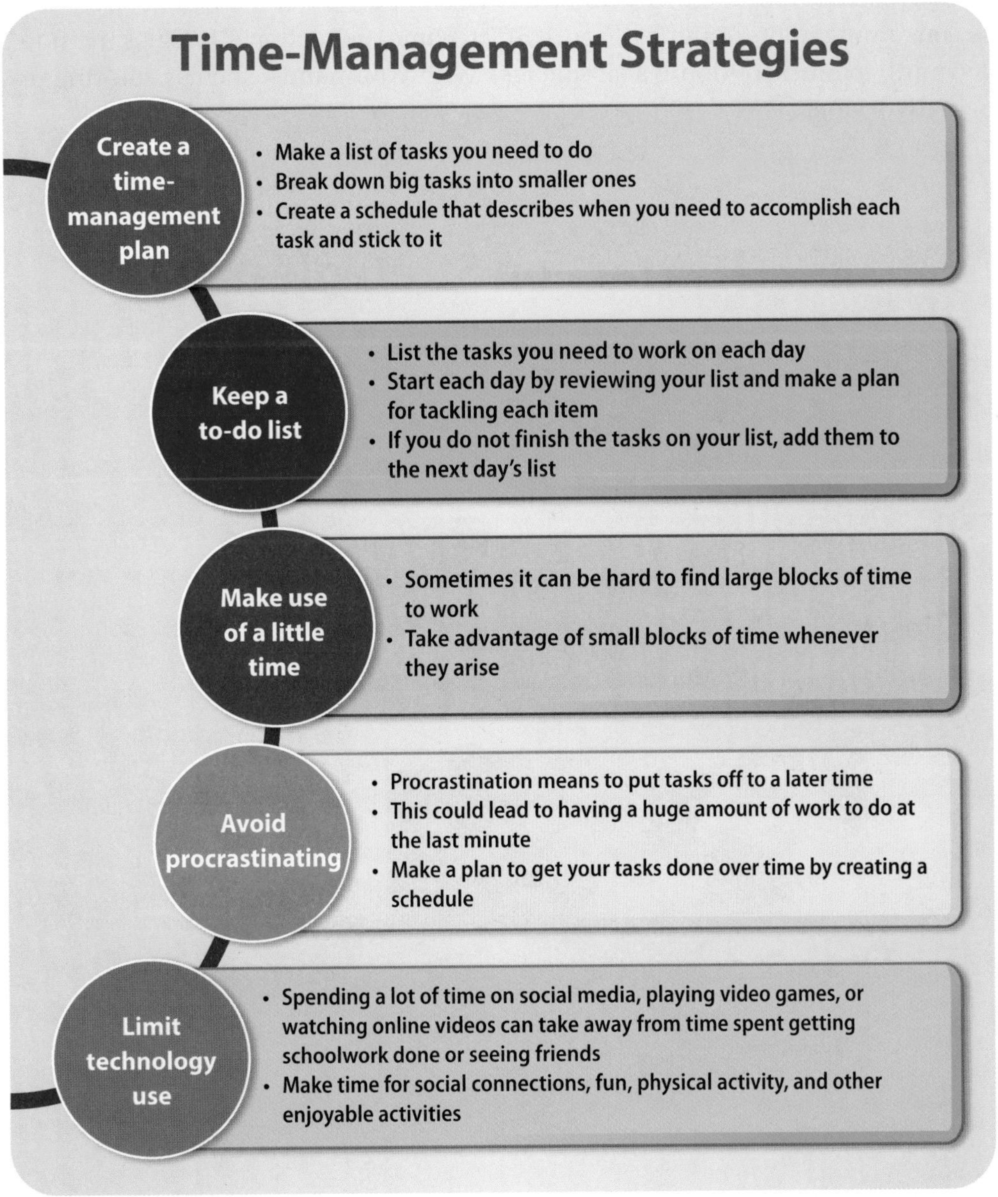

Time-Management Strategies

Create a time-management plan
- Make a list of tasks you need to do
- Break down big tasks into smaller ones
- Create a schedule that describes when you need to accomplish each task and stick to it

Keep a to-do list
- List the tasks you need to work on each day
- Start each day by reviewing your list and make a plan for tackling each item
- If you do not finish the tasks on your list, add them to the next day's list

Make use of a little time
- Sometimes it can be hard to find large blocks of time to work
- Take advantage of small blocks of time whenever they arise

Avoid procrastinating
- Procrastination means to put tasks off to a later time
- This could lead to having a huge amount of work to do at the last minute
- Make a plan to get your tasks done over time by creating a schedule

Limit technology use
- Spending a lot of time on social media, playing video games, or watching online videos can take away from time spent getting schoolwork done or seeing friends
- Make time for social connections, fun, physical activity, and other enjoyable activities

Figure 5.21
Practicing time-management skills such as these can help improve your ability to make the most of your time and accomplish your goals, thereby reducing your stress. *Why do people sometimes take on commitments for which they do not have time or energy?*

One of the best ways to manage your time is to create a time-management plan. First, make a list of everything you need to do. Then break down the big tasks on your list into smaller ones. Create a schedule that describes when you need to accomplish each task and stick to that schedule. This technique is a simple way to keep track of what you have to do and to make sure you get everything done.

Sometimes, people take on commitments they do not have time or energy for because they have a hard time saying *no*. Being helpful to others is good, but committing to many events can create stress when your calendar is already full. Learning to set limits by saying *no* when you know you are too busy can also help you avoid or reduce stress.

Distract Yourself

Many situations that cause stress are either overwhelming or beyond a person's control. These situations may include family financial crises or a family member's serious illness. Intense focus on these types of concerns can increase stress. Finding distractions can be a good way of managing stress that is consuming your thoughts (**Figure 5.22**). Some distraction strategies include listening to music or doing a simple task with your hands, such as coloring or woodworking.

Figure 5.22
People respond differently to stress distractions, so it is important to find the method of distraction that works best for you.

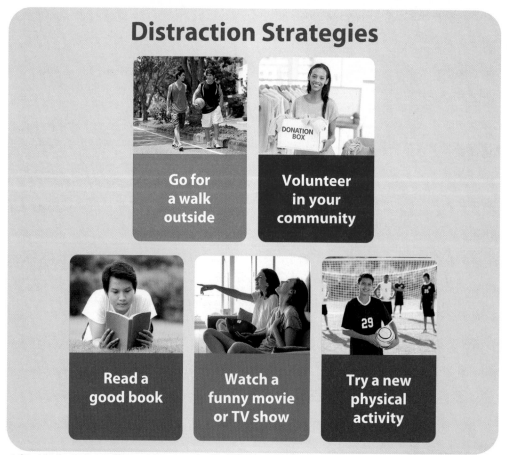

Left to right: Dragon Images/Shutterstock.com; wavebreakmedia/Shutterstock.com; Naypong/Shutterstock.com; Ollyy/Shutterstock.com; Monkey Business Images/Shutterstock.com

Another effective way of managing stress is laughter. Humor may help people cope with stressors by distracting them from their current situation. If you are feeling stressed, watch a funny movie or TV show, or talk to someone who makes you laugh.

These distraction strategies can also help manage stress caused by everyday situations that are beyond your control, such as bad weather. This strategy does not work for all situations, however. For example, if you are anxious about an upcoming class project, developing a time-management plan may be a better way of reducing stress than finding distractions.

Use Relaxation Techniques

Another useful way to manage stress is to change how your body responds to potentially threatening situations. Instead of becoming tense, you can teach your body to relax using several different techniques, such as the following:

- **Visualization.** Some people have success using visualization to reduce stress. *Visualization* is a technique that involves thinking about or imagining being in a pleasant environment. For example, if you find the beach relaxing, you might imagine the sound of waves crashing and the warmth of the sun on your skin.
- **Deep breathing.** *Deep breathing* is a technique that involves taking slow, deep breaths to help your brain and body calm down and relax. Deep breathing can have a number of physical benefits, including lowering your heart rate and decreasing your blood pressure.
- **Progressive muscle relaxation.** *Progressive muscle relaxation* is a technique in which you tense and then relax each part of your body until your entire body is relaxed (**Figure 5.23**). Practicing deep breathing as you relax each part of your body increases the effectiveness of this technique.

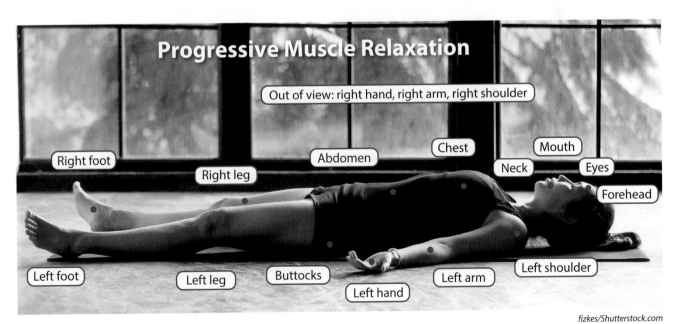

fizkes/Shutterstock.com

Figure 5.23 The model shown identifies the different body parts to tense and relax during progressive muscle relaxation.

- **Mindfulness.** *Mindfulness* involves being present in the moment and paying attention to thoughts and feelings in a nonjudgmental way. By paying attention to the present, you avoid letting your mind wander or shift to ongoing worries and concerns. Mindfulness can be practiced anywhere and at any time. You can also combine mindfulness with other relaxation techniques to practice *mindfulness-based stress reduction (MBSR).*

Seek Professional Help When Needed

Recovery from major stressors—such as experiencing the death of a loved one or starting a new school—can be especially difficult. People experiencing such stressors can become frustrated and discouraged. It is helpful to remember that recovery takes time.

If symptoms of stress last for more than a couple of weeks and interfere with the ability to function in daily life, it is helpful to talk to a mental health professional. These trained professionals diagnose mental health conditions and help people cope with the emotional effects of stress. Professionals who can help include the following:

- psychologists
- social workers
- therapists
- counselors

If you feel you might benefit from this type of professional help, talk to an adult you trust, such as a parent or guardian, teacher, counselor, or doctor. This adult can put you in touch with a professional who can help you. Remember, asking for help is a sign of strength and courage. Seeking help is the first step toward feeling better about your life.

Lesson 5.3 Review

1. What is the difference between eustress and distress?
2. **True or false.** Stress is always associated with negative events or experiences.
3. What are the three stages of the body's response to stress?
4. Visualization and deep breathing are examples of _____ techniques to help manage stress.
5. **Critical thinking.** Name two strategies for managing stress.

Hands-On Activity

Choose one of the stress-management strategies you learned about in this lesson and practice it at home. Then, write an essay describing your experience and the impact it had on your feelings of happiness and level of stress. How well did the stress-management strategy work for you? Would you use this strategy again to help relax? Set three SMART goals for managing stress in a healthy way.

Review and Assessment

Summary

Lesson 5.1 Being Mentally and Emotionally Healthy

- *Mental and emotional health* is your thoughts and feelings. It includes your emotions, mood, feelings about yourself, and way of viewing the world.
- Thoughts and feelings that decrease mental and emotional health are *mental health conditions*. When conditions interfere with daily function for a short time, they are *mental distress*.
- The different parts of your *identity* are physical, social, and psychological. Something a person accepts as true based on experiences, scientific facts, or prior knowledge is a *belief*. *Attitudes* are set ways of thinking or feeling.
- Your *self-image* is your mental picture of yourself, including your appearance, personality, skills and abilities, and weaknesses. Self-image is closely related to *self-esteem*, how you feel about yourself.
- Self-esteem is affected by external (family and friends) and internal (your self-talk) factors.
- People with healthy self-esteem view failures as learning experiences and can adjust when faced with obstacles. People with low self-esteem think negatively about their traits, skills, and abilities.
- Assessing the health of your thoughts and feelings can help improve or maintain your mental and emotional health.

Lesson 5.2 Making Sense of Your Emotions

- *Emotions* are the moods or feelings you experience. These emotions can be pleasant like joy or pride, or they can be unpleasant like guilt or sadness.
- Knowing which emotions you feel, and why, is *emotional awareness*. As you grow up, you can learn to control your emotions by identifying and accepting what you feel, showing self-compassion, and expressing those emotions in healthy ways.
- People with high emotional intelligence (EI) are skilled at understanding, controlling, and expressing their emotions. Having emotional intelligence is necessary to develop close relationships with others.
- People with high EI share similar abilities and characteristics. They are able to control negative emotions, have empathy, and show gratitude and resilience.

Lesson 5.3 Managing Stress

- *Stress* is the physical, mental, and emotional reactions of your body to the challenges you face. *Eustress* can create excitement, add motivation, and help improve performance. *Distress* causes negative feelings and harmful health effects. Factors that cause stress are called *stressors*.
- Generally, your body responds to stress in three stages. In the alarm stage, your body mobilizes to combat a threat via the fight-or-flight response. In the resistance stage, your body devotes energy to maintaining this response. In the exhaustion stage, your body uses its resources by staying in high alert. At this stage, a body is at greater risk for illness.
- *Stress management* is the process of using strategies to reduce stress and handle stressful situations in positive ways. Not everyone will use the same stress-management strategies, so it is important to find the one that works for you.

Check Your Knowledge

Record your answers to each of the following questions on a separate sheet of paper.

1. **True or false.** Mental and emotional health have to do with your external life.
2. Your sex, height, weight, and age are the different attributes that make up your _____ identity.
3. What is the difference between positive self-talk and negative self-talk?
4. **True or false.** People with healthy self-esteem never encounter challenges or experience bad situations.
5. **True or false.** It is possible to feel pleasant and unpleasant emotions at the same time.
6. What are three steps you can take to control your emotions?
7. People who are skilled at understanding, controlling, and expressing their emotions and sensing the emotions of others have high _____ _____.
8. The ability to keep a positive outlook and focus on the good aspects of situations is _____.
9. What is the term for a person's ability to bounce back from stressful or traumatic events?
10. Repeated exposure to severe, chronic stressors can lead to _____ stress.
11. Which of the following statements relates to *eustress*?
    A. It is a negative stress.   C. It is a positive stress.
    B. It can make you lose motivation.   D. All of the above.
12. **True or false.** Taking care of yourself by eating well, getting enough sleep, and regularly getting physical activity can help reduce stress.

Use Your Vocabulary ↗

attitudes	gratitude	self-esteem
beliefs	identity	self-image
distress	mental distress	self-talk
emotion	mental health condition	stress
emotional awareness	optimism	stress management
emotional intelligence (EI)	relaxation response	stressor
empathy	resilience	toxic stress
eustress	self-care	trauma
fight-or-flight response	self-compassion	

13. Draw a cartoon for one of the terms above. Use the cartoon to express the meaning of the term. After you finish your drawing, find a partner and exchange cartoons. Take turns explaining to each other how your cartoons show the meaning of the term you chose.
14. On a separate sheet of paper, list the terms above. Next to each term, list a few words you have learned that relate to the meaning of the term. Then, work with a partner to explain how these words are related. As you discuss the terms, add any new words to your list. Ask your teacher for assistance, if necessary.

Think Critically

15. **Predict.** How do gratitude, resilience, and empathy improve a person's health? Choose one of these character traits and imagine that it became a focus in your life. How would this trait impact your physical, social, and mental health?

16. **Cause and effect.** How does a person's level of self-esteem impact the person's health behaviors and decisions?

17. **Compare and contrast.** Compare and contrast positive and negative stress.

18. **Draw conclusions.** Find and explore a website that claims to provide information about adolescent mental and emotional health. After exploring the site, would you recommend this website to other middle school students? Why or why not?

DEVELOP Your Skills

19. **Accessing information.** Identify a stressor common to teens. Using reliable sources, watch a video, listen to a podcast, or read an article about healthy strategies to manage this stressor. Create a presentation that explains your findings and why these strategies work for this stressor. Then, demonstrate the strategies and have your classmates try it, too. How well did your classmates understand the strategies?

20. **Community advocacy skills.** Develop and implement a campaign for your school community with a mission to increase self-esteem among adolescent students. As you plan, take into consideration the strategies for boosting self-esteem and the importance of healthy self-esteem discussed in the chapter. Reflect on the most common impacts on the self-image of young people. What issues most commonly harm self-esteem? What strategies most effectively build self-esteem?

21. **Stress management and communication skills.** Choose three of the relaxation techniques described in the chapter. Design and create a digital media product that exposes the reader or listener to these short relaxation techniques.

Formats for this product include a blog, website, infographic, and podcast. Present this product to your class.

22. **Stress management and practice health enhancing behaviors.** Use a journal to record your stressors and emotions for a week. Also, record your reactions that occurred and the behaviors you chose as a result of your stressors and emotions. When the week is done, look for trends in your journal. Are the same things causing you stress and strong emotions day after day? Are your reactions under control? Are your behaviors appropriate? Use the information gained from your journal to help you better navigate your stressors and emotions next week.

23. **Communication skills.** Think about the people in your life whom you tend to seek out when your feelings and emotions are strong. Make a list of these people. Then, tell them about the important role they play in your life using informal language. Even if these people already know, by directly stating your feelings, you are keeping the lines of communication open. This helps your mental and emotional health and theirs.

Chapter 6

Understanding Mental Illnesses

Essential Question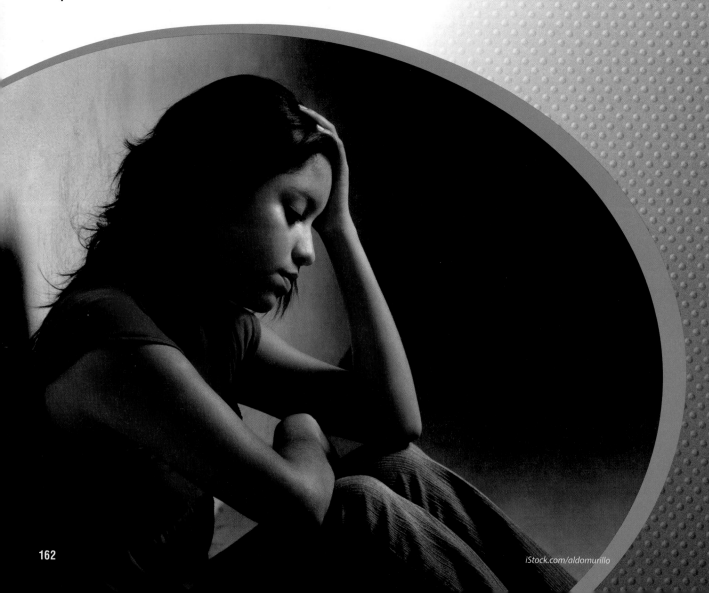

Why is getting help for mental illnesses so important?

iStock.com/aldomurillo

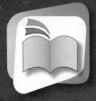

Reading Activity

Before you read the chapter, list any mental illnesses or disorders you have heard about. As you read, make connections between your prior knowledge and the chapter content by looking for references to the illnesses you listed. After reading the chapter, review your list of mental illnesses and write two paragraphs reflecting on your list in light of what you learned in this chapter.

How Healthy Are You?

In this chapter, you will be learning about mental illnesses. Before you begin reading, take the following quiz to assess your habits in regard to getting help for mental illnesses.

Healthy Choices	Yes	No
Do you pay attention to how you are feeling to know if you need help?		
Do you know how to access mental health resources?		
Can you tell the difference between mental health myths and facts?		
Do you tell friends if you are worried about their mental health and offer to help them find help?		
Do you know whom you would talk to if your friends talked about hurting themselves or others?		
Do you intervene if you see someone being bullied?		
Do you know or can you recognize the warning signs of suicide?		
If people talk about suicide, do you take it seriously?		
Do you feel comfortable asking your friends about their feelings and expressing concern?		
Do you know how to get help if you have thoughts of harming yourself?		
Do you listen to and support people who are dealing with loss?		

Count your "Yes" and "No" responses. The more "Yes" responses you have, the more healthy mental health condition prevention and treatment habits you exhibit. Now, take a closer look at the questions with which you responded "No." How can you make these healthy habits part of your daily life? Identify a SMART goal you would like to achieve to help improve your overall health and well-being. Refer to Figure 1.11 to help you set up your SMART goal. If you do not understand the instructions, ask for clarification from your teacher.

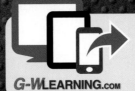

Click on the activity icon or visit www.g-wlearning.com/health to access online vocabulary activities using key terms from the chapter.

Recognizing Mental Illnesses

Key Terms ☞

mental illness mental or emotional condition so severe that it interferes with daily functioning; also known as a *mental disorder*

anxiety disorder condition in which someone responds with extreme or unrealistic fear and dread to certain situations, experiences, or objects

attention-deficit hyperactivity disorder (ADHD) condition in which a person has difficulty paying attention and controlling behavior

major depressive disorder condition characterized by intense negative feelings that do not go away and negatively affect daily life; also known as *clinical depression*

bipolar disorder condition characterized by periods of intense depression that alternate with periods of manic moods

schizophrenia spectrum disorder condition characterized by having irregular thoughts and delusions, hearing voices, and seeing things that are not there

Learning Outcomes

After studying this lesson, you will be able to

- **define** mental illness.
- **explain** possible causes of mental illnesses.
- **identify** the different types of mental illnesses.
- **describe** anxiety disorders.
- **explain** attention-deficit hyperactivity disorder, obsessive-compulsive disorder, and post-traumatic stress disorder.
- **differentiate between** mood disorders and personality and behavioral disorders.

Graphic Organizer

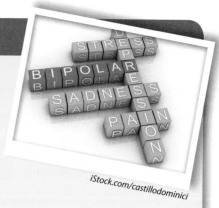

iStock.com/castillodominici

Symptoms of Mental Illnesses

As you listen to your teacher present this lesson, use a table similar to the one shown to list all the mental illnesses you learn about. Include a definition and a list of symptoms for each illness. If multiple illnesses have the same symptoms, highlight each repeated symptom in a different color. An example is provided.

Mental Ilnesses	Symptoms
ADHD	• Difficulty paying attention • Difficulty controlling behavior • Hyperactivity

A s you learned in the Chapter 5, your mental and emotional health involve how you feel about yourself, how well you can control your emotions, and how you can manage the stress in your life. In this lesson, you will learn about factors that can contribute to the development of a mental illness. You will also learn about common types of mental illnesses.

Understanding Mental Illnesses

Almost everyone struggles with feelings of anxiety, sadness, and fear. It is a common part of being human. When these thoughts and feelings decrease mental and emotional health, they are called *mental health conditions*. Short-term feelings and thoughts that interfere with a person's ability to perform daily tasks are called *mental distress*.

A **mental illness** occurs when a mental health condition does not go away and becomes so severe that it interferes with daily functioning. It is also called a *mental disorder*. For example, a person might have a fear of public places. This fear may become so severe that the person avoids going to school or work. The person might even avoid visiting family and friends.

Learning more about mental illnesses will help you understand your feelings and educate other people. It is important to recognize that people are not defined by their mental illness. Like any other health condition, a mental illness is a treatable condition.

What Causes Mental Illnesses?

Causes of most mental illnesses are unknown. Research suggests that a combination of factors contribute to these illnesses, including the following:

- **Family history.** People who have family members with mental illnesses are at a greater risk of developing these illnesses themselves. This is partly due to genetics.
- **Life experiences.** Most experts believe that a person's life experiences play a major role in whether a mental illness develops. For example, a stable and loving home environment may prevent the development of a mental illness. On the other hand, traumatic events and stressors, such as the death of a loved one, financial loss, or divorce, can increase the risk of developing a mental illness. In addition, bullying can increase the risk of mental illnesses (**Figure 6.1**).

Effects of Bullying on Mental Health	
About 20% of students experience bullying	• **Short-term effects** include changes in sleeping or eating habits, low self-esteem, symptoms of anxiety, and poor school performance • **Long-term effects** include increased risk of developing mental illnesses like clinical depression, anxiety disorders, and post-traumatic stress disorder (PTSD)
About 30% of students admit to bullying others	• **Short-term effects** include poor school performance, difficulty maintaining social relationships, and increased risk of substance abuse • **Long-term effects** include risk of substance abuse, antisocial behavior, and the continuation or worsening of violent or risky behaviors into adulthood

Figure 6.1 Bullying can have both short-term and long-term effects on mental and emotional health.

- **Substance use.** People who repeatedly use substances increase their risk of a mental illness. Examples of substances include nicotine, alcohol, and drugs. People who develop an addiction to these substances feel like they cannot stop using a substance, even if they want to.
- **Brain injuries.** People who experience a serious brain injury are at greater risk of developing some mental illnesses. Brain injuries may cause temporary or permanent changes to brain function. Permanent changes can result in depression, anxiety, personality changes, and aggression.
- **Environment during pregnancy.** The environment during pregnancy affects the health of a baby. Certain events and behaviors in a pregnant person's environment increase a baby's risk of developing a mental illness. These include substance use, poor nutrition, stress, trauma, or exposure to viruses or certain chemicals. In addition, signs of mental illnesses during pregnancy also increase the risk in a child developing a mental illness later in life.
- **Unhealthy patterns of thinking.** Having feelings of inadequacy, low self-esteem, anxiety, and anger can contribute to the development of a mental illness. People who have unhealthy patterns of thinking may believe the negative feelings they experience will never go away. Fortunately, people can learn to change unhealthy patterns of thinking and improve their mental and emotional health.

Anxious situations for people with social anxiety disorder include...

meeting new people

eating or drinking in public

performing in front of others

other social situations

Top to bottom: Iconic Bestiary/Shutterstock.com; Visual Generation/Shutterstock.com; Iconic Bestiary/Shutterstock.com; Iconic Bestiary/Shutterstock.com

Figure 6.2 People with social anxiety disorder typically avoid social situations that make them feel uncomfortable.

Types of Mental Illnesses

Mental illnesses affect mental and emotional health. All of these factors influence behavior and daily functioning. Different types of mental illnesses interfere with mental and emotional health in distinct ways.

Anxiety Disorders

Almost everyone experiences anxiety in some situations. Anxiety often involves an increased heart rate, rapid breathing, sweaty palms, and an upset stomach. You may feel this way when you are nervous about something.

A person who has an **anxiety disorder** responds with extreme or unrealistic fear and dread to certain situations, experiences, or objects. These feelings and responses disrupt the person's way of life.

People with *generalized anxiety disorder (GAD)* experience anxiety about parts of their lives that they cannot control. These people may feel anxious about school or work. People with generalized anxiety disorder also experience physical symptoms. These include feeling on edge, difficulty concentrating, and irritability.

People with *social anxiety disorder* feel anxious or afraid of social situations in which they might be judged (**Figure 6.2**). In these situations, a person with social anxiety may worry about being embarrassed or rejected. A person with social anxiety disorder usually avoids social situations. A related mental health condition is *social media anxiety*, in which people feel extremely anxious if they cannot check their social media accounts. You can learn more about how to manage social media anxiety through mindfulness in the infographic on the next page.

Using Mindfulness to Manage Social Media Anxiety

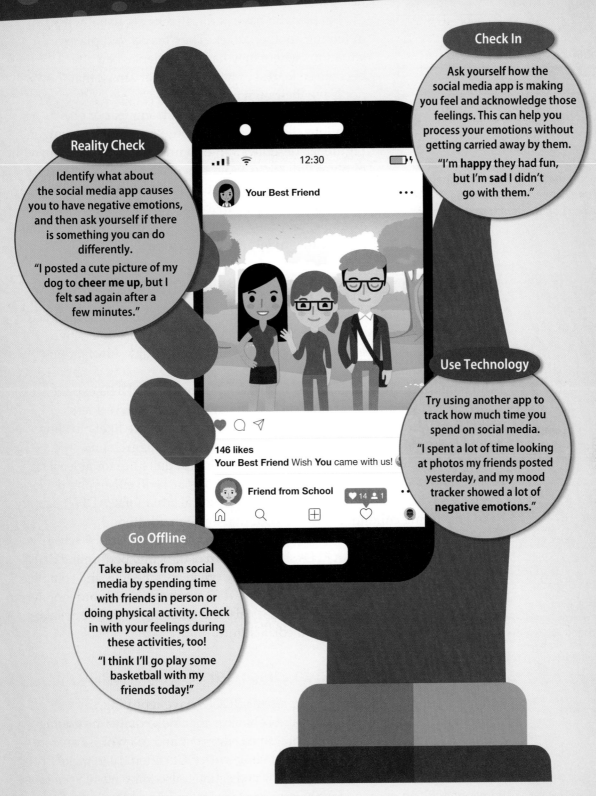

Check In

Ask yourself how the social media app is making you feel and acknowledge those feelings. This can help you process your emotions without getting carried away by them.

"I'm **happy** they had fun, but I'm **sad** I didn't go with them."

Reality Check

Identify what about the social media app causes you to have negative emotions, and then ask yourself if there is something you can do differently.

"I posted a cute picture of my dog to **cheer me up**, but I felt **sad** again after a few minutes."

Use Technology

Try using another app to track how much time you spend on social media.

"I spent a lot of time looking at photos my friends posted yesterday, and my mood tracker showed a lot of **negative emotions**."

Go Offline

Take breaks from social media by spending time with friends in person or doing physical activity. Check in with your feelings during these activities, too!

"I think I'll go play some basketball with my friends today!"

MaDedee/Shutterstock.com; rudall30/Shutterstock.com; Makyzz/Shutterstock.com; cougarsan/Shutterstock.com; Sudowoodo/Shutterstock.com; Art Alex/Shutterstock.com; piggu/Shutterstock.com

Different Types of Phobias

Phobia Name	Fear of...
Arachnophobia	spiders
Ophidiophobia	snakes
Acrophobia	heights
Agoraphobia	open or crowded spaces
Cynophobia	dogs
Astraphobia	thunder/lightning
Claustrophobia	small spaces

Figure 6.3 The word *phobia* is also a suffix for specific conditions, like those listed here. The suffix *-phobia* means "panic or fear of." *What other words can you think of that use the suffix -phobia?*

People with *panic disorder* experience *panic attacks*, or moments of intense fear. These moments of fear occur for no rational reason, and can happen anywhere or anytime without warning. They may also occur due to triggers. Panic attacks include physical symptoms, such as a fast heartbeat, dizziness, trouble breathing, and chest pain.

People who have panic attacks are usually fearful of having another attack. They may avoid places or situations where they have experienced an attack. Some become so fearful of having another attack that they will not leave their own homes.

People with *phobias* have a strong fear of objects or situations that do not really pose much, if any, danger. **Figure 6.3** describes some common phobias. People with phobias will try to avoid the object or situation that they fear. If they are in a situation in which they have to face their fear, they may experience physical symptoms. For example, they may experience shortness of breath, a fast heartbeat, or panic and desire to flee.

Attention-Deficit Hyperactivity Disorder (ADHD)

People with **attention-deficit hyperactivity disorder (ADHD)** have difficulty paying attention and controlling behavior. They also tend to be hyperactive. *Hyperactive* means overly active. People who have ADHD may show various types of symptoms (**Figure 6.4**).

Biological sex influences the symptoms a person with ADHD experiences. Males typically show symptoms such as frequent movement, reckless decision-making, and physical aggression. Females are more likely to show lack of focus, daydreaming, low self-esteem, and verbal aggression.

For people with ADHD, these symptoms disrupt daily life for at least six months and make it difficult to complete everyday tasks like listening in class. It can cause difficulty at home, at school, or in social situations. ADHD usually develops during childhood and can continue through adulthood.

Many symptoms of ADHD are also seen in people with *executive function disorders (EFDs)*. People with EFDs show a pattern of difficulty performing daily tasks. This includes struggling to analyze, plan, organize, schedule, and complete tasks in a timely way. People with EFDs have difficulty working toward long-term goals, identifying the steps to meet these goals, and planning for future events. They tend to focus only on the immediate future.

Obsessive-Compulsive Disorder (OCD)

People with *obsessive-compulsive disorder (OCD)* have repeating, uncontrollable thoughts, feelings, and behaviors that make daily functioning difficult. Uncontrollable thoughts are called *obsessions* and often cause anxiety. An example of an obsession is germs. People with OCD often try to make obsessions go away by engaging in repeated actions, also known as *compulsions*. Someone with an obsession with germs may wash their hands multiple times a day to calm their obsessive thoughts. **Figure 6.5** shows different types of obsessions and compulsions.

People with OCD generally cannot control their compulsions and do not get any pleasure or satisfaction from compulsive behaviors. Obsessive thoughts and compulsive behaviors make it difficult for people with OCD to perform tasks and interact with others.

Post-Traumatic Stress Disorder (PTSD)

People who live through a terrifying event may develop *post-traumatic stress disorder (PTSD)*. The event often involves physical harm or the threat of harm. For example, experiencing war, living through a natural disaster, or surviving a major accident can cause PTSD. People with PTSD experience extreme stress or fear after the danger is over. They may also experience *flashbacks* (vivid memories) of the event, angry outbursts, and nightmares or trouble sleeping.

Mood Disorders

People with *mood disorders* experience serious changes in the way they feel. Some mood disorders can make people feel sad all the time and lose interest in life. Other mood disorders can cause people to go back and forth between feelings of extreme happiness and extreme sadness. Common mood disorders include major depressive disorder, seasonal affective disorder (SAD), and bipolar disorder.

Major Depressive Disorder

Everyone feels sad and depressed at times. These feelings are normal and can help people understand what activities or situations make them happy or upset. These feelings are especially normal during or after stressful

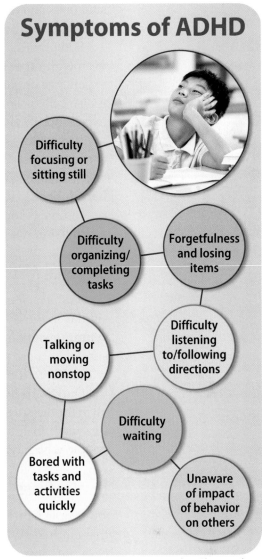

imtmphoto/Shutterstock.com

Figure 6.4 People with ADHD consistently experience various symptoms. *What term associated with ADHD means "overly active"?*

Obsessions and Compulsions

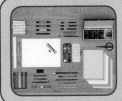

Obsessions
- Contamination and germs
- Order and symmetry
- Bad consequences to actions or inactions
- Safety of loved ones

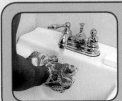

Compulsions
- Washing hands or other cleaning actions
- Arranging and rearranging items
- Checking switches and locks
- Not throwing anything away

Corepics VOF/Shutterstock.com; Margoe Edwards/Shutterstock.com

Figure 6.5 Obsessions are separate thoughts from normal, daily events and concerns. People with OCD often engage in repeated actions, or compulsions, in an attempt to get obsessions to go away. *What does OCD stand for?*

situations and difficult life events, such as the loss of a loved one. Most often, these feelings improve and go away over time.

Sometimes, however, feelings of depression are intense and do not go away, even with time. These feelings negatively affect a person's daily life. People who experience ongoing negative feelings have **major depressive disorder**, which is also called *clinical depression*. People with major depressive disorder may experience the symptoms in **Figure 6.6**.

If symptoms remain untreated, major depressive disorder can have serious consequences. These can disrupt a person's ability to engage in daily life tasks, such as going to school. A person may also be more likely to engage in harmful behaviors and develop various health conditions. People with major depressive disorder often need professional treatment from a mental health specialist to manage the condition and feel better.

Seasonal Affective Disorder

Seasonal affective disorder (SAD) is a mental illness that causes symptoms similar to those of major depressive disorder. People with SAD experience symptoms of depression in the winter months when there is less natural sunlight. These symptoms are severe enough they make it difficult for a person with SAD to function on a daily basis.

Due to the symptoms developing in the winter months, SAD usually goes away in the spring and summer. People with SAD often need professional treatment from a mental health specialist to manage the condition. Some people who have SAD may also benefit from light therapy.

Bipolar Disorder

People who have **bipolar disorder** experience intense symptoms of depression that alternate with *manic* (extremely happy and "up") moods. During periods of depression, any of the symptoms of major depressive disorder may occur. Symptoms of the manic mood include poor judgment, little need for sleep, and hyperactive behavior. A manic mood may also include a lack of self-control.

Figure 6.6 Major depressive disorder is a serious mental illness that has more symptoms than just being sad. *What is another term for major depressive disorder?*

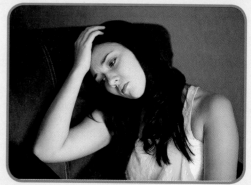

Possible Symptoms of Major Depressive Disorder

- Loss of interest in favorite activities
- Feeling worthless
- Extreme tiredness and loss of energy
- Weight loss or gain
- Difficulty sleeping
- Trouble concentrating
- Irritability, anger, and hostility
- Feelings of guilt
- Feeling like a failure
- Being critical of oneself
- Recurrent thoughts of death

Tracy Whiteside/Shutterstock.com

This can lead to binge drinking, binge eating, or out-of-control spending. To manage the symptoms, people with bipolar disorder need professional treatment.

Personality and Behavioral Disorders

Personality disorders are a category of mental illnesses characterized by consistent patterns of inappropriate behavior. The symptoms of personality disorders interfere with a person's ability to carry out daily tasks and maintain relationships.

Most personality disorders are diagnosed in older teens and adults. Sometimes they may be associated with childhood trauma. When children and younger teens show consistent patterns of inappropriate behavior, they are more likely to be diagnosed with a *behavioral disorder*. In addition to ADHD, two common behavioral disorders are oppositional defiant disorder and conduct disorder.

CASE STUDY

Best Friends: Conor and Julia

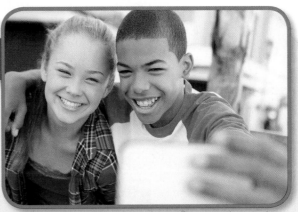
Monkey Business Images/Shutterstock.com

For the last few years, Conor has felt pretty lucky to have the best group of friends in the world. Together, they ride their bikes to the park, listen to music and dance, and always stick together. He loves that he feels like he could tell them anything. His best friend is Julia. They became best friends because they both love playing softball and watching scary movies.

This year, however, Conor notices that Julia is different. She does not come out for batting practice with him anymore and does not want to watch scary movies on the weekends. When she does hang out with their friends, she looks upset. When Conor tries to ask her if something is bothering her, she gives him an annoyed or angry look and huffs, "I'm fine." It is obvious to Conor that she is not fine, but he does not want to push her or call her a liar.

Julia fidgets all the time by rubbing her hands over her arms or legs. Conor has seen her pulling at her skin and sometimes almost pinching it. She will do this under the table in the cafeteria or under her desk in class. He has even seen her pulling at her skin when she is home and thinks no one is looking. Conor can tell she pinches a lot harder when she is particularly nervous or upset. A few weeks ago, he pointed out big bruises on Julia's upper arms. Since then, Julia has started wearing only pants and long-sleeved shirts, even though it is hot outside.

Conor is afraid that he will lose Julia as a best friend if he confronts her about this change in behavior. She seems so on edge about it. He is really worried about her, though, and is afraid she could be hurting herself. Conor does not know what to do.

Thinking Critically

1. What are the signs and symptoms that show Julia may have a mental illness? Which mental illness might she have?

2. Do you think Julia will get help to deal with her mental illness on her own? Why or why not?

3. If you were Conor, what would you do? How could you help Julia?

Oppositional defiant disorder (ODD) is a mental illness usually diagnosed in children. Children with ODD show behaviors that are uncooperative, disobedient, and hostile to other people. Symptoms can include frequent temper tantrums, refusal to obey authority figures, and questioning and arguing. Children with ODD may be easily annoyed by others, speak harshly, and show lots of anger. These behaviors are most common when the child is hungry, tired, or upset.

Conduct disorder is a mental illness that can grow into antisocial personality disorder in adulthood. People with conduct disorder show hostile and sometimes violent behavior toward other people. They ignore other people's feelings and may engage in cruel behaviors such as pushing, hitting, or biting others; hurting animals; and picking fights. People with conduct disorder are also more likely to engage in acts of stealing items or destroying property.

Schizophrenia Spectrum Disorder

People who have **schizophrenia spectrum disorder** typically experience symptoms such as irregular thoughts, delusions, or false beliefs. Schizophrenia can also involve hearing voices and seeing things that are not there. People diagnosed with schizophrenia spectrum disorder may experience paranoia. *Paranoia* is the belief that people are threatening or plotting against you. They may also show inappropriate emotional reactions, such as laughing when they hear someone has died. People diagnosed with schizophrenia spectrum disorder may also appear agitated, talk to themselves, and have difficulty managing personal hygiene tasks.

Lesson 6.1 Review

1. List the six factors that can contribute to a mental illness.
2. A person who has a(n) _____ disorder responds with extreme or unrealistic fear and dread to certain situations, experiences, or objects.
3. What does the acronym *ADHD* mean?
4. **True or false.** All mood disorders make people feel sad all the time and lose interest in life.
5. **Critical thinking.** Describe four different possible symptoms of ADHD. Explain how these symptoms might be disruptive.

Hands-On Activity

Research current mental health apps to better understand the information and features provided by these types of apps. Choose one mental illness to be the focus of your app and design a proposal including the following:
- **Page 1:** name, logo, description, summary of benefits and uses, and target audience
- **Pages 2–4:** three in-app features (drawn or digital) that would be beneficial to your users

Getting Help for Mental Illnesses

Learning Outcomes

After studying this lesson, you will be able to

- **describe** treatment options for mental illnesses.
- **compare** different types of therapy.
- **summarize** barriers to seeking help for mental illnesses.
- **recognize** how to help someone who has a mental illness.

Graphic Organizer

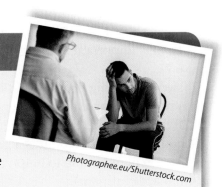

Identifying Resources

Using a graphic organizer like the one shown, identify resources for people who have a mental illness. Write *Resources for People with Mental Illnesses* in the middle oval. As you read the lesson, list resources in the surrounding circles.

Photographee.eu/Shutterstock.com

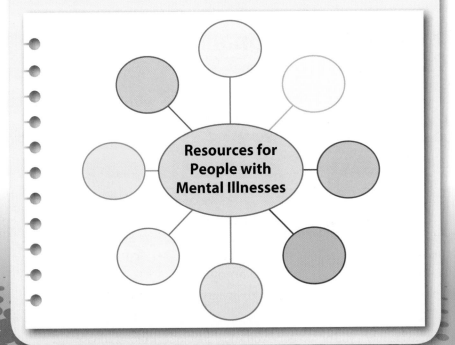

Resources for People with Mental Illnesses

Key Terms

therapy treatment method that focuses on the psychological aspect of mental health

therapist professional who diagnoses and treats people with mental health conditions

individual therapy type of therapy that involves a one-on-one meeting with a therapist to discuss feelings and behaviors

family therapy type of therapy in which all family members meet together with a therapist to build positive, healthy relationships

support groups gatherings in which a therapist meets with a group of people who share a common experience

mental health medication substance that causes changes in the brain to reduce symptoms of a mental illness

inpatient treatment type of treatment that involves staying in a healthcare facility for a period of time

stigma mark of shame or embarrassment that is usually unfair

When mental illnesses interfere with a person's ability to control emotions or cope with daily life, professional treatment from a mental health professional becomes necessary. The mental health professional can then determine which type of treatment will best meet the person's needs depending on the mental illness. Different mental illnesses, and the severity of symptoms, often require different types of treatment.

In this lesson, you will learn about different types of treatment options that are available to treat mental illnesses. You will learn about barriers that may prevent some people with mental illnesses from getting the help they need. You will also learn how you can help someone who has a mental illness.

Recognize When You Need Help

Sometimes, people with mental illnesses do not get the help they need. They may assume their negative feelings will simply go away. Most mental illnesses, however, do not improve without treatment. Knowing when to get help is an essential skill for maintaining your mental and emotional health.

Feeling sad, anxious, or lonely sometimes is a normal part of life for everyone. These feelings will fade over time. Sometimes, however, people need help from a therapist or doctor to manage their feelings. Taking care of your mental and emotional health is just as important as taking care of your physical health. It is important to recognize the signs of needing professional help (**Figure 6.7**).

The next step for getting professional treatment is locating resources. There are many ways young people can get mental and emotional help. One simple resource is talking to a trusted adult such as a parent or guardian, school counselor, school nurse, or doctor. It is a good idea to talk to an adult you trust because this person may be able to help you find a qualified therapist or drive you to and from appointments.

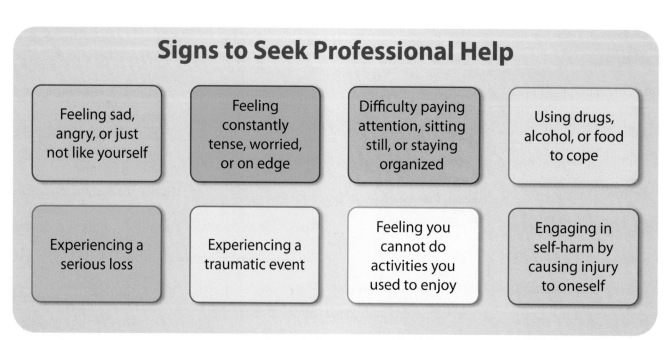

Signs to Seek Professional Help

Feeling sad, angry, or just not like yourself	Feeling constantly tense, worried, or on edge	Difficulty paying attention, sitting still, or staying organized	Using drugs, alcohol, or food to cope
Experiencing a serious loss	Experiencing a traumatic event	Feeling you cannot do activities you used to enjoy	Engaging in self-harm by causing injury to oneself

Figure 6.7 Knowing the signs is important to identify if you or someone you know should seek professional help.

It is also important to understand where you can go to get professional help. Many community agencies and institutions offer some type of mental health counseling. It is possible to find free or low-cost therapy from various locations such as local hospitals, colleges or universities, or mental health clinics.

BUILDING Your Skills

Talking About Mental Health

Onset of many mental illnesses occurs before 24 years of age. Getting early mental health support for adolescents and young adults can help them before conditions interfere with their developmental needs and ability to cope with daily life. Recognizing mental illnesses in yourself and others, and knowing how to seek help, is essential to early treatment of these conditions.

It is essential to create a support system when you are young that encourages your mental health and well-being. This support system will help to guide your decisions and care for you during difficult times. The following activity will help you initiate conversations about decision-making and mental illnesses with a parent, guardian, or trusted adult.

Conversations That Make a Difference

Complete this activity with a parent, guardian, or trusted adult. To begin, choose one of the scenarios below. Then, discuss your ideas about what you would do if you ever faced this situation. Together, create a plan of action. Identify what help you could provide for yourself or your loved one. What treatments may be available for this mental illness? Summarize your conversation and include your plan of action.

Scenarios

- **Scenario 1.** Your friend cannot sit still in class, and is always getting in trouble for being off-topic during class discussions. Your friend also has a hard time paying attention to the teacher's instructions or focusing on an assignment for more than a few minutes at a time.

- **Scenario 2.** You have your highs and lows as a middle school student. At times, you are happy and confident. At other times, you are stressed, insecure, and feel lost. Lately, the negative feelings are coming out more. You hide your emotions well, but sometimes you wish you had someone to whom you could talk.

- **Scenario 3.** Your sibling is always on a roller coaster of emotions. One minute your sibling is so happy it is almost annoying—laughing and talking loudly, running around with endless energy. Then, the next minute, your sibling is withdrawn and tired.

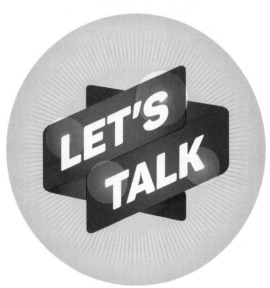

dnd_project/Shutterstock.com

Find Treatment

Researchers are trying to find ways of identifying people who are vulnerable to mental illnesses. These researchers work to better understand how the human brain works and to create new treatments for mental illnesses. The purpose of these treatments is to help people live healthy and productive lives. Treatment may involve receiving therapy, taking medication, or staying in a healthcare facility for a period of time.

Therapy

Therapy is a treatment method that focuses on the psychological aspect of mental health. This type of mental health treatment seeks to change the way a person thinks, interprets information, behaves, and experiences and expresses emotions. Therapy sessions are often conducted by a therapist.

A **therapist** is a professional who diagnoses and treats people with mental health conditions and illnesses (**Figure 6.8**). Therapists include professionals such as psychologists, psychiatrists, social workers, and counselors. Therapists may recommend several different types of therapy, which include the following:

- **Individual therapy** involves a one-on-one meeting with a therapist to discuss feelings and behaviors. The information a patient shares with the therapist is completely confidential in most cases. One exception is if a therapist believes a patient may hurt oneself, or someone else. Then, the therapist may share that information with a parent or guardian. A therapist can also report signs of abuse or neglect.
- In **family therapy**, all members of a family meet together with a therapist. This type of therapy helps families build positive, healthy relationships. Family therapy can also help members of a family support one member with a mental illness.
- In **support groups**, a therapist meets with a group of people who share a common experience. The therapist shares and discusses strategies for managing this common condition with all group members at the same time. Group members also gain information about what strategies were helpful for others. This type of group therapy can be helpful because people feel the other members truly understand their conditions.

What Does a Therapist Do?

Helps people understand their feelings and behaviors in an accepting and nonjudgmental way

Gives specific suggestions for how people can understand their thought processes and help themselves feel better

Helps people learn to cope with difficult thoughts, feelings, and situations in healthy, positive ways

Figure 6.8 A therapist can offer support and treatment for someone with a mental illness. *In addition to therapists, name two other types of professionals who diagnose or treat people with mental illnesses.*

Mental Health Medications

Another form of treatment for a mental illness is medication. Substances that cause changes in the brain to reduce the symptoms of a mental illness are called **mental health medications**. These medications are prescribed by healthcare professionals.

Many researchers believe that mental health medications are most effective when used along with some type of therapy. For example, people with major depressive disorder may take medication and also benefit from therapy. Medication can often effectively manage symptoms of a mental illness. Therapy can help people correct their negative, unhealthy thought patterns.

Different mental health medications reduce the symptoms of various mental illnesses (**Figure 6.9**). Most medications have some possible side effects such as tiredness and weight gain or loss. In some cases, medications can have very serious side effects. For example, some people who take certain types of antidepressants can experience *more* thoughts of suicide. Due to side effects, doctors and mental health professionals frequently monitor people who take mental health medications.

Inpatient Treatment

In some cases, a person's mental illness requires care in a clinic or hospital, or *inpatient treatment*. **Inpatient treatment** is necessary when people are at serious risk of harming themselves or others. People who are depressed and have thoughts of suicide may need to be hospitalized for a period of time to make sure they do not attempt suicide. In the hospital, people receive around-the-clock supervision, medication, and therapy.

Overcome Barriers

Unfortunately, people with mental illnesses do not always get the help they need. Only 44 percent of adults and less than 20 percent of adolescents with mental illnesses get the help they need. Some people may assume their negative feelings will go away on their own. Most mental illnesses, however, do not improve without treatment. Untreated mental illnesses may even get worse and lead to more severe conditions. Some people may face external barriers that prevent them from getting help for their condition. Examples of these external barriers are social stigma attached to mental illnesses and the cost of mental health treatment.

Mental illnesses often carry a social stigma (**Figure 6.10**). **Stigma** is a mark of shame or embarrassment that is usually unfair. Social stigma may cause

Types of Mental Health Medications	
Medication	**Used to Treat**
Antidepressants	Anxiety disorders, major depressive disorder
Anti-anxiety medication	Anxiety disorders
Stimulants	ADHD
Antipsychotics	Schizophrenia spectrum disorder, bipolar disorder, severe depression, ADHD, OCD
Mood stabilizers	Bipolar disorder, major depressive disorder

Figure 6.9
Different kinds of mental health medications can be used to reduce the symptoms of different types of mental illnesses.

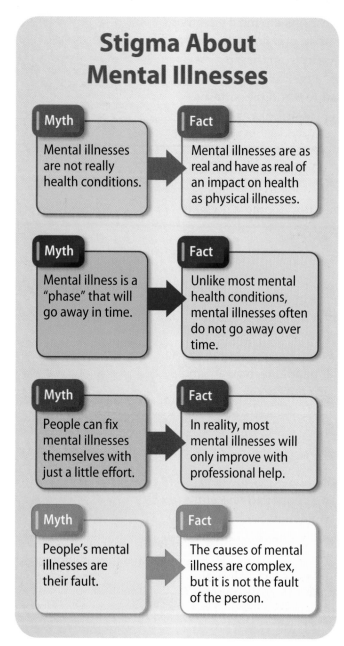

Stigma About Mental Illnesses

Myth	Fact
Mental illnesses are not really health conditions.	Mental illnesses are as real and have as real of an impact on health as physical illnesses.
Mental illness is a "phase" that will go away in time.	Unlike most mental health conditions, mental illnesses often do not go away over time.
People can fix mental illnesses themselves with just a little effort.	In reality, most mental illnesses will only improve with professional help.
People's mental illnesses are their fault.	The causes of mental illness are complex, but it is not the fault of the person.

Figure 6.10 Stigma about mental illnesses can discourage people from seeking help. These harmful beliefs, however, are not true.

people with mental illnesses to avoid seeking help, deny they have a condition, or feel shame and embarrassment. People may also fear they will lose an opportunity because of their condition, such as losing a scholarship or leadership position.

If you feel stigma about having a mental illness, do not let that stop you from getting help. Stigmas may result from a lack of understanding about a mental illness. Learning more about a mental illness will help you understand your feelings and educate other people. Talking to friends and family or joining a support group can help provide support, show that you are not alone, and teach you strategies for feeling better.

Another barrier to mental health treatment is cost. People may worry about being unable to afford treatment. Although mental health professionals do charge for their services, a person's health insurance may cover a portion of the expenses. Some mental health clinics may also provide therapy services at no cost or at a reduced rate.

Helping Someone with a Mental Illness

You may be concerned that someone you care about has a mental illness. Share your concerns with that person in an open and honest way (**Figure 6.11**). Simply saying that you are worried and would like to help lets that person know you are available. You could also offer to find a mental health professional. You may even go with that person to talk to the professional.

Sometimes a person with a mental illness is not interested in seeking help. You must intervene when you suspect people may harm themselves or hurt someone else. In other situations, you need to accept that it is not your responsibility to solve that person's condition. You should not try to protect people from the consequences of their conditions. This type of protection simply enables people to continue having the condition without treatment. For example, if your friend is too depressed to complete homework, doing the homework for your friend just helps hide the seriousness of your friend's condition from people who could offer help.

Remember that sometimes people need more time before they are ready to get help. Take immediate action, however, if you suspect someone has thoughts of suicide. Call 911 or take the person to the hospital right away.

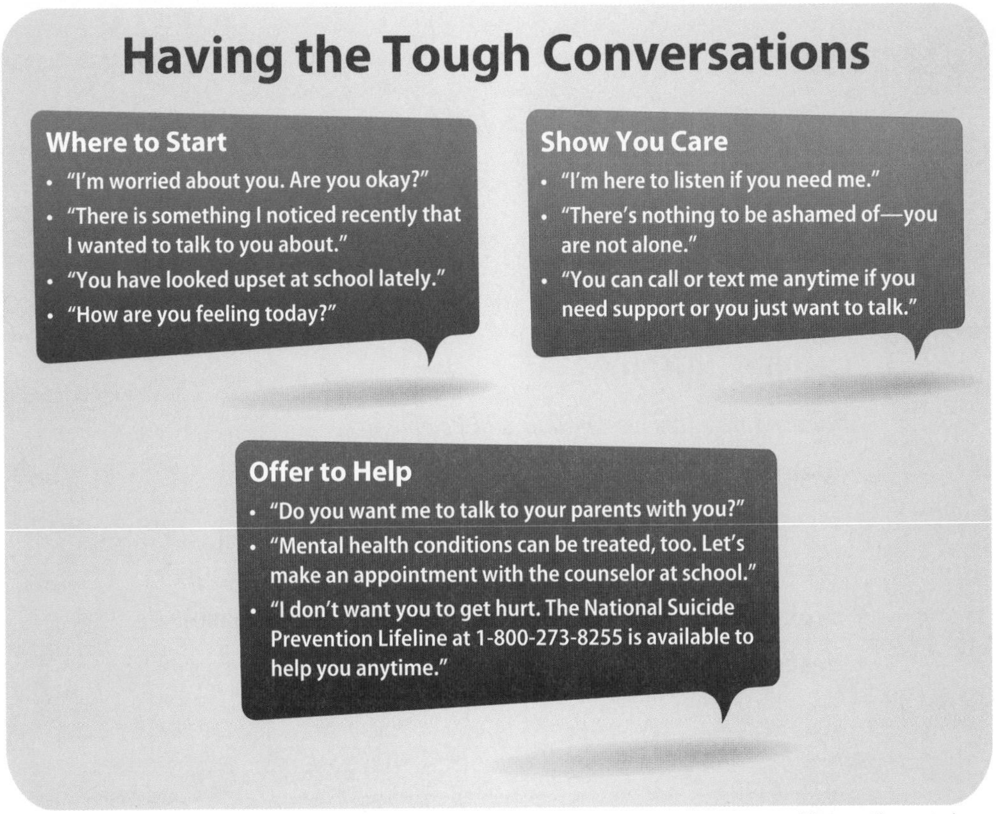

Having the Tough Conversations

Where to Start
- "I'm worried about you. Are you okay?"
- "There is something I noticed recently that I wanted to talk to you about."
- "You have looked upset at school lately."
- "How are you feeling today?"

Show You Care
- "I'm here to listen if you need me."
- "There's nothing to be ashamed of—you are not alone."
- "You can call or text me anytime if you need support or you just want to talk."

Offer to Help
- "Do you want me to talk to your parents with you?"
- "Mental health conditions can be treated, too. Let's make an appointment with the counselor at school."
- "I don't want you to get hurt. The National Suicide Prevention Lifeline at 1-800-273-8255 is available to help you anytime."

Figure 6.11
If a friend opens up to you about personal mental health concerns, do not promise to keep secrets. If your friend becomes a danger to self or to others, you may need to contact a trusted adult without your friend's permission.

RFvectors.Shutterstock.com

Lesson 6.2 Review

1. A professional who diagnoses and treats people with mental illnesses is called a(n) _____.
2. **True or false.** Mental health medications are prescribed by healthcare professionals.
3. Which form of treatment is recommended when people are at serious risk of harming themselves or others?
4. List two barriers for seeking help for a mental illness.
5. **Critical thinking.** List the three types of therapy and explain why each could be helpful for treating a mental illness.

Hands-On Activity

Social stigmas can prevent those with a mental illness from seeking help. Create a flyer to post around school that destigmatizes a mental illness. Raise awareness by using respectful language and accurate information. Encourage those with the condition to seek help. Include the following on the flyer: one mental illness to highlight, information and facts on this mental illness, and treatment options. Include images to support your flyer.

Preventing Suicide

Key Terms 👉

suicide act of taking one's own life

suicide contagion term that describes the copying of suicide attempts after exposure to another person's suicide

suicide clusters series of suicides in a particular community that occur in a relatively short period of time

survivors people who lose a loved one to suicide

Learning Outcomes

After studying this lesson, you will be able to

- **identify** risk factors of suicide.
- **recognize** signs that someone may be at risk of attempting suicide.
- **identify** ways to respond to warning signs of suicide.
- **explain** how treating mental illnesses helps prevent suicide.
- **describe** how suicide affects other people in a person's life.

Graphic Organizer

Myths and Facts About Suicide

Prior to reading, list everything you have heard about suicide—from friends, family members, or the media—and what you already know. List each item as a myth or fact as shown in the example. Compare your table with a partner's table. As you read the lesson, add additional notes and any corrections to your table.

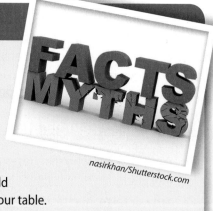

nasirkhan/Shutterstock.com

Myths About Suicide	Facts About Suicide
Talking about suicide or asking someone if they feel suicidal will encourage suicide attempts.	Talking about suicide provides an opportunity for communication for a person in need.

People who consider attempting suicide feel a sense of hopelessness and despair about their lives. They feel like things will never get better. Their emotions become too much to handle. In some cases, mental illnesses may contribute to these feelings.

The good news is that suicide is preventable. Lives and feelings can, and do, get better. Emotions often occur in cycles. There will be times of sadness, but times of happiness may be right around the corner. Treatments are available to help people with mental illnesses feel better. People can learn to recognize the warning signs of suicide and to promote positive mental health to prevent it from happening. By getting the necessary help, people who are thinking about suicide can learn healthy ways to cope with their feelings and eventually lead fulfilling lives.

Recognize Risk Factors of Suicide

The term **suicide** describes when a person takes one's own life. In the United States, suicide is the second leading cause of death for people ages 10 to 34. The most common reason people attempt suicide is severe depression. It can make people believe life is not worth living, the world is better off without them, and no one will miss them. In some cases, a person who attempts suicide has planned to for some time. In other cases, a person who already feels depressed decides to attempt suicide following some negative life event, such as academic failure or a fight with a friend or family member. Many individual and environmental factors affect whether a person attempts suicide (**Figure 6.12**).

Individual Factors

One major individual risk factor for suicide is a previous suicide attempt. If a person attempted suicide before, this person is more likely to make another attempt.

A person's overall mental and emotional health is another individual risk factor. People who consider suicide often do so because of overwhelming sadness and negative thoughts. Sometimes a mental illness causes these symptoms. Anxiety disorders, major depressive disorder, and other mental disorders can cause unhealthy thought patterns. These thought patterns could cause people to consider suicide. It is important to remember, however, that many people with mental illnesses never attempt suicide. Instead, they seek treatment to reduce symptoms and change unhealthy thought patterns to lead fulfilling lives.

Another risk factor for suicide is substance use. Abusing drugs and alcohol can cloud judgment and make people more likely to engage in self-harm or attempt suicide. In fact, people who abuse drugs or alcohol are six times more likely than others to report attempting suicide.

Risk Factors of Suicide

Individual Factors
- Previous suicide attempt
- Overall mental and emotional health
- Genetic makeup
- Unhealthy thought patterns
- Substance abuse

Environmental Factors
- Social environment, including family, friends, and peers
- Community environment
- The media

Figure 6.12   Individual and environmental factors such as these could lead to someone having suicidal thoughts.

Environmental Factors

Environmental factors include your family, friends and peers, community, and the media. People whose family members have a mental illness or attempt or die by suicide may have more risk for attempting suicide themselves. Crises such as financial hardships, death of a close family member, or divorce may strain family relationships and increase risk factors. It is important to remember that many people who face family issues never attempt suicide. They focus on improving and strengthening family relationships. **Figure 6.13** provides some techniques people can use to strengthen family relationships.

People who experience long-term environmental stress have more risk of attempting suicide. This can include exposure to abuse or neglect, racism, or violence. Another example is bullying. Adolescents who are bullied have a greater risk of thinking about and attempting suicide. Bullying can also lead adolescents to develop depression, which increases risk of suicide.

The prevalence of suicide in a community also affects suicide risk. Hearing about a suicide—of a friend, family member, classmate, celebrity, or even a stranger—can increase someone's risk of a suicide attempt. This increased risk after exposure to suicide is called **suicide contagion**. Some communities or groups experience a **suicide cluster**, which is a series of suicides or suicide attempts in a relatively short time. In these clusters, one person dies by suicide, and then other people copy this behavior.

The media can also be a risk factor. For example, after a TV show or movie portrays suicide, the rate of suicide attempts increases in the next few weeks following the release. Media coverage does not lead most people to consider harming themselves, but can trigger a suicide attempt in people who are experiencing a mental health condition or illness. This is similar to a suicide contagion. Due to the increased risk, many media organizations follow careful practices to reduce potential harm (**Figure 6.14**).

Figure 6.13
Healthy relationships within your family can positively affect your mental and emotional health. Following strategies such as these can help you to encourage healthy relationships within your family.

Tips for Strengthening Family Relationships

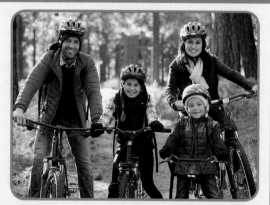

- Always be honest with your family. Lying is a quick way to create conflict with your parents or siblings.
- Participate in new, fun activities together. Watch a new movie, play a board game, or go to the pool. Whatever your family enjoys, do it together.
- Show appreciation for your family and all they do for you. Say "thank you" often. Be helpful around the house in return.

Monkey Business Images/Shutterstock.com

- Laugh together, but not at each other. Laughter helps ease tension and helps family members see one another in a positive way.
- Make an effort to stay calm and be forgiving during times of conflict.

How Media Organizations Cover Suicide

Media Organizations DO Cover:
- Sharing crisis resources
- Encouraging people who are struggling with thoughts of suicide to get help

Media Organizations DO NOT Cover:
- Describing the manner of death
- Showing images of grieving friends and family members

Figure 6.14
Many media organizations are following careful practices to reduce unintended negative consequences of reporting or portraying suicide.

Take Steps to Help Prevent Suicide

Suicide is a tragedy that affects individuals, families, friends and peers, and communities. For example, immediate family members and close friends can grieve intensely after someone close has died from suicide. Other people in a community are also impacted by suicide. People in a person's school, workplace, or neighborhood also grieve, even if they did not personally know the individual who died.

All people can take steps to help prevent suicide—on an individual level and in their communities. This includes recognizing the warning signs of someone who has thoughts of suicide. Promoting positive mental health for oneself and others can also decrease the risk of suicide.

To help prevent suicide, people need to respond to warning signs of suicide. Most people who attempt suicide show some warning signs about their intentions. They often hint at or tell someone about their plans beforehand. Some people may say they feel like they have no reason to live. Others may seem obsessed with death. The infographic on page 184 shows examples of warning signs.

It is very important to always take any thoughts or mention of suicide and any other warning signs very seriously. If you think about hurting yourself, talk to an adult you trust right away. This person can put you in touch with a trained mental health professional.

If a person confides in you about having thoughts of suicide, you cannot keep this secret. Talk to someone who can help immediately. You can also call 911 or a suicide hotline number to reach a trained mental health professional (**Figure 6.15**). If someone (such as a friend) mentions suicide, do not leave that person alone. Stay with the person until help arrives.

Suicide Prevention Resources		
National Emergency Number	Call (and text in certain areas)	911
National Suicide Prevention Lifeline	Call or chat online	1-800-273-TALK (8255) or suicidepreventionlifeline.org/chat
Crisis Text Line	Text	741741
Hope Line	Chat online or e-mail	www.thehopeline.com/gethelp

Figure 6.15
Mental health professionals can provide effective treatment for people with mental health conditions so they can get the help they need to recover.

Watch Out for Warning Signs

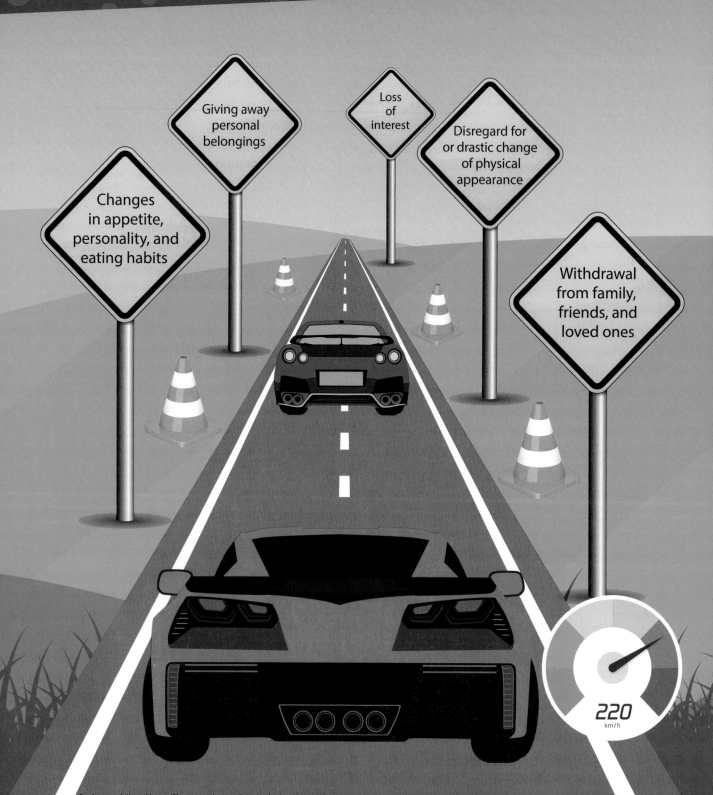

Giving away personal belongings

Loss of interest

Disregard for or drastic change of physical appearance

Changes in appetite, personality, and eating habits

Withdrawal from family, friends, and loved ones

220 km/h

Advocate for Mental Health

The most common cause of suicide is untreated depression. One step to help prevent suicide is to get treatment for a mental health condition and illness and encourage others to get treatment as well. Treatment seeks to reduce negative symptoms, which usually means people no longer consider suicide.

To protect against suicide, you can seek and give support in your relationships, especially if you feel you are struggling. People can find support from family members, friends, and the community (**Figure 6.16**). Simply being able to express feelings and talk with trusted people can be very helpful. In addition, you can help prevent suicide by using skills to build your self-esteem, shift to a positive mind-set, and manage stress. Practicing these skills regularly can help you regulate negative feelings and handle stress in healthy ways.

Stress in the environment is a risk factor for suicide. By improving your environment, you can reduce the risk of suicide and create a supportive environment. For example, students who feel connected to the school community, including other students, teachers, and staff, are less likely to experience mental health conditions and illnesses. They are also more likely to seek help for themselves or their friends.

You can help promote a positive, respectful environment by building supportive, healthy relationships and communicating effectively by showing empathy and respect to others. You can also stand up to inappropriate behavior, such as intervening if you see someone being bullied. Showing tolerance and offering support to your peers can help create a positive school climate, which reduces risk for suicide.

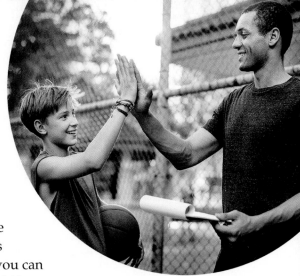

Rawpixel.com/Shutterstock.com

Figure 6.16
Community members, such as a coach of a recreational sports team, can be a source to seek support from if you are struggling with negative thoughts and feelings.

Provide Help for Survivors

The term **survivors** describes people who lose a loved one to suicide. Survivors often feel anger, guilt, and sadness. They may suffer with guilt because they were unable to prevent the death. They may feel rejected and abandoned by the person who died by suicide. Suicide deaths are sudden. This means survivors are unable to prepare themselves for a loss.

Survivors may even feel embarrassed or ashamed by the suicide. Many people are uncomfortable with the topic of suicide. Unfortunately, this means survivors may not get the support they need after their loss.

The good news is that there are ways to help survivors. Some survivors may find support groups or therapy helpful. It is important to let survivors grieve. If you know someone who lost a loved one to suicide, learn about the stages of grief (**Figure 6.17**). Knowing what your friend or family member is going through can help you be more compassionate.

Survivors may not want to talk about their loss right away. When they are ready to talk, however, just listen. Some people feel better when they talk about difficult topics. Listening is a simple way to help survivors overcome their loss.

Figure 6.17
People experience grief
differently and do not
always go through every
stage of grief. Stages
do not necessarily go in
any order. *What term
describes people who
lose a loved one to
suicide?*

Stages of Grief

Stage	Description
Denial	It is normal for some people to deny sad news. People may ignore the facts and try to carry on as though nothing has changed. Not all people experience denial, but those who do are protecting themselves from emotional pain.
Anger	Some people become angry with the person who died. Although this stage is temporary, it may last a long time, and a person's anger may push family and friends away.
Bargaining	People often feel out of control and helpless in the face of death. Some people may try to bargain to feel they have control over the situation.
Depression	Deep sadness comes with the reality of the loss. This depression is normal and can last several months.
Acceptance	As with other stages, not all people experience this stage. When they do, they accept the loss as real and begin to move on knowing that life continues.

Lesson 6.3 Review

1. **True or false.** If a person attempted suicide before, that person is less likely to make another attempt.
2. List two examples of family risk factors that can strain family relationships and could increase the risk of suicide.
3. A(n) _____ _____ is a series of suicides or suicide attempts in a relatively short time.
4. What is the term for a person who has lost a loved one to suicide?
5. **Critical thinking.** List three warning signs that a person may be considering suicide. Explain how you should respond if someone you know is considering suicide.

Hands-On Activity

Create six social media posts that represent the emotional struggles of middle school students. Two of the posts should represent general feelings of sadness. Another two should indicate the signs of a major depressive disorder. The final two should include warning signs of suicidal thoughts. Switch social media posts with a classmate. Take turns explaining whether each post points toward sadness, depression, or suicidal thoughts. Explain how you would respond to the post showing empathy and compassion. Include any actions you would take to help those experiencing emotional struggles.

Review and Assessment

Summary

Lesson 6.1 Recognizing Mental Illnesses

- A *mental illness* is a mental or emotional condition that interferes with daily functioning.
- Family history, life experiences, substance use, brain injuries, environment during pregnancy, and unhealthy patterns of thinking contribute to mental illnesses.
- Anxiety disorders cause extreme or unrealistic fear or dread in response to situations, experiences, or objects.
- Attention-deficit hyperactivity disorder (ADHD) makes it difficult to pay attention or control behavior. Those with obsessive-compulsive disorder (OCD) experience constant and obsessive thoughts, feelings, or behaviors.
- People with mood disorders such as major depressive disorder, seasonal affective disorder (SAD), and bipolar disorder experience extreme changes in the way they feel.
- People with behavioral disorders like oppositional defiant disorder (ODD) or conduct disorder show patterns of inappropriate behavior.

Lesson 6.2 Getting Help for Mental Illnesses

- Treatment for mental illnesses include therapy, medication, or inpatient treatment. Therapists treat people with mental illnesses through individual therapy, family therapy, or support groups.
- Medications, in addition to therapy, can help treat specific mental illnesses. Medication is prescribed by healthcare professionals. Some medications have side effects, so doctors regularly monitor patients on medications.
- People may choose not to seek help due to stigmas of the illness or cost of treatment.
- If you are concerned that someone you care about has a mental illness, share your honest concerns with that person and offer to help the person find treatment.

Lesson 6.3 Preventing Suicide

- *Suicide* describes when a person takes one's own life. Sometimes, a mental illness can lead to suicidal thoughts. Individual and environmental factors such as financial hardship, abuse, or bullying may also lead a person to consider suicide.
- *Suicide contagion* describes how exposure to a suicide or suicide attempt may influence others to attempt suicide. A *suicide cluster* describes a series of suicides or suicide attempts that occur in a community in a relatively short time.
- Most people who attempt suicide show warning signs about their intentions. If you or someone you know experiences thoughts about suicide, talk to a trusted adult immediately.
- Building a support system, having healthy self-esteem, having a positive mind-set, and managing stress can help reduce the risk of suicide. Improving your environment can also decrease the risk of suicide.
- Support groups can be helpful for survivors who often feel anger, guilt, or sadness over the loss of a loved one from suicide. It is important to let survivors grieve.

Check Your Knowledge

Record your answers to each of the following questions on a separate sheet of paper.

1. A mental or emotional condition so severe it interferes with daily functioning is called a(n) _____ _____.

2. Generalized anxiety disorder, social anxiety disorder, panic disorder, and phobias are all examples of _____ disorders.

3. List three common mood disorders.

4. **True or false.** People with seasonal affective disorder (SAD) face depression in the spring and summer when there is more natural sunlight.

5. What are the three types of therapy available to help treat mental illnesses?

6. Who can prescribe mental health medications?

7. **True or false.** Inpatient treatment is necessary when people are at serious risk of harming themselves or others.

8. What could happen if a mental illness remains untreated?

9. How do social stigmas affect people with mental illnesses?

10. Suicide _____ is the term that describes how exposure to a suicide or suicide attempt may influence others to attempt suicide.

    A. cluster

    B. survivor

    C. contagion

    D. risk

11. **True or false.** Most people who attempt suicide rarely show warning signs about their intentions.

12. Give an example of a way someone could provide help for a survivor who loses a loved one to suicide.

Use Your Vocabulary

anxiety disorder	inpatient treatment	suicide
attention-deficit hyperactivity disorder (ADHD)	major depressive disorder	suicide clusters
	mental health medication	suicide contagion
	mental illness	support groups
bipolar disorder	schizophrenia spectrum disorder	survivors
family therapy		therapist
individual therapy	stigma	therapy

13. In teams, create categories for the terms above. Then, classify as many of the terms as possible within the categories your team selected. Share your ideas with another team and discuss your categories. Revise your categories as needed.

14. Write each of the terms above on a separate sheet of paper. For each term, write a word you have learned that relates to the term. In small groups, exchange papers. Have each person in the group explain a term on the list. Work together to properly pronounce the term and take turns until all terms have complete explanations. Ask for assistance, if needed.

Think Critically

15. **Identify.** What are some reasons a middle school student may not seek help for a mental illness? What can be a consequence of not receiving treatment?

16. **Draw conclusions.** How could having a mental illness affect your physical and social health? Give a detailed answer and provide examples.

17. **Determine.** What would you do if you began experiencing depression, thoughts of self-harm, or suicidal thoughts? Identify someone you would talk to and what treatment you would seek.

18. **Compare and contrast.** Compare and contrast the following sets: experiencing mood swings and having a bipolar disorder; feeling anxious and having a generalized anxiety disorder; feeling scared and having a phobia; and being organized and having obsessive-compulsive disorder. Why is it important that only a mental health professional diagnose someone with a mental illness?

DEVELOP Your Skills

19. **Access information and technology skills.** Listen to a podcast featuring a guest who has one of the mental illnesses from this chapter. What symptoms does this person mention? How does this mental illness interfere with this person's daily living? Research local resources and treatment options available in your community to support people with this condition. Create a brochure of your findings to share with the class.

20. **Analyze influences.** Analyze a show or movie to determine how the media displays differences in mental health among fictional characters. Consider the following questions: Is everyone portrayed as happy? If a character has a mental illness, is there a social stigma associated with this condition? Does your show or movie portray it as socially acceptable to have a mental illness? How is the character with a mental illness treated by others? Based on your analysis, reflect on how the media shapes your view on mental illnesses. Present your findings to the class. If you are listening to a presentation, write down questions to ask your classmate after the presentation concludes.

21. **Advocacy and teamwork skills.** With a small group, create a poster to raise awareness of suicide. Consider providing information on the following: potential risk factors, warning signs, how to respond to someone who has thoughts of self-harm or suicide, different treatment options, available community resources, and other pertinent information. Do additional research as needed. With permission, hang the poster in a visible place in the school.

22. **Decision-making and communication skills.** Imagine you hear your friend is considering suicide. Write a hypothetical dialogue explaining what you would do in this situation. What would you say to your friend? What would you do to help? Trade dialogues with a partner and mark any errors, such as those related to pronoun agreement, verb tense, subject-verb agreement, or possessives. Revise your dialogue. Then, practice the dialogue with your partner.

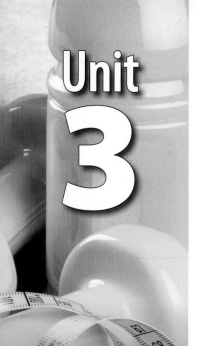

Nutrition and Physical Activity

Chapter 7   Nutrition

Chapter 8   Physical Activity

Warm-Up Activity

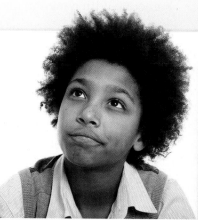

Djomas/Shutterstock.com

Setting Yourself Up for a Healthy Lifestyle

Often, the behaviors you begin today will carry into high school and adulthood. Gaining knowledge on healthy eating and physical activity is the first step to setting yourself up for a healthy lifestyle.

Read the scenario below and decide if Caleb is setting himself up for a healthy lifestyle by making good nutritional choices and engaging in regular physical activity. Then, as a class, answer the discussion questions. When you finish reading the chapters in this unit, review the scenario and determine whether you would change any of your responses to the discussion questions.

Scenario

Ever since Caleb was a baby, he was always a picky eater. As a 13-year-old, Caleb is still hesitant to try new foods. Breakfast is not an issue since Caleb is too busy and rushed in the morning to eat. By lunch, he is starving. School food is okay as long as it is pizza, a corn dog, or chicken nuggets. He will often order potatoes or corn as a side and chocolate milk. After school, he goes on a junk food or snacking frenzy. Caleb's parents work long hours, so dinner can be tough on the family. Luckily, they live three blocks from a burger joint. A cheeseburger, fries, and soda is Caleb's favorite meal there. He loves their milkshakes, but his parents rarely let him get them. To get their daily physical activity, Caleb's family will walk to the restaurant and back. After dinner, it is often time for homework and bed.

Discussion Questions

1. Based on the information provided in the scenario about his current nutritional choices and physical activity, is Caleb setting himself up for a healthy lifestyle?

2. What changes could Caleb make related to his nutritional choices in order to consume a well-balanced diet?

3. Is Caleb getting enough physical activity daily? If he is not, what changes would you recommend?

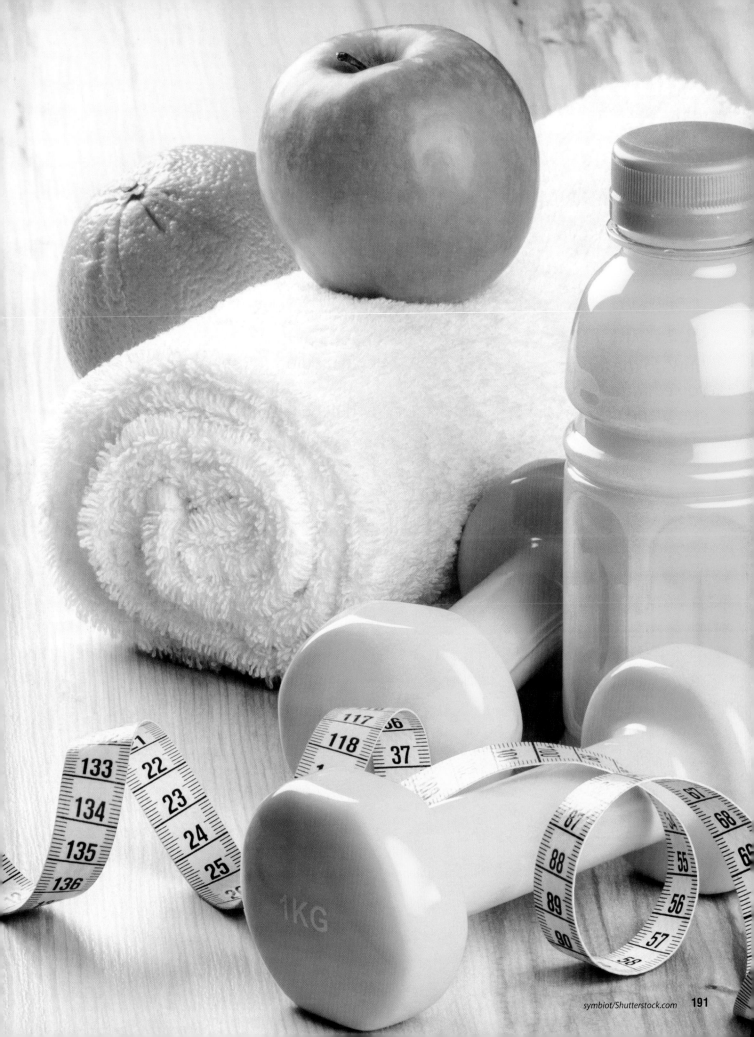

Chapter 7

Nutrition

Essential Question

How do the foods you eat affect your overall health?

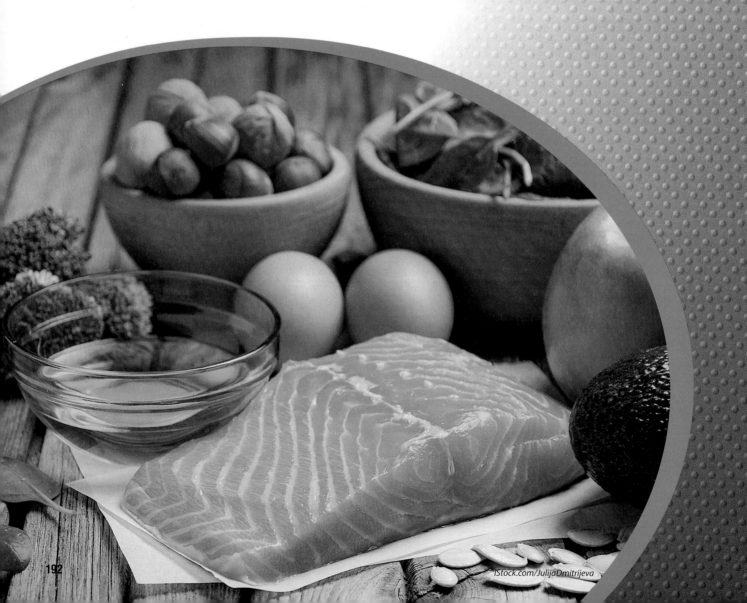

iStock.com/JulijaDmitrijeva

Reading Activity

Imagine you are a nutritionist and your client is using a crash diet to lose weight fast. Write a two-paragraph speech explaining your client's nutritional needs and advice for weight management. Then deliver your speech to a partner. After reading this chapter, team up with your partner again to discuss what you would change about your speech based on any new information you have learned about nutrition. Present your final speech to the class.

How Healthy Are You?

In this chapter, you will be learning about nutrition. Before you begin reading the chapter, take the following quiz to assess your current nutrition habits.

Healthy Choices	Yes	No
Do you eat a nutritious breakfast every morning?		
Do you rarely drink soda or sugar-sweetened drinks?		
Do you eat multiple servings of fruits and vegetables every day?		
Do you rarely, if ever, have feelings of guilt or anxiety when you think about eating certain foods or certain amounts of foods?		
Do you get enough protein in your diet?		
Do you try to limit added sugars, saturated fats, and sodium in your diet?		
Do you drink 8½ to 11½ cups of water per day?		
Do you practice healthy, lifelong eating and physical activity habits?		
Do you stay away from fad diets as quick-fix weight-loss strategies?		
Are you able to identify distorted body image ideals portrayed in the media?		
Do you know about eating disorders and how to prevent them?		

Count your "Yes" and "No" responses. The more "Yes" responses you have, the more healthy nutrition habits you exhibit. Now, take a closer look at the questions with which you responded "No." How can you make these healthy habits part of your daily life? Identify a SMART goal you would like to achieve to help improve your overall health and well-being. Refer to Figure 1.11 to help you set up your SMART goal. If you do not understand the instructions, ask for clarification from your teacher.

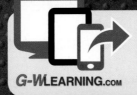

Click on the activity icon or visit www.g-wlearning.com/health to access online vocabulary activities using key terms from the chapter.

G-WLEARNING.com

Getting Enough Nutrients

Key Terms

nutrients chemical substances that give your body what it needs to grow and function properly

carbohydrates major source of energy for the body; found in fruits, vegetables, grains, and milk products

dietary fiber tough complex carbohydrate that the body is unable to digest

protein nutrient the body uses to build and maintain all of its cells and tissues

fats type of nutrient largely made up of fatty acids, which provide a valuable source of energy

saturated fats type of fat found mainly in animal-based foods, such as meat and dairy products

unsaturated fats type of fat found in plant-based foods, such as vegetable oils, some peanut butters and margarines, olives, salad dressing, nuts, and seeds

trans fats type of fat found in foods from animals, such as cows and goats; used to be found in many processed foods, such as packaged cookies and chips

vitamins organic substances that come from plants or animals that are necessary for normal growth and development

minerals inorganic elements found in soil and water that the body needs in small quantities

Learning Outcomes

After studying this lesson, you will be able to

- **identify** the six types of nutrients.
- **explain** the role of each nutrient in the body.
- **identify** sources of each nutrient.
- **describe** the importance of water to good health.

Graphic Organizer

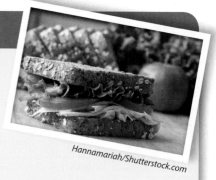

Hannamariah/Shutterstock.com

Overlapping Nutrients

Most healthy foods are good sources of more than one nutrient. As you read the lesson, list your favorite foods that are good sources of protein, carbohydrates, fats, minerals, or vitamins in the diagram shown. Highlight the foods if they contain more than one nutrient. For example, a turkey sandwich on whole-grain bread is a good source of healthy protein and carbohydrates.

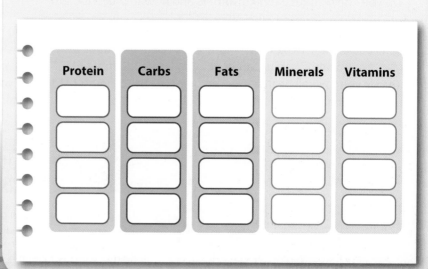

Protein	Carbs	Fats	Minerals	Vitamins

Rei is taller than most of the females and even some of the males in seventh grade. During softball practice, her coach tells her that she throws as far as high school players. She also has not struggled yet with acne. Rei's dad says this is because of the healthy foods they eat as a family. Is Rei's dad correct? Do the foods and beverages they eat and drink affect these aspects of Rei's wellness? The answer to both questions is "yes."

Although you may not think much about the food choices you make, what you eat has a major impact on your overall health. This lesson examines *nutrition* (the processes by which you take in and use food). You will learn about different types of nutrients your body needs and how these nutrients help your body stay healthy.

Types of Nutrients

While it is enjoyable to eat a good meal or a tasty snack, food has a more fundamental role in people's lives. Food is the fuel that powers people's bodies. Food contains **nutrients**, which are chemical substances that give your body what it needs to grow and function properly. There are six general types of nutrients (**Figure 7.1**).

Some of these nutrients provide the energy your body needs to perform daily physical activities, such as playing sports and riding a bicycle. Your body also uses this energy to perform many important functions that go on within your body.

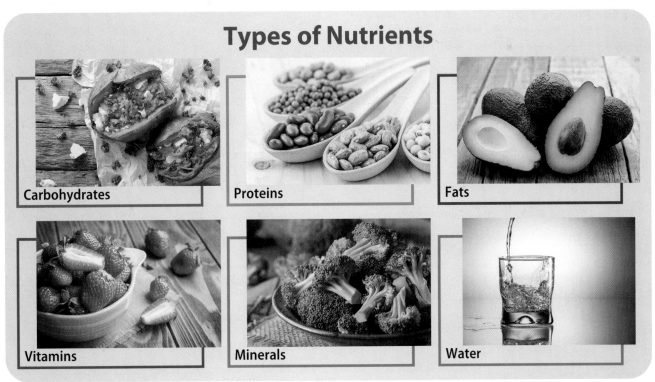

Types of Nutrients

Carbohydrates

Proteins

Fats

Vitamins

Minerals

Water

Figure 7.1 Eat a variety of healthy foods to obtain all the nutrients your body needs.

For instance, your body has to maintain a stable body temperature. It needs to provide energy to the brain and nervous system. It also needs energy to build body tissues.

Other nutrients make it possible for your body to perform certain important functions. For example, your body needs vitamins and minerals to build new cells, strengthen bones, and carry oxygen through your blood. Nutrients also regulate basic processes in your body, such as breathing.

Carbohydrates

Carbohydrates, a major source of energy for the body, are found in fruits, vegetables, grains, and milk products. Carbohydrates are sugars and starches, and are either simple or complex (**Figure 7.2**).

Sugars are *simple carbohydrates*. These simple sugars occur naturally in some foods, including fruits and dairy products. Starches are *complex carbohydrates*. Products made from grains, such as bread, cereal, rice, and pasta, are rich sources of starch. Starch is also found in beans and in some types of vegetables, including potatoes, peas, and corn.

Figure 7.2
Simple carbohydrates are sugars, such as those found in fruit and milk. Complex carbohydrates are starches, such as those found in bread and potatoes. *What is the main function of carbohydrates in the body?*

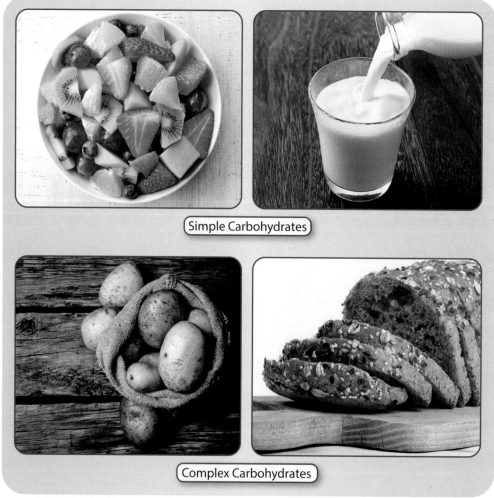

Simple Carbohydrates

Complex Carbohydrates

Left to right: baibaz/Shutterstock.com; NaturalBox/Shutterstock.com; Artem Shadrin/Shutterstock.com; Kodda/Shutterstock.com

Dietary fiber is a tough complex carbohydrate that the body is unable to wholly digest. This type of carbohydrate is found only in plant-based foods. Rich sources of dietary fiber include fruits, most vegetables, whole grains (such as whole-wheat bread or brown rice), and nuts.

Dietary fiber does not provide the body with energy. Still, it does have important health benefits, such as the following:

- **Lowers cholesterol.** Fiber attaches to cholesterol and carries it out of the body during digestion. *Cholesterol* is a type of fat made by the body that is also present in some foods. Having elevated levels of cholesterol in the body increases a person's risk of developing heart disease, high blood pressure, and stroke. A diet that includes enough dietary fiber can reduce the risk of these conditions (**Figure 7.3**).

- **Balances level of glucose.** *Glucose* is the body's preferred source of energy and powers the brain. Glucose enables you to concentrate and pay attention in class. By balancing the level of glucose in the blood, fiber can help control some types of diabetes.

- **Adds bulk to feces.** Fiber helps the digestive system work properly by adding bulk to feces. This can help prevent conditions such as constipation (hard feces) and hemorrhoids. *Hemorrhoids* are swollen veins in the rectum that are caused by straining the muscles to pass hard feces. The condition can be painful.

- **Can prevent overeating.** High-fiber foods take longer to chew than many other types of foods. As a result, people eating a high-fiber meal are inclined to eat less than they would otherwise. Fiber also slows the movement of food out of the stomach and into the intestines. This prevents becoming hungry again soon after eating.

Figure 7.3
Oatmeal is an excellent source of fiber, and it is good for your heart health. You can boost the fiber content even more by adding berries or another fruit.

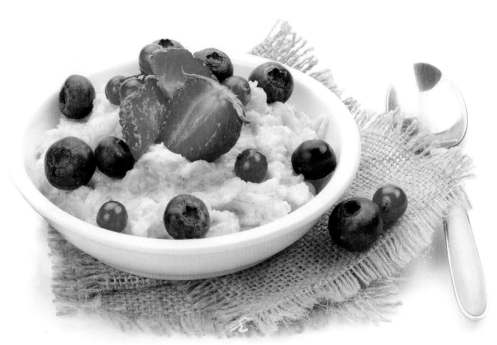

Vitalina Rybakova/Shutterstock.com

Proteins

Protein is a nutrient the body uses to build and maintain all of its cells and tissues. Protein plays a very important role in the body (**Figure 7.4**).

Your body uses up and loses protein every day through many regular activities. For example, when you shower and brush your hair, you are actually losing protein. The shower washes some skin cells off your body. Some hair remains in the brush. Those skin cells and that hair contain protein.

Since you lose protein every day, you need to take in protein to replace it every day. Fortunately, in the United States, many foods that people eat on a regular basis contain protein. In fact, most people eat more protein than they need.

People who do not consume enough protein risk serious consequences. For example, the cells that help the body fight disease are made of protein. People who do not get enough protein are more likely to have weakened immune systems. This means they have an increased risk of developing infections and diseases.

Types of Proteins

All proteins are made up of smaller chemical units called *amino acids*. Twenty different amino acids join in various combinations to make all types of proteins. The body produces some of these amino acids, which are called *nonessential amino acids*. Other amino acids, however, are not produced by the body in sufficient amounts or at all. You can only get them by eating particular foods. This type of amino acid is called an *essential amino acid* because it is essential that your diet includes it. Proteins are divided into two types, depending on whether they include all of the essential amino acids (**Figure 7.5**).

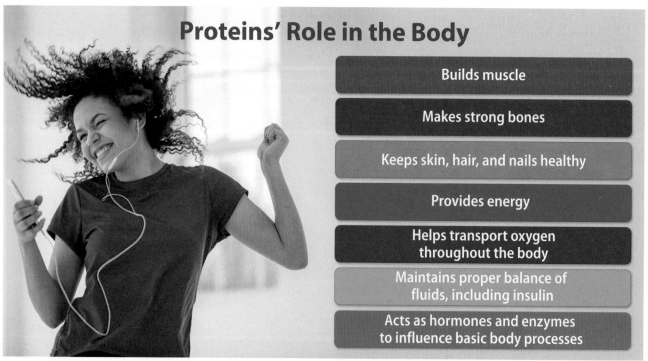

Proteins' Role in the Body

- Builds muscle
- Makes strong bones
- Keeps skin, hair, and nails healthy
- Provides energy
- Helps transport oxygen throughout the body
- Maintains proper balance of fluids, including insulin
- Acts as hormones and enzymes to influence basic body processes

iStock.com/FatCamera

Figure 7.4 Eating proteins every day helps keep your body functioning properly.

Types of Protein Sources

Complete Proteins	Incomplete Proteins
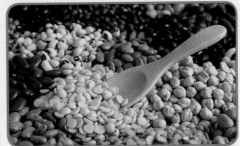	
koss13/Shutterstock.com	Piyaset/Shutterstock.com
Found in animal-based foods, such as meat, poultry, eggs, fish, dairy products, and some plant-based foods such as soybeans.	Found in legumes (dry beans and peas), tofu, nuts and seeds, grains, some vegetables, and some fruits.

Figure 7.5 Complete proteins contain all nine essential amino acids, while incomplete proteins lack one or more of the essential amino acids. *Which type of amino acids does the body produce?*

Proteins and Vegetarians

Some vegetarians avoid eating all (or most) foods from animal sources. This means they must rely on plant-based proteins to meet their needs (**Figure 7.6**). People who eat a vegetarian diet simply have to combine different types of foods that can work together to provide all of the essential amino acids. For example, rice contains essential amino acids that are lacking in red beans and red beans contain essential amino acids lacking in rice. When both rice and beans are eaten, all the essential amino acids are provided.

Types of Vegetarians

Vegans eat only plant-based foods.

Lacto-vegetarians eat dairy products but no meat, fish, poultry, or eggs.

Ovo-vegetarians eat eggs, but no other animal-based products.

Lacto-ovo vegetarians eat dairy products and eggs, but no meat, fish, or poultry.

Figure 7.6 Some vegetarian diets include animal-based foods and others do not.

Fats

Fats are a type of nutrient largely made up of fatty acids, which provide a valuable source of energy. Fatty acids are an important source of energy for muscles. Common fats in the diet include saturated fats, unsaturated fats, and trans fats.

Types of Fats

Saturated fats are found primarily in animal-based foods, such as meat and dairy products. Saturated fats are typically solid at room temperature.

Unsaturated fats are found in plant-based foods, such as vegetable oils, some peanut butters and margarines, olives, salad dressing, nuts, and seeds. Unsaturated fats are liquid at room temperature.

Trans fats used to be found in many processed foods, such as packaged cookies, chips, doughnuts, and crackers. Some trans fats occur naturally and are found in foods from animals, such as cows and goats.

Your body stores excess calories you eat as body fat. Despite the negative publicity that body fat gets, it is important to your body's health. Body fat has important functions, such as the following:

- supply energy to the body when food is unavailable
- act as a cushion to protect internal organs
- provide a layer of insulation to help maintain your body temperature so you do not get too hot or too cold

Fats in the Diet

Although fats are important for the body to function, some fats may be better for you than other fats. Saturated fats tend to be associated with higher levels of cholesterol in the blood. Diets that are high in saturated fats may lead to long-term health conditions (**Figure 7.7**). These conditions may include heart disease, stroke, some types of cancer, and diabetes.

Some scientists believe trans fats pose major health risks as well. Many cities and states have passed laws that require restaurants to limit how much trans fat they use. In 2015, the United States Food and Drug Administration (FDA) declared that trans fats were not "generally recognized as safe." The FDA gave food companies three years to remove artificial trans fats from their food products.

Vitamins

Vitamins are organic substances that come from plants or animals that are necessary for normal growth and development. Different vitamins have different functions in the body.

Your body requires 13 different vitamins. Because your body cannot create these vitamins, you need to absorb them from the foods you eat. Unlike carbohydrates, proteins, and fats, your body requires only very small amounts of vitamins to function properly. Eating a balanced diet that contains a variety of foods can easily provide you with the vitamins you need.

Figure 7.7
Replacing foods high in saturated fats with healthier options can help keep your heart healthy and your weight in check.

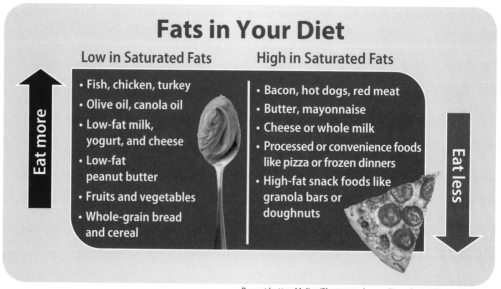

Fats in Your Diet

Low in Saturated Fats

- Fish, chicken, turkey
- Olive oil, canola oil
- Low-fat milk, yogurt, and cheese
- Low-fat peanut butter
- Fruits and vegetables
- Whole-grain bread and cereal

Eat more

High in Saturated Fats

- Bacon, hot dogs, red meat
- Butter, mayonnaise
- Cheese or whole milk
- Processed or convenience foods like pizza or frozen dinners
- High-fat snack foods like granola bars or doughnuts

Eat less

Peanut butter: Melica/Shutterstock.com; Pizza: bestv/Shutterstock.com

Vitamins can be divided into two distinct types—water-soluble and fat-soluble (**Figure 7.8**). *Water-soluble vitamins* dissolve in water. They pass into the bloodstream during digestion and are either used immediately by the body or are removed by the kidneys during urination. The nine water-soluble vitamins are vitamin C and the B vitamins.

Fat-soluble vitamins are absorbed along with dietary fat and dissolve in the body's fats. They are stored in the body for later use. There are four fat-soluble vitamins—vitamins A, D, E, and K.

Types and Functions of Vitamins

Vitamin	Functions	Sources
Water-Soluble Vitamins		
Vitamin B$_1$ (Thiamin)	Helps change carbohydrates into energy	Pork, legumes, enriched or whole-grain products
Vitamin B$_2$ (Riboflavin)	Assists with metabolism	Milk, cheese, leafy vegetables, legumes, tomatoes, almonds
Vitamin B$_3$ (Niacin)	Promotes healthy skin and nerves; improves circulation	Eggs, lean meats, nuts, legumes, avocados, potatoes
Vitamin B$_5$ (Pantothenic acid)	Helps the body use nutrients for energy	Potatoes, sunflower seeds, cooked mushrooms, yogurt
Vitamin B$_6$ (Pyridoxine)	Helps generate energy from food; helps develop brain, nerves, and skin	Avocados, bananas, meats, nuts, poultry, whole grains
Vitamin B$_7$ (Biotin)	Assists in production of hormones and cholesterol; boosts metabolism	Milk, nuts, pork, egg yolks, chocolate
Vitamin B$_9$ (Folic acid)	Helps with cell division and growth; assists production of red blood cells	Leafy vegetables, fortified cereals, bread
Vitamin B$_{12}$ (Cyanocobalamin)	Maintains central nervous system and metabolism; helps form red blood cells	Meat, eggs, dairy products, poultry, shellfish
Vitamin C	Promotes healing within the body; helps maintain healthy teeth and gums	Citrus fruits, broccoli, cabbage, spinach, tomatoes
Fat-Soluble Vitamins		
Vitamin A	Fights infections; promotes eye and bone health	Carrots, kale, broccoli, dairy, meats
Vitamin D	Helps absorb calcium for strong teeth and bones; regulates cell growth; reduces inflammation	Fish, egg yolks, fortified dairy products, cereals, sunlight
Vitamin E	Protects red blood cells from oxidation	Whole grains, leafy greens, nuts
Vitamin K	Assists with blood clotting	Liver, cereals, cabbage

Figure 7.8 Choose a variety of nutrient-rich foods to meet your daily requirements for vitamins. *When you spend time in the sun, which vitamin is your body absorbing?*

Minerals

Minerals are inorganic elements that are found in soil and water. Minerals are absorbed by plants from the soil and water. You then absorb minerals from the plants you eat, the water you drink, or from animal food sources that have absorbed the minerals. Your body needs minerals in small amounts to grow and develop normally.

As with vitamins, each mineral helps with different body processes (**Figure 7.9**). Eating a nutritious and balanced diet generally provides all of

Types and Functions of Minerals		
Mineral	**Functions**	**Sources**
Major Minerals		
Calcium	Promotes muscle, heart, and digestive health; builds bone and teeth	Dairy, eggs, canned salmon or sardines, leafy vegetables, nuts, tofu
Chloride	Assists with balancing bodily fluids	Table salt
Magnesium	Contributes to bone and teeth health	Nuts, soybeans, spinach, tomatoes
Phosphorus	Assists energy processing	Red meat, dairy, fish, poultry, brown rice
Potassium	Assists heart function, muscle contraction, and digestive function	Legumes, potato skins, tomatoes, bananas, dry beans, whole grains
Sodium	Helps with blood pressure and bodily fluid balance	Table salt (sodium chloride), milk, spinach
Sulfur	Promotes metabolism and immune system function	Meats, fish, poultry, eggs, milk, legumes
Trace Minerals		
Chromium	Helps maintain normal glucose levels	Apples, bananas, spinach, green peppers
Copper	Assists metabolism and red blood cell formation	Shellfish, whole grains, beans, nuts, potatoes, dried fruits, cocoa
Fluoride	Prevents dental cavities; stimulates new bone formation	Fluoridated water, most seafood, tea, gelatin
Iodine	Assists thyroid hormone production	Table salt, some fish (cod, sea bass, haddock), dairy products
Iron	Carries oxygen from the lungs to the tissues	Red meat, leafy vegetables, fish, eggs, beans, whole grains
Manganese	Assists bone formation, metabolism, and wound healing; contributes to teeth health	Nuts, legumes, seeds, whole grains, tea, leafy green vegetables
Molybdenum	Helps process proteins	Legumes, grains, leafy vegetables, nuts
Selenium	Protects cells from damage; regulates thyroid hormone action	Vegetables, fish, red meat, grains, eggs, chicken
Zinc	Assists immune, nervous, and reproductive system functions	Beef, pork, lamb, nuts, whole grains

Figure 7.9 Minerals are considered either major minerals or trace minerals. Your body needs major minerals in larger quantities than trace minerals. *Which minerals help build strong teeth and bones?*

the minerals your body needs. Two very important minerals are iron and calcium. The body needs *iron* so that blood cells can carry oxygen throughout the body. It needs *calcium* to build bones and teeth.

Water

Water is necessary for the body to work properly and remain healthy. In fact, although people can live for several weeks, and even months, without taking in food, they can survive only a few days without water.

Your body loses water every day through urination, sweat, and exhalation. For this reason, you need to take in water to replace what your body loses to prevent dehydration. *Dehydration* is a dangerous condition in which the body's tissues lose too much water.

People should drink 8½ to 11½ cups of fluids per day to have enough water in the body. Normally, most people can be sure to have enough water in their body simply by drinking when they are thirsty (**Figure 7.10**).

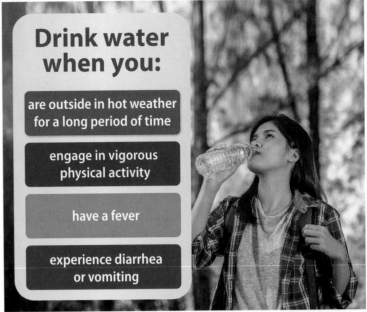

Sunti/Shutterstock.com

Figure 7.10 In certain situations you may need to drink more water for the body to function properly. *What is the name of the condition in which the body's tissues lose too much water?*

Lesson 7.1 Review

1. Sugars are _____ carbohydrates and starches are _____ carbohydrates.
2. **True or false.** Most people in the United States eat less protein than they should.
3. List three common fats in the diet.
4. People should drink _____ to _____ cups of fluids each day to have enough water in the body.
5. **Critical thinking.** What health benefits does dietary fiber provide your body?

Hands-On Activity

Create a plan for your school cafeteria to include healthier food options. For each option you suggest, identify the nutrient(s) the food provides and why these nutrients are important for middle school students. Upon completion, present your plan to the class. Then, as a class, design a plan to advocate for healthier food options.

Following a Healthy Eating Pattern

Dietary Guidelines United States government recommendations for forming patterns of eating that will promote health

nutrient-dense foods foods that are rich in needed nutrients and have little or no solid fats, added sugars, refined starches, and sodium

MyPlate food guidance system United States government system that helps people put the *Dietary Guidelines* into practice

malnutrition condition that results from people not eating the right amounts of nutrients

undernutrition condition that results from people not taking in enough nutrients for health and growth

overnutrition condition that results from people eating too many foods that contain high amounts of added sugar, solid fat, sodium, refined carbohydrates, or too many calories

Learning Outcomes

After studying this lesson, you will be able to

- **explain** the key concepts from the *Dietary Guidelines for Americans*.
- **describe** how poor nutrition can impact health.
- **summarize** recommendations from the MyPlate food guidance system.
- **determine** steps to take to make healthy food choices.

Graphic Organizer

Food Benefits

Think about what you will be eating for lunch today. Fill in a MyPlate graphic organizer like the one shown based on the ingredients of that meal. Do you have foods in every category? Are all your choices nutrient-dense foods? If not, use a different color pen to cross out any foods that are not nutrient dense. Note any foods you could add to or remove from the meal to ensure that it fulfills the nutrition guidelines.

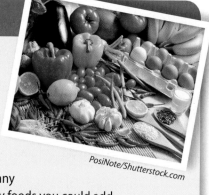

PosiNote/Shutterstock.com

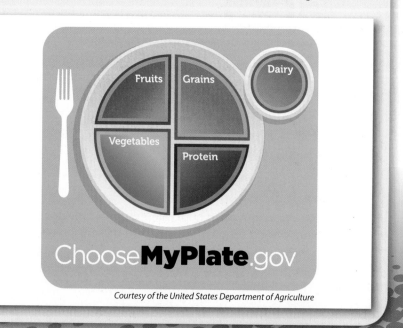

ChooseMyPlate.gov

Courtesy of the United States Department of Agriculture

When you eat healthy foods today, you lower your risk of developing health conditions later in life. These may include heart disease, high blood pressure, type 2 diabetes, stroke, and cancer.

Rei, from the first lesson, helps her dad cook in the kitchen after school almost every day. She is learning what healthy foods to eat and what foods to avoid. Rei understands that an eating pattern full of healthy foods is important for maintaining good health.

In this lesson, you will learn how to make smart food choices and create a balanced eating pattern. You will also learn about the hazards of poor nutrition.

Guidelines for Forming a Healthy Eating Pattern

A healthy eating pattern includes foods that supply the amounts and types of nutrients your body needs to be healthy. Knowing which nutrients your body needs and in what amounts will help you get adequate nutrition.

The United States Departments of Agriculture (USDA) and Health and Human Services (HHS) publish the *Dietary Guidelines for Americans* to help people make good food choices. The USDA and HHS revise these guidelines every five years to make sure the guidelines reflect the most recent research. The **Dietary Guidelines** provides recommendations for forming eating patterns that will promote health (**Figure 7.11**).

A healthy eating pattern requires that the foods you choose are nutrient dense. The *Dietary Guidelines* defines **nutrient-dense foods** as foods that are rich in needed nutrients and have little or no solid fats, added sugars, refined starches, and sodium.

Figure 7.11
The *Dietary Guidelines* are based on nutrition principles that can help make and keep people healthy.

Key Concepts Promoted by the *Dietary Guidelines*

1. Follow a healthy eating pattern throughout your life.

2. Focus on the variety, nutrient density, and the amount of the foods you eat.

3. Limit how much added sugar, saturated fats, and sodium is in your food.

4. Shift to healthier food and beverage choices.

5. Support healthy patterns of eating for others you know.

The added sugars and solid fats found in some foods are called *empty calories*. These sugars and fats are called *empty calories* because they supply few, if any, nutrients to a person's diet.

Calories are a measure of the energy in a given amount of food. It is not bad to eat calories—as long as they come in nutrient-dense foods. Of course, even these good, healthy foods can be harmful to your health if you eat too much of them at a time.

MyPlate Food Guidance System

In 2011, the USDA created the **MyPlate food guidance system** to help people put the *Dietary Guidelines* into practice. The MyPlate graphic is designed to remind people about the proportion of different foods they should eat at a meal (**Figure 7.12**).

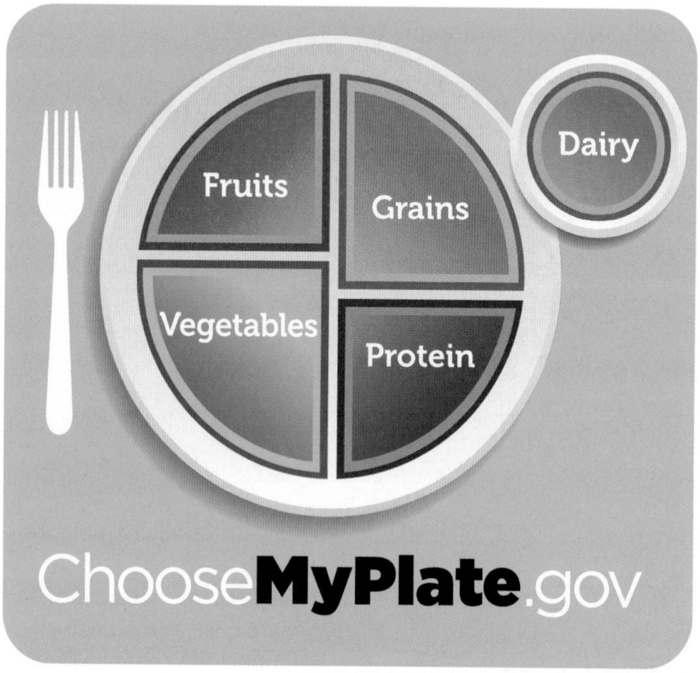

Courtesy of the United States Department of Agriculture

Figure 7.12 MyPlate illustrates the recommended proportions of the different food groups that people should eat in a day. *How does your daily diet align with these suggestions? What food groups should you eat more, or less, of?*

Food Groups

The MyPlate graphic includes the five food groups: fruits, vegetables, grains, protein foods, and dairy. Oils are not included on the MyPlate graphic because oils are not considered a food group. Oils are, however, a necessary part of a healthful diet.

Fruits

Foods in the fruits group are often good sources of fiber, vitamins, and minerals that many diets lack. These foods can be high in vitamin C and folic acid (a B vitamin). Some are rich in the mineral potassium. Fresh, frozen, canned, and dried fruits, as well as fruit juices, are included in this group.

Grains

The grains group includes foods made from wheat, rice, oats, cornmeal, barley, or other cereal grains. Grains provide carbohydrates, vitamins and minerals, and some amino acids. Foods in the grains group are either whole grains or refined grains.

Whole grains contain the entire grain kernel (**Figure 7.13**). *Refined grains* have been processed to produce a finer texture and improved shelf life, and no longer contain the whole kernel. Examples of whole grains are brown rice, oatmeal, whole-wheat bread, and wild rice. Examples of refined grains include couscous, crackers, and white bread.

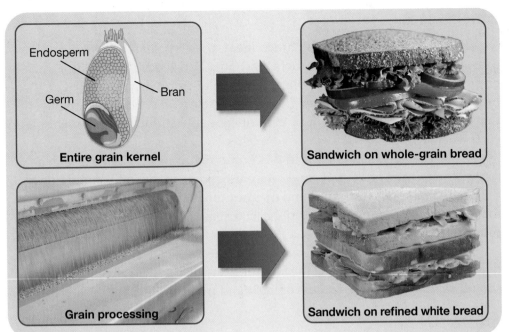

Figure 7.13
Foods that contain the entire grain kernel—the bran, germ, and endosperm—are considered whole grains. During processing, the germ and fiber-rich bran layer present in whole grains are often removed. Foods that do not contain the entire grain kernel are refined grains. *Which of the sandwiches pictured to the left is healthier, and why?*

Left to right: Tefi/Shutterstock.com; Brent Hofacker/Shutterstock.com; Pavel Chagochkin/Shutterstock.com; aperturesound/Shutterstock.com

Vegetables

Most foods in the vegetables group are naturally low in fat and calories. They are important sources of many nutrients such as potassium, fiber, folic acid, and vitamins A and C. Vegetables come in many types and are often very nutrient dense (**Figure 7.14**). Vegetables may be fresh, frozen, canned, dried, raw, cooked, whole, cut up, or juiced.

Dairy

The dairy group includes many foods that are high in calcium. Examples of these foods are milk and milk products, such as cheese and yogurt. You should choose foods in this group that are low-fat or fat-free options. Dairy foods are often good sources of potassium and protein. Many are fortified with vitamin D, which helps the body use calcium.

Calcium-fortified coconut, soy, rice, almond, and cashew milks are included in the dairy group as options for people who are lactose intolerant. *Lactose* is a sugar found in cow's milk. Some people have difficulty digesting milk that has this sugar. In addition to calcium-fortified milk alternatives, people can drink lactose-free cow's milk.

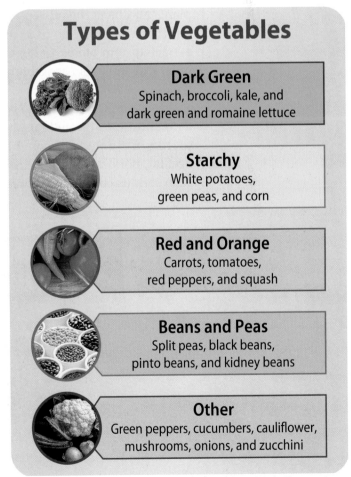

Types of Vegetables

Dark Green
Spinach, broccoli, kale, and dark green and romaine lettuce

Starchy
White potatoes, green peas, and corn

Red and Orange
Carrots, tomatoes, red peppers, and squash

Beans and Peas
Split peas, black beans, pinto beans, and kidney beans

Other
Green peppers, cucumbers, cauliflower, mushrooms, onions, and zucchini

Dark Green: Enlightened Media/Shutterstock.com; Starchy: Brian Mueller/Shutterstock.com; Red and Orange: Gregory Gerber/Shutterstock.com; Beans and Peas: Amawasri Pakdara/Shutterstock.com; Other: Obraz/Shutterstock.com

Figure 7.14 A healthy eating pattern includes eating a variety of vegetable types each week.

Protein Foods

The protein foods group includes meat, poultry, seafood, beans and peas, eggs, processed soy products, and nuts and seeds. Including a variety of protein foods in your meal plan each week improves your nutrient intake and supplies health benefits. The *Dietary Guidelines* recommend that you include at least eight ounces of cooked seafood in your meal plan each week.

In addition to protein, foods in this group may supply vitamins such as niacin, thiamin, riboflavin, B_6, and vitamin E. Some foods in this group have the needed minerals iron, zinc, and magnesium. Some seafood contains fats that may work to reduce the risk of heart disease (**Figure 7.15**). Plant-based proteins are often rich in fiber.

Some animal-based proteins are high in saturated fats. As you have read, these substances may increase the risk for heart disease. For this reason, you should select lean or low-fat cuts of meat and poultry.

Oils

Oils are not considered a food group, but they do provide essential nutrients and must be included in your diet. Oils are naturally present in many plants and fish. The oil is often extracted from a food source and sold as liquid oil. These oils are then used for cooking or flavoring. For instance, olive oil is extracted from olives. Other examples are corn oil and canola oil. Avocados, nuts, and some fish are common sources of oils that are typically included in the diet.

Because they are unsaturated fats, oils are usually liquid at room temperature. Saturated fats, however, are not oils and come from animal sources. Saturated fats commonly found in the diet include butter, milk fat, beef fat, pork fat, and poultry fat. Saturated fat in the diet may contribute to such serious conditions as heart disease.

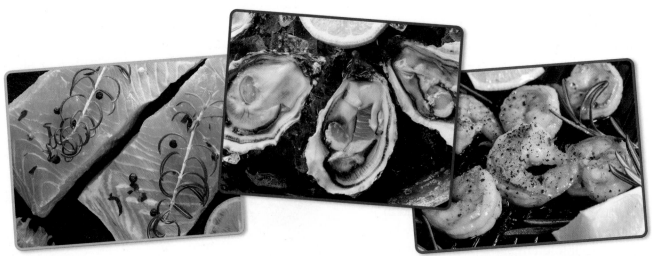

Figure 7.15 According to the MyPlate guidelines, eating about eight ounces of seafood each week can help prevent heart disease. Some popular nutrient-dense seafood choices include salmon, oysters, and shrimp. *Do you get enough seafood in your diet each week?*

Recommended Amounts

The MyPlate food guidance system provides tools to help you develop a personalized daily checklist that shows what and how much you should be eating. This daily checklist outlines the amounts you should consume from each food group (**Figure 7.16**). It also provides information to help you choose nutrient-dense foods.

The amount of food you need from each of the food groups is affected by several factors. These factors include age, sex, height, weight, and level of physical activity.

Nutrition for People Who Are Pregnant

People who are pregnant have special nutritional needs. They have to meet these needs for their own health and for the health of the baby they are carrying.

People who are pregnant or breast-feeding should avoid seafood that is high in mercury. Examples are shark, swordfish, tilefish, and King mackerel. They should also limit canned white tuna (albacore) to less than six ounces per week.

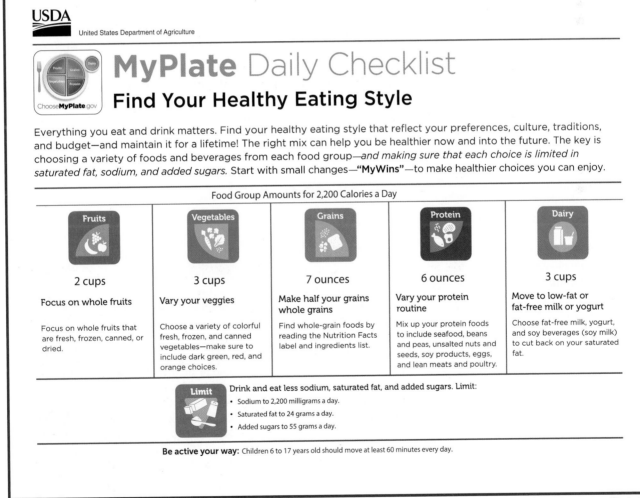

Courtesy of the United States Department of Agriculture

Figure 7.16 Depending on your age, sex, height, and weight, the MyPlate Daily Checklist provides tips for getting the right amount of the best foods for your health.

Poor Nutrition

A healthy eating pattern is an important part of maintaining your health and reducing your risk for certain diseases. A healthy eating pattern can also help you avoid health risks related to poor nutrition, or malnutrition. **Malnutrition** is a condition that results from people not eating the right amounts of nutrients. Undernutrition and overnutrition are forms of malnutrition (**Figure 7.17**).

Undernutrition

One form of malnutrition is undernutrition. **Undernutrition** is a condition that results from people not taking in enough nutrients for health and growth.

Healthy eating is especially important for children and teens. The bodies of children and teens undergo a large amount of growth and development. Children and teens need to be sure to get enough nutrients for that growth and development to be healthy. Children who do not receive enough nutrients may never reach their full height. Undernutrition can also lead to serious and even life-threatening health conditions. Examples are brain damage, vision impairments and blindness, and bone deformities.

Overnutrition

Although many people think about poor nutrition in terms of not getting *enough* nutrients, it can also be caused by eating *too much* of some nutrients. This type of **overnutrition** is often a result of eating too many foods that contain high amounts of added sugar, solid fat, sodium, refined grains, or simply too many calories.

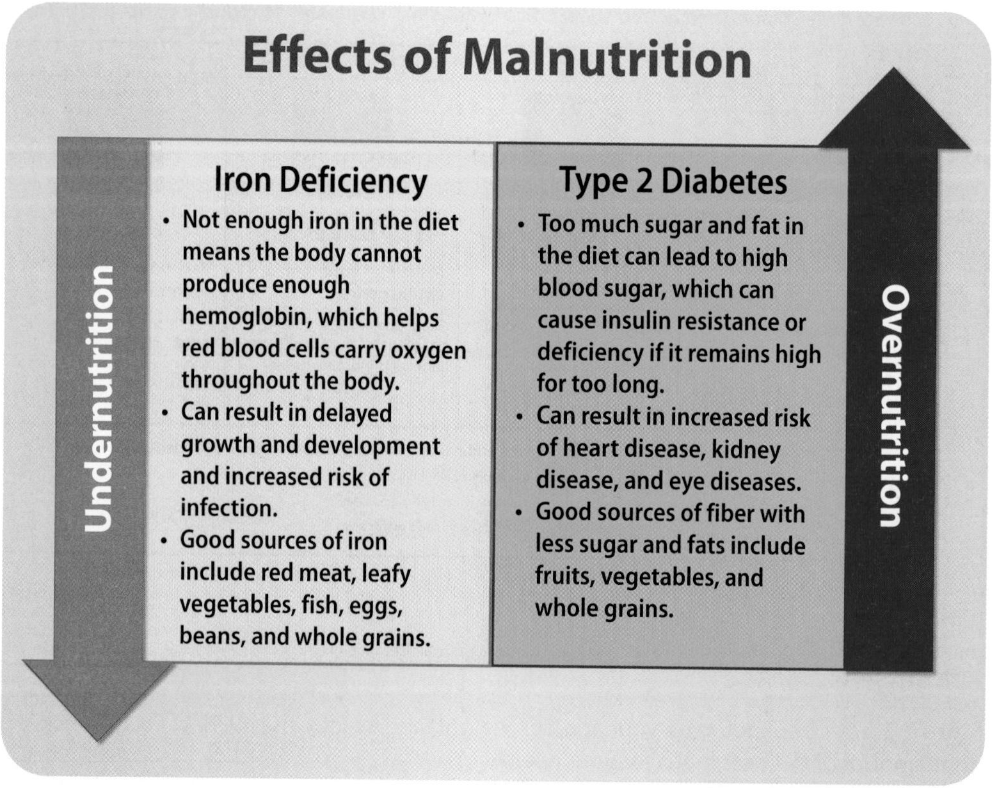

Figure 7.17
Poor nutrition can involve not getting enough of the nutrients your body needs, or getting way more of certain nutrients than your body needs. *What is another name for foods that are rich in needed nutrients and have little or no solid fats, added sugars, refined starches, or sodium?*

Effects of Malnutrition

Undernutrition

Iron Deficiency
- Not enough iron in the diet means the body cannot produce enough hemoglobin, which helps red blood cells carry oxygen throughout the body.
- Can result in delayed growth and development and increased risk of infection.
- Good sources of iron include red meat, leafy vegetables, fish, eggs, beans, and whole grains.

Type 2 Diabetes
- Too much sugar and fat in the diet can lead to high blood sugar, which can cause insulin resistance or deficiency if it remains high for too long.
- Can result in increased risk of heart disease, kidney disease, and eye diseases.
- Good sources of fiber with less sugar and fats include fruits, vegetables, and whole grains.

Overnutrition

Foods high in solid fats, added sugars, refined grains, and sodium are believed to be linked to a variety of health conditions. For instance, as the amount of sodium a person consumes goes down, so does the person's blood pressure. Maintaining a normal blood pressure reduces the risk of heart and kidney diseases.

Skills for Following a Healthy Eating Pattern

To maintain your health, you should follow a healthy eating pattern. The requirements for a healthy eating pattern change across a person's life span. Today, you have different nutritional needs than you did when you were a child. Your nutritional needs also will continue to change as you grow older. The skills in the following sections can help you follow a healthy eating pattern.

BUILDING Your Skills

Making Healthy Food Choices

Following a healthy eating pattern involves making healthy food choices. The foods you choose to eat are important and can have a great effect on your body. Foods nourish your body and help it function properly. Foods give you the energy you need to complete all of your daily activities. Foods can affect all aspects of your physical and mental health.

Many resources are available to help you make healthy food choices. For example, apps are available for tracking food and water intake, setting nutrition goals, and even analyzing food patterns. You can also use online databases to find the nutrient contents of foods.

Evaluating Your Food Choices

For two days, keep track of all the foods, beverages, and amounts you eat. Find a food tracker app to use to record these foods, beverages, and amounts or use a table similar to the one shown. Then, answer the questions to help evaluate your food choices. Set SMART goals to help you improve in areas where you could make healthier choices.

1. Of the foods you ate, which ones were nutrient-dense foods?

2. How did your food choices compare with the MyPlate daily recommendations? Explain.

3. Did you make mostly healthy choices? In what areas do you need to improve?

Daily Food Choices Tracking Form		
Meal or Snack	Day 1—Food/Beverage Amounts	Day 2—Food/Beverage Amounts
Breakfast		
Morning snack		
Lunch		
Afternoon snack		
Dinner		
Evening snack		

Choosing Nutrient-Dense Foods

A healthy eating pattern includes a variety of nutrient-dense foods in appropriate amounts. The foods you eat should provide vitamins, minerals, and other substances that either contribute to adequate nutrient intake or have positive health effects. Nutrient-dense foods have little or no saturated fats, added sugars (sugars that do not occur naturally in foods), refined starches, or sodium (salt). **Figure 7.18** shows ways you can include more nutrient-dense foods in your eating pattern.

Limit Added Sugars, Saturated Fats, and Sodium

Consuming too much added sugars, saturated fats, and sodium can increase risk for heart diseases, obesity, and type 2 diabetes. People should consume less than 10 percent of their calories from added sugars and less than 10 percent of their calories from saturated fats. People should also limit sodium intake to no more than 2,300 milligrams per day and ideally no more than 1,500 milligrams. To compare, most people in the United States consume more than 3,400 milligrams each day.

Eating Breakfast Every Day

Eating a nutritious breakfast every day is very important. People need a morning meal to give them energy, improve concentration, and help provide the nutrients they need to grow. To put together a nutritious breakfast, use whole grains, lean protein foods (like eggs, lean meat, or nuts), low-fat dairy products, and fruits and vegetables. For example, you might make a smoothie, oatmeal with fruit, or a whole-grain tortilla with vegetables and salsa.

Figure 7.18
Following these guidelines can help you include more nutrient-dense foods in your eating pattern.

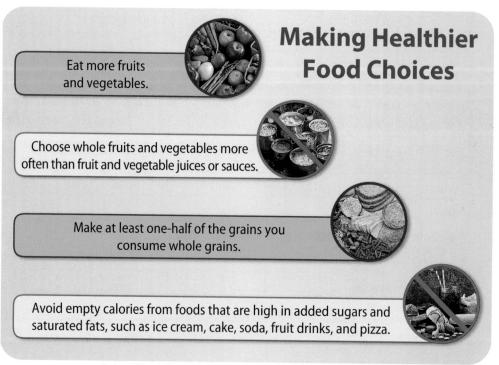

Making Healthier Food Choices

Eat more fruits and vegetables.

Choose whole fruits and vegetables more often than fruit and vegetable juices or sauces.

Make at least one-half of the grains you consume whole grains.

Avoid empty calories from foods that are high in added sugars and saturated fats, such as ice cream, cake, soda, fruit drinks, and pizza.

Fruits and Vegetables: Teri Virbickis/Shutterstock.com; Canned Food: Artem Shadrin/Shutterstock.com; Grains: Stephen Cook Photography/Shutterstock.com; Unhealthy Food: beats1/Shutterstock.com

Understanding Nutrition Facts and Food Labels

To help consumers make good choices about what they eat, the FDA requires any food sold in a package to include a *Nutrition Facts label* (**Figure 7.19**). Nutrition Facts labels show the nutrients in each serving of the food. They also indicate how much of the recommended daily value of that nutrient is in the serving. The information on these labels is scientifically tested and proven so you can rely on it.

Sometimes food packages describe a particular food using a specific claim about its health benefits. For example, a food label might describe a food as "low-fat" or "organic." *Organic* foods are those produced without the use of chemical fertilizers, pesticides, or other artificial chemicals. To use these terms, the food must meet certain criteria established by the FDA and USDA.

Some foods come from *genetically modified organisms (GMOs)*. GMOs are living things that have undergone changes to genetic material (DNA). This technology allows the transfer of certain genes from one organism to another. The goal is to create plants and crops with more resistance to disease, more nutritional benefits, and better taste. Foods produced using this technique are often called *GMO foods*. *Non-GMO foods* are those without genetically modified ingredients. Many countries require the labeling of GMO foods so people know whether the foods they buy have been altered.

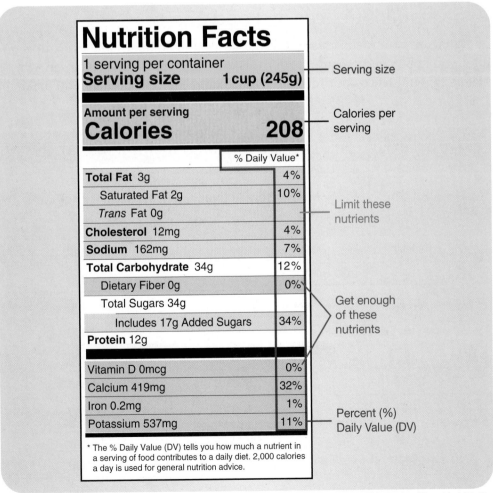

Figure 7.19
A Nutrition Facts label provides information about serving size, calories, nutrients, and how this food can fit into a person's daily eating plan. *Look at the nutrition label on one of your favorite snacks. What is the nutrition value of the item?*

Courtesy of the Food and Drug Administration

Thinking About Calories

Along with nutrients, health experts also look at the calories in food. Remember that calories show the food energy in a food. The number of calories a person should eat each day depends on three factors. These factors include sex, age, and level of physical activity. Generally, males need more calories than females and physically active people need more calories than those who are not active. Adults between the ages of 19 and 30 typically need more calories than middle-aged and older adults need. In fact, adults ages 51 and over need the least number of calories. **Figure 7.20** shows the recommended daily calorie intake for males and females ages 10 through 65.

Eating Healthy Meals Away from Home

You can also make healthy food choices when eating away from home. Start by getting information about the nutrients in restaurant food. Many popular chain restaurants publish information about the nutrients in their foods. People going out to eat can look up this information online. Armed with the facts, they can make healthy food choices.

Some companies that provide food for school lunches also provide nutrition information. You can use this information to make healthy choices. Remember to choose nutrient-dense food options in school.

Analyzing Influences on Food Choices

What are your favorite foods? What tastes do you like? How difficult is it for you to buy and prepare fresh fruits and vegetables? Understanding the factors that influence your food preferences and choices will help you make

Figure 7.20
The amount of calories a person needs to eat during a day depends on many factors, including age and sex. *What is the third factor that can impact how many calories a person should eat each day?*

	Recommended Daily Calorie Intake	
	Male **Moderately Active**	**Female** **Moderately Active**
Age	**Calories**	
10	1,800	1,800
11	2,000	1,800
12–13	2,200	2,000
14	2,400	2,000
15	2,600	2,000
16–18	2,800	2,000
19–25	2,800	2,200
26–45	2,600	2,000
46–50	2,400	2,000
51–65	2,400	1,800

healthy decisions. Your *food preferences* are your opinions about different types of food. **Figure 7.21** shows internal and external factors that influence these preferences.

In addition to food preferences, the availability of food also affects your food choices. A person's income level can affect the variety of food available in a community and in the home. If nutritious foods are not easily available, or if the community has lots of fast-food options, people may find it more difficult to make healthy choices. Most communities have programs and services to help people with low incomes obtain nutritious foods. Some examples of these services are food banks and the Supplemental Nutrition Assistance Program (SNAP).

Knowing what influences affect your food choices can help you identify why you want certain foods. You can then determine whether acting on that desire is a healthy choice. For example, if you are feeling stressed and want to eat ice cream, understanding that mood affects your appetite can help you counteract that craving. You can then choose a healthier, more nutritious option.

Preparing Nutritious Foods

One of the best strategies for making nutritious food choices is preparing your own food. Preparing your own food has many benefits (**Figure 7.22**). For example, when you prepare food at home, you know exactly what ingredients you are using. This makes it easier to limit certain substances and follow a healthy eating pattern.

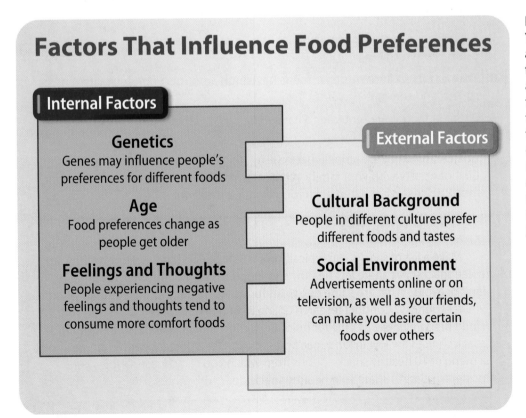

Factors That Influence Food Preferences

Internal Factors

Genetics
Genes may influence people's preferences for different foods

Age
Food preferences change as people get older

Feelings and Thoughts
People experiencing negative feelings and thoughts tend to consume more comfort foods

External Factors

Cultural Background
People in different cultures prefer different foods and tastes

Social Environment
Advertisements online or on television, as well as your friends, can make you desire certain foods over others

Figure 7.21
Your food preferences are influenced by internal factors such as genetics, age, and feelings and thoughts. External factors that may influence your food preferences include cultural background and social environment. *What are some of your favorite foods? How could these factors have influenced your preferences?*

Benefits of Preparing Your Own Food

- Costs less
- Can be made in 30 minutes or less
- Can freeze leftovers to eat later
- Can prepare meals ahead of time
- Is healthier
- Counts as a physical activity
- Can control portion sizes and ingredients used

Figure 7.22 Some of the many benefits of preparing food at home include healthier meals and control over portion sizes and ingredients.

Practicing Food Safety

Sometimes, foods can harm your health if they are not handled and prepared safely. *Food safety*, or safe food handling and preparation, can prevent most foodborne illnesses. *Foodborne illnesses*, or *food poisoning*, refer to illnesses transmitted by foods. Following are food safety strategies you can use to help prevent foodborne illnesses:

- Wash your hands with hot, soapy water for at least 20 seconds before cooking and eating and after handling uncooked meat and poultry.
- Wash counters, tables, dishes, and eating utensils with hot, soapy water.
- Keep hot foods hot (above 140 degrees Fahrenheit) and keep cold foods cold (below 40 degrees Fahrenheit).
- Cook foods to the appropriate temperature.
- Wash fruits and vegetables before preparing them.
- Thaw foods in a refrigerator or microwave. Cook meat or poultry immediately after thawing in a microwave.
- Refrigerate and freeze perishable food and leftovers promptly.
- Wash cooking equipment, utensils, and surfaces after each use.

Lesson 7.2 Review

1. What publication provides recommendations for forming patterns of eating that will promote health?
2. Eating too many foods that contain high amounts of added sugar, sodium, or calories can result in _____.
3. **True or false.** Nutrient-dense foods have high amounts of protein, vitamins, sugars, and sodium.
4. Packaged foods are required to have a _____ _____ label that shows the nutrients in each serving of the food.
5. **Critical thinking.** Describe what healthy food choices you can make at a birthday party with your family. What internal factors might play a role in your food choices? What external factors might be present?

Hands-On Activity

Make a list of snacks you typically like to eat during the day. How healthy are these snacks? Are there less healthy snack options on your list that you should limit or avoid? What are some nutritious foods you could snack on instead when you feel hungry? Conduct research online to find healthy snack ideas that you could prepare ahead of time for quick on-the-go snacks. Make sure that your snack choices are low in fat, sugar, and sodium. Use a poster board to create a menu of 10 healthy snack options from which you can choose. Display your posters in class to share your healthy snack ideas with others.

Managing Your Weight

Learning Outcomes

After studying this lesson, you will be able to

- **describe** ways to determine ideal body weight.
- **explain** how weight affects a person's health.
- **identify** healthy weight-management strategies.

Key Terms

body composition ratio of the various components—fat, bone, and muscle—that make up a person's body

body mass index (BMI) tool used to determine whether a person's weight is healthy for that person's height; BMI = weight (lbs.)/height (in.)$^2 \times 703$

overweight condition of excess body weight from fat, bone, muscle, water, or a combination of these factors

obesity condition of excess body fat or excessive overweight

underweight condition of a body weight that is too low compared with others of the same sex and age

body-fat distribution location of fat deposits on a person's body

fad diets stylish weight-loss plans that promise significant weight loss in short periods of time, often through cutting out food groups or buying premade meals

Graphic Organizer

Healthy Weight Management

As you read this lesson, use a table similar to the one shown to list the strategies for healthy weight management. Then, write one or more summary statements that briefly describes the strategy. Put an asterisk next to the strategy or strategies you believe are most effective. Then, put a check mark next to those you would likely do. Think about other strategies you might use for healthy weight management and add them to your list. An example is provided for you.

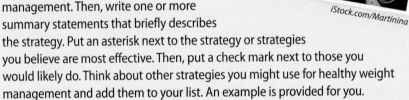
iStock.com/Martinina

Strategies	Summary Statements
Think positively	Remember that permanent change takes time and that everyone has brief slip-ups.

Many people in the United States have difficulty managing their weight. In recent years, rates of obesity in the United States doubled for adults and tripled for children. Approximately 18 percent of children and adolescents, from 2 to 19 years of age, are affected by obesity. As you learn more about this topic, you will understand that weight management is a complex and sensitive issue.

Rei, from the previous lessons, sometimes wishes she weighed more than she actually does. She wants to gain muscle like the professional softball players she watches on TV. When Rei says this to her dad, he tells her that she should not compare her weight to the weight of others. He says that her ideal weight is the weight at which her body is healthy.

Do you agree with Rei's dad's advice? In this lesson, you will learn about what is considered a healthy weight. You will discover how weight affects your health. You will also learn some strategies for weight management.

What Is a Healthy Weight?

Do you ever wish you weighed more or less than you actually do? Do you ever compare your weight to the weight of someone else? Sometimes comparisons with other people influence people's beliefs about how much they should weigh. Perhaps you want to weigh what a friend weighs or what your favorite celebrity or athlete weighs. Comparing your weight to the weight of another person, however, is a bad idea. Your ideal weight is the weight at which *your* body is healthy.

Several factors impact the ideal weight for your body (**Figure 7.23**). Because of these factors, people use several approaches to identify healthy weight ranges. Some of these approaches include the following:

- body composition
- body mass index (BMI)
- body-fat distribution

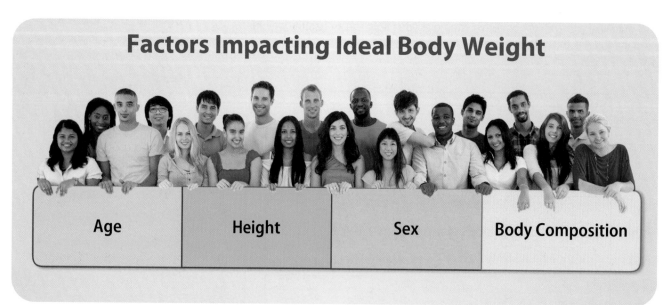

Factors Impacting Ideal Body Weight

| Age | Height | Sex | Body Composition |

Figure 7.23 Ideal body weight differs from one person to the next. Remember to show respect for everyone you meet and to appreciate the differences among people.

Body Composition

Body composition is the ratio of the various components—fat, bone, and muscle—that make up your body. The size and shape of two people who weigh the same, but differ in body composition, can be very different. Genetics, eating patterns, and level of physical activity influence a person's body composition (**Figure 7.24**).

To better understand the concept of body composition, try to envision a brick of metal in comparison to a brick of Styrofoam® of the same size. The metal weighs much more than the Styrofoam. In the same way that metal weighs more than Styrofoam, muscle and bone weigh more than fat. As such, a person with a higher ratio of muscle to fat will weigh more than a person of the same size with a lower ratio of muscle to fat.

Body composition is an important factor in weight. For example, a person may weigh more than others due to being more muscular, not due to being affected by overweight. Athletes often train for long hours, which builds muscle and increases bone density. As a result, athletes often have much lower body-fat averages than nonathletes, even though they may weigh as much or more (**Figure 7.25**).

A person's sex also affects body composition. Male bodies tend to have more muscle than those of females. Female bodies tend to have a greater proportion of fat. On average, adult males have a body-fat percentage of 15 percent and adult females have a body-fat percentage of 25 percent. Females have a higher percentage of body fat than males to support their role in reproduction.

Factors That Influence Body Composition

Genetics
- How much body fat you have and where it is located
- Body type and structure

Eating Patterns
- How much food you eat
- What types of food you eat

Physical Activity
- What types of activities you do
- How much time you spend doing those activities

Figure 7.24 Your body composition is influenced by your genetics, eating patterns, and physical activity.

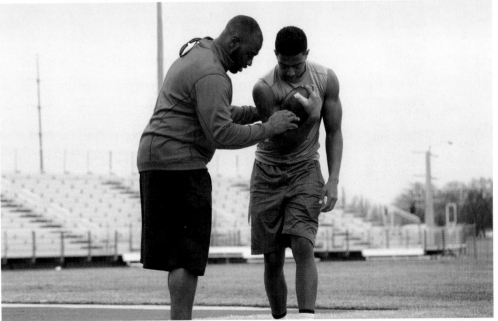

Figure 7.25 Athletes tend to have lower body-fat percentages than nonathletes due to their increased physical activity, muscle content, and bone density. *What is the term for the ratio of fat, bone, and muscle that make up the body?*

iStock.com/digitalskillet

Body Mass Index (BMI)

Body mass index (BMI) is a tool for assessing an individual's weight status. This index is calculated by dividing a person's weight in pounds by height in inches squared. This number is then multiplied by a factor of 703 (**Figure 7.26**).

BMI is calculated in the same way for children, teens, and adults. The resulting number, however, receives different interpretation for different age groups. Because children and teens are still growing, their BMI values are plotted on growth charts based on age and sex. The BMI percentile for children and teens indicates the relative position of the person's BMI compared with others of the same sex and age. (See the *Appendix* in the back of this book to view the BMI charts for boys and girls.)

For children and teens, the Centers for Disease Control and Prevention (CDC) defines **overweight** as having, for a particular height, excess body weight from fat, bone, muscle, water, or a combination of these factors. The CDC defines **obesity** as having excess body fat or excessive overweight. According to the CDC, children and teens who are affected by **underweight** have a body weight that is too low compared with others of the same sex and age. For adults, these weight categories are based on specific BMI values.

BMI calculation is an easy method for assessing weight status, but it is not perfect. For some individuals, BMI is not accurate due to differences in body composition. Because muscle and bone weigh more than fat, people who are highly fit or muscular may have a high BMI, which incorrectly places them in the overweight category. Likewise, an individual may have a body weight in the acceptable range, but a high percentage of body fat to muscle. BMI would inaccurately place this person in the healthy range.

Figure 7.26
The formula for calculating BMI can help indicate if you are within a healthy weight range for your age, sex, and height.

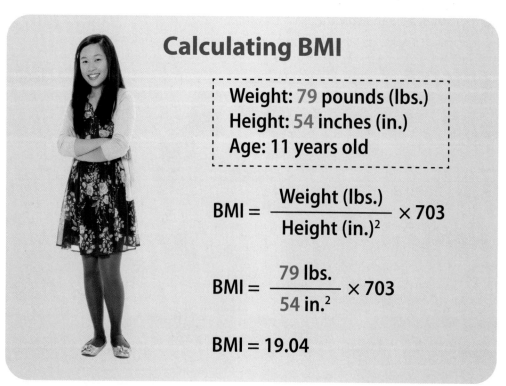

Calculating BMI

Weight: 79 pounds (lbs.)
Height: 54 inches (in.)
Age: 11 years old

$$BMI = \frac{Weight\ (lbs.)}{Height\ (in.)^2} \times 703$$

$$BMI = \frac{79\ lbs.}{54\ in.^2} \times 703$$

$$BMI = 19.04$$

iStock.com/JohnnyGreig

Body-Fat Distribution

Another factor that influences ideal body weight is **body-fat distribution**, or the location of fat deposits on your body (**Figure 7.27**). Body-fat distribution can be as important, if not more important, to your health as how much fat you have. One method for assessing body-fat distribution is to measure your waist size. This measurement is simple to obtain and can be an indicator of excess abdominal fat. You can also use this measurement to monitor your progress toward meeting weight-management goals.

For those affected by overweight, distribution of fat on the body is often a better predictor of physical consequences than actual weight, BMI, or total body fat. People who have *metabolic syndrome* have extra fat around the waist and high blood pressure, blood sugar, and cholesterol levels. This can lead to a greater risk of developing heart disease, stroke, and type 2 diabetes. Males are more likely than females to store fat in the abdomen, which also increases risk for heart disease.

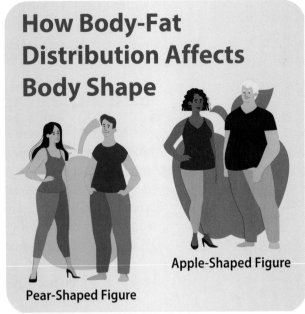

How Body-Fat Distribution Affects Body Shape

Apple-Shaped Figure

Pear-Shaped Figure

Body Shapes: Inspiring/Shutterstock.com; Apple: Fine Art/Shutterstock.com; Pear: Arcady/Shutterstock.com

Figure 7.27 People with apple-shaped figures tend to store extra fat around their waist, or abdomen, and chest. People with pear-shaped figures tend to store extra fat in their lower bodies around their hips, buttocks, and legs.

How Does Weight Affect Your Health?

Your weight has an impact on your health now and in the future. Underweight, overweight, and obesity can cause a variety of negative health consequences.

When people do not take in enough nutrients and experience underweight, they can develop skin, hair, or teeth conditions. They may also feel tired often and are more likely to get sick. This is because their bodies are less able to fight off infections.

Overweight or obesity leads to increased risk of heart disease. It also increases risk for developing high blood pressure, high cholesterol, and type 2 diabetes. In this disorder, the body is unable to utilize blood glucose properly. About 5,000 children under age 20 develop type 2 diabetes each year (**Figure 7.28**). People who are affected by overweight or obesity are more likely to experience respiratory, sleep, and joint conditions and may have trouble getting pregnant.

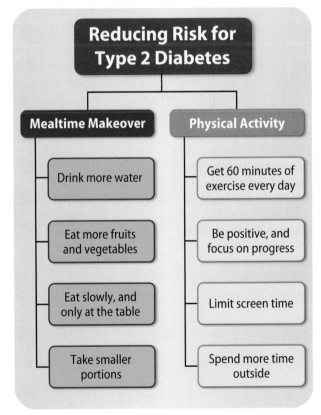

Reducing Risk for Type 2 Diabetes

Mealtime Makeover
- Drink more water
- Eat more fruits and vegetables
- Eat slowly, and only at the table
- Take smaller portions

Physical Activity
- Get 60 minutes of exercise every day
- Be positive, and focus on progress
- Limit screen time
- Spend more time outside

Figure 7.28 Making adjustments to your eating patterns and physical activity level can help reduce your risk for type 2 diabetes.

To avoid the health risks associated with underweight, overweight, and obesity, you need to know how to make good food choices and manage your weight in healthy ways.

Strategies for Healthy Weight Management

Making long-term changes to weight requires a permanent, lifelong change in eating and physical activity habits. To maintain your current weight, you must balance calories you consume with calories used during physical activity (**Figure 7.29**). To lose weight, you must consume fewer calories than you burn, and to gain weight, you must consume more calories. All of these activities require a healthy eating and physical activity plan that fits with your daily life. You can use several healthy strategies to lose, gain, or maintain your weight.

Set and Reward Realistic Goals

One very good strategy for healthy weight management is to set realistic, short-term goals regarding eating and physical activity. For example, you might decide to do the following:

- snack on nutritious foods between meals
- eat an apple instead of chips as a mid-morning pick-me-up
- go for a walk with a friend instead of watching television after school

Setting and meeting short-term goals allows you to feel good about having some success. It inspires you to feel more confident that you can achieve your longer-term goal for overall health. Also, be sure to reward yourself for meeting your short-term goals. For example, after successfully running three miles or substituting water for soda for one month, reward yourself with something you want to do. Avoid using food as a reward.

Figure 7.29
Your body naturally burns calories throughout the day just by keeping up with the functions of the body systems. Additional physical activity should help balance the amount of calories consumed in food and beverages throughout the day.

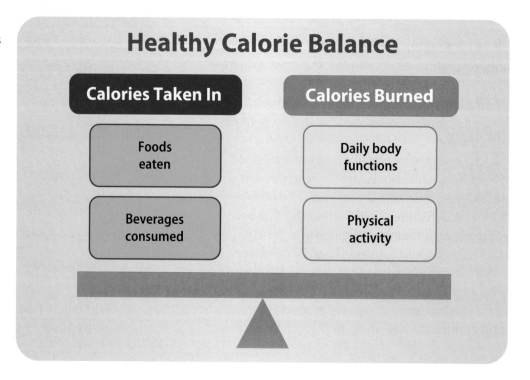

Limit Screen Time

People who spend many hours watching television or playing video games are more likely to be overweight or affected by obesity than those who spend less time in front of screens. In one study, the children and teens who said they have a television in their bedroom watched more TV each day than their peers. They were also more than twice as likely to show higher levels of body fat and larger waist sizes.

Develop a habit that calls on you to limit screentime and be active for a set period of time every day. Find a way to fit the activity into your schedule so you can be sure to do it. Avoid trying to do too much at the beginning. If your goal is to run a mile or two, you might need to build up to it. Try doing a combination of running and walking at first. This will help you develop the staying power to be active longer. Choosing physical activities you enjoy will help you be more likely to stay active. (**Figure 7.30**).

Think Positively

Another way to reach your goal is to think positively about your healthy eating and physical activity habits. First, remember that making permanent changes takes time. Do not attempt to make too many changes all at once. Changing habits gradually is more likely to ensure the habits become permanent. Second, remember that everyone who is trying to create new eating and activity habits will have some slip-ups or lapses. The important thing is to keep these lapses brief. Return to the new habits you are trying to adopt as quickly as possible.

Jacek Chabraszewski/Shutterstock.com

Figure 7.30
Doing physical activities that you enjoy, such as rollerblading, is a fun, healthy way to stay active.

Avoid Unhealthy Strategies

As many as 45 million adults in the United States diet each year. People spend a tremendous amount of money—an estimated $33 billion each year—on weight-loss programs and products. Although these programs and products are highly profitable for the people who sell them, they often promise more than they can deliver.

The amount of weight people lose using any of these programs tends to be small and temporary. As a result, most people who participate in weight-loss programs regain about one-third of any weight lost within one year and return to their initial weight within three to five years.

Some examples of unhealthy weight management are fad diets and the use of appetite suppressants. **Fad diets** often restrict certain types of food groups (such as carbohydrates) and may require the purchase of special, and often expensive, premade meals. The goal of these fad diets is to lose a large amount of weight in a short time. Unfortunately, these types of eating plans can result in muscle loss and nutritional deficits, which is dangerous to your health (**Figure 7.31**). In addition, people often quickly regain any weight lost because the habits that led to the initial weight gain did not change.

The Healthy Weight Journey

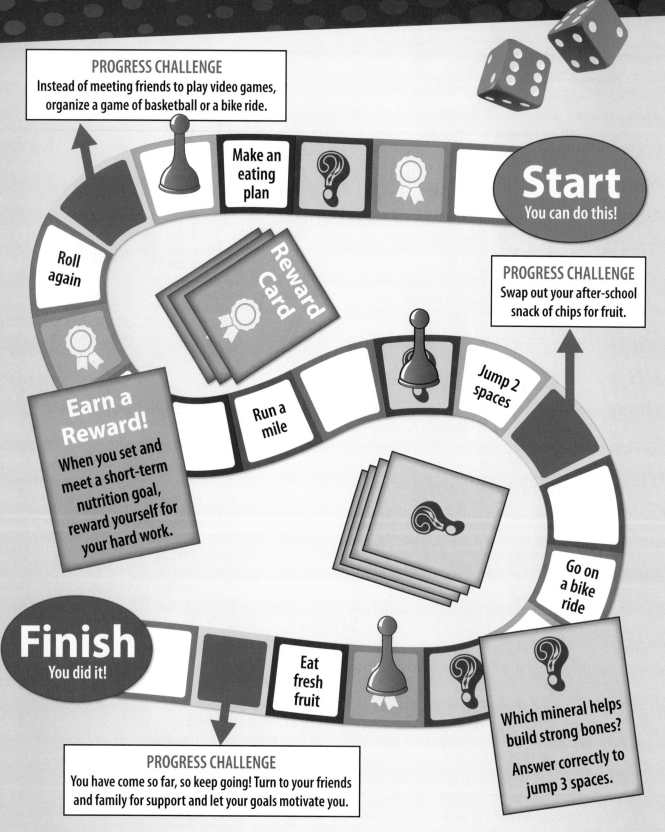

PROGRESS CHALLENGE
Instead of meeting friends to play video games, organize a game of basketball or a bike ride.

Start
You can do this!

Make an eating plan

PROGRESS CHALLENGE
Swap out your after-school snack of chips for fruit.

Roll again

Reward Card

Jump 2 spaces

Run a mile

Earn a Reward!
When you set and meet a short-term nutrition goal, reward yourself for your hard work.

Go on a bike ride

Finish
You did it!

Eat fresh fruit

Which mineral helps build strong bones?

Answer correctly to jump 3 spaces.

PROGRESS CHALLENGE
You have come so far, so keep going! Turn to your friends and family for support and let your goals motivate you.

Board game: EkaterinaP/Shutterstock.com; Pieces: JSlavy/Shutterstock.com; Dice: d-e-n-i-s/Shutterstock.com; Award: Classica2/Shutterstock.com

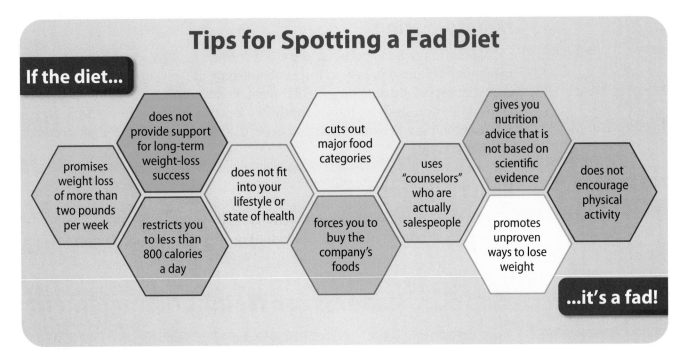

Tips for Spotting a Fad Diet

If the diet...

- promises weight loss of more than two pounds per week
- does not provide support for long-term weight-loss success
- restricts you to less than 800 calories a day
- does not fit into your lifestyle or state of health
- cuts out major food categories
- forces you to buy the company's foods
- uses "counselors" who are actually salespeople
- gives you nutrition advice that is not based on scientific evidence
- promotes unproven ways to lose weight
- does not encourage physical activity

...it's a fad!

Figure 7.31 Fad diets can be easily spotted due to characteristics such as cutting out major food groups and not encouraging physical activity.

Some people use appetite suppressants and diuretics as quick-fix strategies that lead to temporary, short-term weight loss. *Appetite suppressants* trick the body into believing that it is not hungry or that the stomach is full. These drugs increase levels of chemicals in the brain that affect mood and appetite. *Diuretics*, or *water pills*, help the body eliminate salt (sodium) and water, mostly through increased urination. Loss of water causes a drop in weight. The side effects of these drugs—including blurred vision, dizziness, sleeplessness, and irritability—can be so serious that people need medical treatment or hospitalization.

Eat Mindfully

The term *mindfulness* describes being fully focused on the present moment. You can eat mindfully by paying attention to the foods you eat. Mindful eating helps people make healthier food choices, since people focus on the foods they put into their bodies. **Figure 7.32** shows some strategies you can use to practice eating mindfully.

Strategies to Practice Eating Mindfully

Appreciate your food.
- Before starting to eat, take a minute to appreciate the food on your plate.
- Think about the work that went into bringing this food to the table.
- Recognize the different colors, smells, and textures of the food.

Portion out snacks instead of eating straight from the bag or box.

Take small bites so you can better savor the different flavors and tastes.
- Try to identify the different ingredients in each bite.
- Chew each mouthful thoroughly to really taste all the flavors.
- Put your utensils down between bites.
- Fully swallow your food before taking another bite.

Do not skip meals.
- It is hard to practice mindful eating when you are very hungry.
- Eat meals when you are hungry.
- Skipping meals can lead you to overeat just to get something into your stomach.

Figure 7.32 Making sure you take the time to appreciate your food and eat regularly are ways you can eat mindfully.

Monitor Eating

Monitoring when and what you eat is another healthy strategy for managing weight. It is easy to forget about some of the calories you take in each day, especially outside a regular meal. For example, you might eat potato chips while you study or have a candy bar as a quick after-school snack. One way to monitor when and what you eat is to keep a *food diary*, or daily record of what you eat.

Enlist Support

Changing eating and physical activity behaviors is difficult. Having support from others, however, can help (**Figure 7.33**). Simply having a friend

Figure 7.33
Some support systems for weight management include family support and physical activity support services.

Support Systems for Weight Management

Counseling and Psychotherapy Services

Patient-Led Groups	Commercial Groups	Other Community Resources
• Continuing support and encouragement • Most effective when used as a supplement	• Many programs available in communities and online • May offer support services such as workshops, meetings, and online tools	• Educational services in nutrition • Hospital staff dieticians

Family Support

• Participating in the program(s) together
• Making changes in food and eating patterns as a family
• Being encouraging

Online Services

• Access to support groups and commercial groups through their websites
• Social media groups
• Mobile apps that track weight management and overall health

Physical Activity Support Services

• Classes offered at the gym or personal trainers
• Weight management workout plans
• Fitness groups

who will go to the gym or go for walks with you can help (Figure 7.34). Tell friends and family members about your goal and ask them to support or join in your efforts. The best results occur when family members change their own eating habits and provide healthier foods in the home. You can talk to parents or guardians about changing the eating habits and types of foods offered at home.

Some people participate in formal groups to manage their weight. Group approaches are especially effective because they provide social support and healthy competition. It is a good idea to consult with a healthcare professional if you are struggling with weight management. These professionals can help you determine the weight-management strategy best for your health.

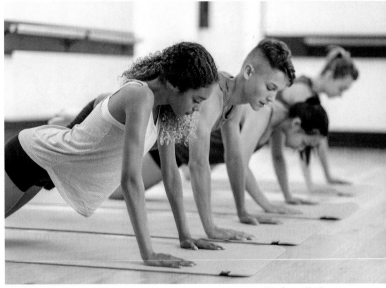

iStock.com/FatCamera

Figure 7.34 Having a friend who will go to the gym or do other physical activities with you can help you stick to adding physical activity to your routine.

Lesson 7.3 Review

1. **True or false.** Fat weighs more than muscle and bone.
2. The healthy range of _____ for children and teens is based on height, age, and sex.
3. List three strategies for healthy weight management.
4. How does mindful eating help people make healthier food choices?
5. **Critical thinking.** Describe the effectiveness of using fad diets to lose weight, especially in a short period of time. What effects do fad diets have on a person's health?

Hands-On Activity

Choose a small piece of fruit that you like and practice eating mindfully by using your senses of sight, touch, smell, and taste. Look at all sides of the food to really see what the food looks like. Feel the weight and texture of the food. What does it really feel like? Carefully smell the food. What smells are present? Place the food in your mouth, but do not chew, to notice what the food tastes like. Now, chew your piece of fruit slowly. Notice how your teeth and tongue work together to make the chewing action happen. Continue to notice the taste of your food. Does it change as you chew? When your body is ready, swallow your food. Try to feel your food going down your esophagus. Notice any aftertastes left in your mouth. What did you enjoy about eating that single piece of food so mindfully?

Having a Healthy Body Image

body image thoughts and feelings about how one's body looks

weight stigma flawed belief that having a thinner body or lower weight is always better

disordered eating range of irregular eating behaviors with negative health consequences

eating disorder mental illness that causes major disturbances in a person's daily diet

purging attempts to rid the body of food

body neutrality focus on what the body can do, rather than how it looks

body positivity appreciation of diverse body types

body compassion feelings of acceptance, care, and kindness toward one's body

Learning Outcomes

After studying this lesson, you will be able to

- **compare and contrast** positive and negative body image.
- **identify** several factors that can influence a person's body image.
- **explain** the difference between disordered eating and an eating disorder.
- **describe** causes, consequences, and signs of eating disorders.
- **explain** approaches for treating eating disorders.
- **demonstrate** skills for improving body image.

Graphic Organizer

Self-Assessment

Everyone struggles with body image issues on some level. As you read this lesson, complete the sentences below on a separate sheet of paper.

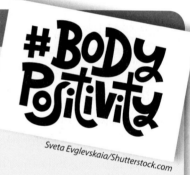

Sveta Evglevskaia/Shutterstock.com

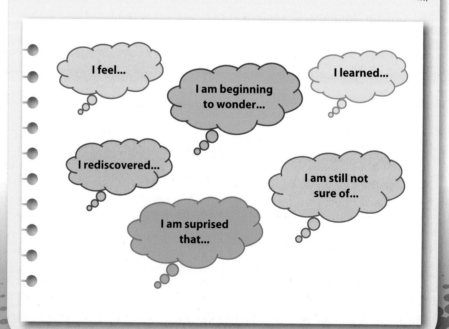

I feel...

I am beginning to wonder...

I learned...

I rediscovered...

I am still not sure of...

I am suprised that...

How do you feel about your body? Do you marvel at its strength and agility? Do you appreciate that the parts of your body do amazing tasks? For example, your heart pumps about 2,000 gallons of blood each day, and your digestive system takes in the nutrients you need from food. Many young people do not think about this when asked how they feel about their bodies. Instead, they worry about body parts they wish they could change. These feelings are part of body image.

Your thoughts and feelings about how you look make up your **body image**. Your body image does not describe what your body *actually* looks like. Your body image refers to how you *think* it looks. How your body actually looks and how you feel about it are not necessarily related (**Figure 7.35**).

People who have a *positive body image* appreciate and value their bodies. They recognize that a person's physical appearance has no impact on value and worth. People with a *negative body image* dislike their bodies and believe their negative perceptions affect their worth and value.

The effect of body image on mental and emotional health can also influence physical and social health. People who have a positive body image are more likely to take care of their bodies. They are also more likely to feel confident in social situations and build healthy relationships.

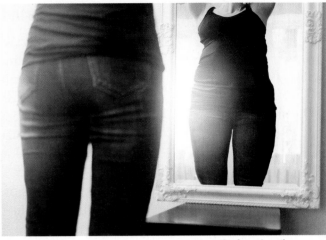

Figure 7.35 A person may think one's body looks differently than it actually does. *What is the term for how you feel about your body and how you think it looks?*

Factors Affecting Body Image

People are not born with a body image. A person's body image develops over time. Factors such as social environment, media and society, race and ethnicity, and athletic activities influence it.

Social Environment

Your *social environment*—which includes the relationships in your life—influences body image. For example, family members can affect body image by valuing certain physical qualities. Friends also influence body image. To fit in with a peer group, young people may feel like they need to look a certain way.

Participation in social media can make pressure from peers worse. Many young people want approval from their friends and only post pictures in which they look good. Some young people even manipulate images using filters and retouching. As a result, young people may feel pressure to always look good and compare themselves to others.

Media and Society

Every day, people see messages communicating ideas about attractiveness. Advertisements associate certain physical traits with attractiveness, wealth, health, success, and happiness. Images in the media are different for female and male bodies. Many of these images are digitally edited and unrealistic.

Female Bodies in the Media

Think quickly: who is the most attractive female TV or film star? Whoever came to mind is almost certainly thin. Media images of celebrities, actors, and models often set unhealthy standards. In one study, women shown female silhouettes of different sizes thought the best body size according to *other* women was thinner than their own best body size. Women also thought the best female body size was thinner than men did. This flawed idea that having a thinner body or lower weight is always better is called **weight stigma** (**Figure 7.36**).

Media images of female bodies also set other unrealistic standards. Female bodies in the media may have large breasts and butts, long legs, a small waist,

CASE STUDY

Asher's Quest—Losing to Win

For as long as Asher could remember, he wanted to be part of the school wrestling program. His dad and grandpa had both wrestled and *won* at the local and state levels. His grandpa even participated on an Olympic wrestling team. Asher was glad to have finally made the middle school team this year.

Asher wanted to continue the tradition of "winning" for his family—but there was an issue. He weighed 117 pounds at the beginning of the school year. Asher knew he would have a better chance of winning in the 106-pound weight class (one of the official weight classes for his state).

Despite his hard work and practice in wrestling, he is not satisfied with how his body is and what it can do. He sees the other wrestlers and notices that their bodies are much more likely to win matches and championships. Asher has seen pictures of his father and grandfather and truly believes that he will never be as successful as them because of his own body shape and size.

During a recent match at a neighboring school, Asher found himself more nervous than he ever had been before. He could not sleep the night before because of it. In fact, he was so nervous that he almost forfeited the match even though he was predicted to easily win. Asher has noticed that he is more self-conscious about his appearance recently, too. He hates being in the locker room with other guys who might notice the imperfections about him.

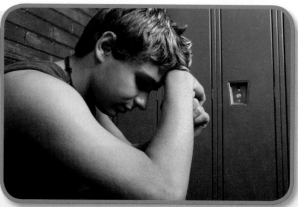

iStock.com/asiseeit

These feelings of anxiety and self-consciousness are all new to Asher and they are impacting his ability to enjoy wrestling. He is also certain that he is letting his dad and grandfather down.

Thinking Critically

1. Does Asher have a positive or negative body image? Explain.

2. Factors in a person's culture and community contribute to that person's body image. What factors may have impacted Asher's thoughts, perceptions, and attitudes about his physical appearance?

3. If you were Asher's friend, what would you do if you noticed these changes in his attitude?

4. What could be done in Asher's school and/or on his team to promote size diversity, body acceptance, and a healthier body image for everyone?

5. Do you think it is possible that Asher is working himself into an eating disorder? Why or why not?

clear skin, little body hair, and perfectly styled light hair. In addition, advertisements and media images almost always show females who are young. Because of standards in the media, many girls and women have negative thoughts about their bodies.

Male Bodies in the Media

Images of male bodies in the media also pressure men to conform to certain standards. In the media, images of male bodies have become increasingly tall and muscular. Many images of male bodies in the media show "six-pack" abdominals, muscular chests, and large biceps. Some also show very thin male bodies. As a result, men and boys may feel insecure about their height and figure.

Media images of male bodies also set standards for other body parts—for example, clear skin and full facial hair. The end result is that often-edited images set a standard that makes many boys and men feel badly about their bodies.

Race and Ethnicity

Images and body types in the media and society reach people from all backgrounds. Unfortunately, media in the United States tends to show mostly Caucasian or light-skinned models. Even when showing different races or ethnicities, the media tends to emphasize light eyes, straight hair, and lack of curves. These traits are more common among Caucasian people.

Not all populations embrace the standards shown in the media to the same extent. Different groups have different values and preferences when it comes to appearance. For example, some research suggests that, compared with Caucasians, African-Americans are less likely to view a very thin female body as best. Research also suggests that people of Hispanic descent tend to value curves more than thinness.

Athletic Activities

Another factor that can influence body image is involvement in some athletic activities. Certain athletic activities emphasize particular body types and features. This can negatively impact young people's feelings about their bodies. For example, dancers, gymnasts, and ice skaters often face pressure to be thin. Other athletic activities emphasize muscle mass or height. This pressure is common in activities such as football, basketball, swimming, volleyball, lacrosse, and ice hockey.

What Is Weight Stigma?

Weight stigma is **discrimination** or **stereotyping** based on a person's weight. Also called *weight bias* or *weight-based discrimination*.

It can increase **body dissatisfaction**, which is a leading risk factor of developing **eating disorders**.

Shaming, blaming, and "concern trolling" (acting in support of someone while actually criticizing them) can happen anywhere—school, home, even at the doctor's office.

Weight stigma is dangerous and can increase risk of **depression, poor body image**, and **binge eating**.

Figure 7.36 Weight stigma is discrimination based on a person's weight, and is dangerous to all aspects of your health. *What is an example of concern trolling? How can you tell?*

In contrast, young people in athletic activities that do *not* emphasize particular body types or features may experience less pressure and feel better about their bodies. They tend to feel good about what their bodies can do—like hit a home run, score a goal, or make a basket.

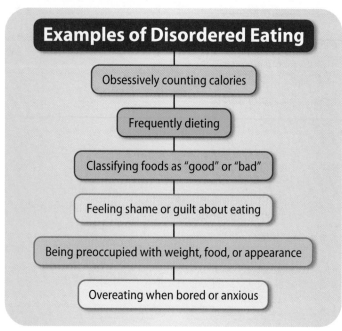

Examples of Disordered Eating

- Obsessively counting calories
- Frequently dieting
- Classifying foods as "good" or "bad"
- Feeling shame or guilt about eating
- Being preoccupied with weight, food, or appearance
- Overeating when bored or anxious

Figure 7.37
Disordered eating can have negative health consequences, and may lead to the development of eating disorders. *What are some factors that may lead to disordered eating?*

Disordered Eating

A healthy diet provides the nutrients your body needs to grow and survive. Not consuming these essential nutrients can hurt health today and in the future. For some people, having a negative body image leads to harmful eating habits.

The term **disordered eating** refers to irregular eating habits that show an unhealthy relationship with body image and food. **Figure 7.37** shows some common examples of disordered eating.

People may develop nutritional deficits from restricting calories or particular foods. They may also lack energy. One example of disordered eating is *orthorexia*. Orthorexia is characterized by an obsession with healthy eating that leads to negative health consequences. Disordered eating behaviors can develop into an eating disorder if they continue.

Eating Disorders

An **eating disorder** is a mental illness that causes major disturbances in a person's eating behaviors. People with eating disorders focus so much on these behaviors that they have difficulty concentrating on anything else. There are several types of eating disorders (**Figure 7.38**).

Risk Factors for Eating Disorders

While experts do not know what exactly causes eating disorders, they know certain factors play a role. Physical risk factors include having a close relative with an eating disorder and having a close relative with another mental illness. A history of dieting also increases risk for developing an eating disorder.

Mentally, having an anxiety disorder increases risk for an eating disorder. *Perfectionism* (feeling the need to meet unrealistically high expectations), rigidity in following rules, and a negative body image are also risk factors.

As you know, media images and societal and family expectations can contribute to a negative or positive body image. Unrealistic portrayals, lack of respect for diversity, and weight stigma are major risk factors for eating disorders. Bullying, teasing, social isolation, and a history of trauma also increase risk.

Types of Eating Disorders

Eating Disorder	Description
Anorexia nervosa	Characterized by severely restricted eating behaviors, intense body dissatisfaction, and low body weight. *Atypical anorexia nervosa* is more common than anorexia nervosa. Atypical anorexia nervosa has the same symptoms and health concerns without low body weight.
Avoidant-restrictive food intake disorder (ARFID)	Characterized by severely restricted eating behaviors without intense body dissatisfaction.
Binge-eating disorder	Characterized by repeated episodes of *bingeing* (consuming large amounts of food quickly and feeling out of control).
Bulimia nervosa	Characterized by repeated episodes of bingeing and *purging* (vomiting or using other methods to rid the body of food consumed).
Otherwise specified feeding or eating disorder (OSFED)	Includes eating behaviors that cause great distress, without meeting criteria for other eating disorders. Examples of OSFEDs are atypical anorexia nervosa, binge-eating disorder and bulimia nervosa of low frequency or duration, purging disorder (purging without binge-eating), and night eating syndrome (frequent episodes of eating at night).

Figure 7.38   In each eating disorder, eating behaviors disrupt daily life.

Health Consequences of Eating Disorders

Eating disorders lead to malnutrition and harmful behaviors. In malnutrition, a person does not consume the right amounts of nutrients needed for health and growth. When the body does not receive the energy it needs from food, it breaks down its own tissues for energy. Early in this process, the body breaks down muscle. This can lead to heart damage and heart failure, which can result in death.

Some eating disorders are also characterized by **purging**, or attempts to rid the body of food. Restricted eating and purging can cause stomach pain, nausea and vomiting, changes in blood sugar, dehydration, blocked intestines, and infections. Vomiting can damage the salivary glands and teeth. Eating disorders can also cause *constipation* (infrequent or delayed hard, dry bowel movements) and life-threatening emergencies such as stomach rupture.

The malnutrition associated with eating disorders can lead to low bone density, dry skin, thin hair, and brittle nails. Lack of nutrition also leads to a weaker immune system and *anemia* (an insufficient number of red blood cells). Anemia is characterized by weakness, fatigue, and shortness of breath. Long-term dehydration can cause kidney failure and death. Some health consequences associated with eating disorders will go away with treatment, but others will not.

Mentally and socially, eating disorders can lead to conflict in relationships, withdrawal from activities, and worsening mental health conditions. Eating disorders are often associated with low self-esteem and *co-occurring disorders* (mental illnesses that occur together). Eating disorders can increase a person's risk for suicide. You learned about how to get help for people having thoughts of suicide in Chapter 6.

Warning Signs of Eating Disorders	
Category	**Warning Signs**
Physical	Changes in weight
	Digestive conditions, such as constipation
	Lack of menstruation in females
	Dizziness, fainting, and weakness
	Feeling cold all the time
	Dental issues, such as cavities or tooth sensitivity
	Yellow skin, lanugo (fine hair all over the body), and discolored hands and feet
	Cuts or calluses on top of finger joints
	Low immune function and healing
Mental and emotional	Extreme focus on appearance, weight, and food
	Discomfort eating around others
	Lack of interest in previously enjoyed activities
	Extreme concern about appearance
	Extreme mood swings
Behavioral	Refusing to eat certain foods
	Not eating or eating very small amounts
	Frequent dieting
	Withdrawal from friends and family
	Frequently checking appearance in the mirror

Figure 7.39
Warning signs of eating disorders may be physical, mental and emotional, and behavioral.

Treating Eating Disorders and Disordered Eating

Eating disorders and disordered eating behaviors rarely go away without treatment, so getting help is important. Eating disorders are mental illnesses and should be treated by a multidisciplinary team of professionals. This most often includes a therapist, doctor, dietitian, and sometimes a psychiatrist. Each professional needs to know about eating disorders and their psychological and physical effects.

Certain warning signs signal that a person is experiencing disordered eating or an eating disorder and needs professional treatment (**Figure 7.39**). It is important to take these warning signs seriously. The earlier a person gets help, the more likely the person is to recover and avoid permanent health consequences.

To start the process of getting help, people can talk with a trusted adult, such as a parent or guardian or school counselor. People can also contact the National Eating Disorders Association Helpline (1-800-931-2237 or myneda.org/helpline) to get support and learn about treatment options. Treatment for eating disorders usually includes individual or family therapy and more advanced treatment, depending on severity.

Improving Your Body Image

You can use certain strategies to improve your body image and health. These strategies focus on developing a positive, realistic body image, which involves valuing and appreciating your body. To improve your body image, you can use the following strategies.

View Media Critically

When you see images of bodies in magazines and advertisements, on TV, or in a movie, ask yourself if the images reflect reality (**Figure 7.40**). For example, when reading a magazine, keep in mind that images in the magazine are carefully posed and constructed. Many young people regularly post edited or filtered images of themselves. To protect yourself from these influences, you can choose media carefully, assess whether images have been edited, and consider the images you share.

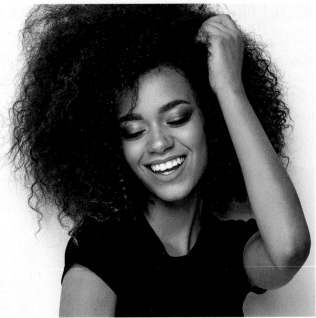

Are images digitally edited or airbrushed to present a more idealized image?

Do they make models appear thinner or more muscular?

Do they fix any facial blemishes or smooth out frizzy hair?

Do organizations that produce the images select models who meet an unrealistic body standard?

Do models represent the average person? Do models represent me?

Figure 7.40 Thinking critically about the images you see can help you determine if images reflect reality or improve your body image.

kiuikson/Shutterstock.com

Value Your Whole Self

Try to focus on the features of your body you like. Also think about what your body can *do*, not just your appearance. This focus on **body neutrality** can help you value your body and the bodies of others for more than just appearance. Part of valuing your whole self is also taking care of your body. This includes eating nutritious foods and getting some type of physical or stress-reducing activity every day.

Acknowledge Diversity

Instead of focusing on whether your body matches the media's artificial standards, recognize that people find many different body features attractive. Acknowledging this diversity and appreciating and valuing your body is called **body positivity**. Body positivity also means understanding and accepting that your body will change over time, due to the natural aging process and personal situations.

Check Your Self-Talk

Another way to adopt a more positive body image is to change how you talk about your body. To assess self-talk, consider what you think to yourself when you see your body in the mirror. If you have a tendency toward negative self-talk, you can improve body image by changing what you tell yourself about your body. This process of developing **body compassion**, or feelings of acceptance, care, and kindness toward your body, takes time and practice (**Figure 7.41**).

Change Your Self-Talk	
Negative Self-Talk	**Body Compassion**
I'll never look like influencers on social media.	This is the body I was born with, and it's attractive too.
I hate my body.	My favorite thing about my body today is my hair.
I look bad in these photos with my friends.	I look happy and loved, and that's what matters!
My legs look gross.	I love my legs for taking me where I want to go on my bike.
This pimple makes me look like such a loser.	My skin will not always be perfect. Acne is totally normal.
I'm getting so fat!	It's natural for my body to grow as I get older.

Figure 7.41 Body compassion is a skill that has to be practiced. Nobody will get it right every time.

Avoid Negative Influences

To promote a positive body image, avoid unrealistic images of people in magazines, on TV, and online whenever possible. You can also avoid negative influences in your daily life. If you have many conversations where your friends talk badly about their bodies, try to shift the discussion to a new topic. In some cases, you may need to walk away or spend less time with friends who focus on appearance.

Advocate for Positive Body Image

To advocate for your own health, remember that you can get help if you have a negative body image or show warning signs of disordered eating or an eating disorder. Talking with a trusted adult or contacting the National Eating Disorders Association can help you get this assistance.

To advocate for a positive body image in your community, you can speak up about idealized images in the media. Let companies, advertisers, and celebrities know how you feel about the images and messages they present. You can also promote a positive body image through campaigns that focus on body neutrality and positivity. Talk to your friends and classmates about starting a positive body image campaign in your school or community.

Lesson 7.4 Review

1. **True or false.** How your body actually looks and what you think your body looks like are always related.

2. What type of disorders can result from family pressure to have a certain body weight and shape?

3. The eating disorder in which people have severely restricting eating and a low body weight is called _____ _____.

4. Why do people need treatment for eating disorders?

5. **Critical thinking.** Name one male and one female celebrity widely considered to be attractive. What influence can seeing these people in the media have on a young person's body image?

Hands-On Activity

Take and print (or draw) a selfie that you really like. Use that picture to create a "self-poster" that includes a word cloud identifying aspects you like about yourself (physically, socially, and mentally), as well as factors that influence your body image. Include key terms from this lesson and everyday language to describe yourself. Share your "self-poster" with a classmate and explain why you chose the words you did. What do you and your classmate notice about the words you chose? What conclusions can you draw about your body image and self-esteem? Discuss your conclusions with your classmate.

Summary

Lesson 7.1 **Getting Enough Nutrients**

- Nutrients allow your body to grow and function properly. These include carbohydrates, fats, proteins, minerals, vitamins, and water.
- Carbohydrates are a major source of energy for the body. Protein helps build muscles, bones, skin, hair, nails, and organs. Fats provide a valuable source of energy.
- Vitamins are necessary for normal growth and development. Minerals are consumed through the plants and animal products you eat and the water you drink.
- You can survive for weeks without other nutrients, but only a few days without water.

Lesson 7.2 **Following a Healthy Eating Pattern**

- The *Dietary Guidelines for Americans* recommend eating patterns that promote health. Using the MyPlate food guidance system helps people put the guidelines into practice.
- *Undernutrition* involves not taking in enough nutrients for health and growth. *Overnutrition* involves eating too many foods with a high content of sugar, solid fat, sodium, refined grains, or calories.
- Healthy food choices can include choosing nutrient-dense foods; limiting added sugars, saturated fats, and sodium; eating breakfast every day; understanding Nutrition Facts and food labels; thinking about calories; eating healthy away from home; analyzing influences on food choices; preparing nutritious foods; and practicing food safety.

Lesson 7.3 **Managing Your Weight**

- *Body composition* is the ratio of the various components—fat, bone, and muscle—that make up your body. *Body mass index (BMI)* is a tool for assessing an individual's weight status.
- Your weight has an impact on your health now and in the future. Underweight can lead to skin, hair, or teeth conditions; increased tiredness; and an inability to fight off infections. Overweight or obesity leads to increased risk of heart diseases, high blood pressure, high cholesterol, and type 2 diabetes.
- Strategies for healthy weight management include setting and rewarding realistic goals, limiting screen time, thinking positively, avoiding unhealthy strategies, eating mindfully, monitoring eating, thinking positively, and enlisting support.

Lesson 7.4 **Having a Healthy Body Image**

- *Body image* is your thoughts and feelings about how you look. Your social environment, race and ethnicity, and athletic activities influence body image. Media and society, which often present unrealistic images of bodies, also have an influence. You can use several skills to improve your body image.
- Irregular eating behaviors that harm health are disordered eating. An eating disorder is a mental illness that causes major disturbances in a person's daily diet. Eating disorders have serious health consequences and rarely go away without professional help.

Check Your Knowledge

Record your answers to each of the following questions on a separate sheet of paper.

1. Name the six general types of nutrients.
2. **True or false.** Vegetarians must get the proteins they need by eating foods from animal sources.
3. What are the two distinct types of vitamins?
4. _____ foods are rich in nutrients and have little added sugars, starches, and sodium.
5. **True or false.** The five food groups included in the MyPlate food guidance system are proteins, carbohydrates, fats, vitamins, and minerals.
6. List three skills for following a healthy eating pattern.
7. What are the three main components that make up body composition?
8. **True or false.** BMI is calculated and interpreted in the same way for each age group.
9. People who experience overweight are at an increased risk for which of the following health conditions?
   A. Type 2 diabetes.
   B. Hearing loss.
   C. Liver damage.
   D. Lung cancer.
10. _____ _____ is a range of irregular eating behaviors that show an unhealthy relationship with body image and food.
11. **True or false.** Eating disorders can lead to heart failure because the body breaks down muscle in the absence of energy from food.
12. Explain the concept of body neutrality.

Use Your Vocabulary ↗

body compassion	eating disorder	overweight
body composition	fad diets	protein
body-fat distribution	fats	purging
body image	malnutrition	saturated fats
body mass index (BMI)	minerals	trans fats
body neutrality	MyPlate food guidance system	undernutrition
body positivity		underweight
carbohydrates	nutrient-dense foods	unsaturated fats
dietary fiber	nutrients	vitamins
Dietary Guidelines	obesity	weight stigma
disordered eating	overnutrition	

13. Working in pairs, locate a small image online that visually describes each of the terms above. Create flash cards by writing each term on a note card and pasting the image on the opposite side. Take turns quizzing each other on the terms.
14. Write the definition for each of the terms above in your own words. Then, read the text passages in this lesson. Double-check your definitions by using the text glossary.

Think Critically

15. **Evaluate.** How do you make decisions about what to eat each day? What internal and external factors have the strongest impact on your decisions?

16. **Make inferences.** What impact does a person's food choices and nutrition status have on that person's academics, activities, social life, and mental health?

17. **Cause and effect.** Does social media usage cause issues with body image? Why or why not?

18. **Assess.** What personality characteristics and social skills do you possess? Do you need to improve to increase acceptance of all body types?

DEVELOP Your Skills

19. **Leadership and advocacy skills.** Examine the lunch offerings in your school cafeteria and look at what students typically choose to eat. Analyze nutrient data on the food labels and compare the food options presented with the *Dietary Guidelines*. Create a new menu that meets the Guidelines and that young people will actually eat. Use the resources on www.choosemyplate.gov to help create your menu plan, such as the "Healthy Eating on a Budget" resources for planning weekly meals and making a grocery list. Ask for clarification if you do not understand the directions.

20. **Communication and practice health enhancing behaviors.** With your family's grocery shopper, discuss what you have learned about nutrition and your family's meals. Then, help plan your family's meals for a week (you can use the meal-planning resources on www.choosemyplate.gov). Create a grocery list that includes healthier foods that you and your family will actually eat for a week. Share this list with your family's grocery shopper and discuss any issues with purchasing these foods. If there are barriers to getting everything on your list, communicate with the shopper to figure out low-cost, healthy solutions that work for everyone. Once you have a grocery list that you are both happy with, help with the shopping and enjoy the food all week.

21. **Advocacy and communication skills.** Write a children's book to promote healthy eating and healthy body image. Include accurate information. Make it interesting with a child-friendly story line and illustrations. Submit your book to a partner for review. Make any spelling or grammatical changes, such as those related to pronoun agreement, verb tense, subject-verb agreement, or possessives. Then, with parents' permission, read your story to children you may know.

22. **Goal-setting skills.** Write a personal plan to improve your nutrition and/or body image. Be sure to include your overall goal and the small steps you will take to achieve it. Also, consider obstacles that may hinder your progress or success, and develop a plan to overcome them.

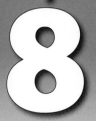

Essential Question

What does it mean to be active and fit?

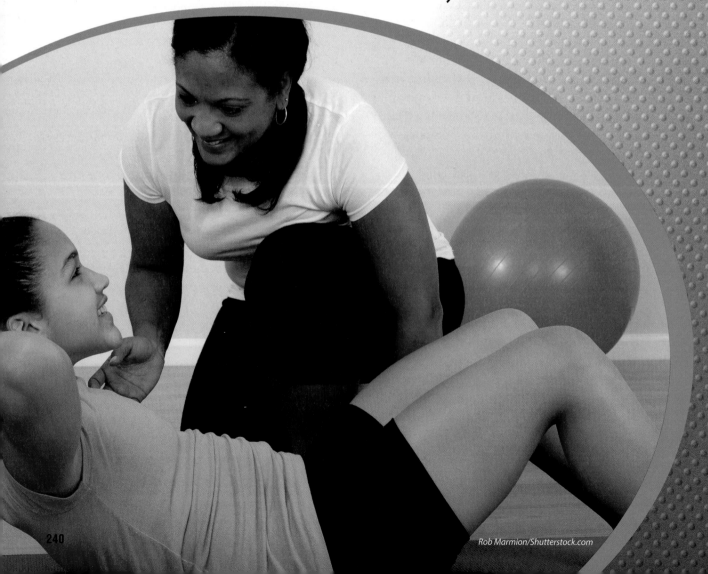

Rob Marmion/Shutterstock.com

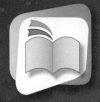

Reading Activity

Arrange a study session to read the chapter aloud with a classmate. Take turns reading each lesson. Stop at the end of each lesson and identify its main points. Take notes of your study session to share with the class.

How Healthy Are You?

In this chapter, you will be learning about physical fitness. Before you begin reading, take the following quiz to assess your current physical activity habits.

Healthy Choices	Yes	No
Do you follow the rules of any physical activity, especially sports, in which you participate?		
Are you physically active for a total of 60 minutes or more each day?		
Do you do cardio activities like playing sports, riding your bike, or taking a dance class?		
Can you balance on one foot, do a handstand, or ride a skateboard?		
Do you drink lots of water before, during, and after physical activity?		
Do you do anaerobic workouts like push-ups, sit-ups, or squats for 20 to 30 minutes, two or three days a week?		
Do you regularly do some type of stretching exercises?		
Do you tend to walk up the stairs instead of taking an elevator or escalator?		
Do you make personal physical activity and fitness plans to improve aspects of your fitness?		
Do you have the energy to perform life's daily activities?		
Do you warm up your muscles before any type of physical activity?		
Do you do a cooldown after physical activity to stretch and help your heart rate return to a normal, lower level?		

Count your "Yes" and "No" responses. The more "Yes" responses you have, the more healthy physical activity habits you exhibit. Now, take a closer look at the questions with which you responded "No." How can you make these healthy habits part of your daily life? Identify a SMART goal you would like to achieve to help improve your overall health and well-being. Refer to Figure 1.11 to help you set up your SMART goal. If you do not understand the instructions, ask for clarification from your teacher.

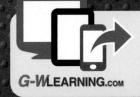

Click on the activity icon or visit www.g-wlearning.com/health to access online vocabulary activities using key terms from the chapter.

Understanding Physical Activity and Fitness

Learning Outcomes

After studying this lesson, you will be able to

- **explain** why engaging in physical activity is so important.
- **describe** the benefits of physical activity.
- **summarize** the key guidelines for children and teens as outlined in the *Physical Activity Guidelines for Americans*.
- **evaluate** how you can improve your health by doing activities you enjoy.

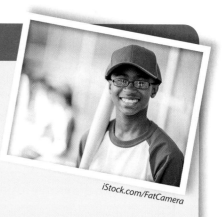

iStock.com/FatCamera

Graphic Organizer

Have Fun Being Active

Prior to reading the lesson, list five physical activities that you enjoy doing in a table like the one shown. While reading the lesson, write down the health benefits from performing each activity. Add additional health benefits that may not have been stated in the text.

Physical Activities I Enjoy	Health Benefits of These Activities
1. Running	• Improves heart and lung function • Helps control weight
2.	
3.	
4.	
5.	

Madison is in sixth grade and loves being active. She walks to school every day. After school, she enjoys riding her bike to her friend Danny's house. Almost every weekend she goes out with her family for a hike or a bike ride.

Madison's friend Danny does not always have the energy for those types of physical activities. He does like to play baseball once a week with friends, and he will occasionally do some push-ups or pull-ups. Lately, however, Danny has noticed that he gets very tired throughout the day. He becomes out of breath quickly when walking up stairs or riding his bike. If he wants to go to the park or to Madison's house, he asks his mom to drive him.

In this lesson, you will discover how leading an active lifestyle can benefit your health and well-being. You will find out how you can promote lifelong health simply by doing physical activities you enjoy.

Engaging in Physical Activity

Physical activity is any action in which the body uses energy. For example, traveling between classes uses energy. Swimming with friends, biking to school, carrying groceries, dancing, playing sports, and lifting weights also use energy.

Many people think exercise is the same as physical activity, but exercise is actually just one type of physical activity. The term **exercise** describes physical activity that is structured, planned, and has the purpose of increasing physical fitness. Examples of exercise include doing sit-ups in PE class, practicing for a sports team, or running to prepare for a half-marathon.

Engaging in physical activity is one of the most important actions you can take to promote lifelong health and well-being. You do not have to participate in structured exercise to experience the benefits of physical activity. Engaging in physical activity for 60 minutes every day can protect your health today and reduce risk factors for various health conditions (**Figure 8.1**).

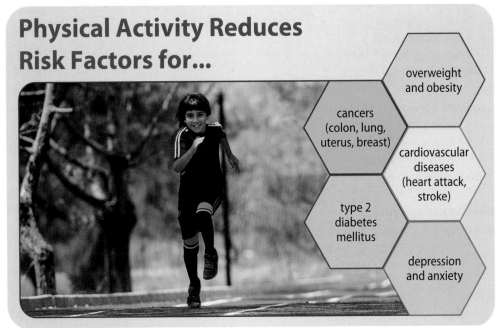

Physical Activity Reduces Risk Factors for...

- overweight and obesity
- cancers (colon, lung, uterus, breast)
- cardiovascular diseases (heart attack, stroke)
- type 2 diabetes mellitus
- depression and anxiety

iStock.com/guvendemir

Figure 8.1
Finding ways to be physically active every day can lead to better health now and in the future.

Physical activity is important for all aspects of your health. Whether you run, bike, dance, swim, or do some other form of activity, you are taking steps to be healthy. Setting SMART goals can help you stay moving and improve your health.

The Benefits of Physical Activity

You do not have to participate in structured exercise to experience the benefits of physical activity. Simply being physically active can protect your health today and in the future. Engaging in physical activity regularly

- lowers your risk of certain diseases, including heart disease, cancer, and type 2 diabetes.
- helps you reach and maintain a healthy weight.
- strengthens your bones and muscles.
- improves your quality of sleep.
- improves mental and emotional health and mood. This happens because engaging in physical activity can cause the brain to release chemicals called **endorphins**, which make you feel good.
- provides an opportunity to spend time with others.
- improves academic performance and concentration.

CASE STUDY

Walk in My Shoes: Jaquan's Story

Thirteen-year-old Jaquan is a good student and does not mind going to school. His parents have high academic expectations for him. As long as he gets good grades, Jaquan can do whatever he wants after school. What he really likes to do is play video games.

For his birthday, Jaquan got a new gaming system and several games. Most days, he will play three to four hours. This often leaves him with little time to do other activities.

Recently, Jaquan has gained a few pounds due to his sedentary behaviors. The increase in his weight makes him feel a little insecure at school. He usually tries to escape these insecurities by retreating to his room to play video games after school.

At times, Jaquan misses hanging out with friends and going to social activities, but does find some companionship with his online gamer friends. His younger sister loves playing soccer and often begs Jaquan to play with little success. She misses hanging out with her brother.

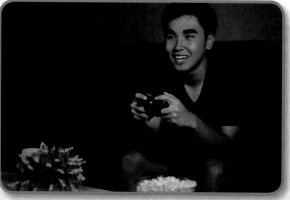

BaLL LunLa/Shutterstock.com

Thinking Critically

1. How could Jaquan benefit from being physically active at his age? Consider how being physically active could positively affect his current physical, mental, emotional, and social health.

2. How could Jaquan enjoy playing video games and achieve health-related fitness?

3. If you were Jaquan's friend, what activities would you recommend to help him stay physically fit, aside from playing team sports?

4. If Jaquan's sedentary behaviors continue, what are the possible long-term health outcomes?

Benefits of Physical Activity on Mental Health

improves your brain's performance. Regular physical activity can keep your memory sharp and boosts creative and mental energy.

reduces symptoms of anxiety and depression, and increases endorphin levels (the chemical in your brain that makes you feel happy).

strengthens your relationships with others when you do physical activity together.

Physical Activity...

helps you get a good night's sleep by regulating your circadian rhythm and increasing your body temperature, which calms your mind.

increases your heart rate, which increases your brain's production of chemicals that improve your mood and help reduce stress levels.

boosts your self-esteem, which helps to build self-confidence.

Running Women, Painting Girl, Sleeping Man: Inspiring/Shutterstock.com; Girl with Arms Crossed, Boy with Dog: Demian_shutter/Shutterstock.com; Children Jumping: Sentavio/Shutterstock.com

Getting Enough Physical Activity

Although the benefits of physical activity are clear, most people do not get enough activity each day. Many people spend much of their day engaging in sedentary behaviors. **Sedentary behaviors** are activities that consist of sitting or lying down and using very little energy. Examples of sedentary behaviors include driving, watching television shows or movies, surfing or chatting online, playing video games, working at a classroom desk, and reading.

The US Department of Health and Human Services (HHS) publishes the **Physical Activity Guidelines for Americans** to guide people in getting enough physical activity. These guidelines recommend that children and teens ages 6–17

- get at least one hour of moderate-to-vigorous physical activity every day.
- spend the majority of that time doing moderate- or vigorous-intensity aerobic activities.
- include muscle-strengthening activities at least three days a week.
- include bone-strengthening activities at least three days a week.

Think about the types of activities you do on a regular basis. Do you jog, swim, or skate? Do you lift weights or do push-ups or sit-ups? Do you ride a bike to school, mow the lawn, or dance around the house? Do you play on a school sports team? How much time do you spend doing activities? Does your current activity level measure up to the 60-minute daily activity guideline for children and teens?

Making physical activity a part of your daily or weekly routine can be challenging at times. The more you do it, however, the easier it becomes. The first, and most important, step is to set aside time each week to be active (**Figure 8.2**). If you are usually inactive, then even as little as 10 minutes of activity at a time is a step in the right direction. Before you know it, physical activity will become part of your daily life.

Types of Fitness Apps

Workout and Exercise Apps

- Allow users to track workouts and weight loss
- Provide users with exercise sets
- Keep track of calories burned and workout routines
- Can be integrated with wearable fitness trackers

Activity Tracking Apps

- Collect data about user's activity
- Track steps taken, distance covered, and other fitness measurements
- Provide users with easy-to-understand charts showing daily, weekly, and monthly activity
- Mostly integrated with wearable fitness trackers

Nutrition Apps

- Help users gain or lose weight and better control healthy eating habits
- Count calorie consumption
- Make recommendations to help follow a healthier diet

Rawpixel.com/Shutterstock.com

Figure 8.2 You can use technology to improve your physical activity habits. Apps can record workouts, set reminders, and track fitness goals. *According to the Physical Activity Guidelines for Americans, how much activity should children and teens engage in each day?*

Choosing Physical Activities You Enjoy

Meeting the daily physical activity guideline for your age group can be easy when you choose activities you enjoy. Some people really enjoy team sports, such as basketball or field hockey. Other people like activities they can do alone, such as walking or lifting weights. Many people enjoy both types of activities.

Think about what you like the most. Do you prefer outdoor or indoor activities? Do you like doing physical activities alone or with other people? Also, consider which physical activities are appropriate for your levels of fitness and development.

If you like to do physical activities with other people, try to find someone who will be active with you. Do you have a friend who would take a brisk walk with you after school? What about going on a bike ride? You could even make new friends by joining a sports team or fitness group. An exercise class might be a good place to meet new people. A pick-up baseball game at a local park could help you meet new people, too.

Many schools and communities provide free or low-cost ways to enjoy physical activities. Community centers often offer dance lessons and sports and fitness programs. Many communities also have places you can use for free or at a reduced cost, such as the following:

- parks and green spaces for playing Frisbee, throwing a baseball, or playing soccer (**Figure 8.3**)
- outdoor sports areas, such as baseball or softball fields and tennis and basketball courts
- indoor sports areas, such as swimming pools, basketball courts, and running tracks
- walking and biking trails and skate parks
- public pools

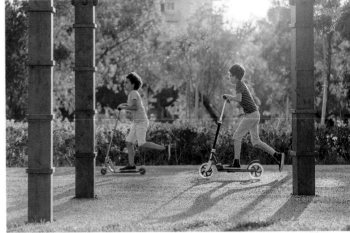

iStock.com/mustafagull

Figure 8.3   Going to a community park is a great, free way to stay active with your friends without spending money on a gym membership.

Lesson **8.1 Review**

1. Why is engaging in physical activity so important?

2. Which of the following is *not* a benefit of physical activity?

   A. Improves quality of sleep.

   B. Improves concentration and mood.

   C. Increases risk of disease.

   D. None of the above.

3. What is the name of the resource that HHS publishes to guide people on how they can improve their health through physical activities?

4. **Critical thinking.** Identify two activities that would be categorized as physical activity and two that would be considered exercise. Explain the difference.

Hands-On Activity

Choose one of the activities you identified in question number four above and do this activity at least three times on three different days. After doing this activity, reflect on how it made you feel. Did you enjoy the activity? How likely are you to keep doing this activity? Write a summary of your findings.

Knowing About Types of Physical Fitness

Key Terms 🔗

health-related fitness type of physical fitness a person needs to perform daily activities with ease and energy

aerobic using oxygen to break down energy for use in the muscles

anaerobic powering the body without the use of oxygen

resistance opposition

endurance ability to continue performing a physical activity over time

skill-related fitness type of physical fitness that improves a person's performance in a particular sport or leisure activity

agility ability to rapidly change the body's momentum and direction

Learning Outcomes

After studying this lesson, you will be able to

- **describe** five parts of health-related fitness.
- **compare and contrast** aerobic activities and anaerobic activities.
- **explain** the two types of endurance.
- **differentiate between** health-related fitness and skill-related fitness.
- **identify** the six aspects of skill-related fitness.

Graphic Organizer

Many Ways to Be Fit

In an organizer like the one shown, identify the five aspects of health-related fitness and the six aspects of skill-related fitness. After each aspect of fitness, offer an example of a physical activity that uses this aspect.

Daisy Daisy/Shutterstock.com

Fitness
- Health-Related Fitness
- Skill-Related Fitness

As people engage in physical activities, they develop some parts of their fitness more than other parts. For example, how fast, and how long, can you run? Are you able to touch your toes? How many push-ups and pull-ups can you do?

Recall from the previous lesson, Madison and Danny's different physical activities. Madison's hiking and biking develop different parts of her fitness than Danny's push-ups and pull-ups. Hiking and biking improve balance or heart and lung strength, while push-ups improve muscle strength and power. These activities represent different types of fitness. In this lesson, you will learn about health-related fitness and skill-related fitness.

Health-Related Fitness

Health-related fitness is the type of fitness you need to perform daily activities with ease and energy. **Aerobic** activities, such as dancing or bicycling, use oxygen to break down energy for use in the muscles. In **anaerobic** activities, such as lifting heavy objects or sprinting, stored energy powers the body without the use of oxygen (**Figure 8.4**).

There are different parts of health-related fitness. These parts include heart and lung strength, muscle strength, endurance, flexibility, and body composition.

Heart and Lung Strength

Your heart and lung strength affects how well you can do physical activities. As you engage in physical activities, your heart beats faster and your breathing quickens. Your lungs must work harder to provide your muscles with oxygen so you can keep moving.

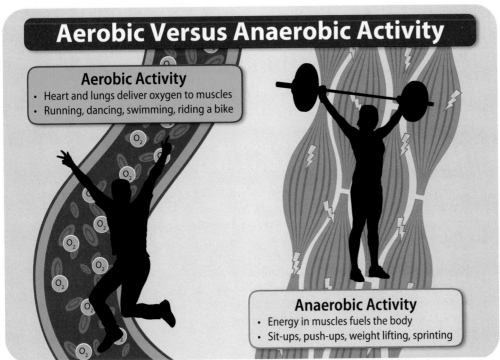

Aerobic Versus Anaerobic Activity

Aerobic Activity
- Heart and lungs deliver oxygen to muscles
- Running, dancing, swimming, riding a bike

Anaerobic Activity
- Energy in muscles fuels the body
- Sit-ups, push-ups, weight lifting, sprinting

Figure 8.4
Aerobic activities use energy that has been broken down by oxygen, while anaerobic activities use energy that is already stored in the muscles. *What is an example of an aerobic activity? an anaerobic activity?*

Most of your 60 minutes of activity each day should be spent doing aerobic activities. Engaging in regular aerobic activity strengthens the heart and lungs. The stronger your heart and lungs become, the more physically fit you become.

Muscle Strength

Muscle strength is the ability of a muscle to exert force against **resistance** (opposition). Imagine you are arm wrestling with a friend. Assume that you have stronger arm muscles than your friend. As you push against your friend's weaker arm muscles, your force will overcome your friend's resistance. This will result in you winning the match.

You can measure your muscle strength in many ways. For example, you can measure how much weight (resistance) you can lift. You can also measure how much weight you can push, and how much weight you can pull.

When you lift weights or do push-ups and pull-ups, you are engaging in anaerobic activities. Anaerobic activities differ from aerobic activities. Anaerobic activities occur in short bursts, while aerobic activities occur over a longer stretch of time. Children and teens can improve their muscle strength by doing anaerobic exercises at least three days each week.

Endurance

Another important part of health-related fitness is a person's endurance. **Endurance** refers to the ability to continue performing a physical activity over time (**Figure 8.5**). There are two types of endurance—aerobic and muscle. *Aerobic endurance* describes a person's ability to engage in cardio activities over a period of time.

Muscle endurance refers to the length of time for which a group of muscles can continue to exert force. Muscle endurance is different from muscle strength.

Figure 8.5
You can judge how hard you are working by how hard you are breathing. The harder you are breathing, the harder you are working. *How can you tell if you are overexerting yourself?*

Your Breathing Can Tell You How Hard You Are Working

Moderate Physical Activity	Vigorous Physical Activity	Overexerting Yourself
• Your breathing gets faster, but you are not out of breath • You develop a light sweat after about ten minutes of activity • You can carry on a conversation, but you cannot sing	• Your breathing is deep and rapid • You develop a sweat after only a few minutes of activity • You cannot say more than a few words without pausing to catch your breath	• You are short of breath • You are in pain • You cannot do the activity for as long as you had planned • Be careful not to overexert yourself; you can always start with lighter activity and build intensity gradually

Muscle endurance has to do with the duration of performance. Muscle strength has to do with the amount of force used to move or lift an object.

Some types of physical activity require high levels of both aerobic and muscle endurance. For example, consider marathon runners who run long distances for hours at a time. These runners must have great aerobic endurance for their hearts to continue pumping at higher-than-normal levels throughout the run. They must also have great muscle endurance for their leg muscles to continue exerting force for such a long time.

Flexibility

People who are flexible are able to fully and easily move their muscles and joints. Some people are very flexible. They are easily able to move their muscles and joints into difficult positions. Ballet dancers and gymnasts are good examples. Other people are not so flexible, and will often have tight or stiff muscles. This can make normal daily activities, such as tying their shoes, difficult to do.

Everyone benefits from having some flexibility. Flexibility helps improve performance in many physical activities. It also lowers the risk of getting an injury. Regularly (and safely) stretching your muscles can increase your flexibility (**Figure 8.6**).

Body Composition

Body composition is an important part of health-related fitness. As you learned in Chapter 7, *body composition* is the ratio of fat, bone, and muscle that naturally make up a person's body. Some people have more muscle than fat, while others have more fat than muscle.

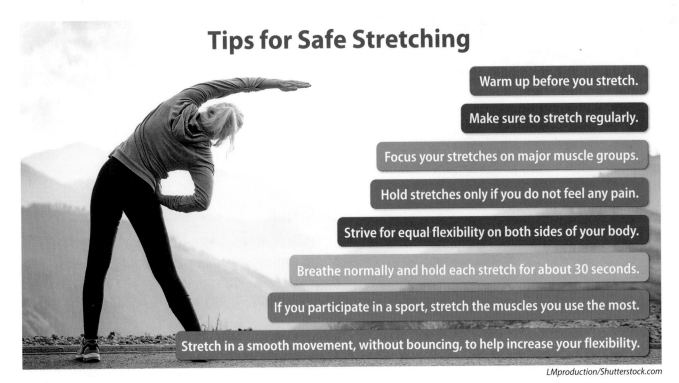

Tips for Safe Stretching

Warm up before you stretch.

Make sure to stretch regularly.

Focus your stretches on major muscle groups.

Hold stretches only if you do not feel any pain.

Strive for equal flexibility on both sides of your body.

Breathe normally and hold each stretch for about 30 seconds.

If you participate in a sport, stretch the muscles you use the most.

Stretch in a smooth movement, without bouncing, to help increase your flexibility.

LMproduction/Shutterstock.com

Figure 8.6 Being flexible is important for your health and well-being, and can be improved over time by safely stretching your muscles.

Engaging in regular physical activity can improve a person's body composition. People who engage in strength training, which includes push-ups, sit-ups, or lifting weights, can increase their muscle mass. Increasing muscle mass and reducing body fat is important to prevent chronic health conditions.

Skill-Related Fitness

Skill-related fitness refers to the kind of fitness a person needs to successfully perform a sport or leisure activity. The different aspects of skill-related fitness include speed, agility, balance, power, coordination, and reaction time.

Speed

If you participate in or watch sporting events, then you know what *speed* is. Many sports require people to be fast. Runners and swimmers must be fast, especially if they are racing short distances. Sprinting requires more speed than long-distance running or swimming. Speed is needed for some leisure activities, too. Sometimes people need to walk quickly to reach a destination on time.

Agility

Another type of skill-related fitness is agility. **Agility** is the ability to rapidly change the body's momentum and direction. This skill involves accelerating in a particular direction from a position of standing still. It can also involve rapidly changing from movement in one direction to movement in another direction. Agility describes a person's ability to go under, over, or around obstacles that the person may encounter (**Figure 8.7**).

Balance

Balance means holding a certain body posture and position on a stable or unstable surface. Balance is very much a part of some sports, such as diving and gymnastics, as well as many leisure activities. Can you do a handstand or ride a skateboard? What about hopping on one foot? These are all examples of activities that involve the ability to balance.

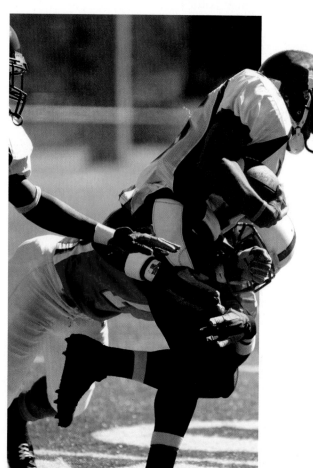

Daniel Padavona/Shutterstock.com

Figure 8.7 A running back on a football team must have agility to move around and away from players on the other team to avoid getting tackled.

Types of Fitness

Start ▶

Choose Your Abilities ▲

Health-Related Fitness

Heart and Lung Strength
Provides oxygen to the muscles to keep you going longer

Muscle Strength
Allows you to lift objects and push against resistance

Endurance
Allows you to be physically active for long periods of time without tiring

Flexibility
Allows you to fully and easily move your muscles and joints

Body Composition
Refers to the amount of muscle and fat in your body

Choose Your Skills ▲

Skill-Related Fitness

Speed
Enables you to move quickly

Power
Enables you to have a mix of strength and speed

Balance
Allows you to hold a certain body posture on a stable or unstable surface

Coordination
Allows you to perform various movements easily and smoothly

Agility
Enables you to rapidly change your body's momentum and direction

Reaction Time
Allows you to respond quickly

Power

Power is a mix of strength and speed. Some people are strong, but not fast. Other people are fast, but not strong. The person who combines strength and speed can be powerful. Power is an important skill in many sports, such as football and baseball. Power is also important in many daily activities, such as carrying groceries or other heavy objects, doing yard work, or walking a dog.

Coordination

Having good *coordination* enables you to perform various movements easily and gracefully. Coordination relates closely to balance (**Figure 8.8**). Some people are naturally more coordinated than others. Practicing activities such as throwing and catching a ball, jumping rope, standing on one foot, or riding a bike can help lead to better coordination.

Reaction Time

Reaction time refers to the quickness of a response. How quickly do you react to someone else's movement? A person's reaction time is important in many activities. You must be able to react quickly to hit a tennis ball, block a soccer ball, or walk on uneven ground.

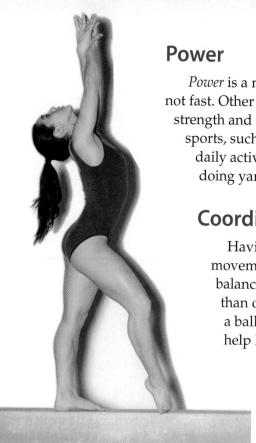

sirtravelalot/Shutterstock.com

Figure 8.8 Gymnastics requires both balance and coordination to perform complex movements. *What is another physical activity that requires good coordination and balance?*

Lesson 8.2 Review

1. **True or false.** Health-related fitness helps you perform daily activities with ease and energy.
2. Name the two types of endurance.
3. Heart and lung strength, muscle strength, endurance, flexibility, and body composition are all parts of _____ fitness.
4. What are the six aspects of skill-related fitness?
5. **Critical thinking.** What is the difference between aerobic activities and anaerobic activities?

Hands-On Activity

Write down each physical activity you perform this week. Make sure to record how long you do each activity. Next to each item, identify whether it is an aerobic activity or an anaerobic activity. Which types of activities do you want to improve? Do you need to improve your aerobic endurance? Do you get enough anaerobic activity? Write a summary describing which types of activities you want to improve.

Staying Safe During Physical Activity

Learning Outcomes

After studying this lesson, you will be able to

- **describe** the importance of following rules and being a good sport.
- **identify** common safety equipment for physical activities.
- **explain** why it is important to start slowly and not overdo it when starting a fitness program.
- **describe** why drinking water is important before, during, and after physical activity.
- **list** steps you can take to ensure your safety when engaging in physical activities in hot or cold weather.
- **compare and contrast** a sprain, dislocation, and fracture.

Graphic Organizer

Staying Safe

This lesson is about preventing fitness-related injuries. Before reading this lesson, make five predictions of safety strategies you think might be included in the lesson. For each prediction, explain why you think this is an important guideline for avoiding injuries. Use your previous personal experience, as well as prior personal knowledge, to fill in a table similar to the one shown. Complete the table from top to bottom, filling in the left column first and then the right column.

kazoka/Shutterstock.com

Safety Strategy	Why Is This Important?
1.	
2.	
3.	
4.	
5.	

Key Terms

hyperthermia serious condition that results when the heat-regulating mechanisms of the body are unable to deal with the heat from the environment, which results in a very high body temperature

hypothermia serious condition that results when a person's body loses heat faster than it can produce it

frostbite injury caused by the freezing of skin and body tissues

sprain injury to a ligament

dislocation serious injury in which bones move out of their normal position

fracture broken bone

concussion type of brain injury that results from a blow or jolt to the head or upper body

As you know, engaging in physical activity is an important part of staying healthy. You probably also know that you cannot engage in physical activity if you are injured. This means that following accepted guidelines and taking the necessary precautions when performing physical activities are critical to your health. This lesson will examine actions you can take to be safe, avoid common injuries, and treat injuries that might occur.

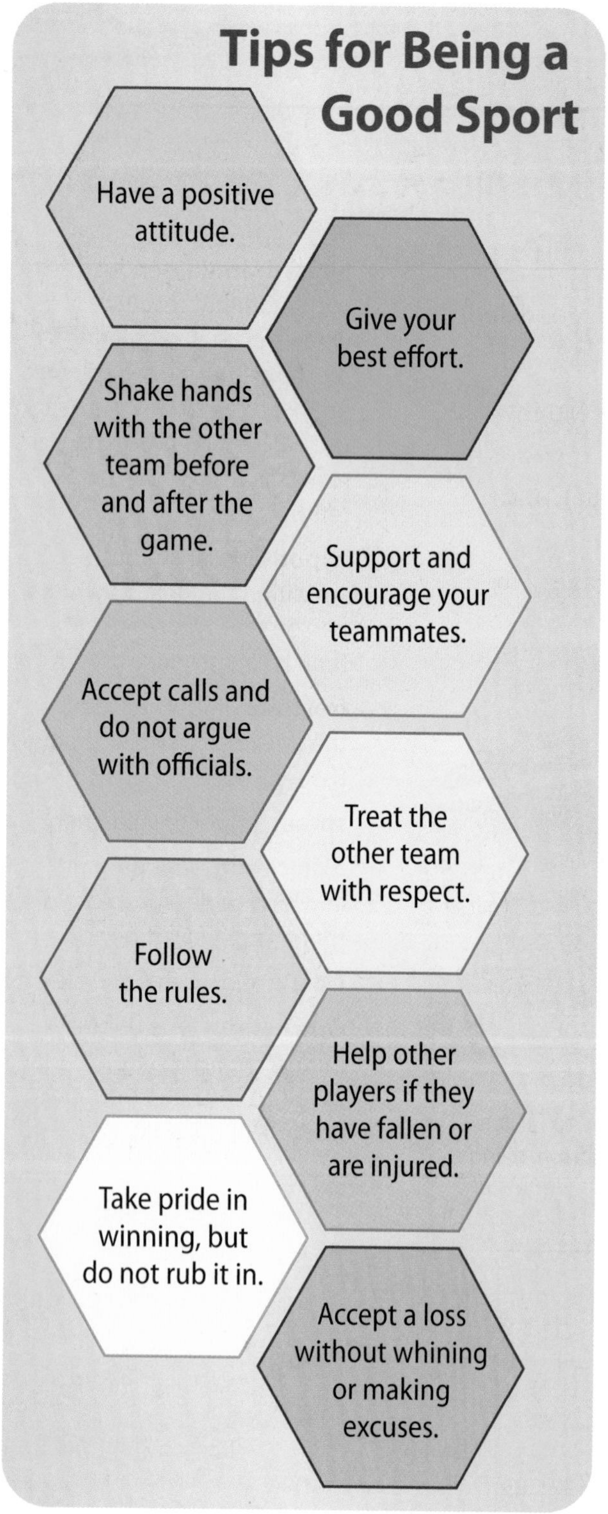

Conduct Yourself Respectfully

Conducting yourself with respect during physical activity involves following rules and being a good sport. Many physical activities, especially sports, have certain rules that people follow to stay safe. Knowing and following the rules of your chosen activity can keep you and others free from injury.

Rules can vary based on the activity. For example, a rule in football or soccer states that all activity on the field must stop when the referee blows the whistle. A rule to obey traffic laws is important for activities such as biking, running, or rollerblading. Because rules can vary for activities, make sure you practice safety by learning the rules of an activity before you participate.

Another aspect of respectful conduct is good *sportsmanship*, or behaviors that a person plays fair and treats people with respect. **Figure 8.9** shows how to be a good sport. Remember that sports is about learning new skills and having fun, not just winning. Treating members of the other team how you would like to be treated shows respect for yourself, your teammates, coaches on both sides, officials, and the game.

Use Proper Equipment

Many physical activities involve wearing proper equipment to prevent injury (**Figure 8.10**). Sometimes, laws even require people doing certain physical activities to wear equipment. In the case of riding a bike, for example, some states require people to wear helmets. In the event of an accident, wearing a helmet can save a person's life.

Tips for Being a Good Sport

- Have a positive attitude.
- Give your best effort.
- Shake hands with the other team before and after the game.
- Support and encourage your teammates.
- Accept calls and do not argue with officials.
- Treat the other team with respect.
- Follow the rules.
- Help other players if they have fallen or are injured.
- Take pride in winning, but do not rub it in.
- Accept a loss without whining or making excuses.

Figure 8.9 Being a good sport means following the rules and giving your best effort, but it also means supporting and helping players from both teams.

Fitness Equipment	
Equipment	**Uses**
Helmets	Organized sports: Baseball, softball, and football Recreational activities: Biking, skiing, and rollerblading
Mouth guards	Lacrosse, ice hockey, football, wrestling, boxing, and kickboxing
Eye protection	Goggles: Swimmers and divers Face masks: Ice hockey, baseball and softball catchers, lacrosse, and football Sunglasses, brimmed hats, or visors: Tennis, golf, beach volleyball, softball, baseball, and biking
Padding for wrists, knees, hips, shoulders, and elbows	Ice hockey, football, soccer, lacrosse, ice-skating, rollerblading, and snowboarding
Reflective gear	Biking or running along the side of the road

Figure 8.10 Safety equipment prevents injuries, which can stop you from getting to play sports or do other physical activities. *What are two kinds of safety equipment that help protect your head?*

When choosing equipment, make sure your equipment fits well. Do not use hand-me-downs or used equipment that is overly worn or the wrong size. Also be sure to take care of fitness equipment and facilities. Fitness equipment is expensive, so you should keep equipment in good condition and store it in a safe place.

Start Slowly and Do Not Overdo It

If you are just starting a fitness program, take care to start slowly (**Figure 8.11**). It can be tempting to exert yourself too much when you first start. You should resist this temptation because doing too much too soon can be harmful. If you overdo any type of physical activity during the first couple of days, you increase your chances of an injury. Then, you will have to wait until you heal before you can get back on track.

Once you feel more comfortable with physical activity, you can increase the time, frequency, and intensity. For example, you could walk, rollerblade, or bike for 30 minutes instead of just 10 to 20 minutes. You could jog instead of walk. Gradually increase the demands on your body. Be patient rather than trying to do too much too soon.

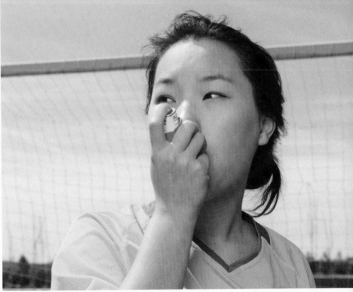

Lopolo/Shutterstock.com

Figure 8.11 People with preexisting conditions, such as asthma or diabetes, should see a doctor before starting any new physical activity. *Why should someone with asthma see a doctor before trying a new physical activity?*

Drink Lots of Water

Your body sweats during physical activity, which decreases the amount of fluids in your body. The loss of too much fluid causes dehydration. This affects your body's ability to function properly. Fluid loss also makes the heart work harder to circulate blood throughout your body. A loss of fluid can also lead to muscle cramps, dizziness, and fatigue. Therefore, drink lots of water before, during, and after physical activity. Remember to drink often to prevent dehydration.

Use Caution in Hot and Cold Weather

Being physically active outside in hot or cold weather can be dangerous if you are not careful. The term *hyperthermia* describes heat-related illnesses and *hypothermia* describes cold-related illnesses. **Hyperthermia** occurs when the heat-regulating mechanisms of the body are unable to deal with the heat from the environment, which results in a very high body temperature. **Hypothermia** is a result of a very low body temperature that occurs from too much exposure to cold weather.

If you are engaging in physical activity outside when it is hot and humid, make sure to drink plenty of water before, during, and after physical activity to avoid dehydration. Wearing light-colored and lightweight clothing can prevent you from becoming too overheated. You can use misting sprays to keep cool, too. Also, be aware of the signs and symptoms of heat-related illnesses (**Figure 8.12**).

Signs and Symptoms of Heat-Related Illnesses

	Heat Stroke	Heat Exhaustion	Heat Cramps
What to Look For	• High body temperature (103°F or higher) • Hot, red, dry, or damp skin • Fast, strong pulse • Headache • Nausea • Confusion • Losing consciousness (passing out)	• Heavy sweating • Cold, pale, and clammy skin • Fast, weak pulse • Nausea or vomiting • Muscle cramps • Tiredness or weakness • Dizziness • Headache • Fainting (passing out)	• Heavy sweating during intense physical activity • Muscle pain or spams
What to Do	• Call 911 right away—heat stroke is a medical emergency. • Move to a cooler place. • Lower your temperature with cool cloths or a cool bath. • Do not drink anything.	• Move to a cool place. • Loosen your clothes. • Put cool, wet cloths on your body or take a cool bath. • Sip water. **Get medical help right away if:** • You are throwing up. • Your symptoms get worse. • Your symptoms last longer than one hour.	• Stop physical activity and move to a cool place. • Drink water or a sports drink. • Wait for cramps to go away before you do any more physical activity. **Get medical help right away if:** • Cramps last longer than one hour. • You are on a low-sodium diet. • You have heart issues.

Figure 8.12 Heat-related illnesses can quickly become dangerous, so it is important to recognize their symptoms and know what you should do to treat them. *What can you do to prevent heat-related illnesses?*

If you are engaging in physical activity outside in very cold temperatures, you need to stay safe. Steps you can take to ensure your safety include the following:

- Check the temperature—including the wind chill factor—carefully before you go outside.
- Dress warmly with several layers of clothing.
- Make sure to protect your head, ears, hands, and feet, which are especially vulnerable to frostbite (**Figure 8.13**). **Frostbite** is an injury caused by the freezing of skin and body tissues. Symptoms of frostbite may include numbness, loss of feeling or a stinging sensation, intense shivering, slurred speech, and a loss of coordination.
- Drink plenty of fluids, just as you would when doing physical activities in hot weather.

Treat Injuries

Sports activities and falls are common causes of injuries. Some of the most common injuries related to physical activities are sprains, dislocations, fractures, and concussions.

A **sprain** is an injury to tissues called *ligaments* that hold joints together. If a joint moves suddenly beyond its normal range of motion, the ligaments stretch and tear. The ankle, knee, and wrist are the most commonly sprained parts of the body. Swelling and pain around the affected area are familiar signs of a sprain.

First aid for a sprain follows the R.I.C.E. treatment (**Figure 8.14**). If a sprain does not improve after two to three days, see a doctor. You may also need to see a doctor if swelling or pain worsens. The doctor may prescribe medication to help reduce the pain and swelling.

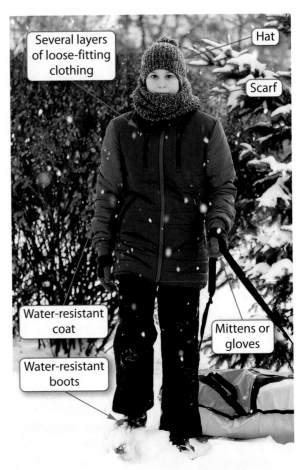

Several layers of loose-fitting clothing

Hat

Scarf

Water-resistant coat

Mittens or gloves

Water-resistant boots

Chekyravaa/Shutterstock.com

Figure 8.13 In cold weather, protective clothing can help prevent hypothermia and frostbite. *Which parts of the body are especially vulnerable to frostbite?*

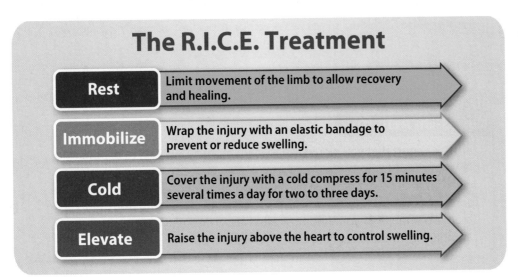

The R.I.C.E. Treatment

Rest — Limit movement of the limb to allow recovery and healing.

Immobilize — Wrap the injury with an elastic bandage to prevent or reduce swelling.

Cold — Cover the injury with a cold compress for 15 minutes several times a day for two to three days.

Elevate — Raise the injury above the heart to control swelling.

Figure 8.14 When following the R.I.C.E. treatment, do all four parts at the same time. *What are the tissues called that stretch and tear when you experience a sprain?*

If you experience a more serious injury, such as a dislocation or fracture, seek medical treatment right away. A **dislocation** is a condition in which bones move out of their normal positions. A **fracture** is a broken bone. Never try to force a bone back into place. This can seriously damage muscles, joints, and nerves.

Always seek medical treatment right away for a concussion, too. A **concussion** is a type of brain injury that results from a blow or jolt to the head or upper body. Contact sports injuries, such as those from football, soccer, wrestling, or hockey, often result in concussions. Concussions are usually temporary, but they can lead to serious permanent complications. Concussions result in the following:

- disorientation
- confusion
- nausea
- weakness
- memory loss
- unconsciousness

If you do experience an injury that requires medical treatment, be sure to follow your doctor's instructions. These instructions could include taking appropriate medications, performing recommended exercises and stretches, or receiving physical therapy. Be sure to follow the doctor's recommendations regarding amount of time to refrain from certain physical activities. Returning to the activity that led to your injury too soon after the injury increases your risk of re-injury.

Lesson 8.3 Review

1. Which of the following is *not* an example of safety equipment for physical activities?

   A. Swim goggles. **C.** Sports jersey.
   B. Reflective gear. **D.** Shin guards.

2. Why is it important to start slowly and not overdo it when starting a fitness program?

3. **True or false.** Drinking lots of water is only important after physical activity.

4. _____ refers to heat-related illnesses, while _____ refers to cold-related illnesses.

5. **Critical thinking.** Compare and contrast a dislocation and fracture.

Hands-On Activity

Pick a sport that you would like to learn more about. Talk to people who play the sport or who know the sport well. You may also choose to watch a live event of the sport on TV. What safety equipment do you need to play the sport? What rules exist to keep players safe and protect them from injury? Create a pamphlet of your findings called *Know the Rules of* _____. Share your pamphlets with the rest of the class.

Developing a Personal Physical Activity Plan

Learning Outcomes

After studying this lesson, you will be able to

- **determine** your current level of physical activity.
- **identify** your personal physical activity goals.
- **explain** what FITT means.
- **determine** your maximum heart rate and your target heart rates for moderate- and vigorous-intensity activities.
- **create** a tracking report to help you achieve your physical activity goals.

Key Terms ☞

pulse person's heart rate

intensity amount of energy the body uses per minute during an activity

FITT acronym used to focus on the key fitness factors of frequency, intensity, time, and type

target heart rate number of heartbeats per minute that is safe and effective for a given intensity

maximum heart rate number of beats per minute a person's heart can achieve when working its hardest; varies by age

sets anaerobic activities done in groups of repetitions followed by rest

Graphic Organizer

Make the Most of Your Physical Activities

In a table similar to the one shown, write the main headings of this lesson. As you listen to your teacher present this lesson, take notes and organize them by heading. Draw a star beside any words or concepts you do not yet understand.

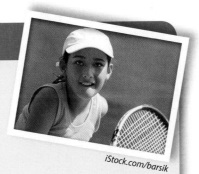

iStock.com/barsik

Checking Your Health-Related Fitness Level
Setting Your Goals
Maximizing Your Workouts

M̲ost people, even those who appear fit, can improve some aspects of their fitness. From the previous lessons, even though he is strong, Danny can improve his heart and lung strength to prevent getting so out of breath. Madison can hike and bike, but she might still have issues with her flexibility or balance. That is why physical activity plans are "personal." You can focus on areas in need of improvement. Madison and Danny's goals may be very different from yours.

In this lesson, you will learn how to create your personal physical activity plan. You are already well on your way. You know how much, and what types of, physical activity you need. You have also had a chance to choose activities you would enjoy doing. The next steps in creating your plan are to check your current level of fitness and set your goals. Then, you will be ready to get moving and experience the benefits of physical activities.

Checking Your Health-Related Fitness Level

To check your current fitness level, you will need to measure the different parts of health-related fitness. This includes your heart and lung strength, muscle strength, endurance, flexibility, and body composition. As you check your fitness level, be sure to record your results. Ask your teacher to look at your results and help you identify the areas in which you may need to improve. Keep your results in a safe place so you can keep track of your progress as you work toward your goals.

To begin, measure the following areas of your health-related fitness:

- Check aerobic fitness by timing yourself to see how long it takes you to briskly walk one mile. Before you start, check and record your **pulse** (your heart rate). Check and record your pulse again after you finish. See **Figure 8.15** for ways to take your pulse.

- Measure your muscle strength and endurance by counting how many push-ups you can do at one time. If you are not very physically active, you may want to do modified push-ups on your knees.

- Check your flexibility by noting how far you can reach forward, toward your toes, while sitting with your legs straight in front of you.

- Measure your waist circumference and determine your body mass index (BMI) using the formula you learned in Chapter 7: *Nutrition*. (Also, see the BMI charts for boys and girls in the *Appendix* at the back of this text.)

Taking Your Pulse

- Find your pulse on the artery of the wrist in line with your thumb.
- Place the tips of your index and middle fingers over the artery and press lightly.
- Start counting on a beat. Count the first beat as zero (not one).
- Count the number of heartbeats for a full 60 seconds. You can also count for six seconds and multiply by 10.

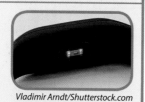
Voyagerix/Shutterstock.com

Heart rate monitors and some *fitness trackers* worn around the wrist can also measure your pulse. These devices measure your pulse by shining a light into the blood vessels in your wrist. The light measures changes in blood volume each time your heart beats and blood is pushed through your body. Less light reflected back into the sensor on your wrist means more blood volume and a faster pulse.

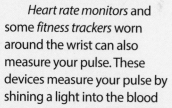
Vladimir Arndt/Shutterstock.com

Figure 8.15 You can check your pulse manually or use a device.

Setting Your Goals

If you currently do not meet the daily physical activity guideline for your age group, you might want to set goals that will help you work toward being more active every day. Perhaps you already get plenty of physical activity, but you would like to perform at a certain level of intensity. **Intensity** is the amount of energy the body uses per minute during an activity. Maybe you would like to set a goal to be physically active at a certain time of day, such as every morning. You might even want to set a goal to join a sports team or take dance lessons.

BUILDING Your Skills

Be SMART, Stay Motivated

Have you ever tried achieving physical activity goals and given up? Perhaps you just never knew where to start. Adopting a more physically fit lifestyle is not easy, and there are often many obstacles to overcome along the way. By setting SMART goals, you are more likely to be successful and stay motivated. Following are examples of SMART goals. Notice that each goal is specific, measurable, achievable, relevant, and timely:

- To improve my endurance, I will ride my bike five miles after school on Monday and Thursday.
- Replace 60 minutes of watching TV with 60 minutes of physical activity on Tuesday, Thursday, and Saturday.
- To prepare for swim team tryouts, swim 30 minutes three days a week starting at the beginning of the summer to increase stamina.
- Join an aerobics class by the end of the month to help lose one pound a week to reach overall weight loss goal.

As you start writing your SMART goal, keep in mind that you are much more likely to be successful when you choose activities you enjoy. Be sure to include both short-term and long-term goals. Your short-term goals should act as stepping stones to the long-term goal. For example, a long-term goal might be to run a five-mile race at the end of the summer. A short-term goal might be to run one mile three times this week.

Setting a SMART Physical Activity Goal

Using the tips above, write your own SMART physical activity goal. Identify the long-term goal and the short term goals you can use to reach your long-term goal. Once you create your goals, design a one-week plan of action. Use Figure 8.17 as an example of a chart you can use. The next step is to get moving. Begin your daily activity plan and fill in your chart. In the comments section of the chart, record your thoughts and feelings related to your progress. After completing your plan for a week, reflect on if you reached your goal and identify any changes you would want to make to your plan. Make any necessary changes and create a new chart for next week. Continue this activity until your behavior becomes a lifestyle.

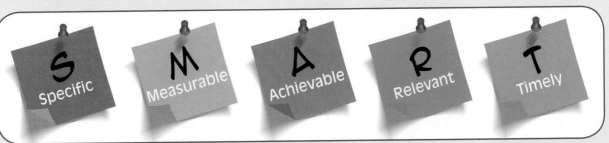

Specific   Measurable   Achievable   Relevant   Timely

WDstocker/Shutterstock.com

As you set your goals, use the acronym *FITT* to keep your focus on key factors. **FITT** stands for frequency, intensity, time, and type. When using FITT factors, consider the following:

- **Frequency.** Frequency involves how often you engage in physical activity. According to the *Physical Activity Guidelines for Americans*, children and teens need to engage in various aerobic activities every day.
- **Intensity.** Intensity is the amount of energy your body uses per minute while engaging in an activity (**Figure 8.16**). You can judge the intensity of a physical activity by how it affects your heart rate and breathing.

Figure 8.16
Different physical activities performed at different intensities affect the number of calories burned. *If you weighed 100 lbs. and ran at a rate of 6 miles per hour for 30 minutes, how many calories would you burn?*

Approximate Calories Burned in 60 Minutes*

Activity	Calories Burned	Activity	Calories Burned
Running: 6 mph (10 min./mile)	480	Hiking	288
Sergey Novikov/Shutterstock.com		*Blend Images/Shutterstock.com*	
Swimming laps (vigorous)	480	Stretching	192
Blacqbook/Shutterstock.com		*Rawpixel.com/Shutterstock.com*	
Jumping rope	480	Volleyball	144
Pressmaster/Shutterstock.com		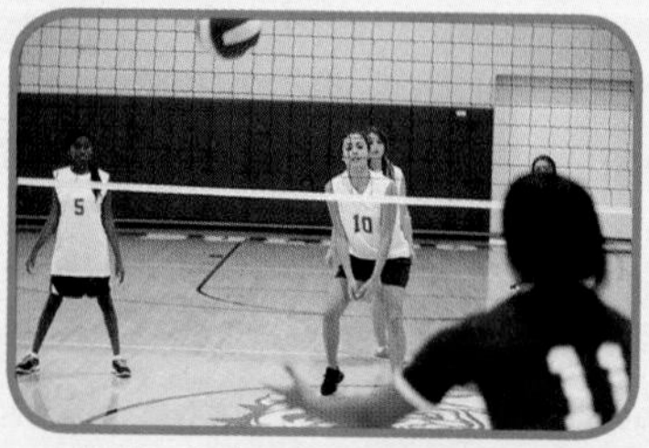 *Monkey Business Images/Shutterstock.com*	
Bicycling: 12–13.9 mph	384	Lifting weights (general)	144
michaeljung/Shutterstock.com		*Rob Marmion/Shutterstock.com*	

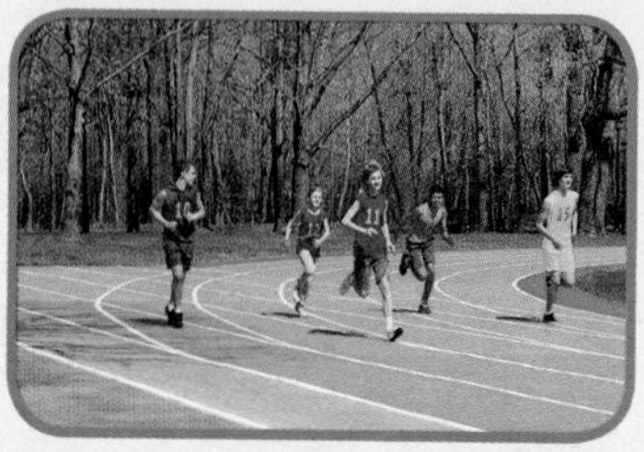

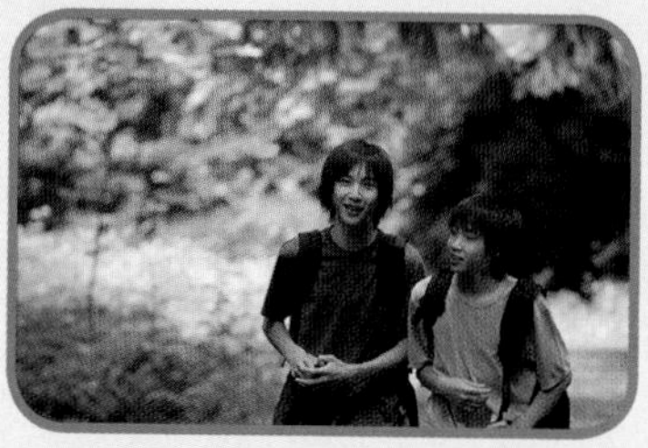

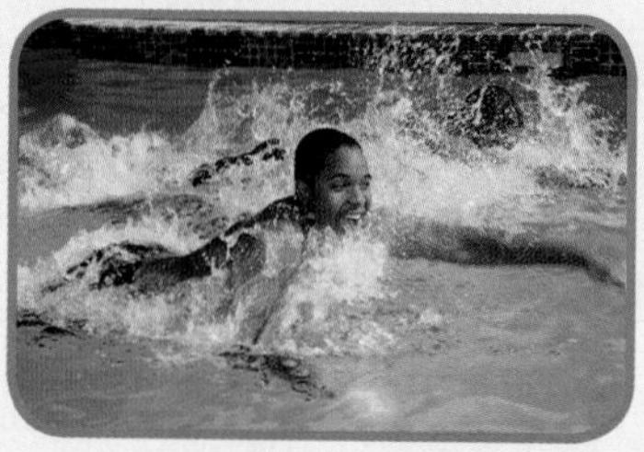

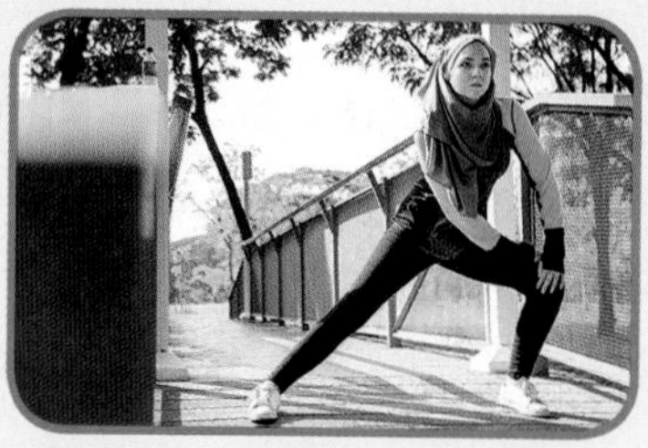

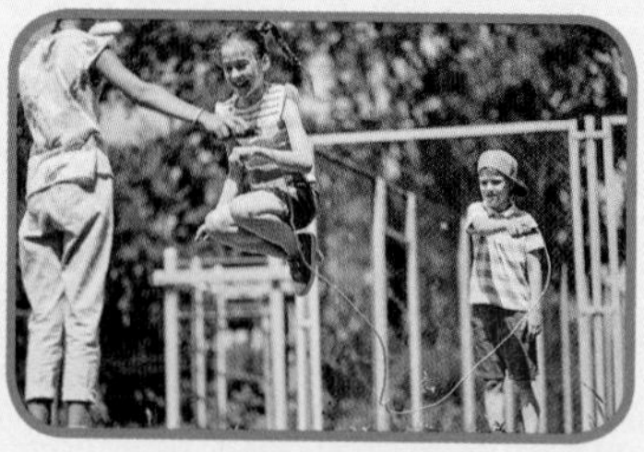

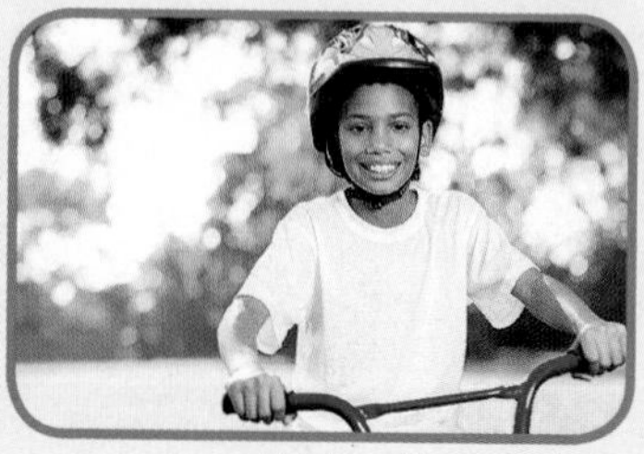

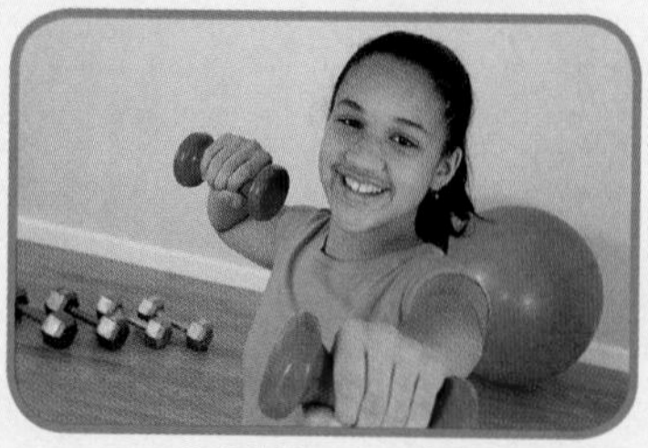

*Based on the average calories burned per hour for a 100-lb. person.

- **Time.** Time refers to the duration of your activity. Children and teens should be active for at least 60 minutes every day. How you choose to use this time depends on your schedule. You may choose to do all 60 minutes at once. Some people, however, prefer to break up their activities into smaller chunks of time. For example, you may do 30 minutes of physical activity in PE class. Then, you may take a 30-minute walk after school.
- **Type.** Type refers to the different activities you do. The types of activities you choose to engage in should be ones you enjoy. Choosing activities that you enjoy helps set you up for success in achieving your goals.

Maximizing Your Workouts

Once you have identified and set your physical activity goals, you are almost ready to get moving. Before you begin, however, figure out how you want to keep track of your progress. You may want to keep an activity log or create a spreadsheet to record your progress. Use whatever tracking method works best for you. **Figure 8.17** shows a sample tracking report.

Recording your workouts will ensure that you stay on track with your goals. If a certain physical activity is not working for you, or a time of day is not good, you may need to revise your plan. Assess your progress regularly and adjust your goals as needed to ensure success.

Sample Tracking Report				
Day	**Physical Activity**	**Time**	**Achievement**	**Comments**
Sunday				
Monday				
Tuesday				
Wednesday				
Thursday				
Friday				
Saturday				

Figure 8.17
This example of a basic physical activity log can help you track your achievements over time. *If your plan is not working for you, what should you do?*

Now that you are ready to start your workout, there are a few important guidelines to remember. In the following sections, you will learn how to make the most of your workouts.

Warm-Ups

No matter what type of physical activity you do, it is important to warm up your muscles before you begin (**Figure 8.18**). A simple 5- to 10-minute warm-up helps get much-needed blood to your muscles. This brief warm-up time helps to prevent injuries.

The warm-up should include the following two distinct parts:

- a low-intensity aerobic activity, such as light jogging, jumping jacks, or brisk walking
- at least 5 minutes of muscle stretching, starting at the top of your body and moving to your lower body

Some experts suggest doing a light version of the activity you are about to do as your warm-up. For example, just before a basketball game, you might shoot some baskets and retrieve missed shots. Before a tennis match, you might casually hit some balls back and forth with a partner.

Aerobic Workouts

To maximize your aerobic workouts, you need to perform aerobic activities at a moderate- or vigorous-intensity level. During an activity of *moderate intensity*, your heart rate and breathing are faster than normal, but you can still carry on a conversation. During an activity of *vigorous intensity*, your heart rate and breathing are much faster than normal. It is difficult to talk during vigorous-intensity activity.

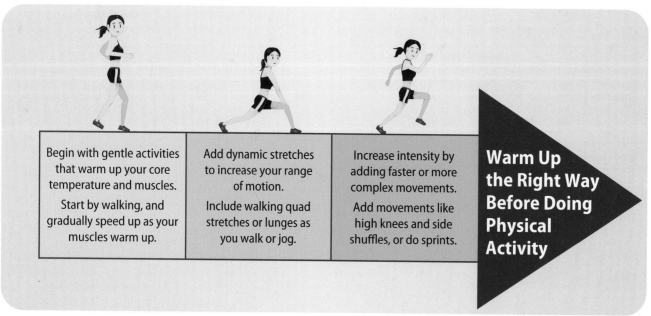

Begin with gentle activities that warm up your core temperature and muscles.

Start by walking, and gradually speed up as your muscles warm up.

Add dynamic stretches to increase your range of motion.

Include walking quad stretches or lunges as you walk or jog.

Increase intensity by adding faster or more complex movements.

Add movements like high knees and side shuffles, or do sprints.

Warm Up the Right Way Before Doing Physical Activity

TORWAISTUDIO/Shutterstock.com

Figure 8.18 Warm-ups should begin with gentle activities and gradually increase in intensity as your muscles warm up and loosen. *Why is it important to warm up before doing physical activity?*

Reaching your **target heart rate** will help you get the best results from your workout. Your target heart rate will vary based on the activity.

- For moderate-intensity activity, a person's target heart rate should be 50 to 70 percent of maximum heart rate.
- For vigorous-intensity activity, a person's target heart rate should be 70 to 85 percent of maximum heart rate.

What is maximum heart rate? Your **maximum heart rate** is the number of beats per minute your heart can achieve when working its hardest. A single, standard maximum does not exist. Maximum heart rate depends on a person's age. There are numerous apps available to help you measure your target and maximum heart rates.

You can also calculate your maximum heart rate by subtracting your age from 220. Once you determine your maximum heart rate, you can calculate your target heart rate for different levels of physical activity. **Figure 8.19** shows how to calculate your maximum heart rate and target heart rates.

Anaerobic Workouts

During anaerobic workouts, you will be performing exercises such as sit-ups, push-ups, pull-ups, and squats. To get the most out of these workouts, do anaerobic exercises for 20 to 30 minutes, two or three times a week. Do not perform any type of anaerobic activity unless you know the proper form for each exercise. Proper form includes holding a position correctly and paying attention to your breathing. Using improper form can lead to injuries and less-than-desirable increases in strength and endurance.

Figure 8.19
Achieving your target heart rate can help you optimize your aerobic workouts.

Calculating Your Maximum and Target Heart Rates

Use the following formula to calculate your maximum heart rate:

220 – age in years = maximum heart rate in beats per minute (bpm)

Example: If you are 13 years of age, you would calculate your maximum heart rate as follows:

220 – 13 = 207 bpm

Multiply your maximum heart rate in bpm by the minimum and maximum levels for moderate- and vigorous-intensity activities to find your target heart rates. Following are the calculations for the example of the 13-year-old:

207 (bpm) x 50% (min. moderate-intensity level) = 103.5

207 (bpm) x 70% (max. moderate-intensity level/ min. vigorous-intensity level) = 144.9

207 (bpm) x 85% (max. vigorous-intensity level) = 175.95

As you can see, a 13-year-old should try to engage in physical activities that cause a heart rate between 104 and 176 bpm. If the goal is moderate-intensity physical activity, this person should maintain a heart rate between 104 and 145 bpm. If the goal is vigorous-intensity physical activity, this person's heart rate should be between 145 and 176 bpm.

The following are some guidelines for achieving anaerobic fitness:

- Start with a 5- to 10-minute warm-up. This includes a low- or moderate-intensity aerobic activity to get blood flowing to your muscles.
- Do two or three **sets** (groups of repetitions followed by rest) of an exercise. For example, you could choose to do three sets of 10 squats.
- As you become stronger, you may choose to do more sets to build muscle endurance.
- Rest your muscles for at least one full day after doing muscle-strengthening exercises. This gives the muscles time to recover.
- Stop right away if you feel sharp pain or experience swollen joints. These are signs that you have done too much. Some muscle soreness is a normal part of doing physical activities. Intense pain, however, indicates a problem.

Cooldowns

A simple 5- to 10-minute cooldown is important after engaging in physical activity. The cooldown helps your heart rate return to a normal, lower level. A cooldown should include some gentle stretching. Stretches help prevent your muscles from feeling stiff and sore the next day. Any light activity can serve as your cooldown. Many people just slow down to low levels of their current activity for a cooldown.

Lesson 8.4 Review

1. Which of the following is a good way to determine your current level of fitness?
   A. Weigh yourself.
   B. Run a marathon.
   C. Test your flexibility.
   D. Take your blood pressure.
2. What does the acronym *FITT* stand for?
3. The maximum _____ _____ is the number of beats per minute a person's heart can achieve when working its hardest.
4. What two parts should be included in a warm-up before physical activity?
5. **Critical thinking.** Why are *FITT* factors important when considering physical activity goals?

Hands-On Activity

Using the formulas in Figure 8.19, calculate your maximum heart rate and target heart rate range. Write these numbers on a piece of paper. Then, engage in aerobic activity for 30 minutes, checking your pulse as soon as you finish. Answer the following questions:

- Was your heart rate within your target heart rate range for moderate- or vigorous-intensity physical activity?
- Do you need to adjust the intensity level to maximize your workout? Why or why not?

Review and Assessment

Summary

Lesson 8.1 Understanding Physical Activity and Fitness

- *Physical activity* is any action in which the body uses energy. *Exercise* describes physical activity that is structured, planned, and has the purpose of increasing physical fitness.
- There are many benefits of physical activity, one of which is lowering your risk of certain diseases, including heart disease, cancer, and type 2 diabetes.
- According to the *Physical Activity Guidelines for Americans*, children and teens should get 60 minutes of physical activity every day.

Lesson 8.2 Knowing About Types of Physical Fitness

- There are two types of fitness: health-related fitness and skill-related fitness.
- The different parts of health-related fitness include heart and lung strength, muscle strength, endurance, flexibility, and body composition.
- *Aerobic* activities, such as dancing or bicycling, use oxygen to break down energy for use in the muscles. In *anaerobic* activities, such as lifting heavy objects or sprinting, stored energy powers the body without the use of oxygen.
- Skill-related fitness is what you need to play sports or other leisure activities. Aspects of skill-related fitness include speed, agility, balance, power, coordination, and reaction time.

Lesson 8.3 Staying Safe During Physical Activity

- Conducting yourself with respect during physical activity involves following rules and being a good sport.
- When engaging in physical activities, wear safety equipment to avoid injury. To avoid dehydration, drink lots of water before, during, and after physical activity.
- Being physically active outside in hot or cold weather can be dangerous if you are not careful. *Hyperthermia* describes heat-related illnesses, and *hypothermia* describes cold-related illnesses, including frostbite.
- First aid for a sprain follows the R.I.C.E. (rest, immobilize, cold, elevate) treatment. For dislocations, fractures, and concussions, seek medical treatment right away.

Lesson 8.4 Developing a Personal Physical Activity Plan

- Checking your health-related fitness level will help you identify areas in which you may need to improve.
- The *FITT* factors of frequency, intensity, time, and type are important to remember when setting physical activity goals.
- Recording your workouts will ensure that you stay on track with your goals. Assess your progress regularly and adjust your goals as needed to ensure success.
- Doing warm-ups and cooldowns are important to help prevent injuries.

Check Your Knowledge

Record your answers to each of the following questions on a separate sheet of paper.

1. Is walking to school an example of exercise or physical activity?
2. People who spend much of their days doing activities that involve sitting and using very little energy are engaging in _____ behaviors.
3. Children and teens should get _____ minutes of physical activity daily.
4. Most of a teen's activity each day should be spent doing _____ (anaerobic/aerobic) activities.
5. **True or false.** Anaerobic activities occur in short bursts, while aerobic activities occur over a longer stretch of time.
6. Which type of fitness refers to the kind of fitness a person needs to successfully perform a sport or leisure activity?
7. What safety equipment is necessary when playing football?
8. The loss of too much fluid from the body causes a condition called _____.
9. A condition in which bones move out of their normal position is called a(n) _____.
10. Which of the following is *not* one of the FITT factors?
    A. Time.
    B. Temperature.
    C. Frequency.
    D. Intensity.
11. Shooting some baskets and retrieving missed shots before you play a game of basketball is an example of a(n) _____ activity.
12. **True or false.** Reaching your maximum heart rate will help you get the best results from your workout.

Use Your Vocabulary ↗

aerobic	fracture	*Physical Activity Guidelines for Americans*
agility	frostbite	
anaerobic	health-related fitness	pulse
concussion	hyperthermia	resistance
dislocation	hypothermia	sedentary behaviors
endorphins	intensity	sets
endurance	maximum heart rate	skill-related fitness
exercise	physical activity	sprain
FITT		target heart rate

13. Write each of the terms above on a separate sheet of paper. For each term, quickly write a word that you think relates to the term. In small groups, exchange papers. Have each person in the group explain a term on the list. Take turns until all terms have complete explanations.
14. Choose four words from the list above. On a separate sheet of paper, write a paragraph correctly using all four of these words. As you write, check the spelling of each word using the glossary in this text or a dictionary. Read your paragraphs in class.

Think Critically

15. **Evaluate.** Based on the information you learned in the chapter, what could you do to make sedentary activities more active? Give a detailed response providing several examples.

16. **Identify.** Identify reasons some teens are physically active while others are not.

17. **Draw conclusions.** Why are teens less likely to follow safety rules such as wearing a helmet while skateboarding or wearing reflective gear at night while biking?

DEVELOP Your Skills

18. **Advocacy and leadership skills.** School districts across the United States have discussed eliminating PE in elementary schools to reduce the school district budget and allow more time for core subjects, such as reading and math. Imagine your former elementary school is considering this change. As a former student, you want to advocate for the younger students who will be impacted. Write a letter to your state senator to voice your concerns. Include the following information in your letter: five or more benefits of physical activity (include ones that are personal to you), the physical activity guidelines for children based on the *Physical Activity Guidelines for Americans*, how you were personally impacted by your PE experience in elementary school, and other relevant information. Present your letter to the class.

19. **Access information and technology skills.** Investigate current fitness-based apps. In small groups, choose one app that you feel is the best one for teens. The app should be fun, increase motivation to be active, and include a variety of activities. Create a presentation about your app highlighting three appealing features and three benefits to using the app. Present it to the class and answer any questions your classmates may have. As you listen to the other presentations, write down the main points and ask for clarification on any details you do not understand.

20. **Communication and goal-setting skills.** Talk with your family about their daily activity habits and health-related fitness. Discuss current obstacles and ways to overcome them. As a family, create a plan to improve family health. This plan may include opportunities to engage in physical activities alone, with one family member, or as an entire family. Display your plan in a visible place in your house.

21. **Decision-making skills.** In the last couple of years, many parents are questioning whether to allow their children to play football due to the short- and long-term effects of concussions. Imagine you are a parent and your child is begging you to play football. Would you allow your child to play? Do additional research about the impact of repetitive concussions and decide if you would let your child play. Write an essay reflecting on the following questions: Would you let your child play tackle football? What is the benefit of playing football? Does the benefit of playing outweigh the risk of concussions? What are the short- and long-term effects of concussions? In your essay, be sure to use transitions and proper paragraph lengths.

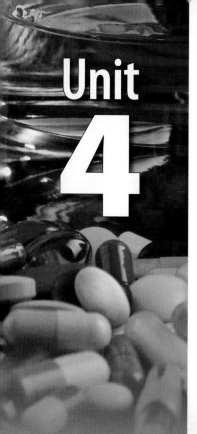

Unit 4

Tobacco, Alcohol, and Other Drugs

Warm-Up Activity

Pros and Cons

While in middle school, you may encounter a situation in which you are asked to try tobacco, alcohol, or other drugs. Read each of the scenarios below. Then, on a separate sheet of paper, list all of the possible pros and cons to each of the scenarios from the person's perspective in the scenario. Consider short-term and long-term pros and cons if this behavior continues. Share your answers with a partner. Add to your pros and cons list based on your partner's responses.

During this unit, you will learn more about tobacco, alcohol, and other drugs. After you finish reading the chapters, revisit these scenarios and add to or change your answers.

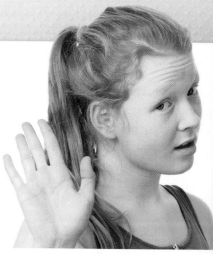

Pete Pahham/Shutterstock.com

Scenario 1
While at overnight camp, one of Maria's roommates pulls out a vape pen from her suitcase. Maria has never tried vaping before and wonders what it would be like.

Scenario 2
Mason's parents trusted him and his friend, James, to stay home while they went to dinner. While Mason plays video games, James explores the house until he finds the liquor cabinet. James breaks the lock and takes two big gulps of liquor, then offers it to Mason. Mason does not want James to tease him for not drinking.

Scenario 3
While at the school dance, several of Kristina's friends invite her to meet in the bathroom to smoke marijuana. Not wanting to be left out, Kristina walks with her friends to the bathroom.

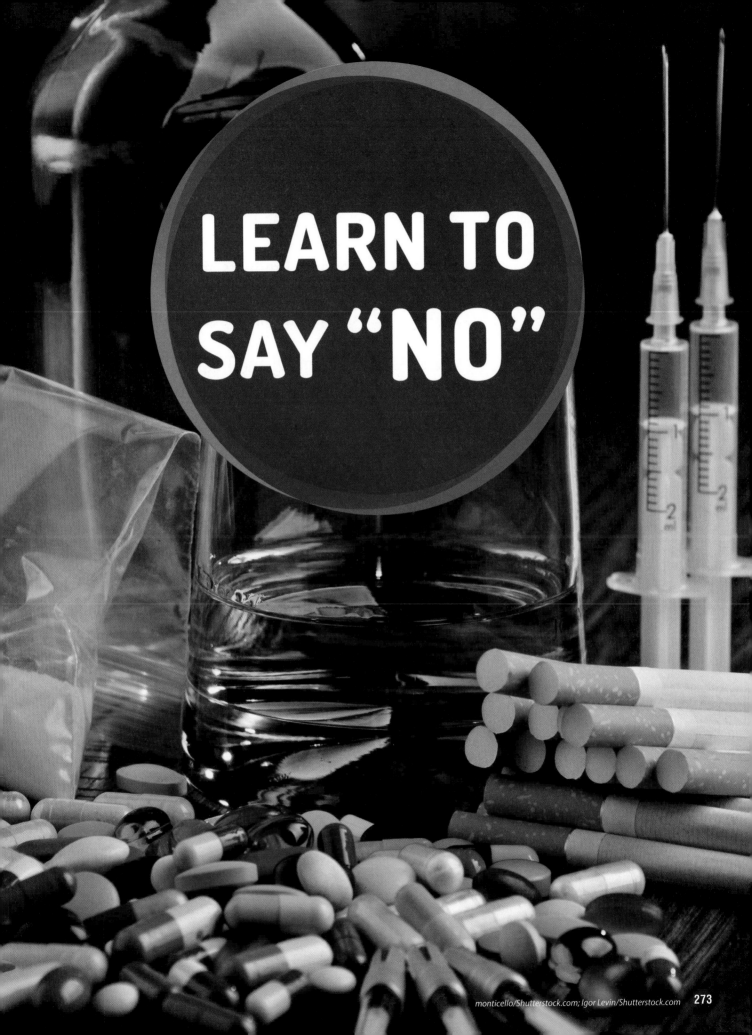

LEARN TO SAY "NO"

Chapter

9

Tobacco and Vaping

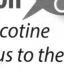

Essential Question

How is nicotine hazardous to the human body?

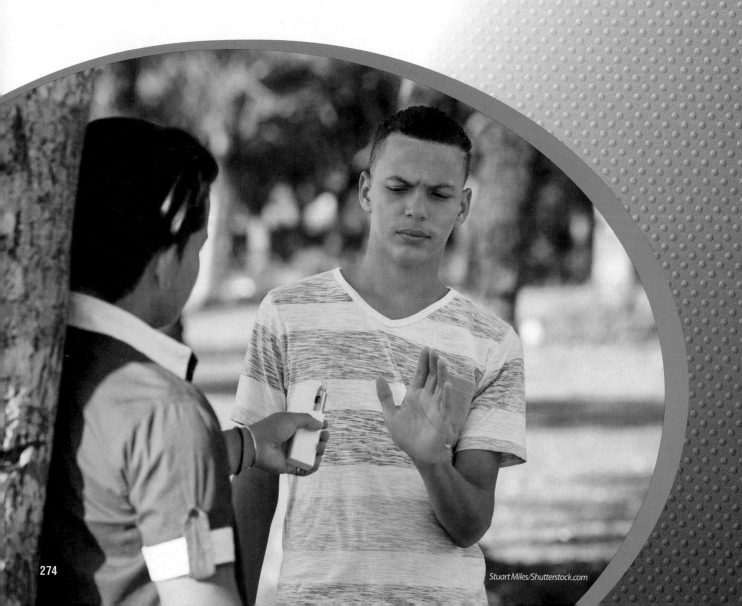

Stuart Miles/Shutterstock.com

Reading Activity

In what ways do you think tobacco products are harmful to your health? Before reading the chapter, write a two-paragraph essay explaining some of the health effects of tobacco products. After you finish reading the chapter, consider what information you might add to your essay. Share your essay and any additions with a partner.

How Healthy Are You?

In this chapter, you will be learning about tobacco products. Before you begin reading, take the following quiz to assess your current tobacco habits.

Healthy Choices	Yes	No
Do you refuse to use tobacco products, such as cigarettes, vaping devices, cigars, pipes, or chewing tobacco?		
Do you avoid exposure to secondhand smoke and aerosol whenever possible?		
Can you identify the many, severe health hazards of using tobacco products?		
Do you understand the social, physical, and mental costs of using tobacco products?		
Are you confident in your ability to say "no" to friends or peers who ask if you want to smoke or vape?		
Can you recognize the signs and symptoms of nicotine addiction?		
Do you understand the danger of beginning to "experiment" with tobacco products?		
Can you identify the symptoms of withdrawal from nicotine?		
Do you know the best techniques for quitting tobacco use?		
Can you evaluate the messages you see in tobacco advertisements and the products sold by tobacco companies to avoid manipulation?		

Count your "Yes" and "No" responses. The more "Yes" responses you have, the more healthy tobacco habits you exhibit. Now, take a closer look at the questions with which you responded "No." How can you replace your unhealthy habits with healthy ones? Identify a SMART goal you would like to achieve to help improve your overall health and well-being. Refer to Figure 1.11 to help you set up your SMART goal. If you do not understand the instructions, ask for clarification from your teacher.

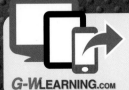

Click on the activity icon or visit www.g-wlearning.com/health to access online vocabulary activities using key terms from the chapter.

Tobacco Products and Your Health

Learning Outcomes

After studying this lesson, you will be able to

- **identify** various forms of tobacco products.
- **assess** the hazardous effects of nicotine on the body.
- **explain** the health risks of cigarettes, vaping devices, and smokeless tobacco.
- **describe** the mental, social, and legal consequences of tobacco use.
- **explain** the health impact of tobacco use on others.

Graphic Organizer

Tobacco Cause and Effect

Create a graphic organizer like the one shown to connect information about tobacco products to the effects they can have on your health and others. Add as much information as you can, and make your columns as long as you need them to be.

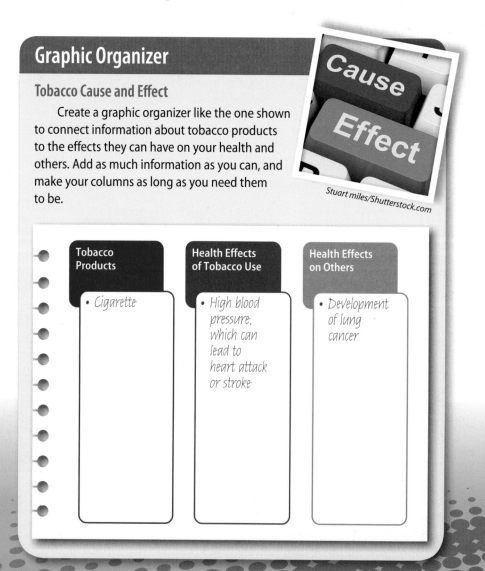

Stuart miles/Shutterstock.com

Tobacco Products	Health Effects of Tobacco Use	Health Effects on Others
• Cigarette	• High blood pressure, which can lead to heart attack or stroke	• Development of lung cancer

U sing any form of a tobacco product increases risk of developing many health conditions. It can also lead to a substance use disorder, which you will learn about in the next lesson. This lesson examines the different types of tobacco products, the effects of tobacco use on the body, and the health impact of being around others who smoke or vape.

Types of Tobacco Products

According to the Food and Drug Administration (FDA), a *tobacco product* is any product made or derived from tobacco and intended for human consumption. **Tobacco** is a plant used to create tobacco-related products such as cigarettes, vape pens, and chewing tobacco. Tobacco leaves contain the chemical *nicotine*. **Nicotine** is a toxic substance that gives tobacco products their addictive quality. Types of tobacco products include cigarettes, vaping devices, and smokeless tobacco.

Cigarettes

A *cigarette* consists of finely cut tobacco, chemical additives, a filter, and a paper wrapping. It is an example of a *combustible* tobacco product, or a product that is burned then inhaled. Someone who smokes a cigarette inhales 7,000 chemicals and **toxic** (poisonous) substances that harm the body (**Figure 9.1**).

Chemicals Found in Cigarettes	
Chemical	**Other Locations**
Acetic acid	Ingredient in hair dye
Acetone	Found in nail polish remover
Ammonia	Common household cleaner
Arsenic	Used in rat poison
Benzene	Found in rubber cement
Butane	Used in lighter fluid
Cadmium	Active component in battery acid
Carbon monoxide	Released in car exhaust fumes
Formaldehyde	Embalming fluid
Hexamine	Found in barbecue lighter fluid
Lead	Used in batteries
Methanol	Main component in rocket fuel
Naphthalene	Ingredient in mothballs
Nicotine	Used as insecticide
Tar	Material for paving roads
Toluene	Used to manufacture paint

Figure 9.1
Cigarettes are made of deadly chemicals that can all cause harm to the body.

The purpose of the filter on a cigarette is to minimize the smoke a person inhales. Modern filters, however, only hold back a small portion of smoke. These filters do not make cigarettes healthier or safer.

Vaping Devices

Historically, cigarettes were the most commonly used tobacco product among young people. Today, vaping devices are the most common form of tobacco product among teens. **Vaping devices** are tobacco products that heat tobacco or synthetic (manmade) nicotine without burning it. These devices are sometimes called *electronic nicotine delivery systems (ENDS)*. **Figure 9.2** shows examples of vaping devices.

Vaping devices contain either tobacco or an **e-liquid**, which is a substance made of nicotine or another drug and other chemicals. E-liquid is also known as *e-juice*, *vape juice*, or *vape liquid*. E-liquids are sometimes flavored with chemicals to taste like peppermint, fruit, or coffee.

A battery is used to heat the e-liquid or tobacco to create a vapor that is inhaled. Many people believe that vaping produces a water vapor. In reality, heating the e-liquid or tobacco creates an **aerosol**, or suspension of fine particles or droplets in the air—like dust, smoke, deodorant spray, or bug spray.

Some people believe vaping devices are safer, healthier, or less addictive than cigarettes. The reality, however, is vaping devices contain nicotine,

Figure 9.2
Vaping devices come in various shapes and forms. *What is a substance made of nicotine and other chemicals that vaping devices contain?*

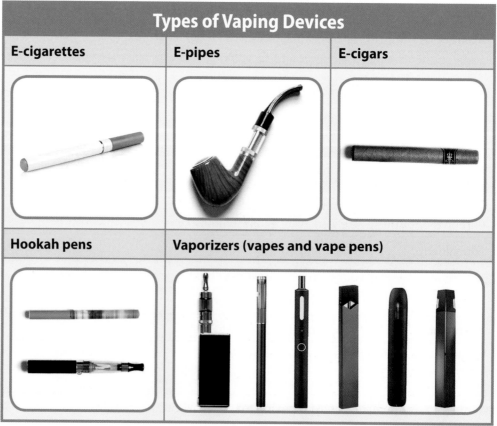

Types of Vaping Devices

| E-cigarettes | E-pipes | E-cigars |

| Hookah pens | Vaporizers (vapes and vape pens) |

E-cigarette: gmstockstudio/Shutterstock.com; All other devices: United States Food and Drug Administration

just like cigarettes. Nicotine, even when vaped, is still a harmful substance that can cause serious health issues and lead to substance use disorder.

Smokeless Tobacco

Smokeless tobacco is a type of tobacco product a person chews, inhales, or dissolves rather than smokes or vapes. It is a *noncombustible*, or not burned, tobacco product. People absorb the nicotine in smokeless tobacco through their mouth tissues. Like cigarettes, smokeless tobacco contains many chemicals and toxic substances that can harm the body. **Figure 9.3** shows forms of smokeless tobacco.

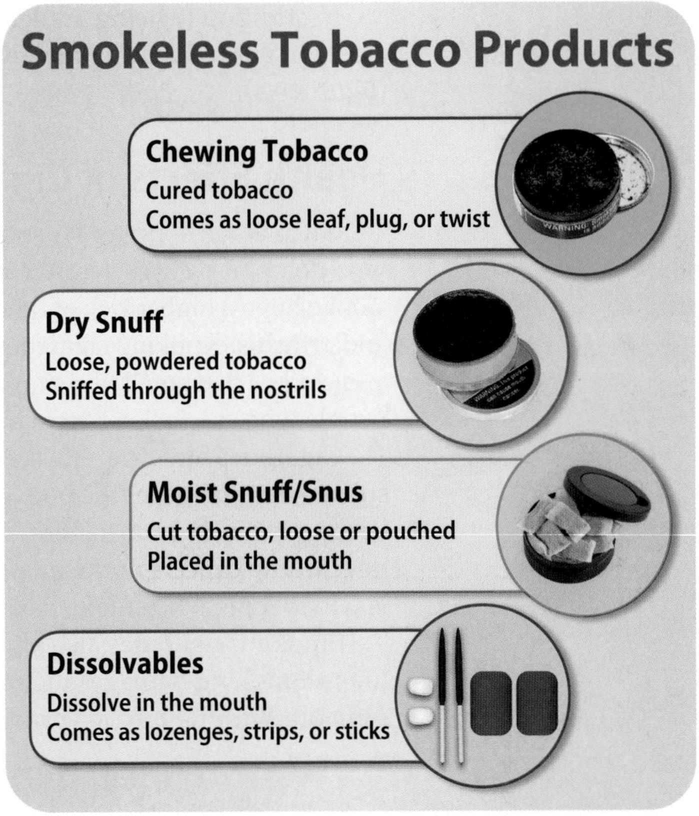

Health Effects of Tobacco Use

Tobacco use increases a person's risk for developing a number of major health conditions. These include cancer, heart disease, and respiratory conditions. In the following sections, you will learn how nicotine affects the body, as well as the health effects of each type of tobacco product.

Smokeless Tobacco Products

Chewing Tobacco
Cured tobacco
Comes as loose leaf, plug, or twist

Dry Snuff
Loose, powdered tobacco
Sniffed through the nostrils

Moist Snuff/Snus
Cut tobacco, loose or pouched
Placed in the mouth

Dissolvables
Dissolve in the mouth
Comes as lozenges, strips, or sticks

Top to bottom: J.A. Dunbar/Shutterstock.com; Rob Hainer/Shutterstock.com; gopixgo/Shutterstock.com; Goodheart-Willcox

Figure 9.3 Smokeless tobacco products include chewing tobacco, snuff, snus, and dissolvables, and can be ingested in a variety of ways.

Health Effects of Nicotine

Tobacco products introduce nicotine into a person's body. Cigarettes, vaping devices, and smokeless tobacco all contain nicotine. Even some e-liquids that claim to be nicotine-free can contain nicotine.

On entering the body, nicotine acts as a stimulant, which increases heart rate, blood pressure, and breathing. It also causes the release of the chemical *dopamine*. **Dopamine** leads to an enjoyable feeling that people crave when using nicotine products. Over time, the body develops a tolerance to nicotine. This means people have to consume higher amounts of nicotine to experience the same effects they felt when consuming lower amounts.

Nicotine is a highly addictive substance, which means it is difficult to stop using. In fact, in 2010, the US Surgeon General identified that nicotine was as addictive as cocaine and heroin. As a result, a person who uses nicotine is at serious risk for becoming addicted and developing a *substance use disorder*. (You will learn about substance use disorder in the next lesson.) Once someone has an addiction to nicotine, that person will experience unpleasant withdrawal symptoms without the substance.

In addition to being addictive, nicotine is toxic and extremely harmful to a person's health. Using nicotine has severe effects on multiple body systems (Figure 9.4).

Health Effects of Cigarettes

On average, long-term users of cigarettes die 13–15 years earlier than people who do not use cigarettes. According to the US Surgeon General, people who smoke have a higher risk of developing type 2 diabetes, vision loss, tuberculosis, and arthritis. Smoking cigarettes leads to stained teeth, sagging skin, and hair and clothes that smell like smoke. It also changes the shape of taste buds. Some people who smoke long-term may lose their appetite and interest in eating.

Cigarettes and cigarette smoke contain thousands of chemicals and toxic substances that harm the body. They also contain more than 70 **carcinogens**, or cancer-causing substances. These carcinogens increase a person's risk for developing cancers of the mouth, throat, esophagus, lungs, and bladder. This is why people who smoke have higher rates of cancer than people who do not.

Smoking cigarettes also affects the respiratory system, which includes the lungs. Smoking damages the respiratory system and makes breathing more difficult. Burning tobacco produces a residue known as **tar**. This substance

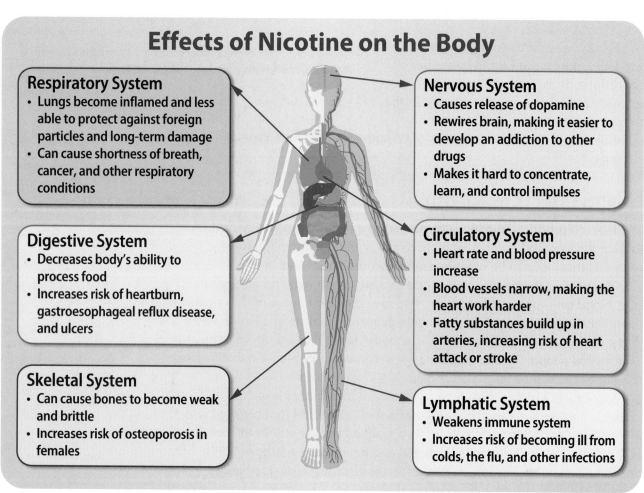

Lilanakani/Shutterstock.com

Figure 9.4 Nicotine is highly toxic to a person's body systems, and its harmful effects are not always reversible.

consists of small, thick, sticky particles. As smoke repeatedly passes through the respiratory system, tar builds up in the lungs. Smoking-related damage to the lungs contributes to the development of chronic respiratory diseases and triggers asthma attacks (**Figure 9.5**).

Health Effects of Vaping Devices

Some people see vaping, or the use of vaping devices, as a harmless alternative to smoking cigarettes. They may also see these devices as less addictive than cigarettes. In reality, vaping is *not* harmless.

Vaping introduces nicotine (or another drug) into a person's body. E-liquids with nicotine contain large amounts of nicotine. For example, one e-liquid pod can contain as much nicotine as a pack of 20 regular cigarettes. Even e-liquids that claim to be nicotine-free contain nicotine.

Most of the time, when people vape, they are consuming an e-liquid made of many chemicals (**Figure 9.6**). Scientists know that inhaling the chemicals in

Respiratory Conditions Caused by Smoking

- **Chronic bronchitis:** ongoing condition in which small tubes in lungs become swollen and irritated
- **Emphysema:** causes airways in lungs to become permanently enlarged and decreases amount of oxygen entering the lungs and bloodstream
- **Asthma:** chronic disease caused by blockages of airflow to and from the lungs; can lead to asthma attack
- **Lung cancer:** abnormal cells grow rapidly along the air passages to form a tumor that affects lungs' ability to transport oxygen to bloodstream

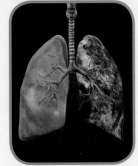
iStock.com/Nerthuz

Figure 9.5 Smoking-related damage to the lungs can have long-term effects on the respiratory system. *What residue from cigarettes damages the lungs?*

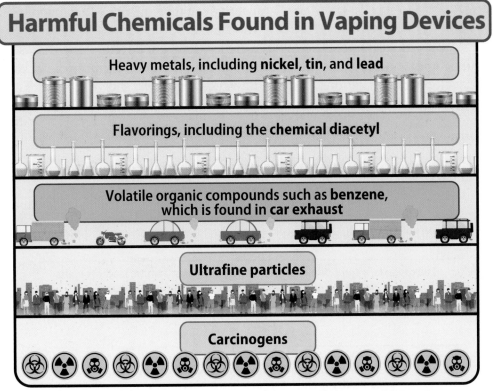

Harmful Chemicals Found in Vaping Devices

Heavy metals, including nickel, tin, and lead

Flavorings, including the chemical diacetyl

Volatile organic compounds such as benzene, which is found in car exhaust

Ultrafine particles

Carcinogens

Figure 9.6 Aerosol created by vaping devices contains many harmful chemicals which are connected to serious health conditions. *What is one rare lung disease related to vaping?*

Top to bottom: Macrovector/Shutterstock.com; Ivan Feoktistov/Shutterstock.com; (vehicles) drical/Shutterstock.com; Antonov Maxim/Shutterstock.com; (signs) ThanasStudio/Shutterstock.com

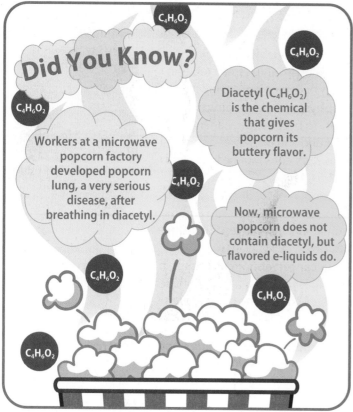

Figure 9.7 begins in the illustration with speech bubbles:

Did You Know?

Workers at a microwave popcorn factory developed popcorn lung, a very serious disease, after breathing in diacetyl.

Diacetyl ($C_4H_6O_2$) is the chemical that gives popcorn its buttery flavor.

Now, microwave popcorn does not contain diacetyl, but flavored e-liquids do.

Popcorn bucket: Finka/Shutterstock.com; Smoke: Arcady/Shutterstock.com

Figure 9.7 The chemical diacetyl ($C_4H_6O_2$), an ingredient in flavored e-liquids, was removed from microwave popcorn because breathing it in caused factory workers to develop a serious disease called *popcorn lung*.

aerosol can lead to respiratory conditions, including inflammation and long-term lung disease. One rare lung disease related to vaping is *popcorn lung*. Diacetyl, a flavoring found in more than 75 percent of flavored e-liquids, causes this disease (**Figure 9.7**). Popcorn lung causes scarring and inflammation in the bronchioles, the smallest airways in the lungs. This can cause coughing, shortness of breath, and wheezing.

Vaping also harms health in other ways. For example, vape battery explosions can cause serious injury and even death. Some people also use vaping devices to consume other drugs such as marijuana.

Health Effects of Smokeless Tobacco

Smokeless tobacco contains nicotine and carcinogens. The harmful effects of these substances are the same as if they were smoked. In fact, because smokeless tobacco is placed directly into the mouth, people who use these products actually absorb even more nicotine than people who smoke.

People who use smokeless tobacco are less likely to develop lung diseases than people who use cigarettes or vaping devices. They do increase their risk of developing other serious diseases, however. **Figure 9.8** shows the health risks of smokeless tobacco.

Figure 9.8 Smokeless tobacco is just as harmful as cigarettes or vaping devices, and can put users at risk for certain cancers, leukoplakia, heart disease, and dental diseases.

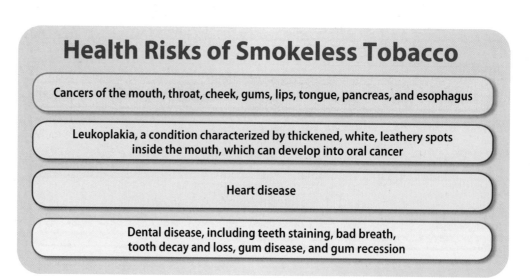

Health Risks of Smokeless Tobacco

Cancers of the mouth, throat, cheek, gums, lips, tongue, pancreas, and esophagus

Leukoplakia, a condition characterized by thickened, white, leathery spots inside the mouth, which can develop into oral cancer

Heart disease

Dental disease, including teeth staining, bad breath, tooth decay and loss, gum disease, and gum recession

The Myths and Facts of Vaping

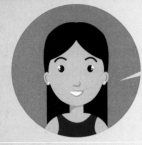

When I vape, I am just inhaling water vapor.

FACT:
Vaping does not create water vapor. It creates an aerosol that can contain harmful substances such as lead.

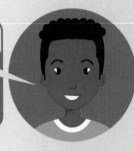

Vaping does not hurt anyone else.

FACT:
Bystanders also breathe in the harmful chemicals in secondhand aerosol exhaled by people who vape.

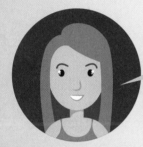

My e-liquid is just flavoring.

FACT:
E-liquids contain harmful chemicals, including some that have been linked to serious diseases.

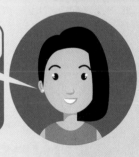

Everyone I follow on social media vapes.

FACT:
Vaping companies sell their products and make money through social media campaigns.

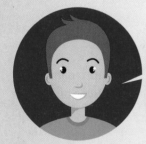

Vaping is not addictive since there is no nicotine.

FACT:
One e-liquid pod can contain as much nicotine as 20 cigarettes. Even nicotine-free e-liquids may contain nicotine.

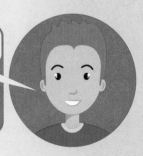

Vaping has nothing to do with cigarettes.

FACT:
Young people who use vaping devices may be more likely to smoke cigarettes in the future.

Studio_G/Shutterstock.com

Mental, Social, and Legal Consequences

Tobacco products do more than affect the human body. They impact a person's mind and social relationships and can lead to legal consequences. The effects of tobacco use are long lasting and can affect your future in serious ways.

Mental Consequences

Most young people believe they can smoke, vape, or chew tobacco occasionally or even regularly for a few years and then easily quit. The reality, however, is most people become dependent on the nicotine. For example, young people are especially sensitive to the effects of nicotine because their brains are still developing until 25 years of age, which makes it easier to develop an addiction. A dependence on nicotine makes it very difficult to stop using tobacco products.

Nicotine makes it harder to learn, concentrate, and control impulses. People who use nicotine are more likely to engage in other risky behaviors, such as sexual activity and illegal drug use. Nicotine can also make mental health conditions and mental illnesses worse if people use nicotine to relieve symptoms instead of seeking professional treatment.

Social Consequences

The use of tobacco can harm a person's social relationships. When people feel dependent on nicotine, getting more of that substance can seem like the only important thing to them. As a result, young people may lie to their parents, guardians, or friends about their use of tobacco products. They may steal money to buy cigarettes, vaping devices or e-liquids, or smokeless tobacco. Lying and theft can cause long-term trust issues.

Because tobacco use harms people's health, people may withdraw from someone who uses tobacco products. A person who uses tobacco products may have to leave a social situation to smoke, vape, or chew. This may cause the person to feel left out or miss special moments.

Legal Consequences

Young people who smoke, vape, or chew tobacco can experience serious legal consequences. In the United States, the federal government recently increased the legal age for buying tobacco products from age 18 to age 21 (**Figure 9.9**). Some cities, such as Beverly Hills in California, have banned the sale of tobacco products altogether.

Some people under the legal age limit try to buy or ask someone else to buy tobacco products for them. If they are caught doing this, they may have to pay fines or perform community service.

Many schools have policies that forbid the use of cigarettes, vaping devices, and smokeless tobacco. Students who bring these products to school or use them in the

Zoart Studio/Shutterstock.com

Figure 9.9 Tobacco products are illegal to purchase under 21 years of age in the United States, including online purchases.

classroom or at school-sponsored events may face disciplinary actions and even suspension. In communities, young people can also face legal consequences for using tobacco products in public places, such as restaurants.

Health Effects on Others

People who use tobacco products are not the only ones at risk for negative health outcomes. Smoking and vaping both release substances into the air other people breathe. **Secondhand smoke** refers to the tobacco smoke released into the environment by people who smoke. People who regularly inhale secondhand smoke because they live or socialize with people who smoke have a greater risk of developing lung cancer or heart disease. Secondhand smoke is especially dangerous for children, as it can cause ear infections, asthma attacks, bronchitis, and pneumonia.

Vaping devices release aerosol that others nearby can inhale. Aerosol inhaled involuntarily by others is called **secondhand aerosol**. Secondhand aerosol from vaping can contain harmful chemicals, such as diacetyl and heavy metals. If you socialize with a person who vapes, you are exposing yourself to similar health risks as if you were vaping.

Thirdhand smoke and aerosol also affect people who are around others who use tobacco products. **Thirdhand smoke** refers to the particles and gases left over after a cigarette is extinguished. Similarly, the particles and gases left over from a vaping device are called **thirdhand aerosol**. The particles in thirdhand smoke and aerosol land and remain on virtually any surface in the area where someone has smoked or vaped (**Figure 9.10**).

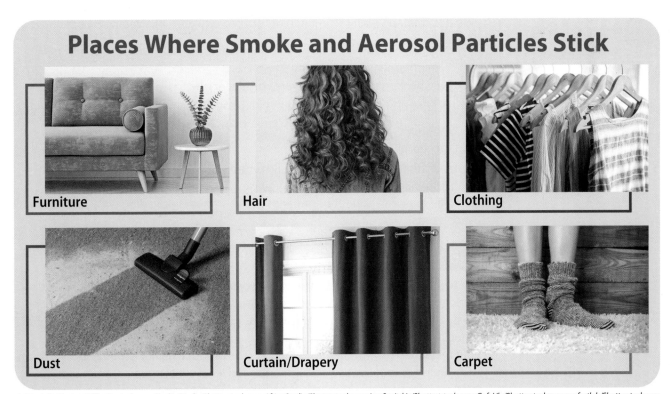

Places Where Smoke and Aerosol Particles Stick

Furniture

Hair

Clothing

Dust

Curtain/Drapery

Carpet

Left to right: Marina_D/Shutterstock.com; Cookie Studio/Shutterstock.com; Africa Studio/Shutterstock.com; Lev Savitskiy/Shuttertstock.com; Gaf_Lila/Shutterstock.com; perfectlab/Shutterstock.com

Figure 9.10 Particles left over from cigarettes and vaping devices can remain on a variety of surfaces.

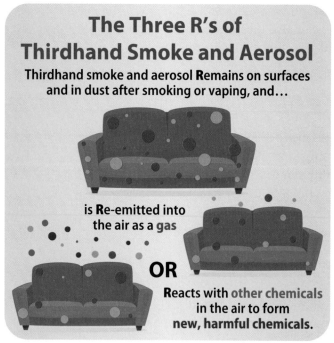

The Three R's of Thirdhand Smoke and Aerosol

Thirdhand smoke and aerosol **Remains on surfaces and in dust after smoking or vaping, and…**

is **Re**-emitted into the air as a **gas**

OR

Reacts with **other chemicals in the air to form new, harmful chemicals.**

Elvetica/Shutterstock.com

Figure 9.11 Thirdhand smoke and aerosol remains on surfaces even after smoking or vaping, and can become harmful as it is re-emitted into the air or combines with other chemicals to form harmful carcinogens.

Exposure to thirdhand smoke and aerosol can lead to serious diseases such as asthma and cancer. These chemicals can even become more dangerous over time. It is very difficult to remove thirdhand smoke and aerosol from spaces. Simple actions such as vacuuming and wiping down surfaces do not eliminate the residue. Particles remain behind, even after the smell fades (**Figure 9.11**). This means that people often are not aware of their exposure to thirdhand smoke and aerosol.

To maintain good health, avoid exposure to secondhand and thirdhand smoke and aerosol whenever possible. Choose restaurants and other public places that do not allow smoking or vaping. If someone is smoking or vaping near you, leave the area or ask the person to stop. If family members or friends smoke or vape, consider explaining the health risks to them and ask them to stop. You might just convince them to quit.

Lesson 9.1 Review

1. What is created when the e-liquid or tobacco is heated in a vaping device?
2. List three major health conditions that a person is at risk of developing through tobacco use.
3. People who smoke have higher rates of cancer due to the _____ in tobacco smoke.
4. Which chemical in vaping aerosol can cause popcorn lung?

   A. Nicotine.

   B. Diacetyl.

   C. Carcinogens.

   D. Nickel.

5. **Critical thinking.** Consider the health effects on your body from secondhand smoke and aerosol. How often are you exposed to secondhand smoke and aerosol? How can you set boundaries about smoking or vaping with your family and friends?

Hands-On Activity

In small groups, create an anti-vaping or anti-tobacco message to encourage students at your school to say "no" to tobacco use. Possible formats include a message for the morning announcements, a poster or flyer, an article for your school newspaper, a brochure, or a social media post. Include the following in your message: harmful chemicals found in the product; health issues associated with vaping or tobacco use; social, mental and legal consequences; and other relevant information and images to enhance your message.

Understanding Tobacco Use

Learning Outcomes

After studying this lesson, you will be able to

- **summarize** individual factors that cause teens to try tobacco products.
- **describe** how family members, peers, and the media are factors that cause tobacco use among adolescents.
- **explain** what is a substance use disorder.
- **analyze** the stages of substance use disorder in relation to tobacco use.
- **give examples** of withdrawal symptoms people with a nicotine addiction may experience.

Key Terms 🔗

peer pressure influence that people your age or status have on your actions

substance use disorder mental illness in which a person continues using a substance despite negative effects on health and life

co-occurring disorder two or more mental illnesses that occur together

tolerance body's need for an increased amount of a substance to experience effects once felt with smaller amounts

dependence effect that occurs when the body needs an addictive substance in its system to function normally or avoid cravings and anxiety

triggers reminders that cause people to feel a strong desire for a substance

addiction physical and psychological need for a substance or behavior

withdrawal unpleasant symptoms that occur when someone with an addiction to a substance tries to stop using that substance

Graphic Organizer

Tobacco Use

Create a KWL chart similar to the one shown. Before reading the lesson, list facts of what you know and what you want to know about people's tobacco use. After reading the lesson, write what you have learned. If you have any question about what you are reading, raise your hand and ask your teacher. Then, team up with a classmate and discuss each other's lists. Are there items you would add to your list?

GrungeElfz/Shutterstock.com

K	W	L
What I Know	**What I Want to Know**	**What I Have Learned**
People may be pressured by friends to use tobacco products.	How does the media influence tobacco use?	Withdrawal describes unpleasant symptoms people experience when quitting.

You learned about health issues and mental, social, and legal consequences associated with tobacco use in the previous lesson. You also learned that secondhand and thirdhand smoke and aerosol puts family members and friends at risk for health conditions. Given these facts, you may wonder why anyone would start to use tobacco products. Despite the health risks, the number of youths who used vaping devices increased by 1.5 million in 2018.

In this lesson, you will learn about several factors that may cause someone to try tobacco products. This lesson also discusses how using tobacco products can lead to a substance use disorder.

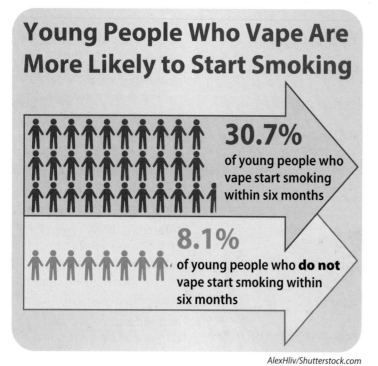

Figure 9.12 Using vaping devices increases the risk of also using cigarettes.

Factors Affecting Tobacco Use

Most young people who begin to smoke, vape, or use smokeless tobacco do plan to quit. They believe that quitting will be easy. They soon find out, however, that tobacco use is very difficult to stop. The majority of young people who use tobacco become adults who regularly use tobacco products (**Figure 9.12**).

Various factors may cause a young person to try a cigarette, vaping device, or smokeless tobacco. These include individual factors and external factors such as family, peer pressure, and the media.

Individual Factors

Individual factors are the factors related to your identity and behaviors. These factors include genetic makeup, mental health, and stage of development. Genetic makeup influences how likely a person is to develop an addiction to nicotine. For example, having a family history of nicotine addiction increases a person's risk for developing an addiction to nicotine.

Some young people smoke, vape, or chew tobacco in an attempt to manage their mental health. They may feel stressed at school and turn to tobacco use as a way to relax. They may also be trying out a new identity. Young people may associate using tobacco with maturity, glamour, rebellion, or toughness. They may also believe that tobacco use will make them seem older or cooler. Mental health conditions can increase the risk of nicotine addiction in young people. Rather than turning to tobacco products, people with mental health conditions and mental illnesses need to seek professional treatment.

Another individual factor that influences risk is stage of development. As you learned in the previous lesson, young people are especially sensitive to the effects of nicotine because their brains are still developing. If a young person uses tobacco at an early age, this person is more likely to develop an addiction to nicotine.

Family

Family members' attitudes and behaviors about tobacco use influence whether young people smoke, vape, or chew tobacco. Young people are much less likely to start using tobacco products if their families set clear expectations, discuss their views on tobacco products, and follow through on consequences for using tobacco (**Figure 9.13**).

Families' attitudes toward tobacco use create an environment that influences young people's behavior. Some families are strongly against the use of tobacco products. These family members do not use tobacco products and may tell guests not to use cigarettes, vaping devices, and smokeless tobacco in the house. In this environment, young people are less likely to use tobacco. Other families are more accepting of tobacco use and may even use tobacco products in the home environment. Young people in this environment are more likely to try using cigarettes, vaping devices, or smokeless tobacco.

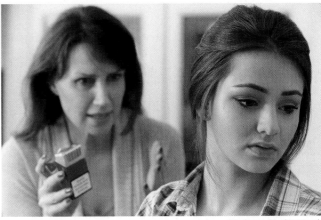

iStock.com/MachineHeadz

Figure 9.13 Parents who set clear rules and consequences to smoking are less likely to have children experiment with smoking.

Peer Pressure

During the school-age years, the influence of friends can be strong. Most young people want their friends to accept them. This may lead them to engage in unhealthy behaviors. The people you spend your time with have a big influence on whether you try tobacco products.

Many young people use their first tobacco product with a friend. Young people with friends who smoke, vape, or chew tobacco are also much more likely to use tobacco products themselves. Young people whose friends smoke or vape are offered a tobacco product much more often than those whose friends do not smoke or vape. It is important to learn how to say "no" when someone offers you a cigarette, a vaping device, or smokeless tobacco. (You will learn more about this in the next lesson.)

Young people may experience peer pressure to use a tobacco product. **Peer pressure** is the influence that people your age or status have on your actions. Peer pressure is negative if used to encourage an individual to do something unsafe, unhealthy, or uncomfortable. Peer pressure is positive if it is respectful and encourages healthy behaviors (**Figure 9.14**).

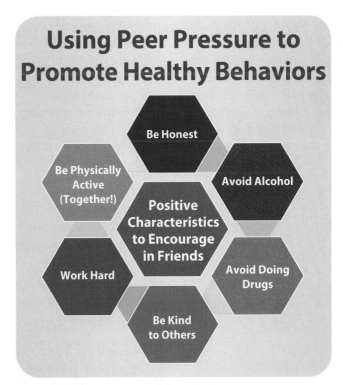

Figure 9.14 There are many ways peer pressure can be used to inspire healthy behaviors. Encouraging your friends not to vape is one example. *Give an example of a time when you influenced someone, or were influenced by someone else, with positive peer pressure.*

CASE STUDY

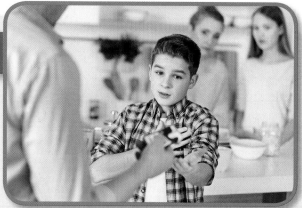

iStock.com/yacobchuk

Kevin's Decision to Vape

Kevin did not think it was that big of a deal when he tried vaping for the first time. It was at the beginning of last school year. He was waiting after school for his mom to pick him up, and an older group of boys dared him to vape. His friend Max was standing next to him and he chose to walk away. Kevin recognized two of the boys from his neighborhood, so he did not think it was a big deal. Secretly, he hoped that he would fit in with the older boys and maybe they would think he was cool.

The older boys did ask Kevin if he wanted to hang out with them several more times during the school year. Kevin always said yes. Sometimes they would just hang out, while other times they would vape or do other stuff that Kevin never would have done with his old friends like Max.

Today, Kevin is grounded and his parents are so disappointed. Kevin and the older boys were caught vaping at school. Upon investigation by school administration, they uncovered that the group of boys were also selling vaping devices at school. Kevin knew it was a bad idea but went along anyway. He was suspended from school and eventually confessed everything to his parents.

Kevin was tired of keeping secrets. If he could go back in time, he would not have given into the pressure to vape. Instead, he would have just walked away with Max.

Thinking Critically

1. Why does experimenting with one risky behavior, such as vaping, often lead to other risky behaviors?

2. Kevin wanted to fit in and be accepted by older boys. What are positive ways to fit in and feel accepted within a group?

3. If you were Max, what could you have said to Kevin before he accepted the dare to vape?

4. What are two ways that Kevin could have respectfully and assertively refused vaping?

Young people may worry that not using tobacco products means others will not like or accept them. If someone pressures you to try a cigarette, vaping device, or smokeless tobacco, that person is not really your friend. Real friends do not want their friends to engage in unhealthy behaviors. You can use positive peer pressure to encourage your friends to practice healthy behaviors.

Media Messages

The media is a factor affecting tobacco use. Originally, tobacco companies advertised their products on television, the radio, and in magazines and newspapers. After scientific data demonstrated the serious health consequences of tobacco use, bans forced tobacco companies to stop these types of advertising.

Today, tobacco companies still cannot advertise on TV or the radio, or in print publications. Instead, they try to avoid these laws by using social media. Some tobacco companies pay *ambassadors* and *influencers* to post content and link followers to tobacco products. Sometimes, posts by influencers do not even mention tobacco, but advertise upcoming events where people promote or give away tobacco products. Young people may see these posts and not even recognize they are sneaky attempts at getting people to try tobacco products (**Figure 9.15**).

People often look to celebrities on social media for ideas about new hairstyles, fashionable clothing, and lifestyle choices, such as using tobacco. Young people also imitate the behaviors of their peers on social media. Social media only tells a small portion of a person's story, however. It may not capture the serious health consequences of tobacco use immediately and in the future. Young people are more likely to try new products after seeing ads or their role models using them.

Television shows and movies also expose many young people to tobacco products. In fact, 26 percent of movies rated G, PG, or PG-13 show tobacco use. It may seem harmless to see smoking or vaping in a TV show or movie. Research shows, however, that young people who see tobacco use in movies are more likely to start smoking or vaping.

Substance Use Disorder

Most people cannot use tobacco products in a casual way. It is much more likely that a person will develop a substance use disorder from using tobacco products. A **substance use disorder** occurs when a person continues consuming a substance, such as nicotine, regardless of its negative effects on the body and areas of a person's life. It involves a person's recurrent use of substances, repetition of behaviors that lead to health issues, and an inability to meet responsibilities at home, school, or work.

A substance use disorder is a mental illness that requires professional treatment to break the addiction. It sometimes occurs with other mental illnesses, such as major depressive disorder and anxiety disorders. Two or more mental illnesses that occur together are called **co-occurring disorders**.

Figure 9.15
Young people are exposed to various forms of advertisements that advertise tobacco products.

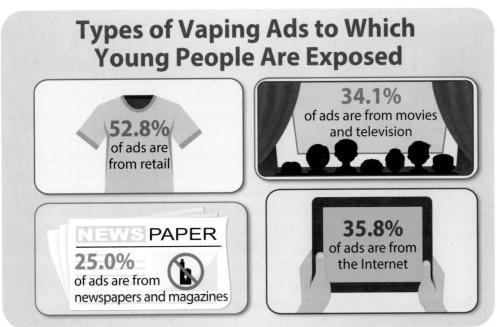

Types of Vaping Ads to Which Young People Are Exposed

52.8% of ads are from retail

34.1% of ads are from movies and television

NEWSPAPER **25.0%** of ads are from newspapers and magazines

35.8% of ads are from the Internet

Shirt: Rvector/Shutterstock.com; Movie screen: Margarita Levina/Shutterstock.com; Newspaper: yekaterinalim/Shutterstock.com; Anti-vape symbol: Siberian Photographer/Shutterstock.com; Tablet: Marish/Shutterstock.com

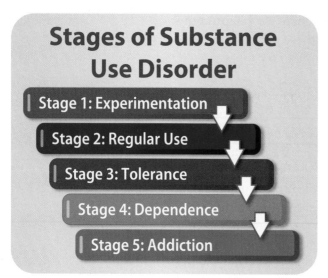

Stages of Substance Use Disorder

| Stage 1: Experimentation |
| Stage 2: Regular Use |
| Stage 3: Tolerance |
| Stage 4: Dependence |
| Stage 5: Addiction |

Figure 9.16 People can move through the five stages of substance use disorder more quickly than they might think.

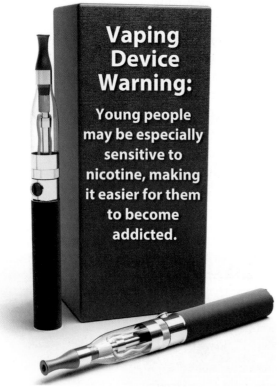

Vaping Device Warning:

Young people may be especially sensitive to nicotine, making it easier for them to become addicted.

Franck Boston/Shutterstock.com

Figure 9.17 Young people are extra vulnerable to many unhealthy habits, including an addiction to nicotine.

Stages of Substance Use

Substances such as nicotine cause changes in the brain and body that negatively affect a person's health. People with substance use disorders often feel like they cannot stop using a substance, even if they want to. The stages of substance use lead to addiction and a substance use disorder (**Figure 9.16**).

Experimentation

People often choose to use a tobacco product "just to try it." This is the stage of experimentation. In this stage, a person is trying a substance. Most substances that lead to substance use disorders cause pleasant feelings, such as happiness and relaxation. These feelings cause a person to want to use more of the substance, which often leads to the regular use of a substance.

Regular Use

After experimentation, people usually increase their substance use. Over time, people may slowly increase the number of times they use a tobacco product per week. They are then likely to develop a regular pattern of using tobacco products, as the pleasant feelings associated with the substance reinforce behavior. For example, people may vape at a certain time of day or while performing a certain activity.

Tolerance

As a person regularly uses a substance like nicotine, the body develops a tolerance for that substance. **Tolerance** describes an increase in how much of a substance the body needs to experience certain effects. The body can quickly develop a tolerance to nicotine and require more of it to achieve the original effect of pleasurable feelings.

For example, during experimentation, a person may smoke one cigarette a week. This may increase to one cigarette each day with regular use. Once a tolerance develops, a person may need to smoke three cigarettes each day to feel the original effects of nicotine (**Figure 9.17**).

A tolerance to nicotine is dangerous because it causes people to use tobacco products more as they pursue the pleasant feelings associated with the substance. This increases the damage done to the body. Even if someone is not feeling the effect of the nicotine, the substance is still entering the body. The more a person uses tobacco, the more damage that person causes.

Dependence

After repeated use, the body becomes dependent on the way nicotine makes it feel. This means the body adjusts to the feelings that nicotine causes. **Dependence** occurs when the body needs an addictive substance in its system to function normally or avoid cravings and anxiety. There are two types of dependence—physical and psychological.

A *physical dependence* occurs when the body adjusts to a substance and requires it to function normally. For example, nicotine causes the release of dopamine, which causes feelings of happiness. Eventually, the brain produces less of these chemicals on its own. This means the body requires nicotine or other substances to reach normal levels of these chemicals. Without the substance in the body, a person feels uncomfortable and even sick.

People can also develop a *psychological dependence*. This causes cravings and anxiety that a person feels when not using or trying to quit the substance. Psychological dependence relates to mental and emotional factors. If a person is unable to use a tobacco product, this person may feel irritable. For example, a person who regularly vapes may feel anxious and irritable if a vape pen is not available when a craving occurs.

People may develop patterns for using a substance, such as vaping after dinner every day. Patterns such as this can connect a substance with certain triggers (**Figure 9.18**). **Triggers** are like reminders that cause people to feel a strong desire for a substance. In this case, the end of the meal becomes the trigger to vape. When people who use tobacco encounter triggers that they connect with tobacco use, they feel a strong psychological need to use a tobacco product.

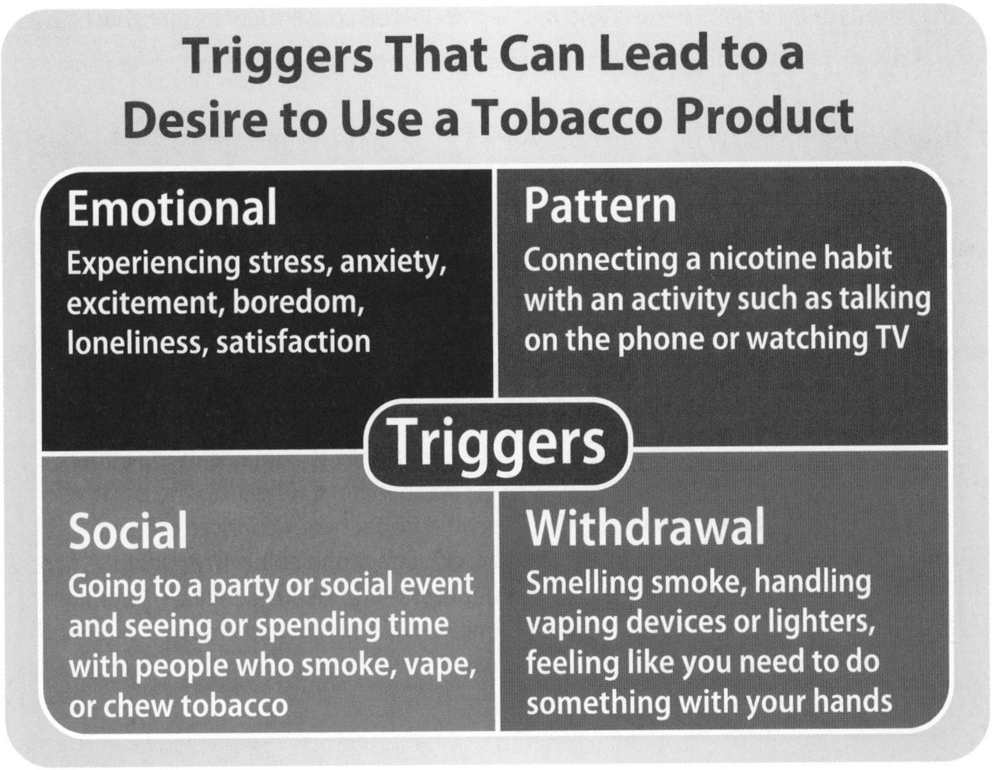

Figure 9.18
People can connect tobacco use mentally with a certain feeling, habit, person, or situation that can increase their desire to smoke, vape, or chew tobacco. *Which type of dependence is related to mental and emotional factors such as stress?*

Triggers That Can Lead to a Desire to Use a Tobacco Product

Emotional
Experiencing stress, anxiety, excitement, boredom, loneliness, satisfaction

Pattern
Connecting a nicotine habit with an activity such as talking on the phone or watching TV

Triggers

Social
Going to a party or social event and seeing or spending time with people who smoke, vape, or chew tobacco

Withdrawal
Smelling smoke, handling vaping devices or lighters, feeling like you need to do something with your hands

Addiction

Addiction develops when a person continues using a substance despite negative effects on health. **Addiction** is the physical and psychological need for a given substance or behavior. For example, people may continue smoking or vaping, even if they experience social isolation or have to turn to other measures to afford the substance. At this point, a person has developed a substance use disorder.

Withdrawal Symptoms

Withdrawal occurs when someone with an addiction to a substance tries to stop using that substance. The term *withdrawal* describes unpleasant symptoms. These symptoms vary based on the addictive substance. People with an addiction to nicotine may experience irritability, difficulty concentrating, fatigue, nausea, and weight gain during withdrawal. They also experience intense cravings for nicotine. This occurs because the body is physically dependent on this substance.

Withdrawal is one of the reasons people who use tobacco have such difficulty quitting. The withdrawal symptoms for tobacco last several weeks or even months. Some people who quit tobacco use have occasional tobacco cravings for years after quitting.

Lesson 9.2 Review

1. List three individual factors that could affect tobacco use.

2. Young people are much _____ (more/less) likely to start using tobacco if their parents or guardians discuss and follow through on consequences for tobacco use.

3. **True or false.** Some tobacco companies pay ambassadors and influencers to post content and link followers to tobacco products.

4. Which of the following is *not* one of the five stages of a substance use disorder?
   A. Regular use.
   B. Tolerance.
   C. Addiction.
   D. Triggers.

5. **Critical thinking.** Compare and contrast a physical dependence and a psychological dependence in the fourth stage of a substance use disorder.

Hands-On Activity

Recall the information that you learned on factors that may cause a young person to try a tobacco product. Based on these factors, reflect on the positive and negative influences in your life that could impact your chances of using tobacco products. Create a two-column chart. Label one column "Positive Influences" and the other "Negative Influences." Write the influences in your life in the appropriate column. Then, write one or two sentences for each influence explaining how you will increase positive influences and reduce the effect of negative influences.

Preventing and Treating Tobacco Use

Learning Outcomes

After studying this lesson, you will be able to

- **identify** skills someone can use to prevent tobacco use.
- **demonstrate** refusal skills.
- **describe** treatment methods for nicotine addiction.

Graphic Organizer

KWL Chart: Preventing and Treating Tobacco Use

Create a table like the one shown. Before you read the lesson, outline what you know and what you want to know about preventing and treating tobacco use. After you have read the lesson, outline what you learned.

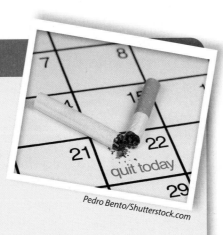

Pedro Bento/Shutterstock.com

K	W	L
What I <u>K</u>now	**What I <u>W</u>ant to Know**	**What I Have <u>L</u>earned**
Nicotine gum or the nicotine patch can help curb withdrawal symptoms for tobacco users.	How can refusal skills help prevent tobacco use?	Using nicotine does not help manage stress. It actually increases stress.

Lesson 9.1 discussed how tobacco products harm the body and negatively affect a person's health, as well as other people's health. In Lesson 9.2, you learned that tobacco products are very addictive, and it can be difficult to quit using them. Quitting is possible, however.

Of course, the best option to prevent tobacco use is never to begin using tobacco products. If someone who uses a tobacco product wants to quit, there are different methods to help with withdrawal symptoms. In this lesson, you will explore ways to prevent tobacco use as well as some strategies for breaking a nicotine addiction.

Preventing Tobacco Use

Did you know that most adults who use tobacco products started this habit when they were teens? Avoiding a lifetime of tobacco use starts now, based on the decisions you make today.

In the United States, smoking costs society an estimated $289 billion a year in healthcare costs. Given the serious threat to public health, both federal and state governments have strategies to regulate the sales, use, cost, and advertisements of tobacco products (**Figure 9.19**). Organizations have created mass media campaigns and public service announcements discouraging

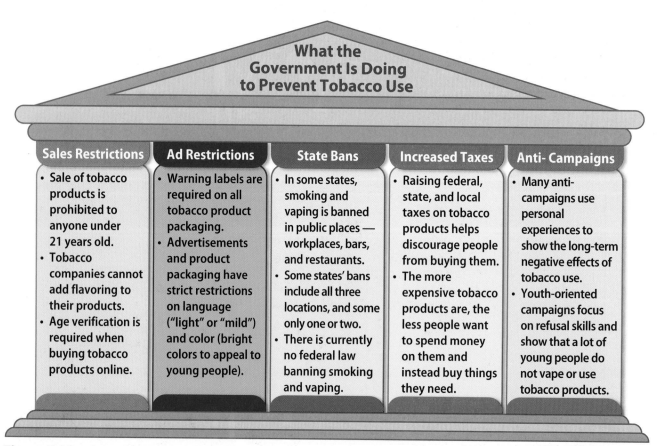

What the Government Is Doing to Prevent Tobacco Use

Sales Restrictions	Ad Restrictions	State Bans	Increased Taxes	Anti- Campaigns
• Sale of tobacco products is prohibited to anyone under 21 years old. • Tobacco companies cannot add flavoring to their products. • Age verification is required when buying tobacco products online.	• Warning labels are required on all tobacco product packaging. • Advertisements and product packaging have strict restrictions on language ("light" or "mild") and color (bright colors to appeal to young people).	• In some states, smoking and vaping is banned in public places — workplaces, bars, and restaurants. • Some states' bans include all three locations, and some only one or two. • There is currently no federal law banning smoking and vaping.	• Raising federal, state, and local taxes on tobacco products helps discourage people from buying them. • The more expensive tobacco products are, the less people want to spend money on them and instead buy things they need.	• Many anti-campaigns use personal experiences to show the long-term negative effects of tobacco use. • Youth-oriented campaigns focus on refusal skills and show that a lot of young people do not vape or use tobacco products.

Figure 9.19 The United States government focuses on preventing nicotine use and helping tobacco users quit by using a variety of methods. *What is the name for media messages that support public health?*

tobacco use. **Public service announcements (PSAs)** are media messages that support public health. Successful campaigns emphasize short- and long-term health effects, strategies for refusing tobacco, and the fact that most young people do not use tobacco. Young people who regularly see these campaigns are less likely to use tobacco products.

The decision about whether or not to use tobacco products ultimately lies with you. You can use several skills to protect yourself from tobacco use. These skills include building healthy relationships, learning to manage stress, thinking critically about the media you see, and using refusal skills.

Build Healthy Relationships

Young people may feel pressured to use tobacco if they have close friends who use these products. Fitting in during social situations if other people are smoking, vaping, or chewing tobacco can be difficult. In healthy friendships, however, your friends respect the choices you make and do not pressure you to engage in unhealthy behaviors. People choose friends because they enjoy spending time with them, not because they use tobacco products.

If your friends do not respect your decision to avoid tobacco products, focus on developing other friendships. Perhaps you have grown apart from some of your other friends. Try to form friendships with people who respect you and accept your choices (Figure 9.20).

In addition to friendships, building healthy relationships with your family can help prevent tobacco use. Have open conversations with family members to know their views of tobacco use. If you have family members who use tobacco, talk to them about the dangers of tobacco on their health and the health of others and offer to help them quit.

Learn to Manage Stress

Some people start using tobacco products to relieve stress, help them relax, or not worry about a difficult situation. Using tobacco actually increases stress, however. A nicotine addiction causes more issues than it solves. It also has negative mental and social consequences. Fortunately, there are many ways of managing stress that are more effective than relying on cigarettes, vaping devices, or smokeless tobacco. Instead of using tobacco products, try using a stress management technique that works

Characteristics of Good Friends Versus Toxic Friends

Good Friends	Toxic Friends
Respect your choices	Do not respect or accept your choices
Do not pressure you to try unhealthy behaviors	Pressure you to try unhealthy behaviors
Trust each other	Talk badly about you to others
Are honest	Lie often
Are attentive	Frequently change your friendship status
Stay loyal through good times and bad times	Spill your secrets
Care about your well-being	Knowingly give you bad advice
Are good listeners	Take advantage of you
Do not judge you	Constantly judge you
Support you	Put you down
Forgive you	Hold long grudges
Are helpful	Are never there when you need them

Figure 9.20 It is important to form friendships with people who show characteristics of a good friend, such as respecting your choices and being supportive.

for you, such as talking with a friend or getting physical activity. You learned about some additional stress management strategies in Lesson 5.3.

Think Critically

Advertisements for cigarettes, vaping devices, and smokeless tobacco try to make these products look attractive. Companies that sell tobacco products cannot advertise on television, the radio, or print publications. Instead, tobacco companies have to use sneaky strategies to persuade people to use their products. Using critical thinking skills can help you recognize the tobacco industry's practices and avoid being tricked.

Today, most people know that cigarettes are dangerous. Since this knowledge is widespread, tobacco companies have changed the types of products they sell to appeal to young people. For example, some tobacco products look like electronic devices, breath strips, and flavored candy.

BUILDING Your Skills

Addiction Prevention

Many factors determine the likelihood that a young person will use tobacco products. Most people form these habits at a young age. One of the most important ways to prevent addiction is never to use tobacco products in the first place.

There will be many negative influences in a young person's life that may influence someone to try vaping or smoking, including peer pressure and representations of it in the media. There are also positive influences that may convince young people *not* to vape or smoke. The power of positive peer pressure can weigh heavily on someone's decision. You have the power to be a positive influence on your friends' (and classmates') decision to say no to tobacco products.

Nicotine-Free Pledge and Personal Promise

Design a Nicotine-Free Pledge and encourage your friends and classmates to sign one, too. See the basic example below to better understand the wording in a pledge. Do additional research to get ideas for what a pledge could look like. In addition to the pledge statement, add the following extra information to make your pledge special:

- an inspirational quote
- at least one image
- at least three harmful effects of tobacco use
- at least two benefits of being nicotine-free
- other relevant information or images (if applicable)

If you are choosing to be nicotine-free, sign the pledge. With teacher permission, hang the pledges at your school to advocate for nicotine-free youth.

Nicotine-Free Pledge

I Am Saying NO to Tobacco Products!

I, _____, pledge to be nicotine-free.
        (person's name)

These products have names that sound like sugary snacks more than addictive tobacco products. To advertise these products, some tobacco companies copy popular social media trends to appeal to young people.

To resist these strategies, use critical thinking skills to analyze tobacco products and the messages from tobacco companies (**Figure 9.21**). People who understand the manipulative nature of tobacco advertisements are able to resist them better. Analyzing advertisements can remind you about the serious consequences of tobacco use.

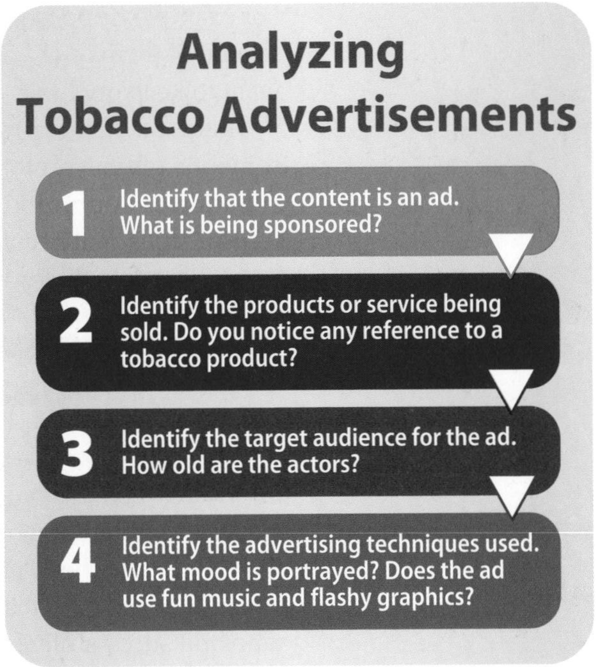

Use Refusal Skills

Resisting pressure to begin smoking, vaping, or chewing tobacco can be challenging. You may feel this pressure from your peers and from the media. Luckily, refusal skills can help you prepare for and respond to situations that may involve tobacco use.

Refusal skills are strategies you can use to stand up to pressures and influences that want you to engage in unhealthy behaviors. These skills can help you in situations when you feel pressured to try tobacco. Strong refusal skills help you stick to your own beliefs and values in the face of peer pressure.

If you do not want to use tobacco products, spend time with people who feel the same. Make sure these people know you do not want to use tobacco products or inhale their secondhand smoke and aerosol. Firmly explain the reasons behind your decision. Then stick to your decision and refuse to give in (**Figure 9.22**).

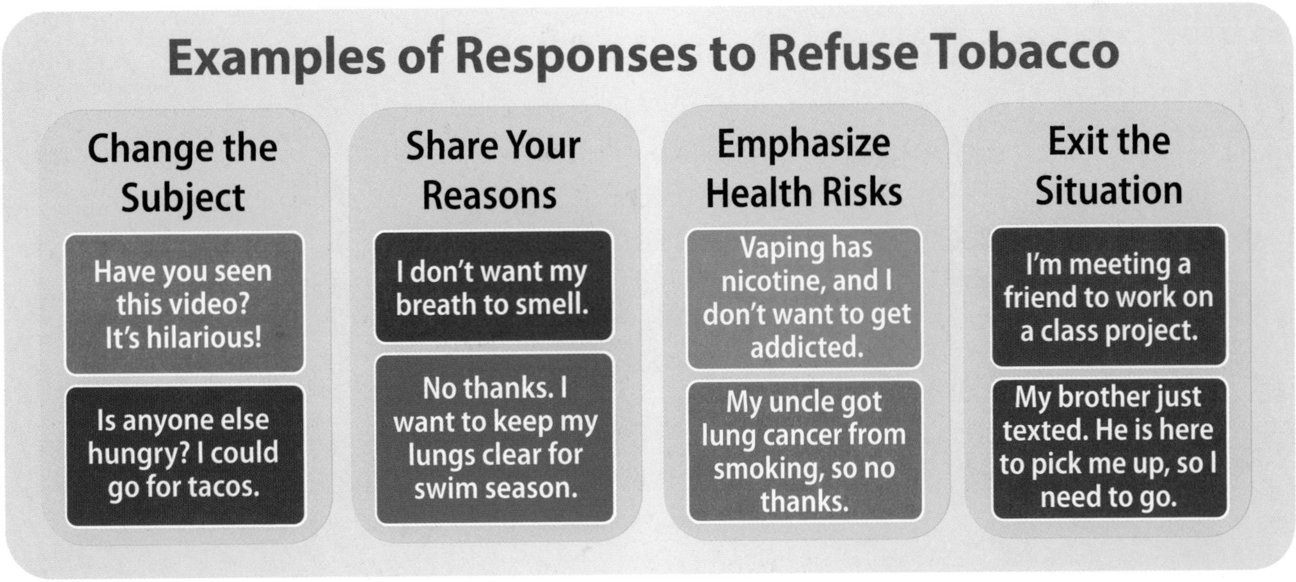

Analyzing Tobacco Advertisements

1 Identify that the content is an ad. What is being sponsored?

2 Identify the products or service being sold. Do you notice any reference to a tobacco product?

3 Identify the target audience for the ad. How old are the actors?

4 Identify the advertising techniques used. What mood is portrayed? Does the ad use fun music and flashy graphics?

Figure 9.21 Smoking and vaping advertisements are designed to make tobacco products appear cool and harmless.

Examples of Responses to Refuse Tobacco

Change the Subject
Have you seen this video? It's hilarious!

Is anyone else hungry? I could go for tacos.

Share Your Reasons
I don't want my breath to smell.

No thanks. I want to keep my lungs clear for swim season.

Emphasize Health Risks
Vaping has nicotine, and I don't want to get addicted.

My uncle got lung cancer from smoking, so no thanks.

Exit the Situation
I'm meeting a friend to work on a class project.

My brother just texted. He is here to pick me up, so I need to go.

Figure 9.22 Saying no to your friends can be extremely difficult, but having a few practiced responses in mind can help when faced with peer pressure. *What skills help a person stand up to peer influences and pressures?*

For example, suppose that when you hang out with a certain group of friends, several of them offer you a vaping device. Your response may be "No thanks. I want to keep my lungs healthy for band."

Remember that practice makes perfect. Imagine situations in which someone offers you tobacco, and then practice your responses. Play out each situation in your mind so you are ready to respond firmly. With time, your refusal skills will become stronger. Eventually, you will feel confident when you tell people that you choose to stay tobacco-free.

Treating Tobacco Use

Because nicotine is addictive, tobacco use can often lead to a substance use disorder. When this occurs, even the threat of serious health conditions often is not enough to make someone stop using tobacco products. More than half of people who have had a heart attack or surgery resulting from lung cancer continue to smoke. Fortunately, it is never too late for someone to stop using tobacco. People who quit successfully experience a number of health benefits (**Figure 9.23**).

Quitting tobacco use is a difficult task to undertake. If you or someone you know is trying to quit tobacco use, the following steps may help:

- Attend individual or group counseling.
- Talk to a school counselor, doctor, teacher, or other trusted adult.
- Call a helpline that provides free counseling to people trying to quit using tobacco.
- Research online resources that have information on quitting.

Although quitting tobacco can be difficult, nicotine addiction is treatable. Treatment strategies include nicotine replacement, medication, and self-management techniques.

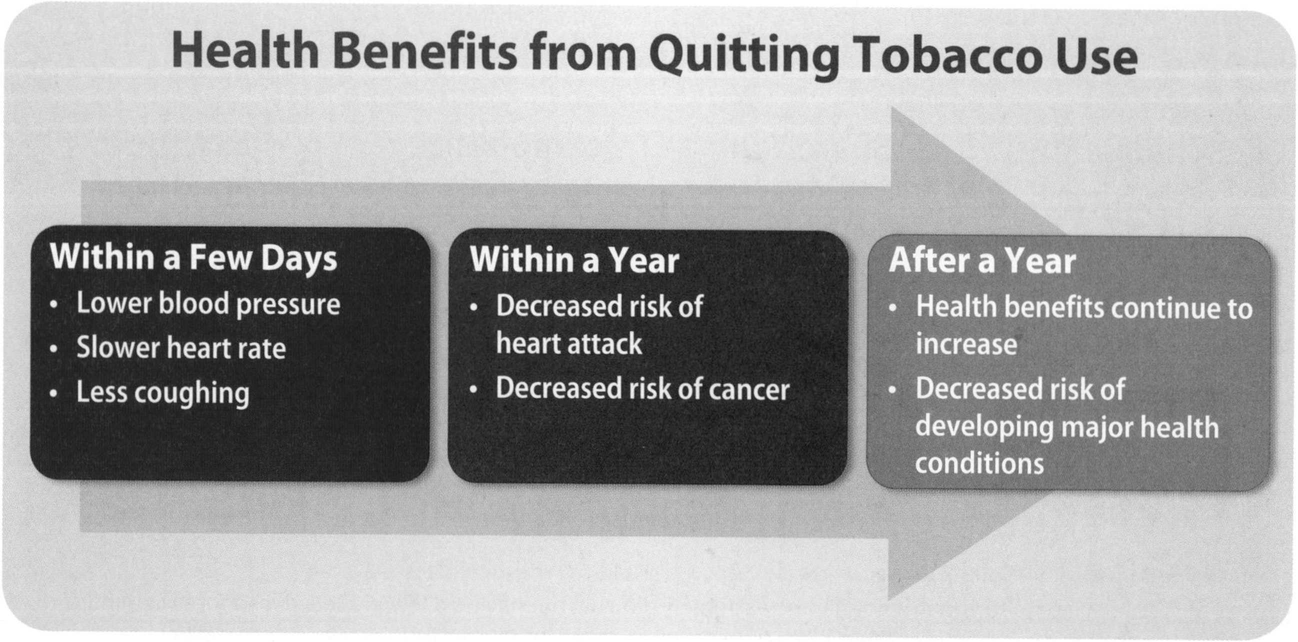

Health Benefits from Quitting Tobacco Use

Within a Few Days
- Lower blood pressure
- Slower heart rate
- Less coughing

Within a Year
- Decreased risk of heart attack
- Decreased risk of cancer

After a Year
- Health benefits continue to increase
- Decreased risk of developing major health conditions

Figure 9.23   The body experiences long-term health benefits when a person quits using tobacco, but it also shows benefits within a few days.

Nicotine Replacement

Some approaches to quitting nicotine rely on nicotine replacement. In **nicotine replacement**, people who use tobacco continue to put nicotine into their bodies. People do not do this, however, through the use of tobacco products. Instead, they typically use *nicotine gum*, *nicotine lozenges*, or the *nicotine patch* as replacements (**Figure 9.24**). These replacements lessen withdrawal symptoms. In this way, nicotine replacement makes tobacco use easier to quit.

Nicotine replacement treatment enables people to gradually use smaller and smaller amounts of the substance. Eventually, people find they are no longer dependent on nicotine.

Companies sometimes market vaping devices such as e-cigarettes as a nicotine-replacement tool for people who want to quit smoking. Unlike nicotine gum, lozenges, and patches, vaping devices have not been approved by the United States government as a successful and safe form of smoking cessation.

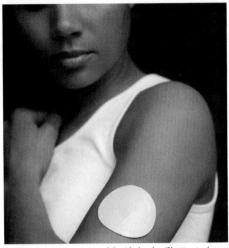

bikeriderlondon/Shutterstock.com

Figure 9.24   Nicotine patches can help tobacco users quit using tobacco products. *What treatment method involves nicotine patches?*

Medications

Sometimes medications prescribed by a doctor help people quit using tobacco. These medications usually simulate dopamine. People who take these medications cope better with withdrawal from nicotine.

Self-Management Strategies

Self-management strategies often involve developing ways to resist temptation (**Figure 9.25**). First, people must identify situations that trigger their desire for tobacco. Once they have that information, they can respond with two techniques—stimulus control and response substitution.

Figure 9.25
If you or someone you know is trying to quit using tobacco, you can take the following steps to use self-management strategies.

Steps to Use Self-Management Strategies to Quit Tobacco

1. Set a "quit date" within the next month and note that date on your calendar.
2. Tell friends and family members about your quit date and ask them to support your efforts.
3. Get rid of tobacco products and their accessories in your environment. Avoid exposure to tobacco advertisements on social media.
4. Develop strategies for coping with nicotine cravings, such as getting physical activity, chewing gum, or keeping busy with other activities.
5. Develop strategies for refusing offers of tobacco products from other people.
6. Remind yourself of the benefits of quitting, including a longer life, more spending money, and increased stamina.
7. Reward yourself for quitting. For example, buy something with the money you saved by not using tobacco.
8. If you slip up, quickly renew your focus on the goal of quitting. Do not let one lapse lead to a return of the unhealthy behavior.

Stimulus control involves trying to avoid tempting situations and managing feelings that lead to tobacco use. Through stimulus control, people learn to avoid or manage each stimulus that causes them to use tobacco. A *stimulus* is a thing or event that causes a specific reaction in the body. In this case, the reaction is a craving for tobacco. The stimulus can be anything from a stressful day to seeing someone else using a cigarette, vaping device, or smokeless tobacco product.

With stimulus control, the goal is to avoid triggers that cause a desire to use tobacco. People may not always be able to avoid their triggers, however. If someone feels triggered to use tobacco, this person can use response substitution.

Through **response substitution**, people learn to respond to difficult feelings and situations with behaviors other than using tobacco. They may use stress management, relaxation, and coping skills. For response substitution to work, the first step is to recognize the stimulus that triggers the desire to smoke, vape, or chew tobacco. Then, a person can respond with an appropriate substitution for the behavior.

Lesson 9.3 Review

1. What are public service announcements (PSAs)?

2. **True or false.** Using tobacco decreases stress.

3. _____ skills are strategies you can use to stand up to pressures and influences that want you to engage in unhealthy behaviors.

4. What are three forms of nicotine replacements people could use to help quit tobacco?

5. **Critical thinking.** Explain how someone can use stimulus control and response substitution to quit tobacco.

Hands-On Activity

On a separate sheet of paper, write refusal responses to the statements below. Then, team up with a partner and share your responses with each other. Practice your responses out loud using clear and assertive language.

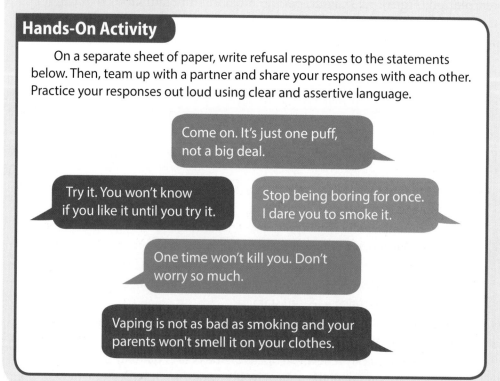

Come on. It's just one puff, not a big deal.

Try it. You won't know if you like it until you try it.

Stop being boring for once. I dare you to smoke it.

One time won't kill you. Don't worry so much.

Vaping is not as bad as smoking and your parents won't smell it on your clothes.

Review and Assessment

Summary

Lesson 9.1 Tobacco Products and Your Health

- *Tobacco* is a plant used to create tobacco products. Tobacco leaves contain the chemical *nicotine*, which is a toxic substance that gives tobacco products their addictive quality.
- Cigarettes are made of 7,000 chemicals and toxic substances.
- *Vaping devices* heat an e-liquid that produces an aerosol containing nicotine and harmful substances.
- Smokeless tobacco is chewed, inhaled, or dissolved but still contains toxic substances.
- Nicotine affects all body systems. Each tobacco product also harms the body. Cigarettes and vaping devices harm the respiratory system. Smokeless tobacco causes oral damage.
- Using tobacco impacts a person's mind and social relationships. Young people who use tobacco can also experience serious legal consequences.
- Secondhand and thirdhand smoke and aerosol release harmful substances into the air that other people breathe. Even brief exposure to the toxins in tobacco can cause health issues.

Lesson 9.2 Understanding Tobacco Use

- Common reasons young people start to smoke include individual factors such as genetic makeup, mental health, and stage of development or external influences such as their family, peers, or the media.
- A *substance use disorder* occurs when a person continues consuming a substance regardless of its negative effects on the body and areas of a person's life. The stages of substance use lead to addiction and a substance use disorder.
- People may develop patterns for using a substance, which can connect a substance with certain triggers, causing people to feel a strong desire for a substance.
- When someone addicted to a substance tries to stop using that substance, they go through withdrawal.

Lesson 9.3 Preventing and Treating Tobacco Use

- To prevent and discourage nicotine use in the United States, federal and state governments have strategies to regulate the sales, use, cost, and advertisements of tobacco products.
- People can use several skills to prevent tobacco use. These include building healthy relationships, learning strategies for managing stress, thinking critically about media messages, and using refusal skills.
- Quitting tobacco can be difficult, but nicotine addiction is treatable.
- Some approaches to quitting rely on nicotine replacement through products such as nicotine gum, nicotine lozenges, or a nicotine patch, which help lessen withdrawal symptoms, or medication. *Stimulus control* and *response substitution* rely on the user developing a way to resist the temptation to smoke.

Check Your Knowledge

Record your answers to each of the following questions on a separate sheet of paper.

1. The toxic substance that gives tobacco products their addictive quality is called ____.
2. What is an e-liquid?
3. The chemical the brain releases in response to nicotine is called ____.
4. **True or false.** The particles in thirdhand smoke and aerosol land and remain on virtually any surface in the area where someone has smoked or vaped.
5. Peer pressure is positive if it is respectful and encourages ____ behaviors.
6. Besides social media and advertisements, what other two forms of media expose many young people to tobacco products?
7. **True or false.** A substance use disorder is *not* considered a mental illness.
8. ____ describes an increase in how much of a substance the body needs to experience certain effects.
9. What is the physical and psychological need for a given substance or behavior?
10. List four examples of skills a person can use to prevent tobacco use.
11. What is the goal of a stimulus control?
12. ____ involves the use of stress management, relaxation, and coping skills as an appropriate substitution for tobacco use.
    - A. Stimulus control
    - B. Response substitution
    - C. Nicotine replacement
    - D. Withdrawal

Use Your Vocabulary ⤤

addiction	peer pressure	thirdhand aerosol
aerosol	public service	thirdhand smoke
carcinogens	announcement (PSA)	tobacco
co-occurring disorder	response substitution	tolerance
dependence	secondhand aerosol	toxic
dopamine	secondhand smoke	triggers
e-liquid	stimulus control	vaping device
nicotine	substance use disorder	withdrawal
nicotine replacement	tar	

13. Working with a partner, write definitions for the terms above based on your current understanding. Then, use the terms to write a summary about what you have learned about tobacco. Team up with another pair of students to discuss your definitions, summaries, and any differences between them. Afterward, discuss the definitions and summaries with the class. Ask your instructor for any correction or clarification.
14. Choose three of the terms above. Use the Internet to locate photos, graphics, or videos that show the meanings of these three terms. Create a digital presentation of these photos, graphics, or videos and show them to the class. Explain how they show the meanings of the terms and answer any questions

your classmates have. While listening to your classmates' presentations, write down any terms or explanations you do not understand.

Think Critically

15. **Predict.** If an adolescent chooses to vape or smoke cigarettes with peers and this behavior continues, predict the impact of this decision on the person's body, family, and future generations.

16. **Identify.** List some reasons a young person might try a vaping device for the first time. Why is it difficult for a young person to just say "no" to risky behaviors like vaping or smoking?

17. **Compare and contrast.** Compare and contrast a cigarette or smokeless tobacco product to a vaping device in terms of health consequences and addiction.

18. **Assess.** Research and calculate the financial cost of a tobacco addiction. How much would it cost to buy two packs of cigarettes every week for one year? What else could you purchase with this amount of money?

DEVELOP Your Skills

19. **Analyze influences.** Think about a time you saw tobacco use being glamorized on television, in social media, in magazines, in movies, or in music. What message about tobacco use was being portrayed? Reflect on the influence of this message and write a summary describing the post, picture, show, movie, or song. Based on what you learned in this chapter, how might this message negatively affect young people?

20. **Communication skills.** Imagine you have a friend or family member who currently smokes, vapes, or chews tobacco. Consider this person's potential reasons for starting and reasons for potentially continuing use. Using basic, everyday language, write a letter to this person about the harmful effects it has on the body, reasons for quitting, strategies used to quit, and the immediate as well as long-term benefits of quitting. As you write, use respectful language and display empathy.

21. **Access information and advocacy skills.** Create a flyer or brochure that provides information on steps for quitting nicotine. In your flyer or brochure, include motivation such as financial and health benefits, behaviors that will help, and local resources that can assist. Consider the difficulty of overcoming nicotine addiction and include strategies for doing so. Include vocabulary from the chapter. Present your flyer or brochure to the class.

22. **Teamwork and advocacy skills.** In small groups, create a public service announcement (PSA) discouraging vaping or tobacco use at your school. Include the following information in the PSA: short- and long-term health effects and strategies to refuse. Emphasize that most young people are not using tobacco. Practice and record a video of your PSA. With teacher permission, request that your PSA be shown during the morning announcements.

Chapter 10

Alcohol

Lesson 10.1 The Effects of Alcohol

Lesson 10.2 Preventing and Treating Alcohol Use

Essential Question ?

What are some health risks of drinking alcohol?

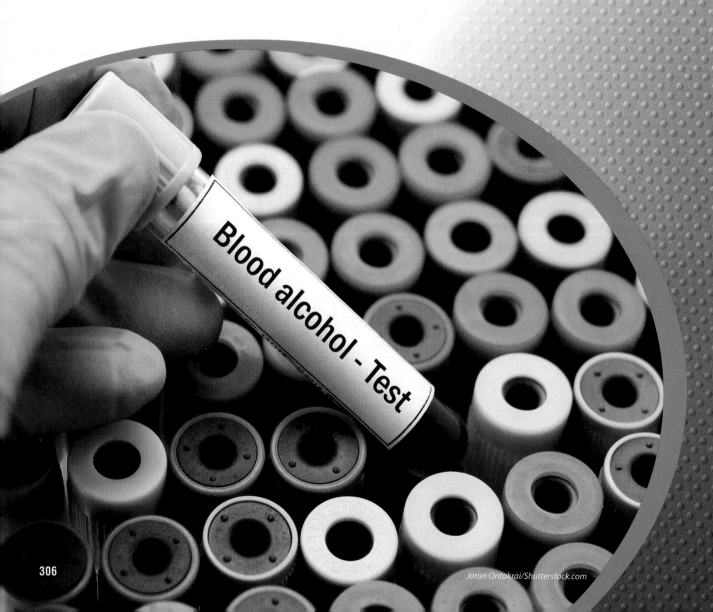

Jarun Ontakrai/Shutterstock.com

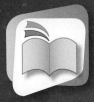

How Healthy Are You?

In this chapter, you will be learning about alcohol. Before you begin reading, take the following quiz to assess your current alcohol habits.

Healthy Choices	Yes	No
Do you understand the health hazards of alcohol use on the muscles, nervous system, and brain?		
Do you understand that alcohol is an addictive substance?		
Do you understand the consequences of underage drinking?		
Do you understand the consequences of consuming excessive amounts of alcohol?		
Do you surround yourself with friends who choose not to drink?		
Do you try to limit your exposure to people drinking in movies and TV shows?		
In social situations where you feel nervous or awkward, do you avoid giving in to peer pressure to drink alcohol?		
Do you stay away from experimenting with drinking alcohol?		
Have you prepared refusal skills to help if you are offered alcohol?		
If you or someone you care about has an issue with alcohol, do you know what help is available?		

Count your "Yes" and "No" responses. The more "Yes" responses you have, the more healthy alcohol habits you exhibit. Now, take a closer look at the questions with which you responded "No." How can you make these healthy habits part of your daily life? Identify a SMART goal you would like to achieve to help improve your overall health and well-being. Refer to Figure 1.11 to help you set up your SMART goal. If you do not understand the instructions, ask for clarification from your teacher.

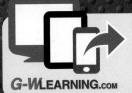

Click on the activity icon or visit www.g-wlearning.com/health to access online vocabulary activities using key terms from the chapter.

The Effects of Alcohol

Learning Outcomes

After studying this lesson, you will be able to

- **differentiate** moderate drinking, binge drinking, and heavy drinking.
- **analyze** the effects of alcohol on the brain.
- **relate** alcohol use to long-term health consequences.
- **explain** the mental, social, and legal consequences of drinking.
- **assess** the role of alcohol in accidents and violence.
- **summarize** how alcohol use can increase the risk of developing an alcohol use disorder.

Graphic Organizer

Alcohol and Your Health

As you read this lesson, use a chart similar to the one shown to organize your notes. If you have any questions about what you are reading, raise your hand and ask your teacher. After reading the lesson, compare your notes with those of a classmate. Discuss similarities and differences between your notes. What items would you add to or delete from your list? Adjust your list, if necessary.

iStock.com/WellfordT

- Alcohol Use
- Health Effects
- Consequences and Risky Behaviors
- Alcohol Use Disorder

Santiago and Priya are in seventh grade together and have the same group of friends. Priya's family is very open about drinking alcohol. Her older siblings are still under 21 years old, but are allowed to moderately drink alcohol at family dinners. Priya herself has tried a small amount of alcohol before at a family party. Her parents also frequently drive home after drinking.

Santiago's family is not this accepting of alcohol. They would never let Santiago drink alcohol until he turns 21, and they would never drive drunk. Santiago's cousin ended up in the hospital last year because of alcohol poisoning from heavy drinking. It opened Santiago's eyes to just how dangerous alcohol can be.

Alcohol is the third leading preventable cause of death in the United States (Figure 10.1). Drinking alcohol has an immediate effect on the body, and can cause lifelong health issues. In this lesson, you will learn about alcohol use and the damaging effect alcohol can have on people's health.

Alcohol Use

Alcohol is an addictive drug that is known as a *depressant*. Alcohol alters a person's brain function. This has an immediate effect on a person's body, thinking, and behavior. Alcohol is found in drinks such as beer, wine, and liquor. In the United States, it is illegal for people under 21 years of age to drink alcohol.

Drinking alcohol can have serious effects on a person's body, decisions, and future. Adults who decide to drink alcohol need to consider the harmful effects.

The best way to avoid the harmful effects of alcohol is not to drink. Some adults, however, choose to consume alcohol despite the harmful effects.

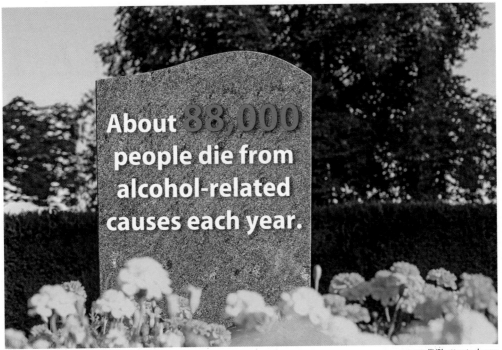

Figure 10.1
Alcohol can lead to death in many ways, including liver failure, car accidents, and alcohol poisoning. *How old does a person have to be in the United States to legally drink alcohol?*

About 88,000 people die from alcohol-related causes each year.

nnattalli/Shutterstock.com

Certain patterns of drinking alcohol can increase or decrease a person's risk of experiencing harmful effects.

Moderate drinking, also called *social drinking*, involves consuming no more than one drink on the same occasion for females and no more than two drinks on the same occasion for males. When experts talk about an alcoholic drink, they are referring to any drink that contains 0.6 ounces (14.0 grams or 1.2 tablespoons) of pure alcohol. **Figure 10.2** shows the one-drink equivalents for different types of alcoholic drinks.

People who drink in moderation do not drink every day. Moderate drinking describes when legal adults *occasionally* consume alcohol. For example, an adult might have a drink at a dinner party or other special event. Moderate drinking is less likely to cause harmful effects, but it could easily lead to binge drinking or heavy drinking.

Binge drinking involves consuming four or more drinks for females and five or more drinks for males on the same occasion and in a short amount of time. The majority of alcohol consumed by underage drinkers is in the form of binge drinking. Binge drinking can result in many harmful effects.

Heavy drinking is drinking eight or more drinks in one week for females and 15 or more drinks in one week for males. Heavy drinking can lead a person to become psychologically and physically dependent on alcohol.

A *psychological dependence* on alcohol is the cravings and anxiety a person feels when not using or trying to quit the substance. This person may feel that drinking alcohol will help with feeling "normal." When somone is *physically dependent* on alcohol, this person needs to consume alcohol for the body to function normally.

Figure 10.2
Although the total liquid ounces are very different in each of the alcoholic drinks shown here, the drinks have exactly the same amount of pure alcohol. *What is the best way to avoid the harmful effects of alcohol?*

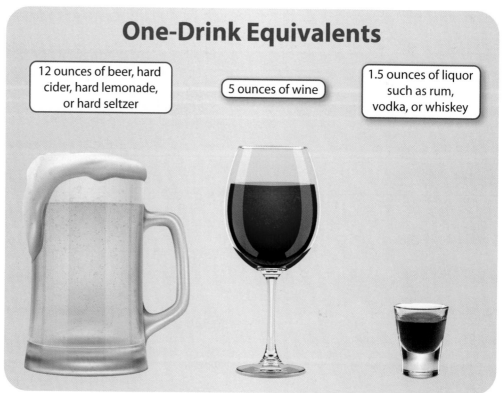

One-Drink Equivalents

12 ounces of beer, hard cider, hard lemonade, or hard seltzer

5 ounces of wine

1.5 ounces of liquor such as rum, vodka, or whiskey

Left to right: Ara Hovhannisyan/Shutterstock.com; VikaSuh/Shutterstock.com; StudioSmart/Shutterstock.com

Health Effects of Alcohol Use

The effects of alcohol vary from person to person, depending on several factors (**Figure 10.3**). Even when people consume small amounts of alcohol, they experience minor effects. When people consume larger amounts of alcohol, they can face life-threatening effects.

Immediate Health Effects

When someone drinks alcohol, the substance is quickly absorbed into the person's bloodstream and is carried to different parts of the body. When someone drinks a lot of alcohol in a short period of time, the body is unable to break down the alcohol fast enough. As a result, the alcohol builds up in the bloodstream. **Blood alcohol concentration (BAC)** is the percentage of alcohol in a person's blood. People who have a BAC of 0.08 or above are considered *legally impaired*, also known as *intoxicated* or *drunk*. A person who is intoxicated shows substantial physical and mental impairments.

Central Nervous System

Alcohol affects every cell in the body and slows down the *central nervous system*. When alcohol enters the central nervous system, it negatively affects many body functions. Certain brain functions slow, chemical changes occur, and a person's inhibition is reduced (**Figure 10.4**). **Inhibition** is the self-control that keeps people from taking dangerous risks.

The more alcohol a person consumes, the more it affects the brain. People who have had one drink may still have some control of behaviors, speak more loudly, and use more body movements. People who consume larger amounts of alcohol, especially in a short period of time, may feel they have less control of behaviors. They may have difficulty thinking clearly and lose coordination in body movements.

Factors That Impact the Effects of Alcohol

- Ethnicity
- Biological sex
- Body weight
- Food consumption
- How fast you drink
- How much you drink

Figure 10.3 Because these factors change from person to person or from day to day, it is hard to predict the effect alcohol will have on a person's body.

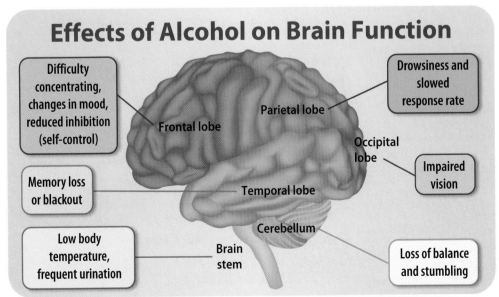

Effects of Alcohol on Brain Function

Difficulty concentrating, changes in mood, reduced inhibition (self-control)

Frontal lobe

Parietal lobe

Drowsiness and slowed response rate

Occipital lobe

Memory loss or blackout

Temporal lobe

Impaired vision

Low body temperature, frequent urination

Brain stem

Cerebellum

Loss of balance and stumbling

Yoko Design/Shutterstock.com

Figure 10.4 Alcohol has many effects on brain function that result in impaired physical and mental abilities. *What is the term for the self-control that keeps people from taking dangerous risks?*

Hangover Symptoms and Alcohol Poisoning

The effects of drinking alcohol can continue in the body—even up to 24 hours—after a person stops drinking. Drinking too much in a short period of time can cause a hangover or even alcohol poisoning, which can be life threatening.

The term *hangover* describes the negative symptoms caused by excessive alcohol consumption in one occasion. Examples of hangover symptoms include the following:

- tiredness, headaches, and muscle aches
- nausea and vomiting
- dizziness and a feeling that the room is spinning
- increased sensitivity to light and sound
- difficulty sleeping
- thirst and dehydration
- shakiness
- depression, anxiety, and irritability
- difficulty concentrating

Alcohol poisoning is a medical emergency that occurs when a large amount of alcohol enters the bloodstream in a short period of time. Alcohol poisoning can result in loss of consciousness, low blood pressure, low body temperature, and difficulty breathing. Extreme levels of alcohol consumption can lead to permanent brain damage or death. Given the serious consequences of alcohol poisoning, you should know the warning signs (**Figure 10.5**). Call 911 immediately if you suspect a person is experiencing alcohol poisoning.

Long-Term Health Effects

Young people who start drinking face serious lifelong health consequences. Alcohol is distributed throughout the entire body, so it affects every single

Figure 10.5
People who have alcohol poisoning may experience life-threatening consequences that require immediate medical attention.

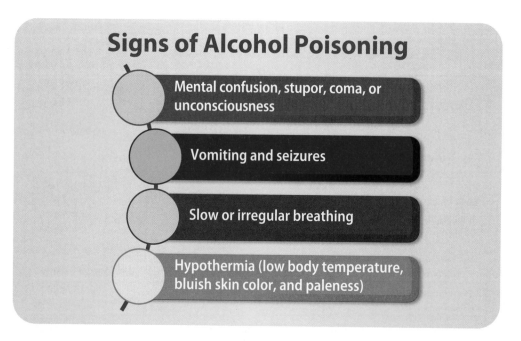

Signs of Alcohol Poisoning

Mental confusion, stupor, coma, or unconsciousness

Vomiting and seizures

Slow or irregular breathing

Hypothermia (low body temperature, bluish skin color, and paleness)

organ and body system. Therefore, regularly drinking large amounts of alcohol is associated with serious and even life-threatening consequences.

Brain Development

Alcohol use has immediate effects on brain function. It also causes long-term effects, especially for young people who start drinking. People who begin drinking early in life experience changes in their brain development. One recent study found that young people who binge drink show permanent changes in their brains, including issues with learning and memory. People who consume large amounts of alcohol on a regular basis can experience issues such as dementia, stroke, difficulty remembering, confusion, and drowsiness.

Binge drinking during adolescence permanently changes how the brain functions. Young people who drink heavily show damage in the *white matter* of the brain, which allows information to travel between different parts of the brain. This can lead to long-term issues with thinking, learning, and memory. Alcohol use also damages the *prefrontal cortex* (found in the frontal lobe), which controls attention, concentration, decision-making, and self-control.

When these parts of the brain are damaged, people find it harder to control their behavior. This increases risk of engaging in dangerous behaviors, such as drinking excessive amounts of alcohol or making unhealthy decisions. This is one reason scientists consistently say "there is no known safe level of binge drinking."

Chronic Diseases

A *chronic disease* lasts three months or more. Over time, drinking too much alcohol can lead to the development of several types of chronic diseases. These may include high blood pressure, heart disease, and certain types of cancer. Another chronic disease associated with heavy drinking is cirrhosis.

Cirrhosis is a buildup of scar tissue in the liver. Heavy drinking often causes liver damage. High levels of alcohol cause fat to build up in the liver, which blocks blood flow. Eventually this lack of blood flow can cause cirrhosis **(Figure 10.6)**.

Alcohol and Pregnancy

When a pregnant person drinks, the alcohol consumed passes from the person's bloodstream to the bloodstream of the fetus. People who drink during pregnancy risk giving birth to babies with *fetal alcohol spectrum disorder (FASD)*. This condition results in lifelong physical and mental effects. For example, babies with FASD often experience poor growth (both in the womb and after birth). They may have decreased muscle tone and poor coordination, as well as heart and facial conditions. Delayed development and issues with thinking, speech, movement, and social skills may also occur.

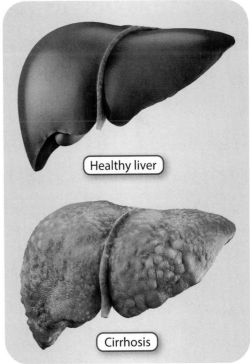

Healthy liver

Cirrhosis

iStock.com/eranicle

Figure 10.6 Cirrhosis of the liver is one of the 15 leading causes of death in the United States. *What often causes liver damage?*

Consequences of Alcohol Use

In the United States, you must be 21 years of age to buy and drink alcohol. Unfortunately, even with this law, many young people experience serious consequences due to alcohol use. In fact, alcohol is the most commonly used and abused substance among youths in the United States. It contributes to the deaths of more than 4,300 Americans younger than 21 years of age each year. Similar to other substances, alcohol use impacts a person's mental health and social relationships. Consuming alcohol can also lead to legal consequences that follow a person throughout life.

Mental Consequences

People may drink alcohol because it makes them feel more relaxed or less self-conscious. This is because alcohol is a depressant and slows down the central nervous system. These feelings from alcohol do not last, however. Once alcohol leaves the body, the feelings that were present before alcohol consumption will return. In addition, alcohol can lead to behaviors a person later regrets and increase feelings of depression. This leaves a person feeling worse than before drinking alcohol. Due to this, alcohol can worsen the symptoms and severity of mental health conditions and negative feelings.

Alcohol use can also lead to mental health conditions. Consuming alcohol can lead to an alcohol use disorder, which you will learn about later in this lesson. Like other types of substance use disorders, an alcohol use disorder worsens existing mental health conditions, harms a person's relationships, and hurts a person's goals.

Young people are largely impacted by alcohol use. Young people who drink alcohol are more likely to start abusing other drugs. Even drinking small amounts can lead to long-term issues with alcohol, such as developing an alcohol use disorder.

Social Consequences

Consuming alcohol can cause strained relationships with family and friends, as well as in the community. Feelings of guilt and fear may result from disappointing loved ones. Friends may become distant if they do not want to drink alcohol. Engaging in risky behaviors can threaten personal and community safety and harm relationships among community members.

Young people who consume alcohol may experience consequences that can negatively impact future educational plans, such as going to a technical school, and school relationships (**Figure 10.7**). Even for adults, alcohol use can impact work performance and relationships. It may result in people missing work, behaving poorly, or being disciplined for alcohol use on the job.

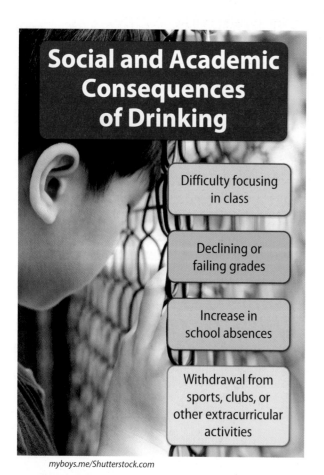

Social and Academic Consequences of Drinking

Difficulty focusing in class

Declining or failing grades

Increase in school absences

Withdrawal from sports, clubs, or other extracurricular activities

myboys.me/Shutterstock.com

Figure 10.7
Drinking alcohol can negatively affect a young person's success in school in many ways.

The Consequences of Underage Drinking

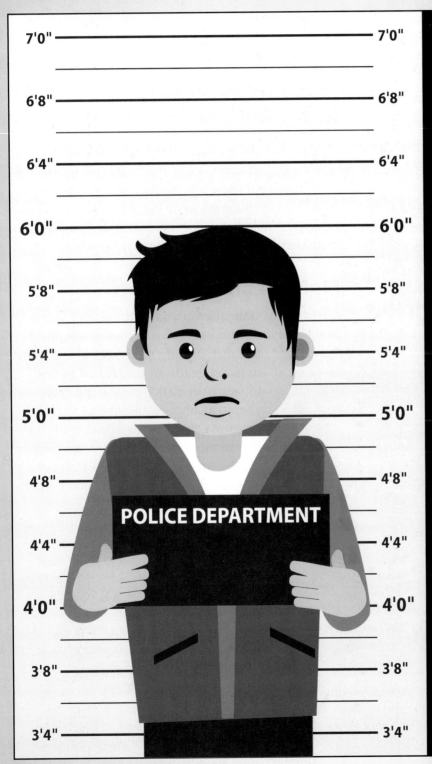

7'0"	7'0"
6'8"	6'8"
6'4"	6'4"
6'0"	6'0"
5'8"	5'8"
5'4"	5'4"
5'0"	5'0"
4'8"	4'8"
4'4"	4'4"
4'0"	4'0"
3'8"	3'8"
3'4"	3'4"

POLICE DEPARTMENT

CHARGES

HEALTH CONSEQUENCES
- Alcohol poisoning
- Changes in mood/behavior
- Hangover
- Increased risk of chronic illnesses

SCHOOL CONSEQUENCES
- Difficulty focusing
- Increased amount of absences
- Declining or failing grades

FAMILY/SOCIAL CONSEQUENCES
- Strained relationships
- Feelings of guilt and fear
- Withdrawal from activities, teams, and hobbies
- Feelings of isolation

LEGAL CONSEQUENCES
- Can be arrested
- Potential for jail time
- Fines and fees
- May have to appear in court
- Offenses can show up on permanent record

Background: Alhovik/Shutterstock.com; Boy: Busyok Creative/Shutterstock.com

Alcohol's Effects on the Central Nervous System

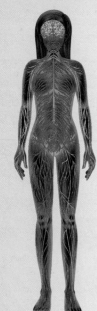

When alcohol slows down the nervous system, the body experiences

- decreased reaction time
- difficulty coordinating movements
- decreased ability to plan or problem solve
- decreased use of good judgment

BlueRingMedia/Shutterstock.com

Figure 10.8 As alcohol filters into the brain and bloodstream, it affects a person's ability to think and move quickly and correctly.

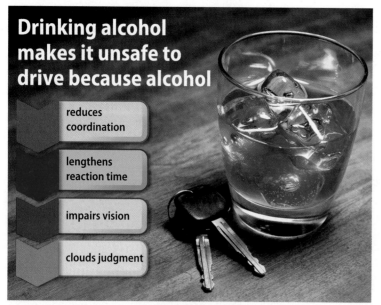

Drinking alcohol makes it unsafe to drive because alcohol

- reduces coordination
- lengthens reaction time
- impairs vision
- clouds judgment

Glass and keys: iStock.com/dehooks

Figure 10.9 Because of alcohol's effects on the body's response time, driving after drinking alcohol frequently results in deadly car accidents. *What is the legal term for a person who has consumed too much alcohol before driving a vehicle?*

Legal Consequences

Alcohol use is illegal for those younger than 21 years of age. If youths are caught using alcohol, this can lead to legal consequences. Young people may be required to pay a fine (as much as $500), take a class about alcohol use, and perform community service. They can also face consequences for trying to purchase alcohol, using a fake identification, or sharing alcohol with another underage person.

Alcohol Use and Risky Behaviors

Alcohol slows down the central nervous system, which affects the body in various ways. **Figure 10.8** shows some of these effects. As a result, people who have been drinking are more likely to engage in unsafe behaviors that often cause accidents. Alcohol may also increase violent behavior in some individuals.

Motor Vehicle Accidents

In every state, there are laws to prevent driving under the influence of alcohol or drugs. Despite this fact, driving after alcohol use leads to many deaths in the United States. In fact, over 10,000 people die each year in alcohol-related motor vehicle crashes. Driving after drinking alcohol is extremely dangerous and can hurt or kill the driver, vehicle passengers, and others in the community (**Figure 10.9**). Therefore, you should never get in a car with a driver who is intoxicated, let alone let them drive at all.

People who drink and drive can face legal consequences for their actions. Adults who drive with a BAC of 0.08 or above are *driving under the influence (DUI)*, which is against the law. In some states, this may also be called *driving while intoxicated (DWI)*. If a driver receives a DUI or DWI, the person's license may be suspended, or taken away for several months. This driver may also have to pay a fine, perform community service, or spend time in jail.

Many states follow a **zero-tolerance policy** for people under 21 years of age. Under this policy, there is no acceptable BAC level for people younger than 21 years of age. Penalties for violating a zero-tolerance policy vary from state to state.

Other Types of Accidents

Alcohol use is also associated with other types of accidents and injuries. Under the influence of alcohol, people experience high rates of the following:

- falls
- burns
- homicides
- suicides
- unintentional firearm injuries
- electrical shocks
- incidents of near drowning
- accidental death while bicycling or swimming

CASE STUDY

Kara's Babysitting Conundrum

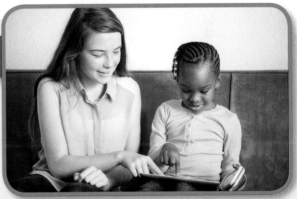

NicolasMcComber/Getty Images

Kara, who is in the eighth grade, frequently babysits for the Patel family. Kara enjoys spending time with children, so babysitting is a perfect job for her.

The Patels live a half mile down the street from Kara's family. When Kara babysits during the day, she often rides her bike to and from the Patel's house. When Kara babysits at night, her parents drop her off and the Patel parents bring her home.

Kara has babysat for the Patels many times without any issues. One evening, however, the Patel parents went to a fancy party. Everything had gone as planned that evening. Kara made dinner and spent time with the children without any arguments. Once the kids were asleep, Kara spent time watching TV, doing a little bit of cleaning up, and periodically checking on the kids. Mr. and Mrs. Patel returned home around midnight as Kara expected. What she did not expect was for them both to have been drinking.

Kara was not sure how drunk Mr. Patel was, but he stumbled when he walked into the house. He was also slow to respond to any of her questions. Mrs. Patel almost immediately fell asleep on the couch. Kara was uncomfortable getting into a car

with Mr. Patel driving, but he was so nice and she did not know how to refuse. Kara decided that it was only a couple of blocks to her house, so she got into the car with Mr. Patel.

Thinking Critically

1. Why was Kara uncomfortable in this situation? What could go wrong on the car ride to her house? Who could get hurt?

2. What other options does Kara have in this situation? How do you think she would feel about these alternative solutions?

3. How might refusing a ride from Mr. Patel affect her relationship with him? Do you think it would be worth it?

4. If you were in a situation like Kara, what would you do?

Violence

People who have been drinking are more likely to behave violently than those who have not been drinking. About 35 percent of people who experience some type of violent attack report that the person who assaulted them was under the influence of alcohol. Alcohol use is also associated with many cases of violence within families, including child abuse and violence between romantic partners. (You will learn more about abuse and violence in Chapter 16.)

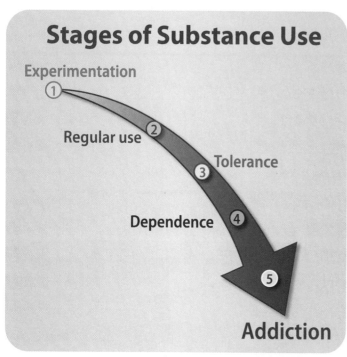

Stages of Substance Use

Experimentation ①

Regular use ②

Tolerance ③

Dependence ④

⑤

Addiction

Figure 10.10 Addiction to alcohol develops gradually through stages.

Alcohol Use Disorder

Like tobacco use, drinking alcohol can be addictive, especially for some people. Alcohol use can increase the risk of developing an alcohol use disorder. An **alcohol use disorder** is a type of substance use disorder in which a person has an addiction to alcohol and continues to consume it despite negative health effects.

No one who drinks alcohol intends to develop an addiction to alcohol. Despite this, drinking alcohol can easily lead to one. People who start drinking before 15 years of age are five times more likely to develop alcohol dependence than those who begin drinking as adults.

Addiction to alcohol develops gradually through a series of stages (**Figure 10.10**). During the *experimentation* stage, people try alcohol and may drink it occasionally. For example, young people may try alcohol after seeing their parents drinking or may feel pressured by their friends.

Some people who experiment with alcohol decide they do not like it and quit drinking. For others, experimentation can lead to *regular use*. During this stage, people consume alcohol on a regular basis. People who engage in moderate drinking limit their alcohol intake to not drink too much. Regular use, however, often causes people to drink more than they should. This results in the development of an alcohol use disorder.

Regular use causes the body to develop a *tolerance* for alcohol. In this stage, a person's body gets use to a certain amount of alcohol (**Figure 10.11**). A person must consume larger amounts of alcohol than previously needed to feel the same effects. This can easily lead to heavy drinking and an alcohol dependence.

Dependence occurs when the user is psychologically and physically dependent on alcohol. Once a dependence on alcohol exists, a person must have the substance in the body for the body to function as it did before alcohol use. If a person tries to stop drinking, withdrawal symptoms may occur. These symptoms may include hallucinations, impaired coordination, and disruptions in brain function.

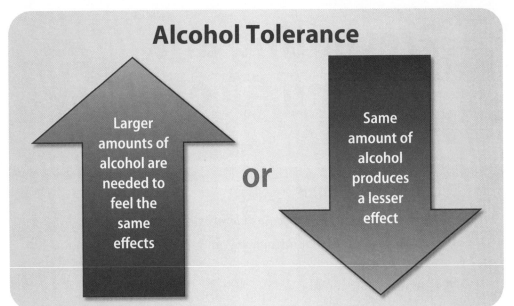

Alcohol Tolerance

Larger amounts of alcohol are needed to feel the same effects

or

Same amount of alcohol produces a lesser effect

Figure 10.11
A tolerance for alcohol means that a person's body has grown used to a certain amount of alcohol. *What stage of substance use causes a person to develop a tolerance for alcohol?*

People with an *alcohol addiction* show a number of symptoms. They may have a strong craving for alcohol and may not be able to limit their drinking. They may also experience memory loss or a *blackout* (forget what happened while drinking). People with an alcohol addiction often continue to drink despite serious issues with their physical and mental health, as well as trouble with their family and friends, school, or other responsibilities.

Lesson 10.1 Review

1. In the United States, a person must be _____ years of age to legally drink alcohol.
2. The majority of alcohol consumed by underage drinkers is in the form of _____ drinking.
3. **True or false.** Changes in the brain, hangovers, and alcohol poisoning are long-term health effects of drinking alcohol.
4. What is the term that describes a type of substance use disorder when a person has an addiction to alcohol and continues to drink it despite negative health effects?
5. **Critical thinking.** How many ounces are equivalent to one drink for beer, wine, and liquor? What does this mean about consumption of these types of alcohol?

Hands-On Activity

In small groups, create an anti-alcohol message to encourage students at your school to say "no" to alcohol. Include the following in your message: consequences related to health, school, family and social relations, and legal. In addition, include other relevant information and images to enhance your message. Possible formats for the message may include a video or script for the morning announcements, a poster or flyer, a brochure, or a social media post..

Key Terms 👉

detoxification process of completely stopping all alcohol use to remove the substance from the body

Alcoholics Anonymous (AA) self-help program for people with an alcohol use disorder to help them change how they think about drinking

enabling encouraging a person's unhealthy behaviors, either intentionally or unintentionally

Alateen support group where young people who have loved ones with an alcohol use disorder come together to share their experiences and learn ways to cope with challenges

Al-Anon Family Groups support group where family members and friends who have loved ones with an alcohol use disorder come together to share their experiences, receive encouragement, and learn ways to cope with challenges

Learning Outcomes

After studying this lesson, you will be able to

- **describe** factors that influence young people's beliefs about alcohol use.
- **demonstrate** methods of preventing alcohol use.
- **explain** treatment methods for an alcohol use disorder.
- **demonstrate** how to help someone who has an alcohol use disorder.

Graphic Organizer

Alcohol Use

Before you hear about the content in the lesson, think about how you would answer the following questions:

- What influences lead young people to try alcohol the first time?
- What are some ways to prevent underage drinking?
- What treatment is available for people with an alcohol use disorder?

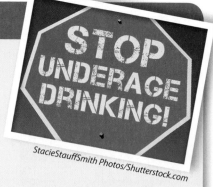

StacieStauffSmith Photos/Shutterstock.com

As you listen to your teacher present this lesson, take notes about these topics using a chart like the one shown. Use the textbook to add any notes you may have missed.

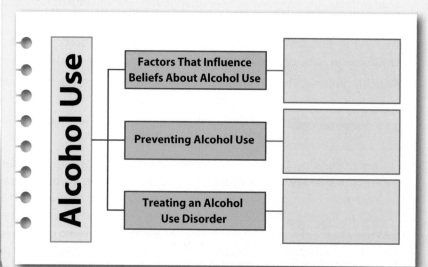

According to the most recent Youth Risk Behavior Survey conducted by the CDC, 15.5 percent of youths drank alcohol for the first time before 13 years of age (**Figure 10.12**). This is an alarming percentage since alcohol use is illegal for people younger than 21 years of age.

Due to her family's openness toward alcohol use, Priya does not see the dangers associated with alcohol as Santiago does. Last week, she even snuck a bottle of her parents' alcohol to share with her friends. Due to Priya's carefree attitude toward alcohol, Santiago may feel peer pressured into drinking by Priya and his other friends. Santiago thinks about telling his parents about Priya's alcohol use, but he does not want to get her in trouble.

This lesson will explore factors affecting alcohol use. You will also learn about strategies for preventing alcohol use and treatment methods to help people overcome an alcohol use disorder.

Factors Affecting Alcohol Use

Similar to tobacco use, several factors may affect someone's views and use of alcohol. These include individual factors and outside factors in an individual's environment such as family, peers, and the media.

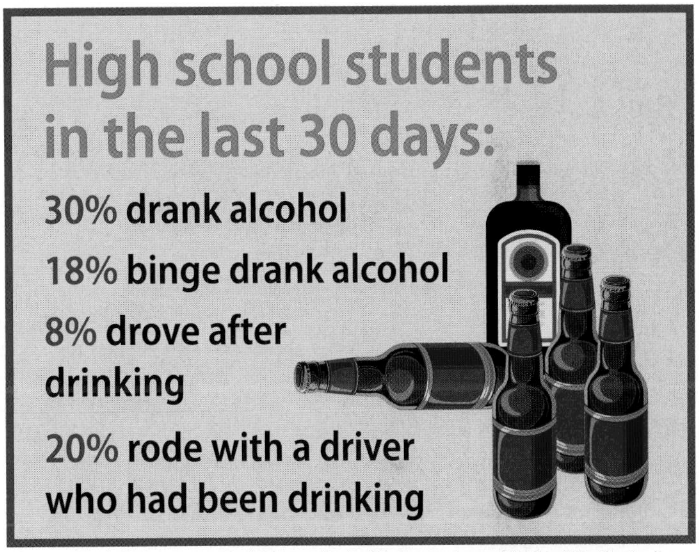

Individual Factors

Two individual factors that could affect someone's alcohol use include genetic makeup and mental health. Research has shown that genetic factors contribute to alcohol use. Some research suggests that people with specific genes have a greater risk of developing an alcohol use disorder. For example, people with a certain gene may be less sensitive to effects of alcohol, which may act as a signal to stop drinking. People who feel less influenced by alcohol may drink more. This pattern can lead to dependence and an alcohol use disorder.

People with mental health conditions also have a greater risk of using alcohol and developing an alcohol use disorder. They may use alcohol to cope with negative feelings (such as anxiety), cheer themselves up, or sleep. Using alcohol to handle these issues is called *self-medication*. Alcohol use can also cause mental health conditions or make existing conditions worse.

High school students in the last 30 days:

30% drank alcohol

18% binge drank alcohol

8% drove after drinking

20% rode with a driver who had been drinking

Alcoholic beverages: Andrii Bezvershenko/Shutterstock.com; SlipFloat/Shutterstock.com

Figure 10.12 Because they fear the consequences of asking an adult for help, young people have a higher likelihood than adults of agreeing to drive under the influence and getting into a car with a drunk driver.

Family

Families have their own attitudes, beliefs, and rules about alcohol use, which influence their children's attitudes toward alcohol. Some families may

Influences on Drinking

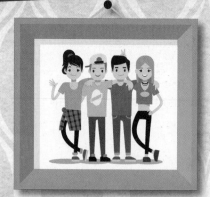

Your "cool," older classmates who you believe are drinking

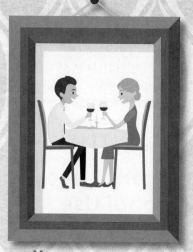

Your parents or guardians who drink during dinner or celebrations

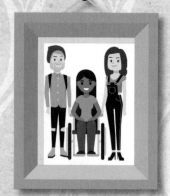

Your older siblings who drink around you and with their friends

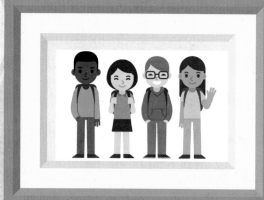

Your friends who want you to try it with them

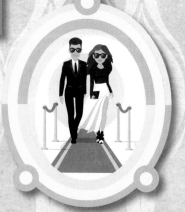

Your favorite celebrity who makes drinking look fun or glamorous

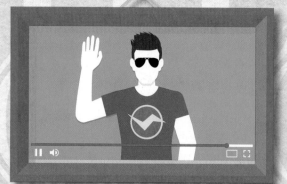

People you see drinking and having fun on social media

keep and drink alcohol in the home, but have rules about alcohol use to protect their children. Other families may have strong beliefs about alcohol use, leading them not to allow any alcohol in the home. Children also learn about occasions for drinking, such as stressful days or celebrations, by watching their family members' drinking habits.

Unfortunately, some young people have parents or guardians with an alcohol use disorder (**Figure 10.13**). This experience may influence young people to either try or avoid alcohol. Young people who have parents or guardians with an alcohol use disorder are more likely to develop one, too. Some young people, however, decide never to try alcohol because of how it affected their parents or guardians.

Siblings can also affect how a young person feels about alcohol use. Young people often look up to older siblings as role models. If a young person's older sibling uses and abuses alcohol, the young person may consider this acceptable and "cool" behavior.

Peer Pressure

Friends can influence a young person's alcohol use. People tend to drink more alcohol when they have friends who drink. This may be due to peer pressure. As you learned in Chapter 9, *peer pressure* is the influence that people your age or status have on your actions. Young people who drink may pressure their friends into trying alcohol. Aggressively pressuring someone to drink alcohol is a form of bullying. Real friends will not pressure you into engaging in unhealthy behaviors.

Peer pressure can be indirect. Young people often believe that their peers are drinking. This may lead them to try alcohol to fit in with the "cool kids" they imagine are drinking. Young people may also view using alcohol as a way to seem older, but teens and young adults do not drink as much as you might think. In fact, many young people are often uncomfortable with alcohol use (**Figure 10.14**).

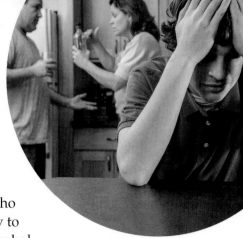

threerocksimages/Shutterstock.com

Figure 10.13
Having a parent or guardian with an alcohol use disorder can cause stress and conflict for young people. It can also increase their risk of developing an alcohol use disorder themselves. *Why might an older sibling influence a young person's personal beliefs about alcohol use?*

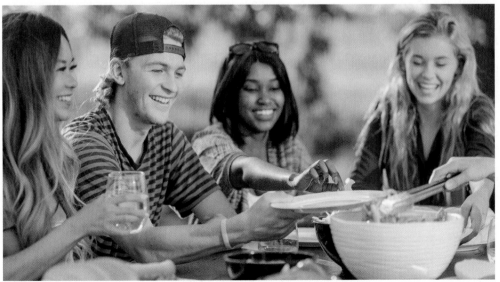

iStock.com/FatCamera

Figure 10.14
Despite common assumptions, most teens and young people do not drink alcohol even with their friends. *What is the term for the influence people your age have on others their age?*

Media Messages

Young people can form attitudes about alcohol use by watching television and movies. Films, even those marketed to young people, frequently show alcohol use. Young people who see drinking in movies tend to view alcohol use more positively. These young people are also more likely to plan to drink alcohol as adults. Advertisements for alcohol products can also influence these attitudes.

In addition, young people may model behaviors and attitudes about alcohol use after their favorite celebrities. Celebrities may drink large amounts of alcohol and post about it on social media. Even seeing social media posts of friends drinking alcohol can shape opinions on alcohol use. Imitating this behavior can lead to negative effects on your health and future.

BUILDING Your Skills

Making Healthy Decisions

Do you know how to make healthy decisions in the best possible way for yourself? Making decisions in the adolescent years is tough. Your parents tell you one thing, while your friends may say something different. Movies, TV, and other media showcase yet another opinion. All the while, your gut may be telling you something very different. So, how should you make *healthy* decisions about alcohol and other health behaviors?

Recall the steps of the decision-making process from Chapter 1. This process is the best way to make healthy and informed decisions.

Step 1	Identify the decision.
Step 2	Brainstorm options.
Step 3	Identify possible outcomes.
Step 4	Make a decision.
Step 5	Reflect on the decision.

When you are making a big decision, about alcohol or something else, it helps to write down your thoughts and brainstorm potential solutions. If the situation is complicated, more than one issue may be involved. Remember that there are usually several possible solutions to any situation. It is okay, and even good, to get ideas for solutions from other people such as the following:

- parents or guardians
- friends
- siblings
- teachers
- coaches
- counselors

When you have come up with some solutions, write a list of the pros and cons for each possible outcome. Be careful though. Just because one option has more pros than another option does not necessarily mean it is the better choice. You have to account for how important each of those pros are to you and how you value them. For example, you may realize that making your parents proud of your decisions or doing well in sports may outweigh all the other pros involved.

Using the Decision-Making Process

Think about a big decision you are facing. On a sheet of paper, use the steps of the decision-making process to help you come up with the best choice.

Preventing Alcohol Use

Making the decision now to not drink alcohol is the best way to protect your brain, body, and mental and emotional health from the effects of alcohol. Various strategies and skills can help people prevent alcohol use. These include education programs, developing refusal skills, and monitoring mental health. In addition, federal and state governments regulate alcohol in several ways to decrease underage use.

Education Programs and Refusal Skills

Schools have developed many education programs to decrease risky drinking, especially in underage drinkers. These programs might mention the health risks and physical effects of alcohol use on the body. They might mention the risk of strained personal relationships, which can occur when a person drinks too much. The programs emphasize the legal consequences of young people possessing alcohol.

Education programs can also disprove the beliefs some young people have about their peers' alcohol use. Young people may believe that using alcohol is the norm among their peers, but the truth is very different. Many studies show that most young people do not drink. In fact, most young people wish there was less drinking in their environment. Educating young people about this fact can encourage them not to drink. For example, some colleges give new students information showing that many of their fellow students are also uncomfortable with how much drinking occurs on campus. Students who receive such information report drinking less alcohol than students who do not receive this information.

Some programs focus on helping young people feel better about themselves. Youths who lack self-confidence may choose to drink alcohol because they do not have the skills to stand up to peer pressure. Prevention programs may build teens' self-esteem and teach strategies for resisting pressure to drink. You must also learn refusal skills. Even if you are aware of the negative consequences of alcohol use and have made the decision not to drink, alcohol may still be present in your environment. Though it is not the norm, some young people do use alcohol. Developing and practicing refusal skills can help when someone offers you alcohol (**Figure 10.15**).

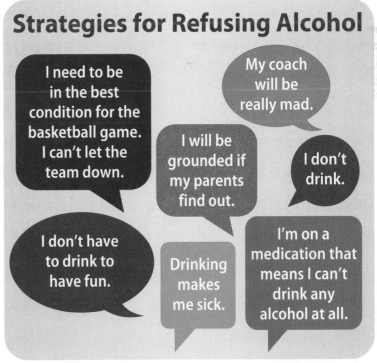

Strategies for Refusing Alcohol

I need to be in the best condition for the basketball game. I can't let the team down.

My coach will be really mad.

I will be grounded if my parents find out.

I don't drink.

I don't have to drink to have fun.

Drinking makes me sick.

I'm on a medication that means I can't drink any alcohol at all.

Figure 10.15 Refusal skills can help you resist pressure to try alcohol. The more you practice your refusal skills, the better prepared you will be to resist peer pressure.

Pay Attention to Mental Health

Paying attention to your mental health is an important part of avoiding alcohol use. People often drink alcohol in an attempt to feel better. Alcohol may temporarily distract people from issues they are facing, but it does not make the issues go away. It can cause even bigger issues.

If you are struggling with negative feelings, stress, or mental health conditions, take steps to build your self-esteem, express emotions, adopt a positive mind-set, and manage stress. Some healthy ways of managing stress might include writing in a journal or spending time with friends. These approaches will help you reduce stress. You can also try to reframe negative events by viewing them as learning opportunities.

If you are struggling with a mental health condition or illness, do not try to self-medicate. Instead, seek help from a mental health professional. Talk to a trusted adult for help in finding this type of resource.

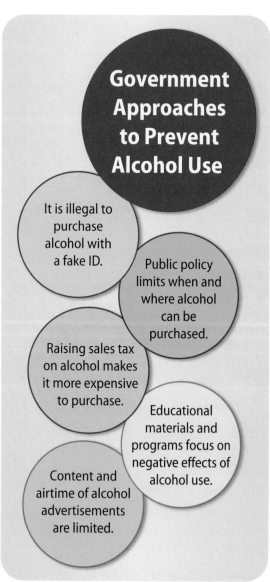

Figure 10.16 Governments use various restrictions to discourage and protect people from harmful effects of alcohol.

Government Approaches

The government seeks to make it difficult for young people to access alcohol. One of the most obvious and effective government approaches is setting the minimum legal drinking age at 21. Forbidding people who are younger than 21 years of age from purchasing alcohol makes it more difficult for young people to have access to alcohol. Additional methods used by the government are shown in **Figure 10.16**.

Treating an Alcohol Use Disorder

People with an alcohol use disorder are often physically and psychologically addicted to alcohol. Although breaking this addiction is difficult, there are a number of strategies that can help people quit drinking.

Detoxification

One of the first steps in recovery from an alcohol use disorder is **detoxification**. This is the process of completely stopping all alcohol use to remove the substance from the body. Detoxification is a necessary step in recovering from an addiction to alcohol. This process, which is sometimes called *drying out*, may take up to a month. The process may or may not include time spent in the hospital. Detoxification can include severe withdrawal symptoms, such as intense anxiety, tremors, and hallucinations. A doctor may prescribe medications to lessen these symptoms.

Support Groups

Community support groups can be helpful tools for those overcoming an alcohol use disorder. *Support groups* are groups of people with a common struggle who share the obstacles they faced and examples of overcoming them.

Alcoholics Anonymous (also known as *AA*) is the most well known and widely used self-help program for people with an alcohol use disorder. The program includes a support group element. The goal of AA is to help people with an alcohol use disorder change how they think about drinking. This program involves going through 12 distinct steps, which are a set of guiding principles designed to help people recover from addiction.

According to AA, when a person with a severe alcohol use disorder consumes even a small amount of alcohol, the presence of alcohol in the bloodstream leads to an irresistible craving for more alcohol. Thus, the goal for recovery is never to drink any alcohol again.

During AA meetings, group members share with other group members any alcohol-related struggles they have experienced. This process of sharing their experiences may help people stop drinking. In addition, group members may work with a *sponsor* who provides support, empathy, and accountability.

Self-Management Strategies

Many programs that help people with an alcohol use disorder also teach self-management skills. First, these programs focus on helping people become aware of why they drink. Understanding the motivations that lead someone to drink is an important first step in learning how to avoid alcohol.

Next, people develop skills for managing the situations that lead them to want to have a drink (**Figure 10.17**). People can use these types of self-management skills in combination with other treatments for an alcohol use disorder. Other treatments may include attending AA meetings or undergoing detoxification.

Helping Someone with an Alcohol Use Disorder

Loving and caring about someone with an alcohol use disorder can be very difficult. People who have loved ones or know someone with an alcohol use disorder may feel ashamed, angry, afraid, and guilty. Other people feel so overwhelmed by their loved one's alcohol use disorder that they just deny the issue and pretend that nothing is wrong.

If you care about someone who has an alcohol use disorder, you must first get support for yourself. Try to find an adult you can talk openly and honestly

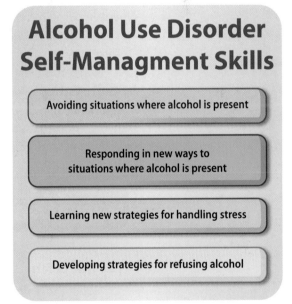

Alcohol Use Disorder Self-Managment Skills

- Avoiding situations where alcohol is present
- Responding in new ways to situations where alcohol is present
- Learning new strategies for handling stress
- Developing strategies for refusing alcohol

Figure 10.17 Learning how to manage their own behaviors in situations where alcohol is present can help people with an alcohol use disorder avoid alcohol.

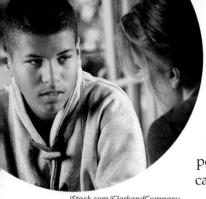

iStock.com/ClarkandCompany

Figure 10.18
Hiding someone's alcohol use disorder can allow that person's behavior to continue. To help a loved one, it is best to speak to a trusted adult. *Who would you feel comfortable talking to about an alcohol use disorder?*

with about the issue. This trusted adult may be a family member, school counselor, school nurse, doctor, religious leader, or coach (**Figure 10.18**).

Some people feel they should try to solve or fix their loved one's alcohol use disorder. They may try to punish, threaten, beg, or bribe their loved one to stop drinking. They may try to make the person feel guilty about their alcohol use. The first step to alcohol recovery, however, is for a person to recognize that an issue exists. The person has to want to change. You cannot force a person to stop drinking.

People may also try to hide their loved one's alcohol use. They may cover up the issues caused by the person's drinking or hide evidence of the drinking. These actions simply help the person avoid the natural consequences of the behavior. Hiding a person's alcohol use is an enabling behavior. **Enabling** involves encouraging a person's unhealthy behaviors.

Many young people who have family members with an alcohol use disorder find joining support groups helpful. These groups can help young people learn how to cope with the difficulties of their loved one's alcoholism. Support groups can also be comforting because they show that other people are facing the same challenges.

Young people who have loved ones with an alcohol use disorder may find Alateen to be helpful. **Alateen** members include young people whose lives have been affected by someone else's drinking. In Alateen meetings, young people come together to share their experiences, gain encouragement, and learn various ways to cope with challenges. In Alateen, young people can find other people their age who have the same concerns and worries.

Alateen is part of the Al-Anon Family Groups organization. In **Al-Anon Family Groups**, family members and friends who have loved ones with an alcohol use disorder come together to share their experiences, receive encouragement, and learn methods to cope with challenges.

Lesson 10.2 Review

1. List four factors that may influence young people's beliefs about alcohol use.
2. **True or false.** Most young people experiment with drinking alcohol.
3. What three strategies can a young person use to prevent alcohol use?
4. Encouraging a person's unhealthy behaviors, such as an alcohol use disorder, is called _____.
5. **Critical thinking.** Compare the three strategies described in this lesson for treating an alcohol use disorder.

Hands-On Activity

Conduct informal interviews with your parents or guardians, older siblings, and/or grandparents about any alcohol use disorder they may know about in your family. Find a time to talk openly and honestly with them. How was this conversation—easy or difficult? What did you learn? What questions would you still like to have answered?

Summary

Lesson 10.1 The Effects of Alcohol

- *Alcohol* is an addictive drug found in drinks that can cause a person to act and feel differently. Depending on the amount consumed, drinking alcohol can be considered moderate drinking, binge drinking, or heavy drinking.
- *Blood alcohol concentration (BAC)* is the percentage of alcohol in a person's blood. People with a BAC of 0.08 or above are considered intoxicated.
- The central nervous system slows down when people consume alcohol. This causes brain functions to slow, chemical changes to occur, and a decrease in inhibition.
- Most people who drink too much will experience a hangover. Symptoms may include headaches, muscle aches, vomiting, dizziness, and sensitivity to light and sound.
- *Alcohol poisoning* is a medical emergency that results from too much alcohol in the bloodstream. Extreme cases can lead to permanent brain damage or death.
- Drinking alcohol long-term is associated with serious consequences, including permanent issues with learning and memory and chronic diseases such as cirrhosis.
- Alcohol is the most commonly abused drug among youth in the United States. People who drink alcohol may experience various mental, social, and legal consequences. Drinking alcohol also puts people at greater risk for accidents and other risky behaviors.
- An alcohol use disorder occurs when the use of alcohol causes issues that interfere with a person's health and responsibilities. People with an alcohol addiction continue to drink despite these consequences.

Lesson 10.2 Preventing and Treating Alcohol Use

- A person's genetic makeup and overall mental health are individual factors that can affect a person's alcohol use.
- Young people are more likely to experiment with alcohol use if their parents or older siblings use or abuse alcohol. Their friends and peers may also try to pressure them into trying alcohol. The messages young people see in the media, such as TV commercials, social media, or in magazines, can also influence this decision.
- Education programs can help disprove the beliefs young people have about drinking as well as build self-esteem. These programs also help them learn the physical, social, and mental consequences of alcohol use. Refusal skills can also help young people avoid drinking alcohol.
- Paying attention to mental health and managing negative feelings and stress is an important part of avoiding alcohol use.
- People with an alcohol use disorder can use detoxification, support groups such as Alcoholics Anonymous, and self-management strategies for treatment. Enabling a person's unhealthy behaviors by covering up their challenges will not treat the alcohol use disorder.

Check Your Knowledge

Record your answers to each of the following questions on a separate sheet of paper.

1. Alcohol is a type of a drug known as a(n) _____.

2. For moderate drinking, how many alcoholic drinks can males and females consume on the same occasion?

3. **True or false.** Drinking eight or more drinks in one week for females and 15 or more drinks in one week for males can lead a person to become dependent on alcohol.

4. A person with a BAC of _____ or above is considered intoxicated or drunk.

5. **True or false.** Alcohol affects and is associated with health issues in every single organ and body system.

6. What is the name of the disorder in which a person has an addiction to alcohol and continues to consume it despite negative health effects?

7. **True or false.** A person's parents or guardians, siblings, peers, and celebrity idols do not have much of an influence on whether the person decides to use alcohol.

8. Developing and practicing _____ skills can help you say "no" when someone offers you alcohol.

9. What is the most obvious and effective government approach to prevent alcohol use among young people?

10. Which of the following is *not* an effective treatment method for an alcohol use disorder?
    A. Support groups.
    B. Detoxification.
    C. Enabling.
    D. Self-management.

11. The most well-known and widely used support group for people with alcohol use disorder is _____.

12. What is the sub-group of AA that helps young people come together to share their experiences of having been affected by someone else's drinking?

Use Your Vocabulary ⟑

Al-Anon Family Groups	alcohol use disorder	enabling
Alateen	binge drinking	heavy drinking
alcohol	blood alcohol	inhibition
Alcoholics	concentration (BAC)	moderate drinking
Anonymous (AA)	detoxification	zero-tolerance policy

13. With a partner, choose two terms from the list above. Create a Venn diagram to compare the two terms. Write one term under the left circle and the other term under the right circle. For each term, write descriptions in each respective circle. Where the circles overlap, write three characteristics the terms have in common.

14. In small groups, create categories for the terms above and classify as many of the terms as possible. Then, share your ideas with another pair and discuss your categories.

Think Critically

15. **Assess.** Why are rules and laws about alcohol use needed? What are the intentions behind a minimum legal drinking age, laws against drinking and driving, or zero-tolerance policies?

16. **Compare and contrast.** Many factors influence a person's decision to use alcohol. Which influences do you think impact young people the most? Why?

17. **Predict.** If an adolescent decided to drink alcohol and this behavior continues, predict the impact the decision will have on the person's health and social relations. Support your prediction with information learned from the chapter, as well as any additional resources.

18. **Identify.** What are the different options for treating alcohol use disorders? Use valid resources to identify three treatment facilities or programs in your community.

DEVELOP Your Skills

19. **Conflict resolution and communication skills.** Imagine that someone you know is showing signs of an alcohol use disorder. How would you address this issue? What if this person does not agree with your thoughts and is adamant that the alcohol use is safe and under control? What would you do?

20. **Decision-making and advocacy skills.** Create a public service announcement (PSA)—print, audio, or video—targeted toward students in your school. Focus your PSA on the promotion of having fun without drinking alcohol and healthy alternatives to drinking alcohol. Mention the dangers of alcohol use and information about how students can access help for an alcohol use disorder. Present your PSA to the class. If listening to a presentation, provide feedback to the presenter to show your understanding.

21. **Refusal and communication skills.** Write at least three statements that clearly express your desire not to drink alcohol. An example includes "I'm not interested in drinking because I have alcoholism in my family."

22. **Refusal and communication skills.** With a classmate, role-play a situation in which one person is pressuring another to go to a party where "everyone" will be drinking alcohol. Discuss familiar topics like your thoughts as well as unfamiliar topics like the health effects of alcohol use. Make sure to demonstrate your effective refusal skills.

23. **Access information.** Find a news story from the last six months that involves adolescent alcohol use. In a presentation to the class, summarize the article and discuss the accuracy of the facts about alcohol presented. How well were you able to understand the story? What can a teen learn from this situation, and what questions may remain? Properly cite the news story.

24. **Decision-making skills.** Go to the Al-Anon Family Groups' website and click on the self-quiz for teens. On a sheet of paper, write your answers to the quiz questions. Use your decision-making skills to determine whether Alateen is a group that might be helpful to you.

Chapter

11

Medications and Drugs

Essential Question 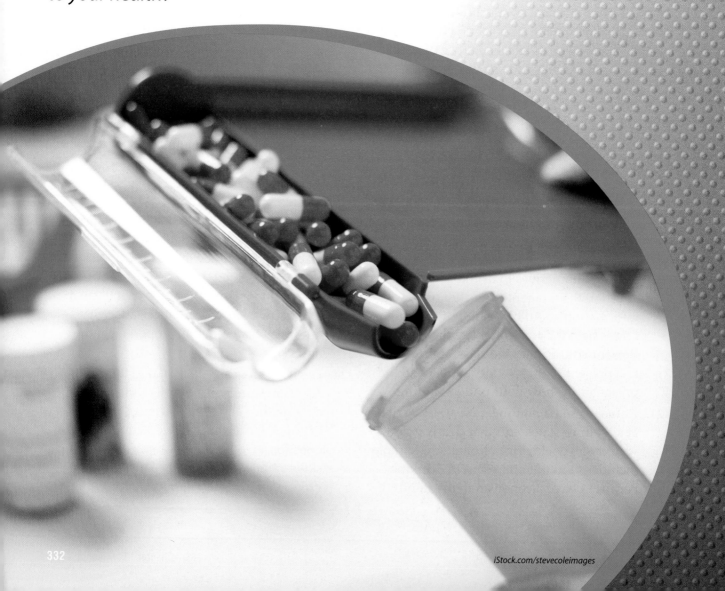?

How do your decisions about drugs and medications relate to your health?

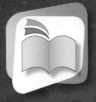

Reading Activity

Before reading the chapter, look at the illustrations and write a prediction about how the image illustrates a text concept. As you read the chapter, write notes about what information the text gives regarding these illustrations. After you finish reading the chapter, compare your predictions with your notes.

How Healthy Are You?

In this chapter, you will be learning about medications and drugs. Before you begin reading, take the following quiz to assess your current medication and drug habits.

Healthy Choices	Yes	No
Are you aware of the possible side effects of any medication you may take?		
Are you aware of the health risks caused by your medication interacting with other medications, dietary supplements, foods, or drinks?		
Are you aware of any allergies you have to medications?		
Do you always carefully read and follow the instructions for taking medication?		
Do you refuse to take medicine prescribed for someone else?		
Do you only use medication for the purposes and in the doses intended?		
Do you refuse to consume illegal drugs, including heroin and club drugs?		
Do you understand the serious health risks, especially to adolescents, of using marijuana?		
Do you avoid self-medicating with drugs to treat mental health conditions?		
Do you feel confident that you could refuse a friend's offer to try drugs?		
Do you avoid going to parties where drugs are present?		
Do you know about the resources at your school, in your community, and online that can help educate you about the dangers of abusing medications and drugs?		

Count your "Yes" and "No" responses. The more "Yes" responses you have, the more healthy medication and drug habits you exhibit. Now, take a closer look at the questions with which you responded "No." How can you make these healthy habits part of your daily life? Identify a SMART goal you would like to achieve to help improve your overall health and well-being. Refer to Figure 1.11 to help you set up your SMART goal. If you do not understand the instructions, ask for clarification from your teacher.

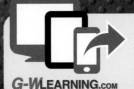

Click on the activity icon or visit www.g-wlearning.com/health to access online vocabulary activities using key terms from the chapter.

Medication Use and Abuse

Learning Outcomes

After studying this lesson, you will be able to

- **differentiate between** over-the-counter and prescription medications.
- **explain** health risks of taking medications.
- **list** strategies for using medications safely.
- **identify** possible consequences of medication misuse.
- **describe** the negative health consequences of abusing medications, such as depressants, opioids, stimulants, diet pills, and performance-enhancing drugs (PEDs).

Graphic Organizer

Safe Medication Use

In a graphic organizer like the one shown below, write eight statements about strategies for using medications safely. As you read the lesson, note any health benefits of safe medication usage not previously known.

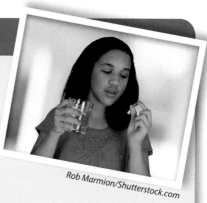

Rob Marmion/Shutterstock.com

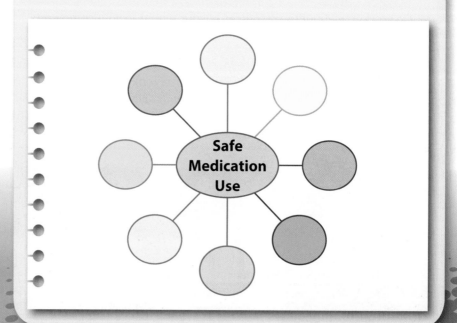

Safe Medication Use

Jamal is 12 years old. He has to stay home from school today because he is sick. His dad gives him an ibuprofen to treat his low-grade fever and tells him to get some sleep. Jamal has a hard time resting, however, because of his cough. When it starts to become painful, Jamal's dad drives to the drugstore and buys some over-the-counter cough syrup and cough drops to help soothe his throat. Jamal takes one dose of cough syrup and another one after his two-hour nap. He did not read the label, so he does not know that he is only supposed to take one dose every four to six hours.

Ibuprofen and cough medicine are examples of medications people like Jamal can take to treat symptoms of an illness or prevent a disease. These medications come with specific instructions, however, that must be followed.

Defining Medications and Drugs

When you hear the terms *medications* and *drugs*, would you define them in the same way? Sometimes, you might say they are the same. At other times, you would not. A **drug** is any substance that causes a physical or psychological change in the body. Drugs can have medical or nonmedical purposes. **Medications** are substances used to treat symptoms of an illness or to cure, manage, or prevent a disease. According to these definitions, all medications are drugs. Not all drugs, however, are medications.

If used properly and for their intended purpose, medications can have many benefits. Incorrect medication use and drug use, however, can have serious, negative consequences on physical, mental and emotional, and social health.

Types of Medications

There are two different types of medications people take to improve their health. These types include over-the-counter medications and prescription medications. Both types come in many different forms (**Figure 11.1**).

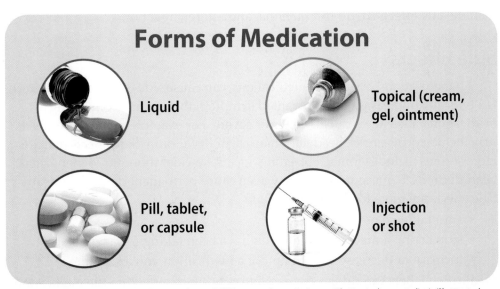

Forms of Medication

Liquid

Topical (cream, gel, ointment)

Pill, tablet, or capsule

Injection or shot

Figure 11.1
The form of medication a person needs depends on the type of condition being treated.

Clockwise from top left: Africa Studio/Shutterstock.com; Triff/Shutterstock.com; Enriscapes/Shutterstock.com; studiovin/Shutterstock.com

Types and Functions of Prescription Medications

Types	Functions
Antibiotics	Kill or slow the growth of bacteria
Anesthetics	Eliminate or reduce pain
Vaccinations	Work with the body's natural immune system to reduce the risk of developing an infection or disease
Opioids	Reduce pain, often after surgery
Depressants (also called *sedatives* or *tranquilizers*)	Reduce anxiety and help people relax, stay calm, and sleep
Stimulants (available both with a prescription and over-the-counter)	Increase energy, alertness, and attention

Figure 11.2 The types of medications listed in the table above can only be purchased by having a prescription from a doctor. *What is the name of a store that sells both OTC and prescription medications?*

Over-the-Counter Medications

People can purchase **over-the-counter (OTC) medications** without a doctor's prescription to treat the symptoms of many minor health conditions. Your family may keep certain OTC medications at home in case someone gets sick. These medications can treat headaches, fevers, and the common cold.

The most commonly used OTC medications are pain relievers, such as aspirin, acetaminophen, and ibuprofen. Other OTC medications include fever reducers, cold medicines, cough medicines, and certain allergy medications.

Prescription Medications

People can only purchase **prescription medications** with a prescription from a doctor (**Figure 11.2**). When the doctor gives a patient a prescription, the person can take it to a pharmacy to get the medication. A *pharmacy* is a store that sells both OTC and prescription medications. If more of the prescription medication is needed, the person must get approval for a refill from the doctor.

Health Risks of Taking Medications

Taking OTC and prescription medications can be beneficial to your health. Using these medications, however, can also carry some risks. These include side effects, drug interactions, and allergic reactions.

Side Effects

All medications, even OTC medications, can cause side effects. A **side effect** is a typically unpleasant and unwanted symptom that occurs from taking a medication. Side effects can be minor or severe. For example, minor side effects may include drowsiness, headache, nausea, or dry mouth. Side effects that are more serious include stomach bleeding, ulcers, suicidal thoughts, or abnormal heart rhythms. Some side effects may even cause permanent damage or death. Side effects are more likely to occur if you

- start taking a new medication
- stop taking a medication that you have been taking for a while
- increase or decrease the amount of a medication you are taking

Medication labels should list the possible side effects of taking the medication.

Medication Interactions

Some medications cause health risks by interacting with other drugs, dietary supplements, foods, or drinks. These health risks can be minor. For example, you may need to take a medicine with food. If you take the medicine without eating anything, you may get an upset stomach. Other health risks from drug interactions are serious and can be life threatening.

If two medications work together to increase overall effect (called *synergism*), the effect on the body can be too strong. For example, taking sleep medications and pain relievers together can lead to serious health risks, including death (**Figure 11.3**).

Sensitivities and Allergic Reactions

Sometimes the same medication can have different effects on different people. For example, a person who has a *drug sensitivity* is more likely to experience negative side effects using a specific medication. If a person has a *drug allergy*, the body responds to a certain medication as if it is harmful. People are most often allergic to antibiotics. Allergic reactions from a drug allergy can range from rashes and itching to swelling, breathing issues, and even death. If you have any sensitivities or allergies, tell your doctor and pharmacist and read medication labels carefully.

Medication Tolerance and Withdrawal

Using a medication for a long time can make the body need more of the medication to feel an effect. This is called *tolerance*. As tolerance builds, the body needs larger amounts of the medication. Not taking a medication after a long time can cause *withdrawal*. During withdrawal, the body craves the medication. Symptoms can include depression, anxiety, fatigue, sleeplessness, seizures, and hallucinations. The best way to avoid these risks is to use medications safely and only as directed.

Strategies for Using Medications Safely

Carefully reading and following prescription and OTC usage instructions can help people make sure they are taking medications safely. The instructions

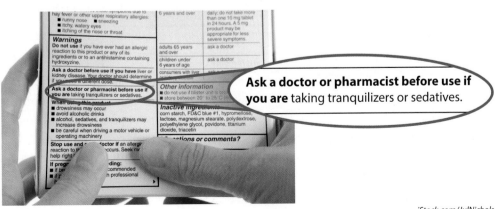

Figure 11.3
OTC medication labels will list any potential drug interactions. Read the label carefully before taking any medicines.

should be on the medication label, box, or container. **Figure 11.4** shows the usage instructions on a prescription medication label and an over-the-counter label. Always make sure you understand the usage instructions before taking any medication. If you have any questions about a medicine, consult your doctor or pharmacist.

Other strategies for using medications safely include the following:

- Always tell your doctor or pharmacist about any drug allergies or sensitivities you have and any medications or drugs you are taking. Ask any questions you have about the instructions or side effects.
- Follow the directions for taking a medication exactly as written. An app may help remind you. Pay attention to any warnings on the label.
- Use OTC medications that have only the ingredients needed to treat the condition or symptoms.
- Check the expiration dates on medications. Dispose of medications by dropping them off at a *drug take-back location*. Follow the instructions on the label or prescription to dispose of medications at home.
- Store medications carefully in a dry, cool area on high shelves or in locked cabinets where children cannot reach them.
- Do not give OTC medications intended for adults to infants or children.

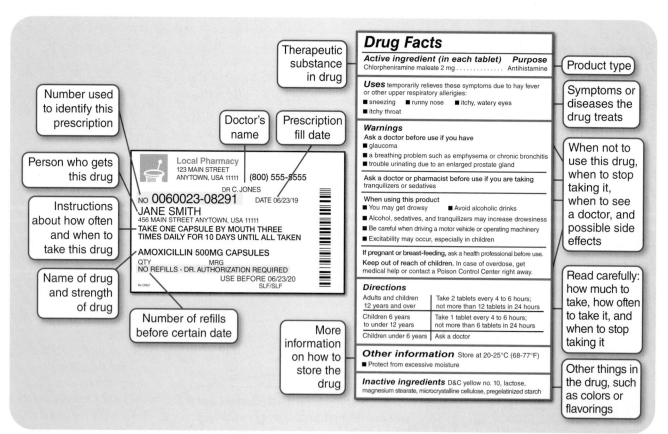

Figure 11.4 Both prescription and OTC labels provide instructions about when to use the drug, when not to use the drug, when to stop taking it, and possible side effects. **Who should you consult if you have any questions about a medicine?**

- Never use a medication prescribed for someone else or let someone else use a medication prescribed for you. Prescriptions are given specifically for one person, based on that person's symptoms, age, weight, and height, and cannot be used safely by anyone else.
- See a healthcare professional if a health condition does not go away after using OTC medication. Also see a healthcare professional if you feel worse after taking a medication or develop symptoms such as a rash, vomiting, or difficulty breathing.

Medication Misuse

Not following a medication's instructions is **medication misuse**. Using medications incorrectly can cause serious health consequences. Misused medications may not be effective. They can increase health risks, such as unpleasant side effects, and may result in serious illness or even death. To avoid medication misuse, follow the directions for taking medications and ask questions if unsure what to do.

Medication Abuse

When you think about hazardous substances, you probably think of illegal drugs and alcohol. The reality is that, after marijuana, prescription and OTC medications are the most commonly abused substances among teens (**Figure 11.5**). **Medication abuse** includes

- using medications for purposes that are not prescribed or stated on the label
- sharing a prescription medication with someone else

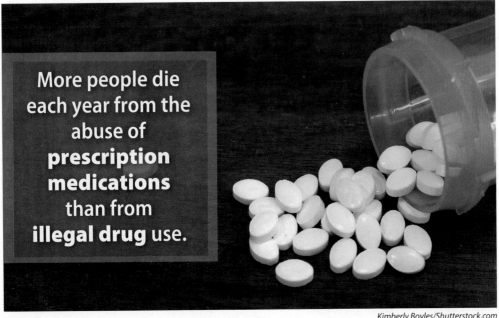

More people die each year from the abuse of **prescription medications** than from **illegal drug** use.

Kimberly Boyles/Shutterstock.com

Figure 11.5
The most commonly abused medications are opioids, depressants, and stimulants. *Why do doctors typically prescribe opioids?*

Drug Facts

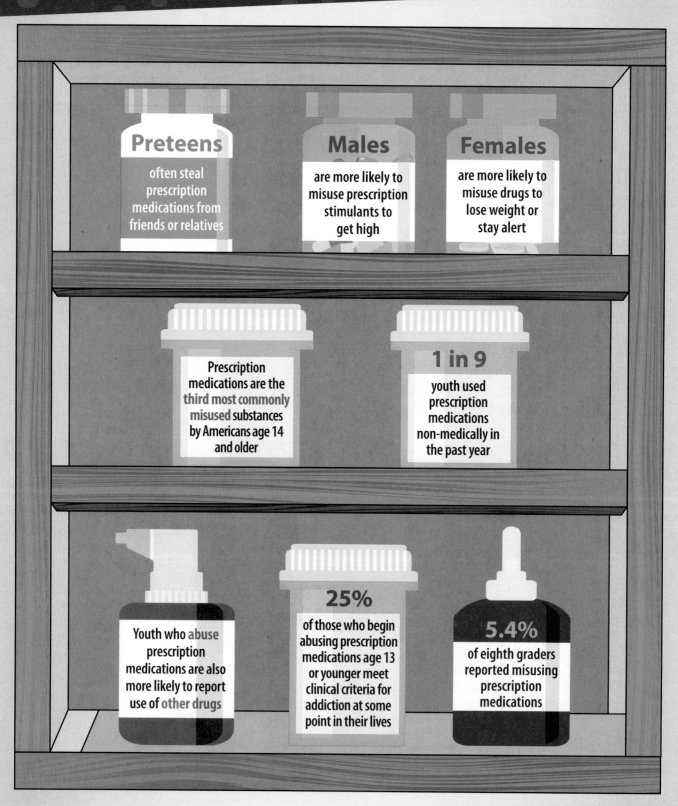

Preteens often steal prescription medications from friends or relatives

Males are more likely to misuse prescription stimulants to get high

Females are more likely to misuse drugs to lose weight or stay alert

Prescription medications are the **third most commonly misused** substances by Americans age 14 and older

1 in 9 youth used prescription medications non-medically in the past year

Youth who **abuse** prescription medications are also more likely to report use of **other drugs**

25% of those who begin abusing prescription medications age 13 or younger meet clinical criteria for addiction at some point in their lives

5.4% of eighth graders reported misusing prescription medications

Bottles top, bottom: Krylovochka/Shutterstock.com; Bottles middle, bottom middle: Neonic Flower/Shutterstock.com

- selling a prescription medication
- taking more than the prescribed or recommended amount of a medication
- combining medications without a doctor's approval

Health Effects of Medication Abuse

Abusing prescription and OTC medications can have serious consequences, including death. Some medications stimulate the brain to release *dopamine*, a chemical that causes pleasant feelings. Some medications, such as prescription opioids, cause a rush of dopamine and endorphins. This rush can lead to an intense high. If someone abuses a medication for this high, the body develops tolerance and then dependence. This can lead to a substance use disorder.

Medication abuse can harm other parts of the body, including the liver. It can also lead to a fatal overdose. An **overdose** occurs when a person consumes more of a medication than the body can handle at one time. An overdose can happen in minutes and lead to death within hours. Overdoses that do not lead to death can cause permanent brain damage and other health complications (**Figure 11.6**).

Medication abuse can lead to many mental changes. People who abuse medications may become agitated, anxious, or depressed and are more likely to attempt suicide. Socially, medication abuse can harm relationships. People who abuse medications may lose the trust of family members and feel like others are disappointed in them. Breaking laws about medication abuse can cause legal consequences or expulsion from school.

Commonly Abused Medications

Commonly abused medications include both prescription and OTC medications. Examples include depressants, opioids, stimulants, diet pills, and performance-enhancing drugs (PEDs).

- **Depressants.** Depressants trigger the brain to release chemicals that slow the nervous system, breathing, and heart rate. This reduces anxiety and helps a person relax, stay calm, or sleep. Abusing depressants can lead to slowed breathing, slurred speech, lack of coordination, and death by overdose if the nervous system slows down too much.
- **Opioids.** Opioids are strong medications that relieve pain and stimulate the brain to release endorphins and dopamine (**Figure 11.7**).

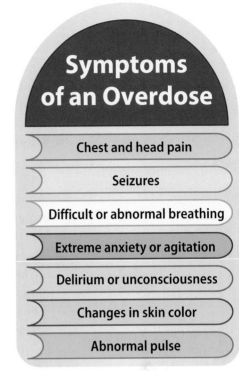

Symptoms of an Overdose

- Chest and head pain
- Seizures
- Difficult or abnormal breathing
- Extreme anxiety or agitation
- Delirium or unconsciousness
- Changes in skin color
- Abnormal pulse

Figure 11.6 Someone who is experiencing an overdose needs immediate medical attention. *What should you do if you think someone has overdosed?*

Examples of Prescription Opioids

Opioid	Description
Codeine	Typically prescribed to treat pain and coughing; abuse can produce a high and lead to tolerance and dependence.
Morphine	Treats severe pain; produces a strong high, which contributes to tolerance and dependence.
Methadone	Treats severe pain, including withdrawal symptoms; used to treat people with addictions to other opioids.
Fentanyl	Treats extreme pain; is 50 to 100 times more powerful than morphine.

Figure 11.7 Some people who abuse opioids get them in these forms from a doctor. Other people buy opioids from criminals who sell them without a prescription.

When a person abuses opioids, the brain stops producing endorphins and dopamine on its own. This causes physical dependence. Opioid abuse can also cause weakness, nausea, and confusion. People who abuse opioids can easily lose consciousness and die from overdose. In recent years, there has been an alarming increase in opioid overdoses in the United States. Opioid overdose has become the 10th leading cause of death, killing more people than suicide. This has been called the *opioid epidemic*.

- **Stimulants.** Stimulants increase energy, alertness, and attention. Abusing stimulants, including OTC stimulants, or stimulant supplements like caffeine, can be dangerous and life threatening. Stimulants can cause physical dependence and lead to cognitive impairment, depression, delusions, hallucinations, paranoia, and other health conditions.
- **Diet pills.** Some people use diet pills in an attempt to lose weight. Using these pills without supervision from a doctor can be extremely dangerous. Abusing diet pills can lead to digestive issues, heart failure, respiratory failure, anxiety and panic attacks, depression, and addiction.
- **Performance-enhancing drugs (PEDs).** Some people use performance-enhancing drugs to improve strength, speed, and stamina. These drugs have many health risks. For example, abusing *anabolic steroids* can lead to permanent disability or infertility, liver disease, aggression, depression and paranoia, and addiction.

Lesson 11.1 Review

1. Substances used to treat symptoms of an illness or to cure, manage, or prevent a disease are called _____.
2. **True or false.** It is safe to take sleep medications and pain relievers together.
3. Unintentionally not following a medication's instructions is medication _____.
4. How does physical dependence develop when people abuse opioids?
5. **Critical thinking.** What factors do you think explain why people abuse medications, despite the negative consequences?

Hands-On Activity

Create a list of risky behaviors related to medication use, misuse, and abuse. Write each risky behavior on a sticky note, and arrange the notes in order from *least* risky to *most* risky. In a small group, compare answers and discuss why you ranked the risky behaviors in a particular order. Based on collaboration with your partner, change your ranking order, if needed, and add to your list of reasons. Lastly, choose one of the behaviors and create an illustrated digital poster to raise awareness about the negative long-term effects of this behavior. Present your digital poster to the class.

Drug Abuse

Learning Outcomes

After studying this lesson, you will be able to

- **explain** the short-term and long-term effects of drugs on the brain and body.
- **identify** mental, social, and legal consequences of drug abuse.
- **describe** the health risks of commonly abused drugs.

Graphic Organizer

Negative Effects of Drugs

As you read this lesson, use a table like the one shown below to list the types of drugs and include a list of negative side effects. Highlight the negative effects the drugs have in common. An example is provided for you.

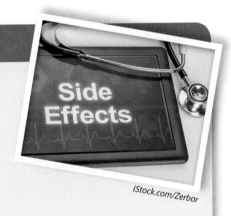

iStock.com/Zerbor

Drug Name	Negative Effects
Inhalants	Slurred speech, memory issues, lack of coordination, muscle spasms and tremors, dizziness, hallucinations

Key Terms

drug abuse use of addictive, illegal drugs

marijuana drug made up of dried parts of the cannabis plant

cocaine drug that usually comes in the form of white powder made from the leaves of the coca plant

methamphetamine stimulant that speeds up brain functions

hallucinogens drugs that alter the way people view, think, and feel about things, causing hallucinations

heroin illegal opioid that has dangerous side effects and is very addictive

fentanyl prescription opioid more powerful than morphine; sometimes cut with heroin

club drugs several different types of drugs that young people may abuse at parties, bars, and concerts

inhalants chemicals that people breathe in to experience some type of high

I n the previous lesson, you learned that *medications* are substances used to treat symptoms of an illness or to cure, manage, or prevent a disease. In this lesson, you will be learning about drugs that are not medications.

Jamal, from the first lesson, does not mess around with illegal drugs. He is even generally pretty careful with the prescription medications he uses. His cousin tried cocaine when he was younger, and Jamal remembers the way the drug took over his cousin's life. She sold all of her things to make money to buy more drugs, and she stopped going to school or hanging out with her friends. Eventually, she got arrested. Jamal never wants that for himself, so he promised that he would never take illegal drugs.

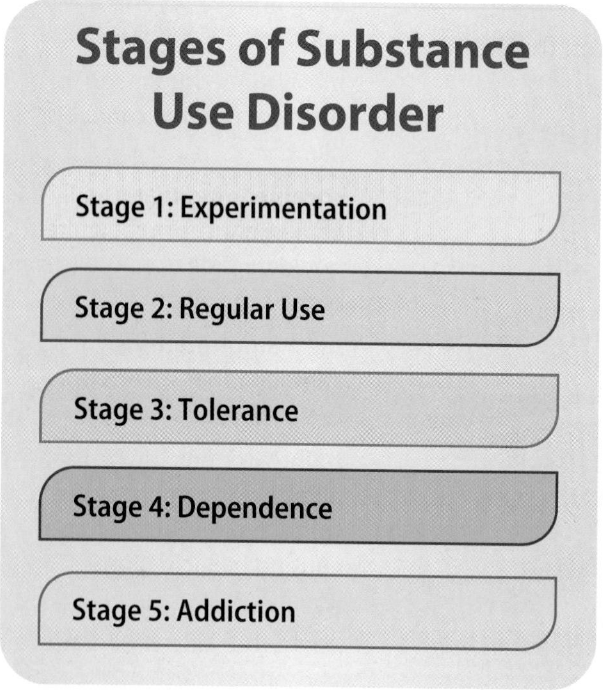

Stages of Substance Use Disorder

Stage 1: Experimentation

Stage 2: Regular Use

Stage 3: Tolerance

Stage 4: Dependence

Stage 5: Addiction

Figure 11.8 Continuing drug abuse can lead to the development of a substance use disorder.

Health Effects of Drug Abuse

As you know, *drugs* are substances that cause physical and psychological changes in the body. These substances are often illegal and can cause serious health consequences.

Drug abuse occurs when a person uses addictive, illegal drugs. People take them to experience a high, fit in with friends, or escape from reality or negative feelings. Drug abuse can lead to *substance use disorders*, which you learned about in Chapter 9 (**Figure 11.8**). The more a person uses a drug, the more the person is at risk of developing a dependence on the drug. A person with a substance use disorder uses a drug despite harmful or negative consequences.

How Drugs Affect the Brain

People often think it is harmless to experiment with drugs, but this is untrue. Experimentation can lead to regular use and addiction.

Many drugs cause a high by triggering the brain to release lots of *dopamine*, a chemical that causes feelings of pleasure. In response, the brain starts producing less dopamine naturally, leading to less motivation and pleasure without the drug. The body develops tolerance and then physical dependence. In this way, using drugs easily leads to addiction and a substance use disorder.

Many illegal drugs interfere with the brain region that regulates self-control. As a result, people who abuse drugs have difficulty thinking. They are more likely to engage in risky behaviors. Drug abuse also impairs a person's ability to drive, causing more accidents.

Other Health Effects

Because many drugs cloud thinking and judgment, people who abuse drugs are more likely to get certain diseases. For example, *human immunodeficiency virus (HIV)* and *hepatitis* can be contracted through needle injection or sexual activity. Over time, hepatitis can cause severe, permanent liver damage. HIV can suppress the immune system to the point of death.

Vaping drugs can lead to lung damage, since e-liquids for vaping devices contain harmful chemicals. You learned about these chemicals in Chapter 9. Drug abuse also causes long-term damage to the body's organs. People who use drugs have a risk of *overdosing*, or taking more of a drug than the body can process. Overdoses can kill someone within hours or minutes.

Mental, Social, and Legal Consequences

Like medication abuse, drug abuse can lead to mental changes. Drug abuse interferes with people's goals and makes people more likely to engage in risky behaviors. Drug abuse also makes mental health conditions and illnesses worse. When people use drugs to handle symptoms of mental illnesses, they

CASE STUDY

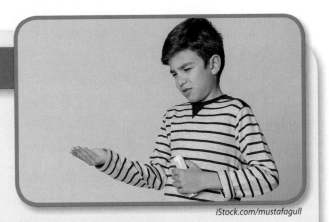

iStock.com/mustafagull

Mateo's Risky Behavior

Mateo did not think it was that big of a deal—just a couple hits of marijuana. He felt so free. All his thoughts and worries disappeared. He laughed with his friends that day, but mostly just chilled. When Mateo returned home, his parents were still yelling at each other, and his responsibilities as a big brother felt overwhelming.

Days passed and Mateo remembered craving the feeling of getting high. Tension continued to escalate in his family, and his grades were dropping. He promised himself that he would never vape marijuana again. Mateo's cousin used to make straight A's in high school and had such a promising future until she started vaping marijuana all of the time. Mateo was not sure why she vaped so much considering she did not have any of the stress he did. Mateo thought to himself, "I have real problems, and it feels like no one sees me or hears my voice."

Mateo resisted for weeks, and then gave in and vaped with a group of friends—once again, feeling free and happy. He vaped about once a week during the school year. His home life never got better, and his grades continued to decline throughout the school year.

Finally, school was out for the summer. Mateo's parents allowed him to attend a graduation party

with a small group of friends. While at the party, one of Mateo's friends pulled out a handful of pills and offered them to the group. No one seemed interested. Neither was Mateo—although he was a little curious. His friend said it was Xanax and that the pill would make him feel relaxed. Mateo had promised himself that he would never move onto another drug.

Thinking Critically

1. How is drug use molding Mateo's future?

2. If you were Mateo's friend, what advice would you give him to cope with his stressful family life? List at least four healthy strategies that Mateo could use to relieve stress and anger.

3. Do you think Mateo will take the Xanax? Why or why not? Defend your answer.

4. Predict whether you think that knowing the consequences will help Mateo to stop using drugs. Defend your answer.

The Consequences of Medication and Drug Abuse

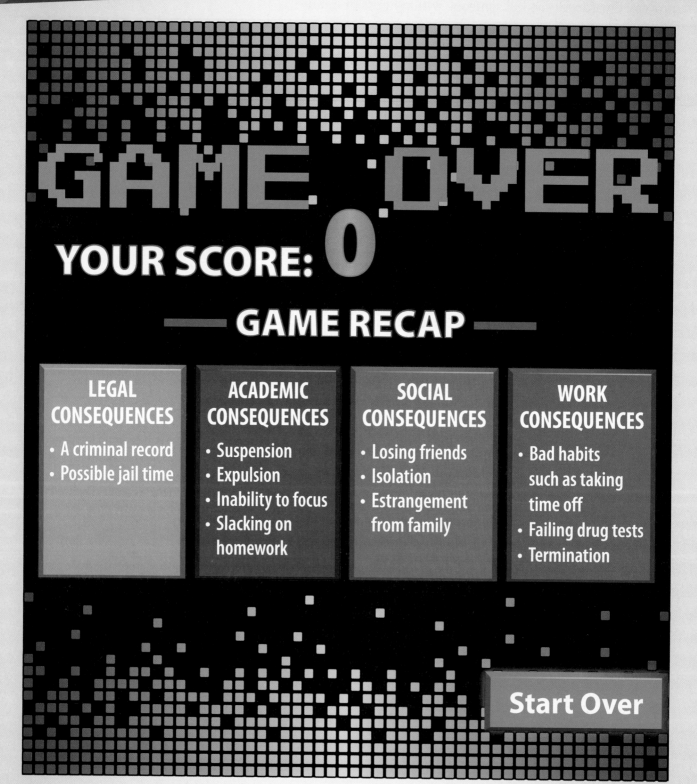

GAME OVER

YOUR SCORE: 0

— GAME RECAP —

LEGAL CONSEQUENCES
- A criminal record
- Possible jail time

ACADEMIC CONSEQUENCES
- Suspension
- Expulsion
- Inability to focus
- Slacking on homework

SOCIAL CONSEQUENCES
- Losing friends
- Isolation
- Estrangement from family

WORK CONSEQUENCES
- Bad habits such as taking time off
- Failing drug tests
- Termination

Start Over

Background: Untashable/Shutterstock.com; Game over: nikiteev_konstantin/Shutterstock.com

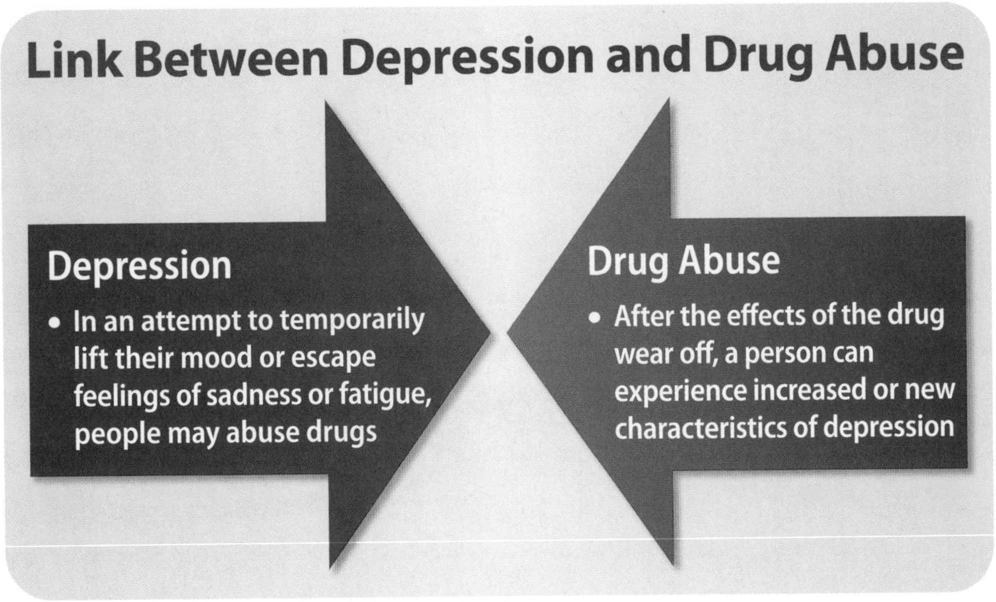

Link Between Depression and Drug Abuse

Depression
- In an attempt to temporarily lift their mood or escape feelings of sadness or fatigue, people may abuse drugs

Drug Abuse
- After the effects of the drug wear off, a person can experience increased or new characteristics of depression

Figure 11.9
People who are depressed may use drugs to treat their mental health condition, but drugs can increase feelings of despair, exhaustion, and sadness. *What is the only way to successfully treat a mental health condition?*

are not treating the real issue. Lack of treatment and the consequences of drug abuse cause more symptoms (**Figure 11.9**).

People who abuse drugs may also experience
- legal consequences, such as getting arrested
- academic trouble, such as being suspended or expelled from school
- work trouble, such as not coming to work, failing drug tests, and getting fired
- financial difficulty
- social consequences, such as losing friends, having conflict with family, or experiencing violence due to criminal activity

The National Institute on Drug Abuse estimates drug abuse costs United States society approximately $700 billion each year. Because of drug abuse, the criminal justice system spends time and resources handling drug-related crimes. Businesses suffer from productivity loss and theft. Unemployment and homelessness are other potential issues that stem from drug abuse.

Commonly Abused Drugs

In the following sections, you will learn about some commonly abused drugs. You will also learn about the harmful effects these drugs can have on all aspects of a person's health.

Marijuana

According to the National Institute on Drug Abuse, marijuana is the most commonly used drug in the United States. **Marijuana** is an addictive drug made up of dried parts of the cannabis plant (**Figure 11.10**). People may smoke or vape marijuana. They may also brew marijuana in tea or consume it as an *edible* (food mixed with marijuana). Taking marijuana in tea or food affects the brain more slowly, which can make someone consume more. Slang terms

Figure 11.10

Parts of the cannabis plant are dried to create the drug marijuana. *What is the name of the mind-altering chemical that is the active ingredient in marijuana?*

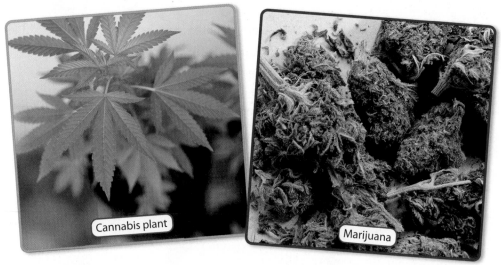

Cannabis plant

Marijuana

Cannabis plant: iStock.com/MStudioImages; Marijuana: Courtesy of the Department of Justice, Drug Enforcement Administration

for marijuana include *weed, pot, dope, hash, herb, Mary Jane,* and *Aunt Mary. Synthetic cannabinoids* (sometimes called *synthetic marijuana*) do not come from cannabis, are manmade, and are even more dangerous than marijuana.

The active ingredient in marijuana is a mind-altering chemical called *THC.* Upon entering the bloodstream, THC travels to the brain and causes a high. THC affects the parts of the brain that control pleasure, memory, thinking, concentration, sensory and time perception, and movement. Another chemical in the marijuana plant is *CBD.* CBD is similar to THC, but does not affect thinking or cause a high.

Marijuana can be manufactured to have up to four times the concentration of THC. This is called *marijuana concentrate,* or *THC extraction.* Slang terms for marijuana concentrate include *wax, honey oil,* and *dabs.* Marijuana concentrate is similar in appearance to honey or butter, and is usually smoked or vaped.

Negative Health Effects

Using marijuana may lead to addiction and a substance use disorder. Marijuana is commonly called a *gateway drug.* This is because people who use it are more likely to abuse other drugs.

People who use marijuana experience negative health effects. These may include poor coordination, difficulty thinking and solving problems, and issues with learning and memory. For this reason, certain tasks, like driving, can be very dangerous while a person is under the influence of marijuana. The effects of marijuana on learning and memory can last for days or weeks after the immediate effects wear off.

Marijuana use can lead to issues with the heart and blood vessels and increase heart rate. A person's risk of a heart attack in the first hour after using marijuana is five times higher than usual.

People who smoke or vape marijuana may experience the same respiratory conditions as people who smoke or vape nicotine. Minor respiratory issues include a daily cough, chest illnesses, and an increased risk of lung infection. Like tobacco smoke, marijuana smoke contains carcinogens, which increase risk for developing cancer.

Legalization of Marijuana

Until recently, marijuana was illegal to sell, buy, and use across the United States. Today, many states and the District of Columbia allow adults with a doctor's prescription to legally buy and use marijuana in that state for medical purposes only. Marijuana can ease the symptoms of various medical conditions, including seizures, muscle spasms, and the nausea caused by chemotherapy treatments for cancer.

Although marijuana is still illegal according to the federal government, in 2014, Colorado became the first state to allow those over age 21 to buy a limited amount of marijuana for nonmedical use. During the 2016 election, California, Nevada, Maine, and Massachusetts also legalized recreational marijuana use and sale. Ten states and the District of Columbia have now legalized marijuana for recreational use for adults over age 21. Several conditions still limit use in these states. Some states regulate how much marijuana people can possess at one time. In some states, using marijuana is legal for residents, but not for nonresidents.

There is much debate about whether marijuana should be legal. Scientists continue to conduct research about medicinal uses for marijuana. The majority of people in the United States who use marijuana do so illegally.

Cocaine

Cocaine is a highly addictive stimulant that comes from the leaves of the coca plant (**Figure 11.11**). People who use cocaine inhale it through the nose, dissolve it in water and inject it, or smoke or vape it. Some people may process this illegal drug into a solid form, known as *crack cocaine*, which they smoke, vape, or inject. Slang terms for cocaine include *blow, bump, coke, crack, flake, candy, rock,* and *snow*.

Cocaine causes a fast, intense high. The high wears off quickly, however, and the user feels nervous and depressed. Cocaine is addictive because its high does not last very long. A person is likely to use cocaine more than once to achieve that intense high again. The more a person uses cocaine, the more dangerous it becomes.

Cocaine can have both short- and long-term negative effects on the body. These effects include high body temperature, increased heart rate, high blood pressure, headaches, organ damage, severe depression, abdominal pain and nausea, paranoia, and loss of sense of smell. Using cocaine just one time can lead to sudden death due to a heart attack or stroke.

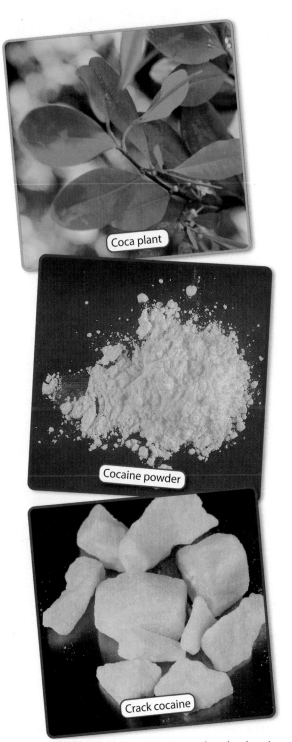

Coca plant

Cocaine powder

Crack cocaine

Coca plant: iStock.com/mtcurado; Cocaine powder and crack cocaine: Courtesy of the Department of Justice, Drug Enforcement Administration

Figure 11.11   The leaves of the coca plant are manufactured into a white powder, called *cocaine*, or into a solid form, which is known as *crack cocaine*.

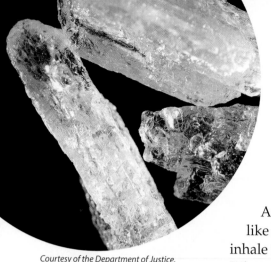

Figure 11.12
The clear crystal chunks of crystal meth is a form of methamphetamine that is very powerful and addictive.

Methamphetamine

Methamphetamine is an extremely addictive stimulant that speeds up brain function. Like cocaine, it causes an intense high. Once the high wears off, a person craves the drug. Some people develop addictions the first time they use this drug. Slang terms for methamphetamine include *meth, ice, crank, crystal,* and *speed.*

Some people take methamphetamine in powder or pill form. A common form of methamphetamine is *crystal meth,* which looks like clear crystal chunks (**Figure 11.12**). People may smoke or vape it, inhale through the nose, inject, or swallow crystal meth.

When people use methamphetamine, they feel energized. They can often engage in continuous activity without stopping for sleep. Users also experience irregular heartbeats, high blood pressure, loss of appetite, sweating, blurred vision, and dizziness. Methamphetamine's short- and long-term health effects include the following:

- violent and unpredictable behavior and mood swings
- difficulty thinking and memory issues
- hallucinations, severe anxiety, and paranoia
- broken or rotten teeth known as *meth mouth* (**Figure 11.13**)

Long-term use of crystal meth can lead to brain damage, malnutrition, tooth decay, skin sores, coma, stroke, and death. Using too much methamphetamine at one time can also result in brain damage, coma, stroke, and death.

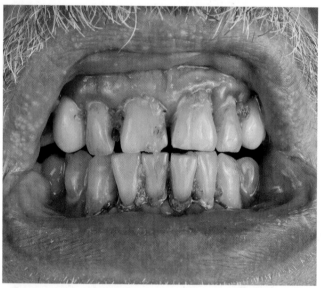

vilax/Shutterstock.com

Figure 11.13 One of the more visible side effects of abusing crystal meth is damaged, blackened teeth. *What is the nickname for this condition?*

Hallucinogens

Hallucinogens are drugs that alter the way people view, think, and feel about situations, thereby causing hallucinations. *Hallucinations* are things that seem real, such as a sound, image, or smell, but do not really exist.

The most common hallucinogen is *LSD,* which is a colorless, odorless substance that is often soaked into pieces of paper. People lick or swallow this paper to take the drug. People may also swallow hallucinogens as pills or tablets.

People who use hallucinogens experience negative short-term health effects. These include trouble sleeping, panic, increased blood pressure and breathing rate, and paranoia. Long-term negative health effects include memory loss, difficulties with speech and thinking, and seizures. People may also experience *flashbacks,* or recurring effects of these drugs. Flashbacks can happen suddenly, without warning, within a few days, or more than a year after using the drugs. In some cases, even a single use of a hallucinogen can lead to death.

Heroin

The drug known as **heroin** comes from *morphine*, a prescription opioid. Slang terms for heroin include *smack*, *horse*, *big H*, *brown sugar*, and *hell dust*.

Pure heroin is a white powder, but people often mix or "cut" it with other substances. Some substances used to cut heroin may be poisonous. People may not know what is in the heroin they use. For example, heroin cut with **fentanyl** (a prescription opioid 50 to 100 times more powerful than morphine) can cause sudden death due to overdose (**Figure 11.14**).

People usually inject, snort, vape, or smoke heroin. Some people mix heroin with crack cocaine, called *speedballing*. By mixing heroin, an opioid, with crack cocaine, a stimulant, people hope to achieve a more intense high and avoid the negative effects. In reality, speedballing is extremely dangerous and often leads to death by overdose.

Once a user takes heroin, the drug rapidly enters the brain. Users feel a sudden, intense "high" that quickly wears off. Many negative short-term health effects soon follow the high. These include dry mouth, flushed skin, difficulty thinking, and semiconsciousness. Heroin is highly addictive. People experience constant cravings for the drug, making it difficult to stop using heroin.

People who have addictions and try to stop using heroin experience severe withdrawal symptoms. These symptoms can begin within a few hours after taking the drug. Symptoms may include vomiting, cold flashes, uncontrollable leg movements, muscle aches, sleep issues, and severe cravings for the drug.

Many long-term negative health effects occur from using heroin (**Figure 11.15**). Death can occur, even after one use, if a person takes too much heroin. This is because heroin is a type of opioid and can slow breathing until it stops. The lack of oxygen to the brain can cause a coma, permanent brain damage, or death.

Long-term effects of heroin use include heart infection, liver and kidney conditions, pneumonia, and depression. HIV or hepatitis may result from using an infected needle.

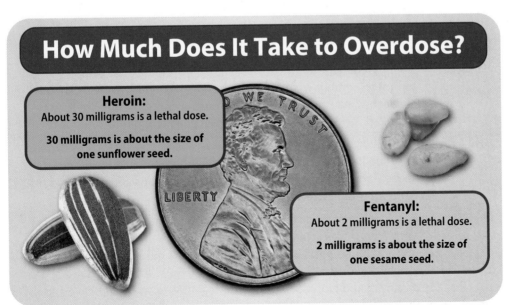

How Much Does It Take to Overdose?

Heroin:
About 30 milligrams is a lethal dose.

30 milligrams is about the size of one sunflower seed.

Fentanyl:
About 2 milligrams is a lethal dose.

2 milligrams is about the size of one sesame seed.

Figure 11.14
Opioids are especially dangerous because it only takes a small amount to be lethal.

Sunflower seeds: EM Arts/Shutterstock.com; Penny: Spiroview Inc/Shutterstock.com; Sesame seeds: schankz/Shutterstock.com

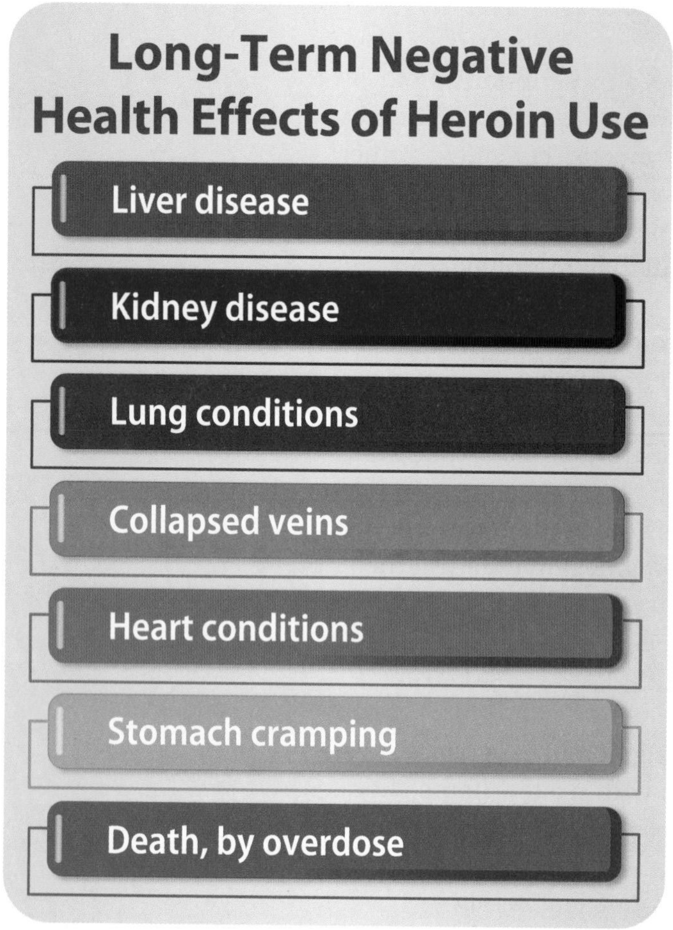

Long-Term Negative Health Effects of Heroin Use

- Liver disease
- Kidney disease
- Lung conditions
- Collapsed veins
- Heart conditions
- Stomach cramping
- Death, by overdose

Figure 11.15 Heroin use can cause negative health effects in many parts of the body, including the heart, lungs, kidneys, and stomach.

Club Drugs

The term **club drugs** refers to several different types of drugs young people may abuse at parties, bars, and concerts. These drugs include Rohypnol® (*roofies*), GHB (gamma hydroxybutyrate), and MDMA (*ecstasy*, or *Molly*). Club drugs often come in capsule, tablet, liquid, or powder form. Some types may also be ground and inhaled or injected into the body.

Club drugs often have no smell or taste. Sometimes, people may slip these drugs into someone else's food or drink without the person knowing. This can lead to highly dangerous situations. For example, these drugs are known as *date rape drugs* because criminals sometimes use them to commit sexual assaults. Club drugs have many short- and long-term health effects (**Figure 11.16**).

Inhalants

Inhalants are chemicals that people breathe in to experience some type of high. Common inhalants are often substances found in the home (**Figure 11.17**). These substances are inhaled into the nose or mouth in several ways. Chemical fumes may be sniffed or snorted from a container, which is called *huffing*. Chemicals can also be sprayed directly into the nose or mouth. Slang terms for inhalants include *whippets*, *poppers*, and *snappers*.

Figure 11.16
Some criminals use club drugs to help them commit sexual assaults. *What is another name for club drugs when this type of dangerous situation occurs?*

Effects of Club Drugs	
Rohypnol	Rohypnol makes people unable to move or respond to events that are happening. After the drug wears off hours later, the person cannot remember what happened. Short-term health effects include headaches, nausea, dizziness, and confusion. Long-term effects may include difficulty breathing and depression. Rohypnol is addictive.
GHB	GHB is a drug that slows the processes in the brain. It causes an intense high and hallucinations. Short-term health effects include dizziness, nausea, and vomiting. The drug may cause unconsciousness. Using GHB can result in death.
MDMA	MDMA is a manmade chemical that is the main ingredient in ecstasy. MDMA increases activity of chemicals in the brain that increase heart rate and blood pressure and affect a person's mood, sleep, and other functions. Short-term side effects include muscle tension, nausea, dizziness, and high body temperature. MDMA can be addictive and may lead to permanent brain damage, organ failure, or death.

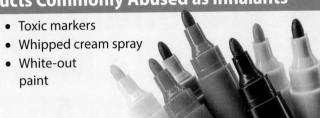

Household Products Commonly Abused as Inhalants

- Air freshener
- Cooking spray
- Gasoline
- Hairspray
- Nail polish remover
- Paint thinner
- Spray deodorant
- Spray paint
- Toxic markers
- Whipped cream spray
- White-out paint

Lunatictm/Shutterstock.com

Figure 11.17
Products commonly found in households can be very dangerous when used for purposes other than their intended uses. *Why do people abuse common household products as inhalants?*

Inhalants cause a high that lasts just a few minutes, so people tend to use them more than once to maintain the feeling. Inhaling chemicals can decrease the body's supply of oxygen. This damages the body's cells, especially brain cells. Other side effects of using inhalants include slurred speech, memory issues, lack of coordination, muscle spasms and tremors, dizziness, and hallucinations.

Inhalant use can also cause serious, permanent side effects. These include hearing loss and damage to the brain, central nervous system, liver, and kidneys. Using inhalants—even once—can cause death due to heart failure or suffocation.

Lesson 11.2 Review

1. _____ is a drug that comes from the cannabis plant, and the drug _____ comes from the coca plant.
2. Which type of drug involves experiencing sounds, images, or smells that do not really exist?
3. Heroin cut with fentanyl can lead to sudden death due to _____.
4. **True or false.** The health outcomes a person will face due to drug abuse are the same for all drugs.
5. **Critical thinking.** Name three types of illegal drugs and explain the negative short- and long-term health effects associated with each.

Hands-On Activity

The decision to use drugs can cost you more than you know—so much more than just money. In small groups, choose one of the drugs described in Lesson 11.2. Research how this drug can negatively affect social, mental and emotional, and physical health, along with the monetary costs of the drug or addiction over time and the legal consequences. Use presentation software to create your group's report. Include pictures that support your findings, and be sure to credit the sources. Present your report to the class. To aid your understanding while you listen to the other presentations, write down the main points you hear. Then write a brief summary of the information from each presentation.

Preventing and Treating Medication and Drug Abuse

Key Terms 📲

rehabilitation program treatment for substance use disorders that may involve detoxification, medications, or time spent in a rehabilitation facility

residential treatment program plan for helping people get through the early stages of breaking an addiction in an inpatient environment with lots of support and few distractions

outpatient treatment program provides drug education or counseling without requiring a hospital stay

medication-assisted treatment (MAT) use of medicinal and behavioral treatment together

relapse occurrence when a person takes a medication or drug again after deciding to stop

skills-training program plan that teaches people skills for dealing with peer pressure and for handling stressful events without relying on medications or drugs

sober living communities alcohol- and drug-free living environments that reduce some of the temptation and pressure people may feel to use alcohol and drugs

Learning Outcomes

After studying this lesson, you will be able to

- **identify** factors that affect why people abuse medications and drugs.
- **explain** strategies for preventing medication and drug abuse.
- **demonstrate** refusal skills to resist peer pressure to abuse medications and drugs.
- **describe** several treatment methods for substance use disorders.
- **explain** how you can help someone with a substance use disorder.

Graphic Organizer

Prevent Drug Addiction

This lesson is about preventing medication and drug abuse. After reading this lesson, write two summary statements for each of the headings found in the graphic below. Team up with a partner and discuss each other's lists.

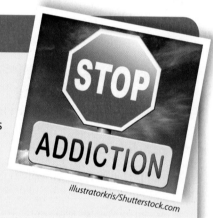

illustratorkris/Shutterstock.com

Why Do Some People Abuse Medications and Drugs?
- •
- •

Preventing Medication and Drug Abuse
- •
- •

Treating Medication and Drug Abuse
- •
- •

Helping Someone with a Substance Use Disorder
- •
- •

n the previous lessons, you learned about the negative health effects associated with medication and drug abuse. Despite the negative effects, some people continue to abuse medications and drugs.

The best way to avoid medication and drug abuse is never to abuse medications or try drugs, like Jamal from the previous lessons. Strategies exist to prevent medication and drug abuse and refuse drugs. In this lesson, you will learn about those prevention strategies. Despite the peer pressure, Jamal is always open and honest with his friends about not wanting to do drugs. Because they are his friends, they respect Jamal's choices and do not bully him.

In this lesson, you will learn how people like Jamal's cousin can get help to treat a substance use disorder. When her family found out about her addiction, they looked into rehabilitation programs for her. You will also learn how you can help and support someone who is trying to stop using or abusing medications and drugs. Jamal and his family only want to show his cousin that they want what is best for her and to support her in her recovery.

Why Do Some People Abuse Medications and Drugs?

Choosing not to abuse medications and drugs can be challenging for young people. This is especially true when their environment exposes them to drugs and the pressures of trying them (**Figure 11.18**). For example, if a young person's family member, friend, or role model abuses medications or drugs, the person may copy that behavior.

Often, young people have an incorrect picture of how medications and drugs will make them feel or affect their lives. For example, young people may believe that drugs will help them think more clearly, become popular, and be better artists or athletes.

During the adolescent years, peers have a strong influence. Young people may feel pressured to abuse medications or drugs if they attend parties where substances are present. They may not want to feel left out, or they may think they will enjoy the party more if they join in. Young people whose friends abuse medications and drugs are more likely to do so themselves.

Some young people may believe that medication and drug abuse can help them feel better. For example, young people who have mental health conditions, such as depression or anxiety, may use drugs to cope with their symptoms. The only way to successfully treat their conditions, however, is to seek professional help.

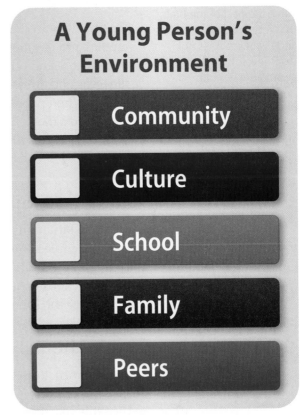

Figure 11.18 The people and communities in a young person's life have the biggest influence on whether or not the person decides to abuse medications or drugs.

It is important to remember that abusing a medication or drug just one time can cause serious health conditions. That single use can also lead to long-term abuse, addiction, and a substance use disorder.

Preventing Medication and Drug Abuse

Medication and drug abuse have serious health consequences and can lead to substance use disorders. Abusing these substances changes brain function, and a young person's brain is still developing (**Figure 11.19**). Preventing early medication and drug abuse can help prevent serious health consequences.

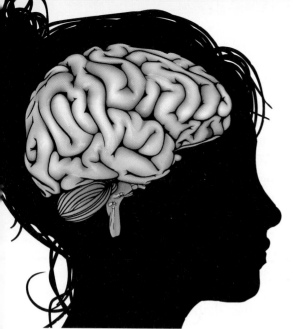

Christos Georghiou/Shutterstock.com

Figure 11.19
Since the part of the brain that regulates emotions and impulses does not stop developing until about age 25, young people are more likely to engage in dangerous, risky behaviors such as abusing medications or drugs.

Promote Mental Health

One way to prevent medication and drug abuse is to care for your mental and emotional health. Poorly managed stress can lead to anxiety, depression, and other health conditions. Mental health conditions and illnesses and stress increase a person's risk for medication and drug abuse. When people abuse medication or drugs to deal with mental health conditions, they only make them worse. When substance use disorders occur together with other mental illnesses, they are called *co-occurring disorders*.

Avoid Risky Situations

Certain situations carry more risk for abusing medications or drugs. For example, people sometimes use drugs at parties. Spending time with someone who abuses medications or drugs can also put you at risk. To avoid these situations, choose not to go to parties where drugs are present. Make friends with people who share your values about avoiding medication and drug abuse.

Think Ahead

Sometimes it can be hard to say *no* when someone offers you drugs. In a surprise situation, you might forget what you want to say. Planning ahead can reduce this risk. Before you get into this situation, plan how you will say *no*. What will you say? What will you do if the person keeps asking you? What will you do to get out of the situation? Talking through this plan with a trusted adult can help.

As you think ahead, consider how you can protect yourself from accidental exposure to medication and drugs. Only accept medications from your parent or guardian, doctor, or pharmacist. At parties, do not let anyone else pour you a drink and do not leave your drink alone. At home, store medications in their original, closed containers and talk with your parent or guardian before taking a medication.

Staying Drug-Free

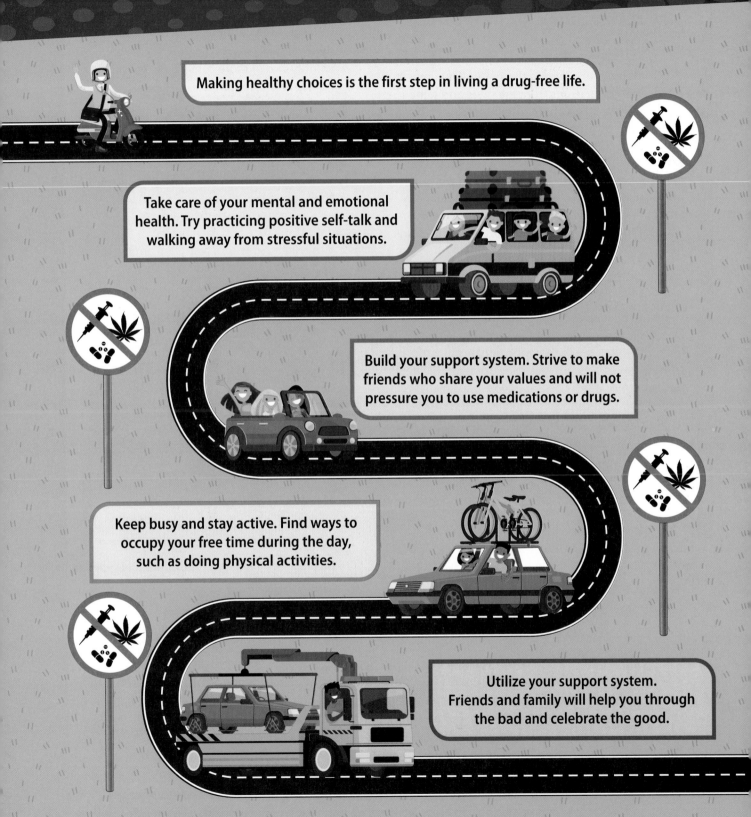

Making healthy choices is the first step in living a drug-free life.

Take care of your mental and emotional health. Try practicing positive self-talk and walking away from stressful situations.

Build your support system. Strive to make friends who share your values and will not pressure you to use medications or drugs.

Keep busy and stay active. Find ways to occupy your free time during the day, such as doing physical activities.

Utilize your support system. Friends and family will help you through the bad and celebrate the good.

Road: Victor Metelskiy/Shutterstock.com; Grass: Mironova Iuliia/Shutterstock.com; Vehicles: tynyuk/Shutterstock.com; Sign: Aleksandar Levai/Shutterstock.com

The Opioid Epidemic: Advocating for a Drug-Free Life

Students often receive their education about medications and drugs from teachers and family. Your ability to advocate for the benefits of a drug-free life can positively influence your peers and others. In fact, your peers may be more likely to listen to you than to some adults. The power of positive peer pressure and peer education can make such a difference in the decision making of young people. This activity requires you to take a leadership role to educate and advocate for drug-free youth.

Educating Your Peers

Be an advocate for a healthy, drug-free life by creating an opioid-awareness presentation to educate your peers about the negative consequences of abusing opioids. To begin, divide into groups of three. Then, assign responsibilities to each group member for creating your presentation. Refer back to the chapter and do additional research as needed. Your presentation should do the following:

- include current statistics about the opioid epidemic (opioid abuse and deaths due to overdose)
- give examples of opioids
- identify three or more harmful short-term and three or more harmful long-term effects of opioid abuse
- identify two or more convincing ways to refuse opioid abuse
- express at least three ways to get "high on life" without abusing medications or drugs
- summarize at least two benefits of remaining drug-free
- share personal short- and long-term goals for choosing to be drug-free

After your group finishes creating the presentation, practice and then present it to the class. With teacher and administration approval, deliver your presentation to another classroom of peers.

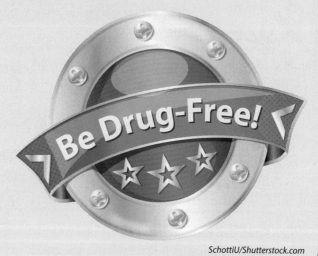

SchottiU/Shutterstock.com

Using Refusal Skills

As you learned in Chapter 9, refusal skills are strategies you can use to stand up to pressures and influences that want you to engage in unhealthy behaviors. Knowing how to respond and what to say if someone offers you medications or drugs can help you avoid them (**Figure 11.20**). For example, one good strategy for refusing drugs is to be direct and say in a firm, but polite way, "No thanks, I don't use drugs." Another strategy is to provide an excuse, such as "I don't want to try drugs because my parents will ground me if I do."

If you continue to feel pressure to use drugs, you might ask the person pressuring you to stop. Remember that real friends respect each other's choices. Let the person know that you need friends who will respect your decision.

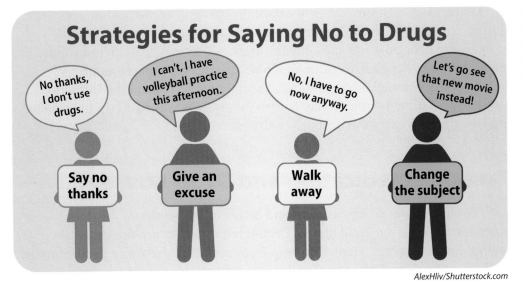

Strategies for Saying No to Drugs

AlexHliv/Shutterstock.com

If the person refuses to accept this, you may need to stop spending time with that person.

You may feel pressured to use drugs because it seems like everyone is doing it, but this is not true. Many young people have never tried drugs and have committed to living a drug-free lifestyle. A good rule is to make friends with people who share your values. You may want to make new friends by getting involved in activities that promote health and wellness.

Educate and Advocate

Unfortunately, many young people do not understand how quickly abuse can lead to addiction. Educating young people about health hazards can help prevent medication and drug abuse.

Schools play a role in preventing medication and drug abuse. Many schools have substance-abuse prevention programs to help educate students. Studies show that medication and drug abuse are less common among students who participate in these programs. Substance-abuse prevention programs explain the short- and long-term effects of medication and drug abuse. In addition, school policies and regulations exist to eliminate drug use on school property.

Certain government groups and programs increase public awareness about medication and drug abuse. For example, the CDC and the National Institute on Drug Abuse (NIDA) create public service announcements (PSAs) for TV, radio, and the Internet. A *public service announcement (PSA)* is a media message to support public health. You may have seen some PSA videos on TV, in movie previews, or on the Internet.

The *AWARxE Prescription Drug Safety Program* spreads awareness about prescription medication abuse. The program teaches people valuable skills, such as how to use, store, and dispose of medications safely (**Figure 11.21**).

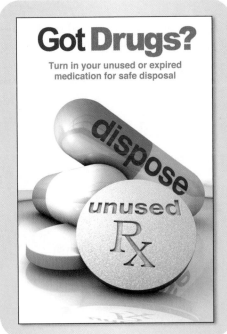

Courtesy of the Department of Justice, Drug Enforcement Administration

Figure 11.21
In addition to the AWARxE program, many community resources help prevent medication misuse by collecting and safely disposing of unused or expired medications.

Media campaigns are also important for preventing medication and drug abuse. The "Above the Influence" campaign seeks to help young people stand up to peer pressure and other influences that may lead them to abuse medications or drugs. This campaign reaches young people through TV commercials, Internet advertising, and social media. "Above the Influence" encourages young people to stay true to themselves and stand up to those who may want them to try medications or drugs.

Treating Medication and Drug Abuse

People who abuse medications and drugs often develop a substance use disorder, which is a mental illness. People with a substance use disorder cannot fix themselves. They need help from family, friends, and professionals, such as counselors. Even after breaking an addiction, many people struggle to manage their addiction throughout their lives.

Often, the first step in treating a substance use disorder is getting help from a **rehabilitation program**. In these programs, healthcare professionals begin treatment by overseeing the process of *detoxification* (which clears all medications or drugs from a person's body). Programs may be residential or outpatient (**Figure 11.22**). In **residential treatment programs**, people get through the early stages of breaking an addiction in an inpatient environment with lots of support and few distractions. An **outpatient treatment program** may provide education or counseling without requiring a hospital stay.

Professionals typically use medicinal and behavioral treatment for substance use disorders. *Medicinal treatment* may include medications that help lessen withdrawal symptoms. *Behavioral treatment* focuses on teaching people how to handle cravings. When these strategies are used together, they are called **medication-assisted treatment (MAT)**.

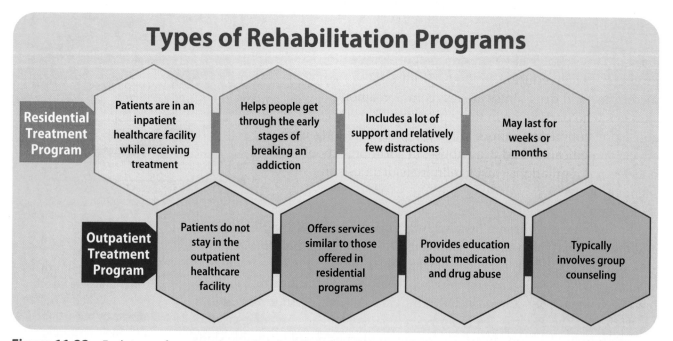

Types of Rehabilitation Programs

Residential Treatment Program
- Patients are in an inpatient healthcare facility while receiving treatment
- Helps people get through the early stages of breaking an addiction
- Includes a lot of support and relatively few distractions
- May last for weeks or months

Outpatient Treatment Program
- Patients do not stay in the outpatient healthcare facility
- Offers services similar to those offered in residential programs
- Provides education about medication and drug abuse
- Typically involves group counseling

Figure 11.22 Each type of program has a slightly different approach to helping a person overcome a substance use disorder. *What term describes when a person takes a drug again after deciding to stop?*

A **relapse** occurs when a person takes a medication or drug again after stopping. It is important to have a good support system, as well as professional help, if a relapse occurs. People who are recovering from substance use disorders can take advantage of the following programs to avoid relapse and move on:

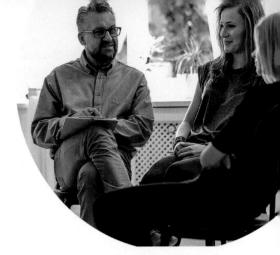

- **Skills-training programs.** **Skills-training programs** help people recognize and avoid situations that lead them to abuse medications or drugs. People learn positive ways of dealing with peer pressure and handling stressful events without relying on medications or drugs.
- **Support groups.** People with a substance use disorder come together and discuss the challenges they face (**Figure 11.23**). Sharing struggles with people who understand can help those with substance use disorders. Narcotics Anonymous is an example of a support group for drug abuse.
- **Sober living communities.** **Sober living communities** are alcohol- and drug-free living environments for people who are trying to stay away from substance use. These environments reduce some of the temptation and pressure to use alcohol and drugs and provide social support.

Photographee.eu/Shutterstock.com

Figure 11.23
Sometimes, people come together in a group to overcome a challenge together, sharing advice and emotional support. *What is an example of a drug abuse support group?*

The Substance Abuse and Mental Health Services Administration (SAMHSA) provides a locator tool people can use to find treatment options. It may also be helpful to talk to a trusted adult, such as a parent or guardian, doctor, school counselor, or school nurse.

Helping Someone with a Substance Use Disorder

Addiction is a serious and sometimes scary situation. If you want to help someone you know who has a substance use disorder, you should first get support for yourself. Talk to a parent or guardian, doctor, school counselor, or school nurse. These trusted adults can often provide advice and guidance for helping someone who has an addiction.

How do you know if someone is abusing medications or drugs? Possible warning signs are shown in **Figure 11.24**.

If you know that your friend is addicted to drugs, express your concern. People with an addiction can often feel alone and isolated. Tell your friend that you care, and that you will be available to help. Knowing that you care and are concerned can help the person understand the seriousness of the issue. Offer to help the person find someone to talk to about the

Warning Signs That Someone May Be Abusing Medications or Drugs

- Loss of interest in school
- Change in mood or personality
- Trouble concentrating in class
- Change in sleeping habits
- Change in eating habits
- Hanging out with a new group of friends who abuse medications or drugs
- Stealing money or selling belongings to get money for medications or drugs

Figure 11.24 Being alert to the warning signs of potential medication and drug abuse can increase the chances that you can help a friend or loved one with a substance abuse disorder.

addiction. A person must want to break the addiction. You may need to wait for your friend to admit that an issue exists.

Once a friend has decided to stop abusing medications or drugs, you can support your friend in various ways. You can offer to go with your friend to a meeting with a counselor. Offer your friend encouragement and praise for staying drug-free. Your friend may want to avoid parties where drugs are present. To support your friend, you can avoid those parties and spend time together. In addition, you may want to attend a support group for relatives and friends of someone with a substance use disorder. This can help you get the support you need.

If you notice your friend starting to relapse, talk to a trusted adult. This does not mean you are a tattletale or a snitch. Instead, this means you are concerned about your friend and want the person to get help.

Lesson 11.3 Review

1. Why are young people more vulnerable to changed brain function due to medication and drug abuse?

2. **True or false.** Most young people have tried or would like to try drugs.

3. When a person takes a medication or drug again after deciding to stop, it is called a(n) _____.

4. Which type of program helps people recognize and avoid situations that lead them to use drugs?

5. **Critical thinking.** What can you do to help someone who has a substance use disorder? Explain actions you can take before the person gets help, once the person decides to get help, and if you notice a relapse.

Hands-On Activity

Standing up to peer pressure can be very difficult. Practicing what you will say in difficult situations can help. Imagine that you are at a party and someone is pressuring you to take a drug. You are immediately uncomfortable and want to say *no*. With a partner, practice your refusal responses to the following pressure lines using the skills you have learned:

| Take the pill. My mom takes them for her back pain and she is fine. | Everybody vapes. One hit of marijuana is not a big deal. | If you want to hang out with us, you have to smoke this. | Pop this Molly and you will feel so good. |

Once you and your partner are confident with your responses, choose one or two to role-play for the class. Listen to your partner's intonation and sound patterns to know when and how to respond. What suggestions does the class have for making your refusals stronger?

Review and Assessment

Summary

Lesson 11.1 Medication Use and Abuse

- *Medications* are substances used to treat symptoms of an illness or to cure, manage, or prevent a disease. *Drugs* are medications and other substances that change the way the body or brain functions. Medications can be prescription medication or over-the-counter (OTC) medication.
- Medications can cause side effects. Some medications can also cause health risks by interacting with other drugs, dietary supplements, foods, or drinks. Some people are allergic to certain medications and develop tolerance.
- Carefully reading and following usage instructions can ensure that people are taking medications correctly. *Medication misuse* involves taking medication in a way that does not follow the instructions, which can be on accident. *Medication abuse* is purposely taking a medication in a way other than its intended use. Depressants, opioids, stimulants, diet pills, and performance-enhancing drugs are commonly abused.

Lesson 11.2 Drug Abuse

- Drug abuse is the use of addictive, illegal drugs. Drugs impact the brain and can lead to a substance use disorder. They cause long-term damage to the body and also have severe mental, social, and legal consequences.
- Examples of commonly abused drugs include marijuana, cocaine, methamphetamine, hallucinogens, heroin, club drugs, and inhalants.

Lesson 11.3 Preventing and Treating Medication and Drug Abuse

- To prevent medication and drug abuse, you can practice positive alternatives by taking care of your mental health. You can avoid risky situations and plan ahead.
- Refuse drugs by saying "no" in a direct and firm, but polite, way. Real friends will respect your choices and will not pressure you to do something you do not want to do.
- School and government programs increase awareness about the health effects of medication and drug abuse. PSAs help teach young people to stand up to peer pressure.
- Treatment for a substance use disorder usually involves medicinal treatment and behavioral treatment. Using these two methods together is called *medication-assisted treatment (MAT)*.
- Treatment usually begins with a rehabilitation program, which may be residential or outpatient. Programs that support recovery include skills-training programs, support groups, and sober living communities.
- If you know a person who has a substance use disorder, express your concern and offer to find help. Wait for your friend to admit an issue exists. Support your friend through treatment. If you notice a relapse, talk to a trusted adult.

Check Your Knowledge

Record your answers to each of the following questions on a separate sheet of paper.

1. **True or false.** All drugs are medications, but *not* all medications are drugs.
2. Which type of medications can be purchased without a doctor's order?
3. In a drug _____, the body responds to a certain medication as if it is harmful.
4. What are the health risks of abusing diet pills?
5. Which of the following is a potential health effect of marijuana use?
   - **A.** Improved memory.
   - **B.** Anxiety and panic attacks.
   - **C.** Improved coordination.
   - **D.** Clear problem solving.
6. What is involved in the condition "meth mouth" from the use of meth?
7. **True or false.** Heroin is often cut with other dangerous substances.
8. How does positive mental health protect against medication and drug abuse?
9. What is the name for a media message that supports public health, such as an anti-drug commercial?
10. What are the two types of treatment for drug addiction?
11. **True or false.** In a residential treatment program, a person will stay at a healthcare or rehabilitation facility while receiving treatment.
12. Which of the following is a sign of medication and drug abuse?
    - **A.** Regular sleeping habits.
    - **B.** Changing eating habits.
    - **C.** Interest in school.
    - **D.** Steady personality.

Use Your Vocabulary 📇

club drugs	medication misuse	prescription medications
cocaine	medication-assisted treatment (MAT)	rehabilitation program
dopamine		relapse
drug abuse	medications	residential treatment program
drugs	methamphetamine	
fentanyl	outpatient treatment program	side effect
hallucinogens		skills-training program
heroin	overdose	sober living communities
inhalants	over-the-counter (OTC) medications	
marijuana		
medication abuse		

13. The spelling of English words often follows set rules or patterns. Applying these rules will result in words spelled correctly. Write a paragraph about medication and drugs. Make an effort to spell each word correctly.
14. Choose one of the terms on the list above. Then, use the Internet to locate photos that visually show the meaning of the term you chose. Share the photo and meaning of the term in class. Ask for clarification if necessary.

Think Critically

15. **Identify.** Marijuana and OTC and prescription medications are widely abused among teens. Identify reasons the use of these substances is so popular.

16. **Draw conclusions.** What are reasons some teens choose to abstain from drug use while others choose to use drugs?

17. **Analyze.** What do you think causes some people to develop an addiction while others use, but are able to quit?

18. **Make inferences.** Since some drugs are illegal, should schools allow random drug testing among students with legal consequences for positive results? Defend your answer.

DEVELOP Your Skills

19. **Decision-making skills.** Imagine it is Friday night, and you are home with your family watching a movie. Several of your friends are at a party, and one of your friends posts a picture on soical media with the following caption:

    "Come over! No adults are here, just us and some high school kids. Everyone brought pills and alcohol. I even took a Xanax and drank a little."

    You are immediately concerned about her safety. What should you do? Write a paragraph describing how you would respond to this situation.

20. **Communication skills.** Imagine that you attend a "punch-bowl party" where kids are taking pills from a large bowl and ingesting them. The pills are multicolored without any identifying marks. You have no idea what kind of pills are in the bowl. Your best friend tells you that she is going to close her eyes, select two, and swallow them. How would you respond to convince her not to do it? Write your response in essay form. Then, share and discuss your responses with the rest of the class.

21. **Advocacy, access information, and technology skills.** In groups of three, review Lesson 11.3 and do additional research on ways to help a friend who is using or addicted to drugs. Then, create a public-service announcement (PSA). Use school-approved video creation software to create a video highlighting at least six ways to help and be a supportive friend. In addition, include information on local resources available in your community, and add pictures or video footage that support the content in your video PSA. Share your video in class or post it to the class website for peer and teacher review.

22. **Access information and technology skills.** Some people have to take medicine weekly, daily, or even several times throughout the day. Research what kinds of apps are available for people who take medications. These apps can help people take medication correctly and decrease the risk of abuse. Choose one and create a presentation about your app highlighting three appealing features and two benefits to using the app. Present it to the class.

Unit 5

Protecting Your Physical Health and Safety

Warm-Up Activity

Reducing Risks

As you grow up, you will become more and more responsible for managing your health, safety, and environment. Part of managing these factors is identifying and reducing *risks*, or potential threats. For example, during the winter season, your classmates may catch the flu. When you hang out with friends at the mall, a stranger may make you uncomfortable. You may cough when there is smog in the air. In all of these situations, you can take certain actions to reduce your risks.

The pictures below illustrate situations that have different risks. Look at these pictures and work with a partner to list actions you could take to reduce the risks present. Write these actions on a separate piece of paper. After reading this unit, revisit your list and add or change actions based on what you learned.

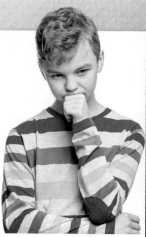

VaLiza/Shutterstock.com

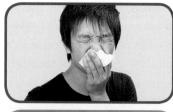
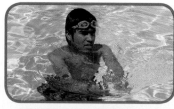
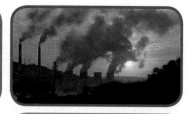
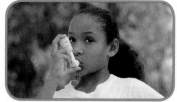
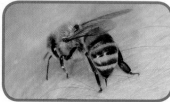
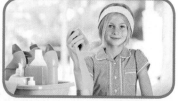

Left to right: leungchopan/Shutterstock.com; juan carlos tinjaca/Shutterstock.com; Tatiana Grozetskaya/Shutterstock.com; sirtravelalot/Shutterstock.com; Mirko Graul/Shutterstock.com; Africa Studios/Shutterstock.com

Chapter

12

Understanding and Preventing Diseases

Essential Question

What causes communicable and noncommunicable diseases, and how can you prevent them?

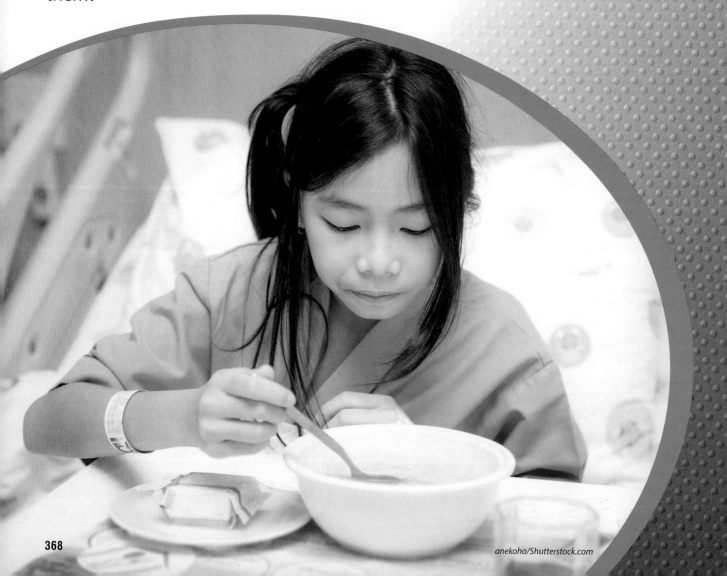

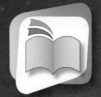

Reading Activity

Skim through this chapter from top to bottom and from left to right and list all of the headings you see. Note key terms with which you are unfamiliar and scan through the chapter to find their definitions. After reading, write a "topic sentence" and brief summary for each heading. After you read this chapter, write a new topic sentence and summary for each section, outlining the main points you learned and using the key terms you have defined.

How Healthy Are You?

In this chapter, you will be learning about diseases and how to prevent them. Before you begin reading, take the following quiz to assess your current disease prevention habits.

Healthy Choices	Yes	No
Do you take medications prescribed to treat diseases exactly as ordered by your doctor?		
Do you regularly wash your hands with soap and water?		
Do you practice respiratory etiquette, including covering your mouth and nose with a tissue or your sleeve when coughing or sneezing?		
Do you avoid going to school sick?		
Do you make sure that any meat you eat has been cooked thoroughly?		
Do you wash fruits and vegetables before eating, peeling, or cutting open?		
Do you receive the recommended vaccines, including an annual flu vaccine?		
Do you know your family's history of noncommunicable diseases?		
Do you eat a healthy diet, engage in regular physical activity, and avoid tobacco and alcohol to prevent heart disease?		
Do you know the modifiable risk factors for different types of common cancers?		
Do you get regular screenings and physical examinations to increase the possibility of treating diseases in their early stages?		

Count your "Yes" and "No" responses. The more "Yes" responses you have, the more healthy disease prevention habits you exhibit. Now, take a closer look at the questions with which you responded "No." How can you make these healthy habits part of your daily life? Identify a SMART goal you would like to achieve to help improve your overall health and well-being. Refer to Figure 1.11 to help you set up your SMART goal. If you do not understand the instructions, ask for clarification from your teacher.

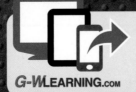

Click on the activity icon or visit www.g-wlearning.com/health to access online vocabulary activities using key terms from the chapter.

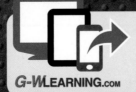G-WLEARNING.com

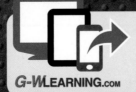

Communicable Diseases

communicable disease condition someone can develop after coming into contact with living things or objects infected with the disease; also called *infectious disease*

pathogens microorganisms that cause communicable diseases

method of transmission way a disease gets from one organism or object to another; may be direct or indirect

influenza viral infection of the respiratory system; also known as *the flu*

mononucleosis common viral infection that spreads through kissing or by sharing certain objects; also known as *mono* and *the kissing disease*

tonsillitis bacterial or viral infection that affects the tonsils

conjunctivitis viral or bacterial infection that causes inflammation of part of the eye; also known as *pinkeye*

antibiotics substances that target and kill pathogenic bacteria

Learning Outcomes

After studying this lesson, you will be able to

- **understand** the nature of communicable diseases.
- **explain** the types of pathogens that can make you sick.
- **describe** the different methods of disease transmission.
- **understand** common communicable diseases.
- **describe** treatment methods for communicable diseases.

Graphic Organizer

Understanding Communicable Diseases

Create a graphic organizer like the one shown to increase your knowledge and awareness about pathogens that cause communicable diseases. As you read this lesson, list three key points about each type of pathogen identified in the organizer. Then, list a disease that each may cause.

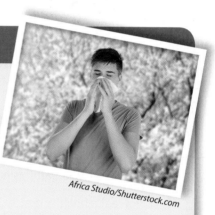

Africa Studio/Shutterstock.com

Bacteria
1.
2.
3.

Viruses
1.
2.
3.

Fungi
1.
2.
3.

Protozoa
1.
2.
3.

The term *communicable* means "able to be transmitted." If a disease is *communicable*, that means it can be transmitted to you. In other words, a **communicable disease** (also called an *infectious disease*) is a condition you can develop after coming into contact with living things or objects infected with the disease.

Twelve-year-old Dakota knows that communicable diseases such as the flu are different from diseases such as heart disease that he might inherit from his parents or grandparents. A communicable disease is one that he can "catch." When his friend Tavon came to school with the flu last month, for example, Dakota ended up sick, too. Dakota cannot, however, catch heart disease.

In this lesson, you will learn about the causes of communicable diseases. You will also learn about common communicable diseases that you may encounter in your life. Finally, you will learn possible treatment methods for communicable diseases.

Understanding Communicable Disease

Common living things that you can see are called *organisms*. You, your teacher, your dog, and the trees outside are all examples of organisms. Many living things, however, are too small to see with the naked eye. These *microorganisms* are so small that you cannot even see them without the use of a microscope. Certain microorganisms, known as **pathogens**, can cause communicable diseases (**Figure 12.1**). The term *pathogen* is a more scientific way of describing *germs*.

Pathogens are everywhere. They are so small, however, that you cannot see them. Pathogens are only visible with a microscope, which magnifies them, or creates a bigger image of them. These microscopic organisms influence human lives in many ways. Pathogens include bacteria, viruses, fungi, and protozoa.

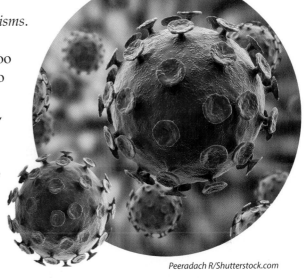

Peeradach R/Shutterstock.com

Figure 12.1
Pictured here is an example of a pathogen. Pathogens are disease-causing microorganisms. Specific pathogens cause different communicable diseases. ***Can you see microorganisms with the naked eye? Why or why not?***

Bacteria

Bacteria are single-celled organisms that live in almost every place where life can thrive. Bacteria even live inside the human body. In fact, so many bacteria live in the body that, of the several trillions of cells that make up your body, 90 percent are bacterial cells.

You may find it scary that bacteria are nearly everywhere. The good news is that most bacteria are helpful. For example, the bacteria found in your body help the digestive system function efficiently. These bacteria also prevent harmful bacteria from thriving in your body. The bad news is that certain varieties of bacteria can cause different kinds of illnesses. Some of these illnesses may be minor, while others can be quite serious and even deadly.

One type of bacteria that can cause disease is *E. coli*. *E. coli* bacteria typically live in healthy people's and animals' intestines. There are different varieties of *E. coli* bacteria, however. Some varieties are harmless, while others can cause food poisoning. Exposure to harmful *E. coli* bacteria can occur from eating

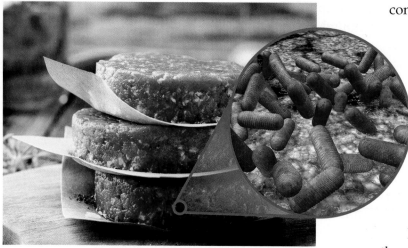

Beef: istetiana/Shutterstock.com; E.coli: bluecrayola/Shutterstock.com

Figure 12.2 Undercooked ground beef can contain *E. coli*. If consumed, *E. coli* can cause food poisoning.

contaminated food, such as undercooked ground beef, or drinking contaminated water (**Figure 12.2**). If you get sick from food poisoning, you may develop symptoms such as diarrhea, nausea, fever, and vomiting.

Another common type of bacteria, *S. aureus*, is present in about 30 percent of people's nasal passages. The bacteria *S. aureus* often does not cause any harm. It can, however, spread to others through contact with contaminated hands. Sometimes, *S. aureus* causes *staph infections* (skin and soft tissue infections). Anyone can get a staph infection, especially if you have a cut or scratch. People with chronic diseases and weakened immune systems are at greater risk of developing a more serious staph infection.

Viruses

Viruses are very different from bacteria or cells in your body. Viruses are much smaller than bacteria, and they are completely incapable of doing anything cells can do on their own. Viruses depend entirely on other cells for reproduction and growth. In fact, every virus must live inside a cell and use that cell's resources and energy to grow and reproduce.

Viruses must be inside another living organism to thrive. Though viruses can stay on surfaces for a short time, they will die quickly if they do not find an organism in which to live. Once inside the body, a virus invades a person's cells and multiplies quickly. The result of a virus multiplying is an illness (**Figure 12.3**).

Fungi

Fungi (singular—*fungus*) are multicelled, plant-like microorganisms that thrive in damp, warm places. These microorganisms are much more complex than bacteria and viruses. Examples of fungi include mushrooms, molds, and yeast. A fungus cannot produce its own food, so it receives nourishment from plants, foods, and animals.

Like bacteria, few fungi cause disease, and many are beneficial. For example, the mold known as *Penicillium notatum* makes the life-saving drug penicillin,

Figure 12.3
Some common viral illnesses are influenza, the common cold, measles, chicken pox, West Nile virus, and mumps.

Common Illnesses Caused by Viruses

Influenza (the flu)	Common cold	Measles	Chicken pox	West Nile virus	Mumps

an antibiotic that controls bacterial infections. Other fungi, however, damage crops and stored foods. A few fungi cause infections, or *mycoses*, in humans. Ringworm, athlete's foot, and jock itch are common fungal infections. People with weakened immune systems may be more likely to contract a fungal infection.

Protozoa

Protozoa are single-celled organisms that live nearly everywhere, and only a few cause diseases. Many kinds of protozoa form the basis of food chains, providing nutrients for other organisms. Certain protozoa, however, cause some of the world's most feared diseases. These include *malaria*, a dangerous flu-like illness, and *dysentery*, a severe intestinal infection. Protozoa thrive in moist environments, and typically spread through contaminated water.

Common Communicable Diseases

For a disease to be *communicable*, it must be able to transmit from one source to another. Pathogens causing communicable diseases may travel by various methods of transmission (**Figure 12.4**). A **method of transmission** is simply the way a disease gets from one organism or object to another. Methods of transmission are either direct or indirect, depending on how the transmission occurs.

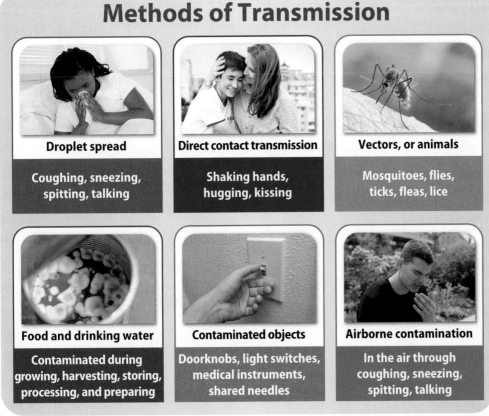

Methods of Transmission

Droplet spread	**Direct contact transmission**	**Vectors, or animals**
Coughing, sneezing, spitting, talking	Shaking hands, hugging, kissing	Mosquitoes, flies, ticks, fleas, lice
Food and drinking water	**Contaminated objects**	**Airborne contamination**
Contaminated during growing, harvesting, storing, processing, and preparing	Doorknobs, light switches, medical instruments, shared needles	In the air through coughing, sneezing, spitting, talking

Figure 12.4
Communicable diseases are spread among people, animals, and objects. Different diseases spread through different methods of transmission. For example, the common cold is transmitted through droplet spread and direct contact. West Nile virus is usually transmitted through mosquitoes acting as vectors. *Which method of transmission involves medical instruments and shared needles?*

Left to right: Andrey_Popov/Shutterstock.com; Olesya Kuznetsova/Shutterstock.com; frank60/Shutterstock.com; Jana Behr/Shutterstock.com; Alexey Rotanov/Shutterstock.com; Michael Moloney/Shutterstock.com

Direct transmission is the movement of a pathogen from a person with a communicable disease to a susceptible person. A person who is *susceptible* to a disease is likely to be easily affected or harmed by it. A person who has a weak immune system may be more susceptible to a disease than someone with a healthy immune system. *Indirect transmission* is the movement of a pathogen to a susceptible person through a source that acts only as a disease carrier. In this case, the carrier is simply moving a pathogen from one source to another.

There are many examples of communicable diseases. You will likely encounter one or more communicable disease during your life. Some common communicable diseases include influenza, mononucleosis, tonsillitis, and conjunctivitis.

Influenza

Influenza, also known as *the flu*, is a viral infection of the respiratory system. This means the virus infects the nose and lungs. It also causes other symptoms throughout the body. The flu moves from person to person through droplet spread, and sometimes through contact with an object touched by someone with the flu. **Figure 12.5** shows common flu symptoms. The best treatment for the flu is to get lots of rest, drink plenty of liquids, and see a doctor, if needed.

Mononucleosis

Mononucleosis, also called *mono*, is a very common viral infection. This infection is often known as *the kissing disease* because it typically spreads through direct contact such as kissing. Mononucleosis may also spread when people share objects such as cups, toothbrushes, and lip gloss.

Symptoms of mononucleosis include fatigue, fever, sore throat, loss of appetite, and sore muscles. Some people experience mild symptoms.

Figure 12.5
Common symptoms of the flu are headache, fever, stuffy nose, sore throat, muscle aches, and dry cough. *How does the flu move from person to person?*

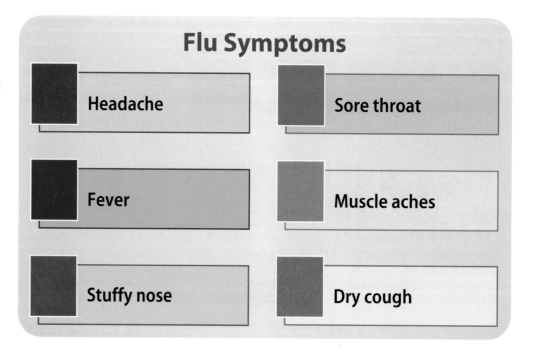

Flu Symptoms

Headache

Sore throat

Fever

Muscle aches

Stuffy nose

Dry cough

Others experience no symptoms at all. A person experiencing any combination of these symptoms should see a healthcare provider for diagnosis and treatment.

Tonsillitis

A virus or bacterium may cause **tonsillitis**, which is an infection that affects the tonsils (**Figure 12.6**). The tonsils usually protect the body from infection. Sometimes, however, the tonsils become infected.

Symptoms of tonsillitis include sore throat, fever, painful swallowing, and voice changes. If you think you have tonsillitis, you should contact a doctor. Often, the best treatment for tonsillitis is getting lots of rest and drinking plenty of fluids.

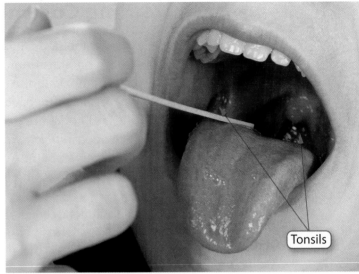

BravissimoS/Shutterstock.com

Figure 12.6 Tonsillitis is an infection of the tonsils, which are located at the back of the throat. When the tonsils are infected, they become *inflamed*, or swell and turn red.

Conjunctivitis

Conjunctivitis, also known as *pinkeye*, is a viral or bacterial infection that causes inflammation of the conjunctiva in the eye. The *conjunctiva* is the tissue that covers the eye and inner surface of the eyelid. Inflammation of the conjunctiva results in itchiness and a red or pink appearance, which gives this condition its name (**Figure 12.7**).

If pinkeye is the result of a bacterial infection, treatment typically involves the application of antibiotic drops to the affected eye. If the infection is viral, however, antibiotics will not work. A viral infection will run its course and go away as the body fights it.

Figure 12.7
Itchiness and red or pink eyes are symptoms of pinkeye. *What does the conjunctiva cover?*

Symptoms of Pinkeye

- Eye itchiness
- Red or pink appearance of the eye
- Swelling of the eye
- Discharge, or liquid, from the eye

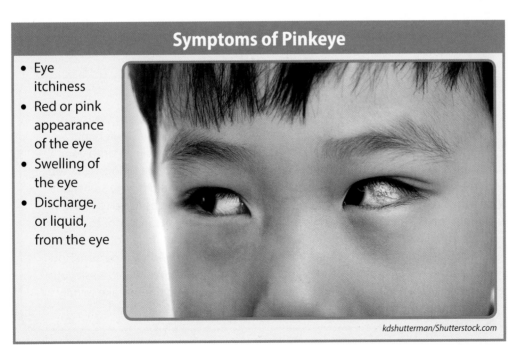

kdshutterman/Shutterstock.com

Treating Communicable Diseases

Treatment methods for infections vary depending on the type of infection. To treat bacterial infections, many doctors prescribe antibiotics such as penicillin or amoxicillin. **Antibiotics** are substances that target and kill *pathogenic*, or harmful, bacteria.

While antibiotics are generally very effective, some pathogenic bacteria have developed *antibiotic resistance*. This means certain antibiotics are ineffective against them. Antibiotic resistance is a growing issue. The best way to avoid contributing to it is to take antibiotics exactly as instructed by a doctor.

While antibiotics generally work well to treat bacterial infections, they do not work against viruses, fungi, and protozoa. Medications cannot cure a virus infection, but some medications can help treat the symptoms, such as a fever and body aches. The best treatment methods for viral infections include rest, good nutrition, and fluids to strengthen the body so it can fight the virus.

To treat fungal infections, doctors often prescribe antifungal ointments or creams that are applied directly to the infected area. Doctors may also prescribe medications to treat infections caused by protozoa. These medications are determined on a case-by-case basis, depending on the type of illness and the person's symptoms and overall health.

Lesson 12.1 Review

1. What is a pathogen?
2. **True or false.** Bacteria are multicelled, plant-like microorganisms that thrive in damp, warm environments.
3. List two methods of disease transmission.
4. List four communicable diseases.
5. **Critical thinking.** What are antibiotics? For what communicable diseases are antibiotics most effective?

Hands-On Activity

One of the best ways to lessen the spread of communicable diseases is to wash your hands regularly. To see how important hand washing is, put a small amount of hand lotion on your hands. Before spreading it into your hands, dump a small amount of single-colored glitter on the lotion. Now, rub the lotion into your hands as usual. Your classmates should do the same, but with a different color glitter. Go on with your class period as usual (passing out papers, sharing writing utensils, working together, etc.). Try not to pay any attention to the glitter on your hands. At the end of class, take notice of how many different colored glitters are on your belongings and your person. How does this relate to the spreading of communicable diseases? Now, wash your hands. Try first with just water, then add soap. How long does it take to fully wash your hands?

Noncommunicable Diseases

Learning Outcomes

After studying this lesson, you will be able to

- **understand** terms associated with noncommunicable diseases.
- **explain** the risk factors for noncommunicable diseases.
- **identify** five common noncommunicable diseases that are important health concerns in the United States.
- **describe** risks that noncommunicable diseases pose to your health.

Graphic Organizer

Risk Factors for Noncommunicable Diseases

Create a graphic organizer similar to the one shown to visually organize your notes as you listen to your teacher present this lesson. In the large circle on the left, write "Noncommunicable Diseases." In the circles on the right, list the types of noncommunicable diseases you learn about in this lesson. In the space around each circle, list two risk factors (lifestyle, heredity, or environment) that can increase the likelihood for developing that disease.

klenger/Shutterstock.com

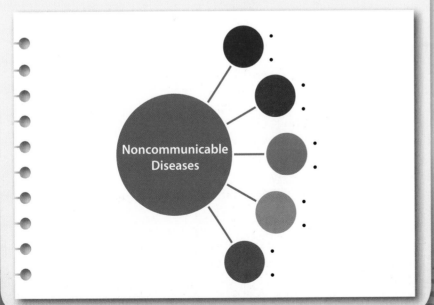

Key Terms

noncommunicable diseases medical conditions that cannot be spread among living things and objects, but develop as a result of heredity, environment, and lifestyle factors; also known as *noninfectious diseases*

heart attack medical emergency in which flow of blood to the heart is restricted, causing the heart to beat irregularly and inefficiently

stroke medical emergency in which blood flow to part of the brain is interrupted, injuring or killing brain cells

cancer complex disease that typically involves an uncontrolled growth of abnormal cells

tumor mass of abnormal cells

diabetes mellitus disease resulting from the body's inability to regulate glucose; commonly known as *diabetes*

autoimmune disease disease that causes the body's immune system to attack and damage healthy body tissues

arthritis condition that results in inflammation of the joints, causing pain and stiffness

What Is a Noncommunicable Disease?

Communicable disease
- Infectious disease
- A disease that can be spread

Noncommunicable disease
- Noninfectious disease
- A disease that cannot be spread

Figure 12.8 Noncommunicable diseases are different from communicable diseases in that they are not caused by pathogens and cannot be spread among living things and objects.

Recall in the first lesson of this chapter, Dakota and Tavon both developed cases of the flu, which is a communicable disease that people can "catch." In this lesson, you will learn how people develop noncommunicable diseases. *Noncommunicable diseases* are diseases that cannot be transmitted (**Figure 12.8**). Tavon, for example, has asthma, which is not something that Dakota can catch from him.

In most countries, more people die from noncommunicable diseases than from communicable diseases. If these diseases are not transmitted, how do they develop? Understanding noncommunicable diseases is important to reducing the number of deaths they cause.

Understanding Noncommunicable Diseases

Noncommunicable diseases, also called *noninfectious diseases*, cannot be spread among living things and objects. Instead, a person may inherit the possibility of developing a noncommunicable disease. A person's environment and lifestyle choices may also contribute to its development. **Figure 12.9** shows common noncommunicable diseases.

Many noncommunicable diseases are *chronic* illnesses. This means they are long-term diseases that may not heal for years. In fact, they might even cause permanent disability or health complications.

When evaluating a patient with a noncommunicable disease, doctors may give a prognosis. A *prognosis* is a prediction (educated guess) of how likely a person is to recover from the disease. A prognosis means something is

Figure 12.9 Common noncommunicable diseases include heart disease, stroke, cancer, high blood pressure, lung diseases, and arthritis. *Can noncommunicable diseases spread between people? Why or why not?*

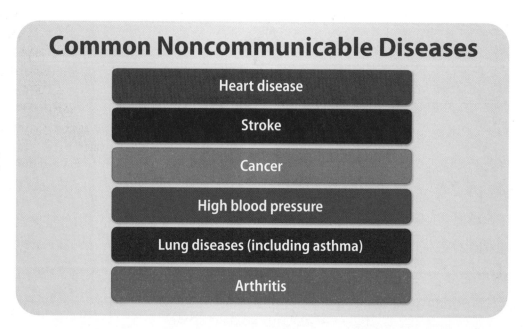

Common Noncommunicable Diseases

- Heart disease
- Stroke
- Cancer
- High blood pressure
- Lung diseases (including asthma)
- Arthritis

likely to happen, but it is not a sure guarantee that it will. Prognosis includes the chances for full recovery, disability, or death. Diseases that will end in death are *terminal*.

Sometimes, a disease enters *remission*, which is a time without signs and symptoms associated with that disease. Remission may last for weeks, years, or an indefinite period. The term *relapse* refers to the recurrence of a disease, in which signs and symptoms return after a period of remission (**Figure 12.10**). Certain cancers can return after remission in an even more severe way than before. A *complication* is a new condition or second disease that arises in a person who already has one disease. For example, a serious complication of diabetes is loss of eyesight.

Risk Factors for Noncommunicable Diseases

Noncommunicable diseases develop as a result of heredity, environment, and lifestyle factors. *Heredity* is the passing of characteristics or diseases from one generation to the next. Heredity and family history are important factors in a person's risk of developing noncommunicable diseases. For example, some genetic disorders can develop due to heredity, even without environmental or lifestyle factors. In contrast, for heart disease and some types of cancer, heredity mainly affects risk. Inheriting an increased risk for these diseases is not a guarantee someone will develop them.

Environment can play a role in the development of some noncommunicable diseases. Living in a major city with lots of pollution can increase your risk of developing chronic lung diseases. Exposure to secondhand smoke and aerosol may also increase your risk of developing breathing conditions.

A person's lifestyle choices and behaviors can increase or decrease risk of developing a noncommunicable disease. For example, behaviors such as using tobacco products, being physically inactive, and eating an unhealthy diet can lead to breathing conditions, heart disease, and cancer.

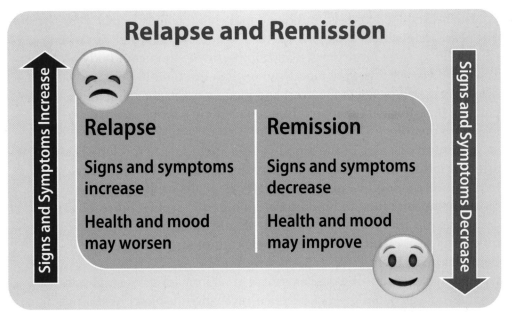

Relapse and Remission

Signs and Symptoms Increase

Relapse

Signs and symptoms increase

Health and mood may worsen

Remission

Signs and symptoms decrease

Health and mood may improve

Signs and Symptoms Decrease

Figure 12.10
Some noncommunicable diseases have symptoms that come and go. Symptoms subside during remission and return during relapse. *Does relapse occur before or after remission?*

ober-art/Shutterstock.com

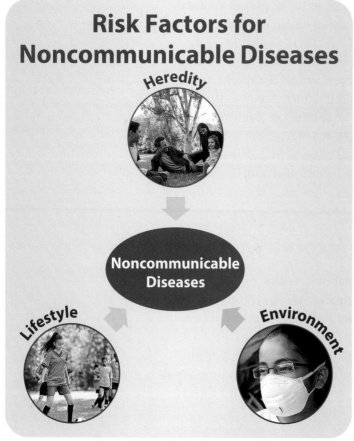

Risk Factors for Noncommunicable Diseases

Heredity

Noncommunicable Diseases

Lifestyle

Environment

Clockwise from top: Monkey Business Images/Shutterstock.com; iStock.com/VikramRaghuvanshi; iStock.com/Steve Debenport

Figure 12.11 Heredity, environment, and lifestyle choices all contribute to a person's likelihood of having a noncommunicable disease. *Is diet a hereditary, environmental, or lifestyle-related risk factor?*

In most cases, a combination of lifestyle factors, environment, and heredity determines a person's overall risk for developing certain types of noncommunicable diseases (**Figure 12.11**). As a result, you can reduce your risk of developing some of these diseases. Although family history is an important risk factor, behavior and environment also often contribute to risk. Changing your lifestyle and behaviors can potentially reduce your risk of developing certain noncommunicable diseases.

Common Noncommunicable Diseases

Heart disease, cancer, chronic lung disease, diabetes, and arthritis are important health concerns in many countries, including the United States. In the following sections, you will learn about the risks these diseases pose to your health. Gaining knowledge about these diseases can help you make lifestyle choices that promote optimal health both now and in the future.

Heart Disease

The heart, blood vessels, and blood make up the body's *circulatory system*. The heart adapts to the changing needs of your body. It speeds up when your body requires more oxygen and slows down when your body is at rest. The blood vessels transport blood and oxygen throughout your body. Heart disease causes damage to the heart and blood vessels, meaning they cannot perform their normal functions. This can result in serious health outcomes, including death.

Common diseases of the blood vessels include atherosclerosis and arteriosclerosis. In *atherosclerosis*, fatty deposits called *plaque* develop in the walls of blood vessels. These fatty deposits can build up and block the normal flow of blood through blood vessels (**Figure 12.12**). In *arteriosclerosis*, the walls of the blood vessels thicken, harden, and become inflexible. As a result, the blood vessels cannot stretch to allow blood to pump through them.

Atherosclerosis and arteriosclerosis can result from tobacco use, physical inactivity, and an unhealthy diet. Nicotine can change the blood vessels, making them more likely to develop fatty deposits. Physical inactivity and an unhealthy diet

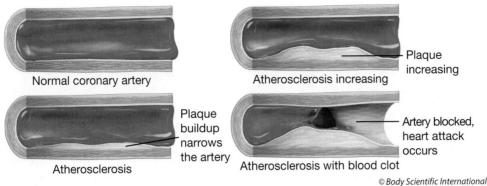

Figure 12.12
Atherosclerosis refers to the narrowing of blood vessels. Plaque builds up in the walls of blood vessels, restricting blood flow. Complete blockage of blood flow in coronary arteries (blood vessels that deliver blood to the heart) can lead to a heart attack.

Normal coronary artery

Atherosclerosis increasing

Plaque increasing

Plaque buildup narrows the artery

Atherosclerosis

Atherosclerosis with blood clot

Artery blocked, heart attack occurs

© Body Scientific International

can lead to obesity, which contributes to heart disease in various ways.

The blockage of important blood vessels can stop the flow of blood to the heart. When blood flow to the heart stops, and the heart cannot get enough oxygen, a **heart attack** occurs. During a heart attack, the heart beats irregularly and inefficiently. Pain arises partly because the heart is not receiving enough oxygen. A heart attack is a medical emergency, and immediate help can save lives (**Figure 12.13**).

A blockage of blood vessels can also cause a **stroke**. During a stroke, blood flow to a part of the brain is interrupted, injuring or killing brain cells. A stroke can result in paralysis, inability to speak, and disability. Lifestyle choices that contribute to atherosclerosis increase a person's risk of experiencing a stroke.

There are several treatment options for heart disease. One option is surgery to insert a *stent*, a small tube made of a fine mesh that pushes aside fatty deposits. Doctors may also prescribe blood-thinning medications to increase blood flow.

Cancer

Cancer is a complex disease, and different forms of the disease have different characteristics. All forms of cancer involve an uncontrolled growth of abnormal cells. Healthy cells control their growth, dividing only when needed. Cancerous cells divide rapidly and produce abnormal cells that do not function like normal cells. Scientists call a mass of abnormal cells a **tumor**. Tumors fall into two categories—malignant and benign. *Malignant* tumors are cancerous, while *benign* tumors are not.

There are more than 100 forms of cancer, but certain forms are more common than others. Cancers of the skin, lung, breast, and colon are some of the most common types of cancer (**Figure 12.14**). Together, these four types of cancer make up most of the reported cases in the United States.

Signs of a Heart Attack

Lightheadedness, nausea, and vomiting

Pain in the jaw, neck, or back

Arm or shoulder discomfort or pain

Pain or discomfort in the chest

Shortness of breath

vector illustration/Shutterstock.com

Figure 12.13 If you or someone you know shows signs of a heart attack, call 911 right away. Signs may differ between males and females. For example, females are more likely to have shortness of breath, dizziness, and pain in the back or abdomen.

Common Types of Cancer

Skin Cancer

- Caused by UV radiation, which comes from sunlight and tanning beds
- Melanoma is a very serious type that spreads from skin cells to other cells in the body if it is not caught early
- Can monitor changes in the skin with the ABCDE method (asymmetry, border, color, diameter, evolution)

Lung Cancer

- Leading cause of cancer death in the United States
- Main cause is tobacco smoke
- Symptoms include a cough that gets worse with time, chest pain, difficulty breathing, coughing blood, fatigue, and weight loss

Breast Cancer

- Group of diseases that affect breast tissue
- More common in females
- Risk for developing breast cancer increases with age
- Signs and symptoms include a lump in the breast or armpit, thickening or swelling of breast tissue, and irritation or pain in breast tissue or nipple

Colon Cancer

- Second leading cause of cancer death in males and females
- Polyps (abnormal growths) develop in the colon or rectum and can become cancerous
- Sometimes, no symptoms may be present

As with other noncommunicable diseases, heredity, environment, and lifestyle are all risk factors that can increase a person's chances of developing cancer. For example, some people inherit the risk of developing cancer from their parents and grandparents. Environmental exposure to carcinogens, such as those found in tobacco smoke, may also increase your risk of developing cancer. Physical inactivity can lead to obesity, which can cause certain types of cancer. Making healthy lifestyle choices and forming healthy habits now can reduce your risk of developing cancer later in life.

Early detection of cancer allows for early treatment and better chances for recovery and survival. There are common signs and symptoms of cancer, which are summarized by the acronym *C.A.U.T.I.O.N.* (**Figure 12.15**). Other symptoms of cancer include tiredness, easy bruising, ongoing pain in a part of the body, and loss of appetite or unplanned weight loss.

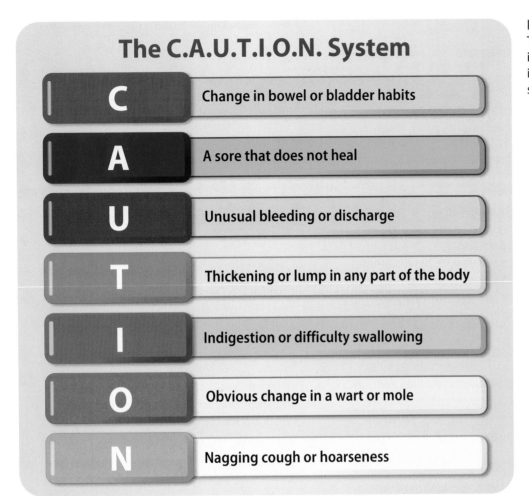

The C.A.U.T.I.O.N. System

C — Change in bowel or bladder habits

A — A sore that does not heal

U — Unusual bleeding or discharge

T — Thickening or lump in any part of the body

I — Indigestion or difficulty swallowing

O — Obvious change in a wart or mole

N — Nagging cough or hoarseness

Figure 12.15
The C.A.U.T.I.O.N. system is used to detect changes in the body that may signal cancer.

People who have cancer often see a doctor who specializes in cancer care, called an *oncologist*, for treatment. Cancer treatment may include specific methods, which include the following:

- **Surgery.** Doctors remove the cancerous tissue from a person's body.
- **Radiation therapy.** Machines deliver powerful X-rays to the part of the person's body affected by cancer. The goal is to shrink cancerous tissues or eliminate them completely. Side effects include fatigue, nausea, and vomiting.
- **Chemotherapy.** Medicines are delivered to patients through an IV, by mouth, or by injection to kill cancer cells. Side effects include weight loss, hair loss, nausea, and loss of appetite.
- **Immune therapy.** Medicine is delivered into the body to stimulate the body's defense to attack the cancer.

Treatments are tailored to specific cancers and the needs of individual patients, since each patient and type of cancer are different. A combination of treatments is often more effective than any one treatment. For example, chemotherapy and radiation both shrink the amount of cancerous tissue in a person's body. Surgery is more likely to be effective if the cancer is confined to a small area. Therefore, a patient may receive chemotherapy or radiation therapy before surgery, to make the surgery simpler.

CASE STUDY

Sawyer Copes with Cancer

Sawyer is a middle school student who loves school. Her teachers often describe her as someone who "loves learning and works hard to achieve her goals." Sawyer always tries to answer questions in class, even when she is not sure of an answer. If she answers incorrectly, Sawyer does not get upset, but considers it a learning opportunity.

Sawyer also gets along well with her classmates. She is kind to others and always willing to help when needed, but is not bossy, mean, or snobby. Her classmates think she is friendly and enjoy working with her.

Although she is not perfect, Sawyer is aware of positive health behaviors and she tries to take care of herself. She eats healthy foods, gets enough sleep, does not let stress overwhelm her, and gets some sort of physical activity every day. When she is sick, she stays home to recover and keeps her germs to herself.

It came as a shock to everyone when Sawyer was out of school for an extended length of time. People were starting to spread rumors about her being kicked out, about her moving, or about her being very sick. Unfortunately, the last rumor was true. Sawyer was diagnosed with cancer. Not a cancer that had anything to do with choices she or her family made; just a cancer that happens. Fortunately, Sawyer's cancer was detected early. She has been receiving treatments in a nearby city that

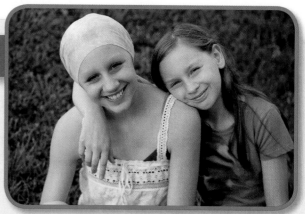

iStock.com/jessicaphoto

make her feel terrible, but she remains optimistic about her future. Despite her illness, and the fact that she does not feel great, Sawyer wants to come back to school, and she does.

Thinking Critically

1. What can Sawyer do to ensure her mental and emotional, physical, and social health throughout her illness and treatment?

2. How should Sawyer's classmates and friends treat Sawyer? What questions could they ask Sawyer to help them better understand the situation?

3. If you were Sawyer, what would you do? How much information about your illness would you want your classmates to know?

4. Why do you think remaining optimistic and hopeful are important characteristics during treatments for noncommunicable diseases such as cancer?

Chronic Respiratory Diseases

The *respiratory system* includes the nose, throat, voice box, windpipe, and lungs. Chronic respiratory diseases cause damage to these structures, meaning that they no longer work properly. Although respiratory diseases can damage all structures of the respiratory system, they are often called *chronic lung diseases* for short. Examples of chronic lung diseases include the following:

- asthma
- chronic obstructive pulmonary disease (COPD)
- respiratory allergies

Asthma

Asthma is a chronic disease in which a person's airways constrict and fill with mucus, making it difficult to breathe (**Figure 12.16**). Membranes in the airways also swell, blocking airflow even more and trapping stale air in the lungs. This triggers the wheezing that often occurs in asthma. Asthma cannot be cured, but medications can reduce the amount and severity of attacks. It may develop due to genetics or environment.

Chronic Obstructive Pulmonary Disease (COPD)

Chronic obstructive pulmonary disease (COPD) is a group of lung diseases that limit the amount of air that can flow through the lungs. These diseases include emphysema, chronic bronchitis, and asthma. (To review information on emphysema and chronic bronchitis, see Chapter 9.)

People with COPD often experience breathlessness, as well as a cough that lasts a long time and produces a lot of mucus. Causes of COPD include tobacco use, air pollution, and exposure to dusts or chemicals in the workplace. Goals of COPD treatment include managing the condition and its symptoms, as well as preventing the condition from getting worse.

Respiratory Allergies

Respiratory allergies are those that specifically affect a person's ability to breathe. The main example of a respiratory allergy is *allergic rhinitis*, commonly known as *hay fever*. Hay fever occurs when someone breathes in a substance that the person is allergic to, known as an *allergen*. This causes inflammation and swelling inside the nose. Indoor and outdoor allergens can cause hay fever (**Figure 12.17**). Hay fever usually goes away on its own, but it can cause irritating symptoms that may require medication.

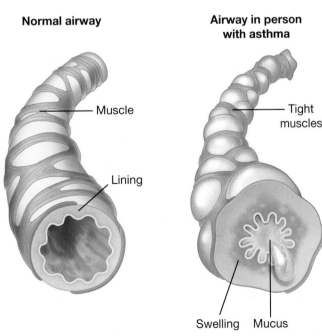

Normal airway

Muscle

Lining

Airway in person with asthma

Tight muscles

Swelling   Mucus

© Body Scientific International

Figure 12.16
In asthma, a person's airways swell and become clogged with mucus. The buildup of mucus makes breathing difficult. *Is asthma a long-term or short-term disease?*

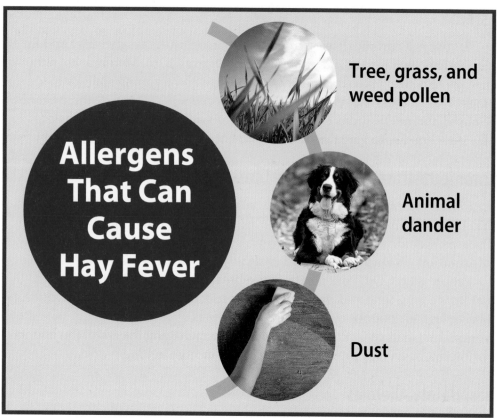

Top to bottom: tomertu/Shutterstock.com; DragoNika/Shutterstock.com; Photographee.eu/Shutterstock.com

Diabetes

Diabetes mellitus, commonly referred to as *diabetes*, is a disease that results from the body's inability to regulate glucose. *Glucose* is a sugar found in foods that the body converts into energy. In someone who does not have diabetes, glucose enters the bloodstream through food. The pancreas, an organ that helps with digestion, creates a hormone called *insulin* that transports glucose to the body's cells. Diabetes disrupts this process.

There are two types of diabetes—type 1 diabetes mellitus (often called *juvenile diabetes*) and type 2 diabetes mellitus. Each type disrupts the body's use of glucose in a different way. Both types result in high blood sugar, which can lead to other health conditions. Some potential long-term health complications of diabetes may include heart disease, nerve damage, vision damage, hearing impairment, foot damage, and kidney damage.

Type 1 Diabetes Mellitus

Type 1 diabetes mellitus is an **autoimmune disease**, or a condition that causes the body's immune system to attack and kill healthy tissues. In type 1 diabetes, the immune system attacks the pancreas and kills cells that make insulin. This means there is no insulin to transport glucose to the body cells. Instead, glucose stays in the blood, resulting in a high blood sugar level. Type 1 diabetes can occur at any age, but usually first appears between 10 and 14 years of age.

The main risk factor for type 1 diabetes is family history of the condition. The most common symptoms include excessive urination, thirst, hunger, and weight loss (**Figure 12.18**).

Diabetes by the Numbers

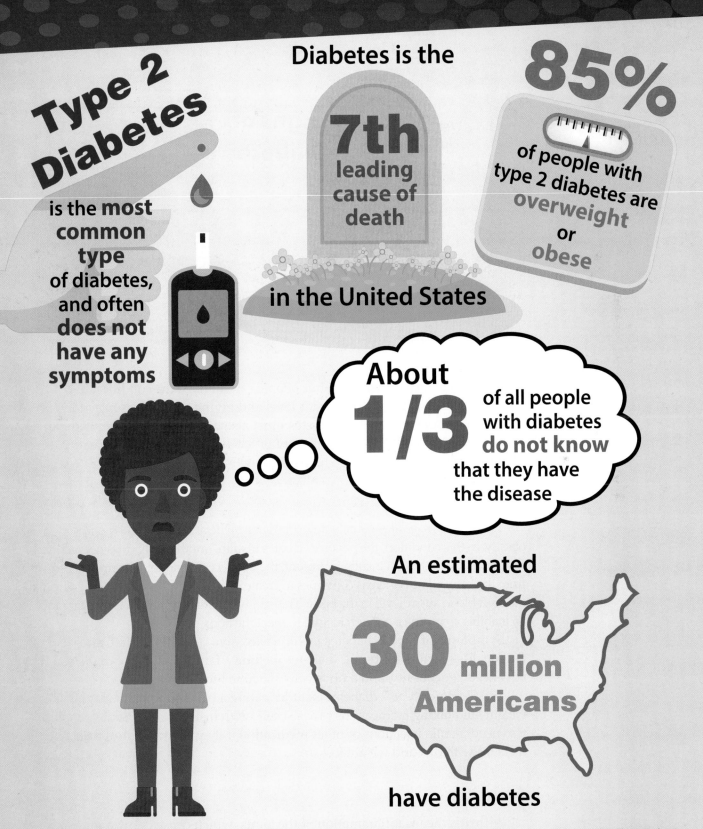

Type 2 Diabetes is the **most common type** of diabetes, and often **does not have any symptoms**

Diabetes is the **7th** leading cause of death in the United States

85% of people with type 2 diabetes are **overweight** or **obese**

About **1/3** of all people with diabetes **do not know** that they have the disease

An estimated **30 million Americans** have diabetes

Map: chrupka/Shutterstock.com; Girl: Visual Generations/Shutterstock.com; Speech bubble: Vector.design/Shutterstock.com; Scale: VAZZEN/Shutterstock.com; Tombstone: jabkitticha/Shutterstock.com; Diabetes test: HelgaMariah/Shutterstock.com

Figure 12.18
Diabetes causes symptoms in multiple systems of the body. It also causes changes in the eyes and breath and weight loss.

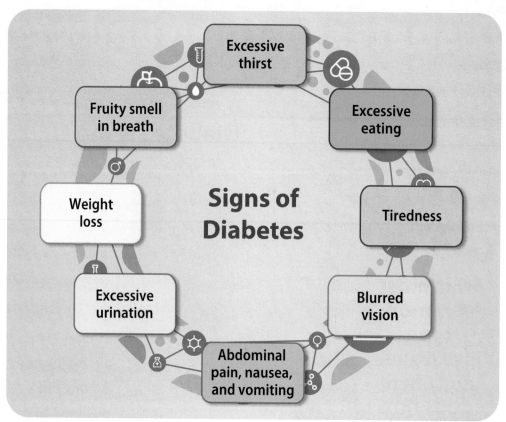

Signs of Diabetes

Excessive thirst

Excessive eating

Tiredness

Blurred vision

Abdominal pain, nausea, and vomiting

Excessive urination

Weight loss

Fruity smell in breath

ananaline/Shutterstock.com

Type 1 diabetes is incurable, but people can manage the condition by regularly checking their blood sugar level and giving themselves injections of insulin. People with type 1 diabetes must also control the amount of sugar in their blood by controlling the amount of food and the sugars they eat. Moderate physical activity also helps regulate blood sugar.

Type 2 Diabetes Mellitus

Type 2 diabetes mellitus usually develops later in life and is associated with obesity. In this condition, the pancreas creates insulin, but the body does not respond to it normally. Although insulin is present, the body's cells cannot take up glucose from the blood. The pancreas continues to create insulin, however, because it detects the high blood sugar level in the body. This can wear out the pancreas, resulting in an inability to produce enough insulin to meet the body's needs.

Symptoms of type 2 diabetes include excessive urination, thirst, and fatigue. Risk factors for type 2 diabetes include a family history of diabetes, advanced age, obesity, and a physically inactive lifestyle.

Treatment for type 2 diabetes includes eating a balanced diet, managing weight, and taking medications to assist cells with insulin usage. Some people also need insulin injections or other medication if they cannot control their diabetes with diet and weight loss.

Arthritis

Arthritis means inflammation of the joints, which causes slow and stiff movement. Multiple joints within the body can be affected by arthritis (**Figure 12.19**). Two common types of arthritis include osteoarthritis and rheumatoid arthritis. Each type of arthritis has different causes, treatments, and outcomes.

Osteoarthritis is the most common form of arthritis among adults. It is caused by the wearing down of cartilage that pads the surfaces of bones that meet at the joints. The bones then come into contact with each other, triggering pain, swelling, and stiffness. Osteoarthritis can be treated with anti-inflammatory medicine, pain relievers, and mild physical activity. Severely damaged joints may require surgery or replacement with an artificial joint.

Rheumatoid arthritis is an autoimmune disease in which the body's immune system attacks and damages the joints, causing severe arthritis. In rheumatoid arthritis, the same joints often swell painfully on opposite sides of the body. The pain and swelling often come and go, repeatedly becoming worse, then improving. Over time, the damage from this disease causes crippling deformities in the joints and even affects other organs in the body.

Treatment for rheumatoid arthritis includes anti-inflammatory medication, pain relievers, and mild physical activity. Certain medications target the immune system and block its attack on the joint tissues.

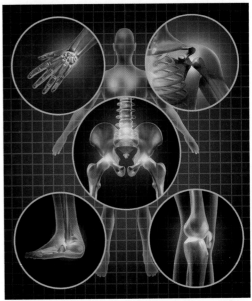

Lightspring/Shutterstock.com

Figure 12.19 Arthritis can cause inflammation in many different joints and often affects joints in the hands, shoulders, back, hips, knees, and feet. *How does arthritis affect the movement of joints?*

Lesson 12.2 Review

1. List three factors that contribute to the development of a noncommunicable disease.

2. The heart, blood vessels, and blood make up the body's _____ system.

   A. respiratory   **C.** reproductive

   B. circulatory   **D.** lymphatic

3. A mass of abnormal cells is called a(n) _____.

4. What is arthritis?

5. **Critical thinking.** Contrast the risk factors for type 1 diabetes and type 2 diabetes.

Hands-On Activity

With a partner, choose one noncommunicable disease discussed in this chapter. Review information about the disease's causes, signs and symptoms, and treatments. Find an additional valid and reliable source of information about this disease to enhance your knowledge. Then, create a flowchart that illustrates this information. Your flowchart should start with the causes of the disease and end with treatment options. For each step in the flowchart, include a related image. Be sure to cite the sources you used on your flowchart. Share your completed flowchart with the class.

Preventing Diseases

Key Terms 🖝

respiratory etiquette
practice of covering your
mouth and nose with a tissue
while coughing or sneezing,
or sneezing into your sleeve

food sanitation food safety
practices that maintain the
safety of food you handle and
eat; includes refrigerating
and freezing certain foods,
cooking meat thoroughly, and
washing vegetables and fruits

vaccine substance that
contains a dead or nontoxic
part of a pathogen that is
injected into a person to train
that person's immune system
to eliminate the live pathogen

Learning Outcomes

After studying this lesson, you will be able to

- **demonstrate** proper hand washing to prevent communicable diseases.
- **describe** respiratory etiquette practices to prevent communicable diseases.
- **give examples** of food sanitation practices that maintain the safety of food you handle and eat.
- **explain** the purpose of vaccines in disease prevention.
- **summarize** how to reduce your risk of noncommunicable diseases.

Graphic Organizer

Focus on Disease Prevention

Create a table similar to the one shown. Include as many rows as you need. As your teacher presents the lesson, list the main topics and ways to prevent or reduce the risk of communicable and noncommunicable diseases. Identify as many details as you need for each prevention method and include information with which you are familiar and unfamiliar. (An example is provided for you.) Then, team up with a classmate to discuss each other's lists. Did you and your classmate draw the same conclusions from the lesson? What items do you need to add? If there is anything about the lesson you do not understand, seek clarification from your teacher.

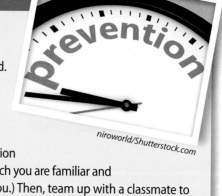

niroworld/Shutterstock.com

Preventing Communicable Diseases	Preventing Noncommunicable Diseases
Cover your mouth and nose with a tissue while coughing or sneezing.	Eat a healthy diet to reduce the risk of heart disease, cancer, and diabetes.

The previous lessons introduced you to how diseases develop. Some diseases develop after contact with pathogens, such as the flu that Dakota and Tavon had. Others, such as Tavon's asthma, develop due to family history, behavior, and environment. No matter what the cause, prevention methods exist for all types of disease. In this lesson, you will learn steps you can take to prevent communicable diseases. You will also learn about lifestyle changes that can help prevent and manage noncommunicable diseases.

Preventing Communicable Diseases

As you learned, microorganisms called *pathogens* cause communicable diseases. Bacteria, viruses, and other pathogens can travel among living things and objects (**Figure 12.20**). How can you protect yourself from something you cannot even see? The task may seem impossible, but you can use a few simple actions to ensure microorganisms do not make you sick. You can prevent communicable diseases by washing your hands frequently, using respiratory etiquette, practicing food sanitation, and getting regular vaccines.

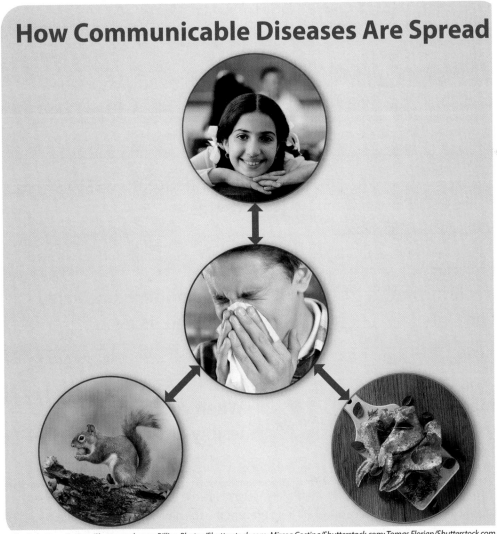

How Communicable Diseases Are Spread

Top to bottom: Zurijeta/Shutterstock.com; Billion Photos/Shutterstock.com; Mircea Costina/Shutterstock.com; Tomas Florian/Shutterstock.com

Figure 12.20
Communicable diseases can be transmitted among living things and objects. *What are disease-causing microorganisms called?*

Hand Washing

What have you touched today? Nearly everything you touch, from doorknobs to your pet, contains pathogens that transfer to your hands. Now think about everything you do with your hands. When you eat with dirty hands, pathogens you pick up from other objects enter your body with the food. Washing your hands on a regular basis, and in certain situations, can eliminate pathogens and prevent communicable diseases. **Figure 12.21** lists occasions to wash your hands.

Hand washing is the most important method of preventing many communicable diseases. Washing your hands is a simple action you can take to prevent germs on your hands from making you sick. Always use running water and soap to wash your hands. Rub your hands together, scrubbing every surface, for 20 seconds. To make sure you are washing your hands for at least 20 seconds, hum or sing the "Happy Birthday" song twice. After 20 seconds of scrubbing, rinse your hands under warm running water. Then air-dry your hands or pat them dry with a clean towel.

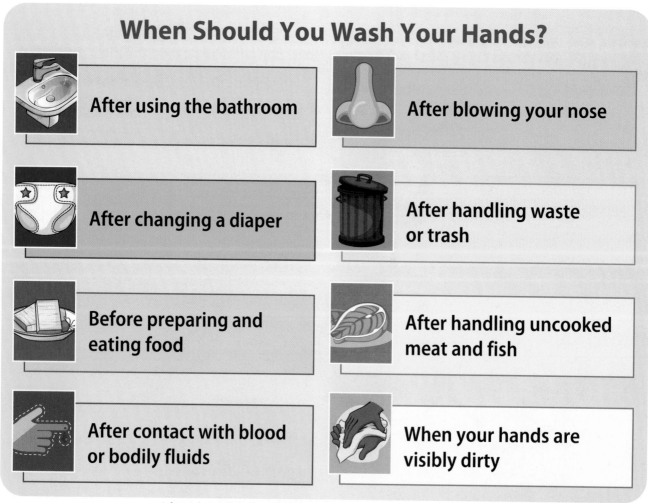

When Should You Wash Your Hands?

- After using the bathroom
- After blowing your nose
- After changing a diaper
- After handling waste or trash
- Before preparing and eating food
- After handling uncooked meat and fish
- After contact with blood or bodily fluids
- When your hands are visibly dirty

Figure 12.21 Washing your hands on all of these occasions will help prevent the transmission of communicable diseases.

How to Wash Your Hands

1. Wet hands

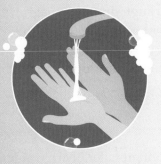

2. Use soap

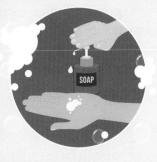

3. Begin timing 20 seconds

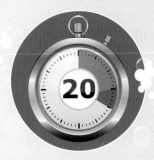

4. Or you could hum "Happy Birthday" twice

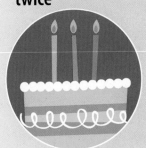

5. Rub palm to palm

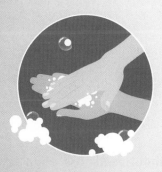

6. Back of hands

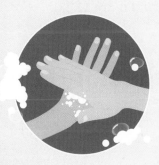

7. Rub fingernails

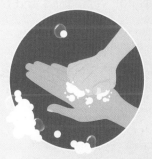

8. Fingers interlaced

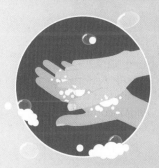

9. Base of thumbs

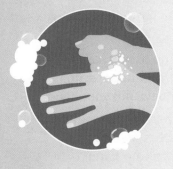

10. Rub wrists

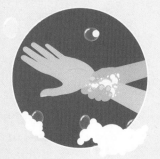

11. Rinse hands

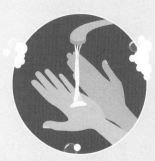

12. Dry hands

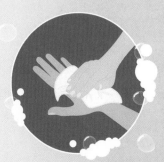

Washing hands: Pro_Vector/Shutterstock.com; Birthday cake: vannilasky/Shutterstock.com; Timer: Aleksandr Bryliaev/Shutterstock.com

Alcohol-based hand rubs, or hand sanitizers, are very effective when soap and water are unavailable. Visibly dirty hands, however, need to be washed first for an alcohol rub to work. Alcohol-based sanitizer dispensers are often located in stores and other public places. Although use of hand sanitizers is convenient, prolonged use can dry out a person's skin.

Respiratory Etiquette

In Lesson 12.1, you learned that communicable diseases, such as the common cold and flu, can infect people through droplet spread. Droplet spread occurs when pathogens travel in droplets of fluid created by coughing, sneezing, and talking. Doctors recommend that people practice respiratory etiquette to prevent spreading diseases through droplet spread. **Respiratory etiquette** is the practice of covering your mouth and nose with a tissue while coughing or sneezing, or sneezing into your sleeve (**Figure 12.22**). Use respiratory etiquette when you are sick to help the people around you avoid getting sick.

Food Sanitation

The indirect transmission of pathogens through contaminated food, water, and surfaces can cause some dangerous communicable diseases. You can adopt certain food safety practices, known as **food sanitation**, to maintain the safety of the food you handle and eat. Food sanitation practices include refrigerating and freezing certain foods, cooking meat thoroughly, and washing vegetables and fruits (**Figure 12.23**).

Figure 12.22
Respiratory etiquette helps prevent the spread of communicable diseases through droplets in the air. *What are some examples of diseases that can infect people through droplet spread?*

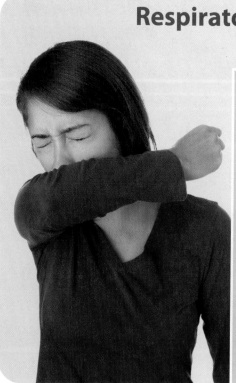

Respiratory Etiquette

- Cover your mouth and nose when you sneeze or cough. This prevents droplets from spreading.
- Cover your nose and mouth with a tissue when coughing or sneezing. Do not reuse or store the tissue.
- If you have no tissues, cough or sneeze into your upper arm, sleeve, or elbow, not your hands.
- Wash your hands after using a tissue, or after sneezing and coughing into your hands.

iStock.com/sebarnes

Food Sanitation Practices

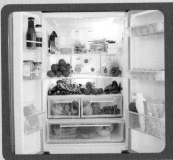

Refrigerate and Freeze Perishables

Refrigeration and freezing slows or stops the growth of pathogens. Food that can spoil should be kept cold or frozen. Remember, however, that refrigerating and freezing foods does not kill pathogens.

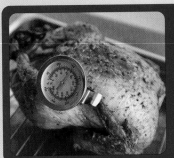

Cook Meat Thoroughly

Cooking meat thoroughly will kill pathogens. Instant meat thermometers have a scale noting safe temperatures for various types of meat. Always use a meat thermometer or cook meat until its juices no longer run pink.

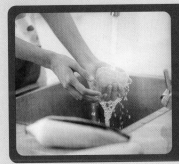

Wash Vegetables and Fruits

The outer coverings of fruits and vegetables often contain pathogens. Therefore, it is important to wash vegetables and fruits under running water before eating. Fruits you peel or cut open should be washed before cutting.

Top to bottom: Andrey_Popov/Shutterstock.com; Africa Studio/Shutterstock.com; Pumz/Shutterstock.com

Figure 12.23
Practicing good food sanitation includes refrigerating and freezing perishables, cooking meat thoroughly, and washing vegetables and fruits.

Vaccines

Vaccination is the only proven method of successfully getting rid of a communicable disease. For example, the highly contagious, deadly viral infection *smallpox* was eliminated by vaccination. In the next few years, vaccines will probably conquer *polio*, which has caused paralysis in many people throughout history.

A **vaccine** is a substance that contains a dead or nontoxic part of a pathogen that is injected into a person to train the immune system to eliminate the live pathogen. A doctor or another healthcare worker will administer a vaccine through an injection. When injected into a person, the vaccine causes an immune response in the body. This means the person's body produces white blood cells, proteins, and chemicals that fight infections. The vaccine is the body's first encounter with the pathogen. The body's immune response to the vaccine is like a rehearsal for when the body encounters the real pathogen.

Common Vaccines for Adolescents

Vaccine	Effect
Human papillomavirus (HPV) vaccine	The HPV vaccine helps prevent cancers caused by HPV, a common sexually transmitted infection (STI). It is recommended for males and females around age 11 or 12.
Influenza (flu) vaccine	The flu vaccine (commonly called the *flu shot*) is given yearly and protects against infection with the flu. If a vaccinated person does get the flu, symptoms are milder.
Meningococcal vaccine	Meningococcal vaccines protect against diseases caused by the *Neisseria meningitidis* bacteria. These bacteria can cause severe infections around the brain and spinal cord. The vaccine is recommended at age 11 or 12 and again at age 16.
Tdap vaccine	The Tdap vaccine protects against three diseases: tetanus, diphtheria, and pertussis (also called *whooping cough*). The vaccine is recommended around age 11 or 12.

Figure 12.24 Most vaccines are given during childhood. The vaccines in this table are recommended for adolescents. *Which vaccine is given yearly?*

The dead pathogen or part of a pathogen in the vaccine cannot cause an illness, but it makes the person's body familiar with the illness. After getting a vaccine, a person's body will recognize the pathogen included in the vaccine. If a person encounters the real, disease-causing pathogen, the immune system will respond strongly and quickly. When exposed to a pathogen after vaccination, the body knows how to react to the pathogen.

Because vaccination activates the immune system, it is also called *immunization*. Vaccines are safe and effective, and they prevent many types of communicable diseases (**Figure 12.24**). Some vaccines are effective for nearly a lifetime, others for many years. Some vaccines require follow-up injections, called *boosters*, to restimulate the immune system.

Preventing Noncommunicable Diseases

Pathogens do not cause noncommunicable diseases. Instead, family history, environment, and lifestyle choices contribute to the development of noncommunicable diseases. People cannot avoid conditions such as heart disease, cancer, chronic respiratory disease, and diabetes through hand washing or food sanitation. Making healthy lifestyle choices early in life can help you prevent noncommunicable diseases (**Figure 12.25**).

Figure 12.25
Your health now impacts your health in the future.

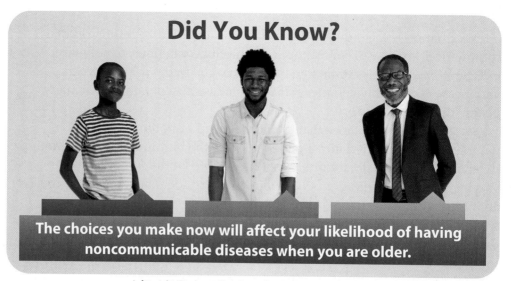

Did You Know?

The choices you make now will affect your likelihood of having noncommunicable diseases when you are older.

Left to right: iStock.com/Yuri_Arcurs; Rawpixel.com/Shutterstock.com; Rawpixel.com/Shutterstock.com

Family History

Noncommunicable diseases are caused by lifestyle choices, your environment, and the genes passed down to you by your biological parents. Your genes determine many of your traits, including your eye color, hair color, and likelihood of having certain noncommunicable diseases. Because of this, some noncommunicable diseases run in families. For example, if a grandparent had heart disease, you may be at an increased risk for having heart disease when you are older.

To see what noncommunicable diseases run in a family, doctors often ask questions about *family history*, which is a biological family's history of disease. A family history typically includes information about your biological parents, siblings, and extended family, and should list diseases such as heart disease, cancer, diabetes, and asthma.

Charting Your Family's History of Disease

Knowing your family's history of noncommunicable diseases can help you take action to prevent diseases in your future. For example, if your family has a history of type 2 diabetes, you can reduce your risk factors for that disease. To chart your family history, begin by meeting with your parents or guardian. Draw a family tree like the one below and fill in the names of your biological parents, siblings, and grandparents. If you do not have access to this information, talk with your teacher. For each person on your family tree, write down any noncommunicable diseases the person has or had. Talk with your parents or guardian about the noncommunicable diseases that run in your family and make a list of five actions you could take to reduce your risk of these diseases in the future.

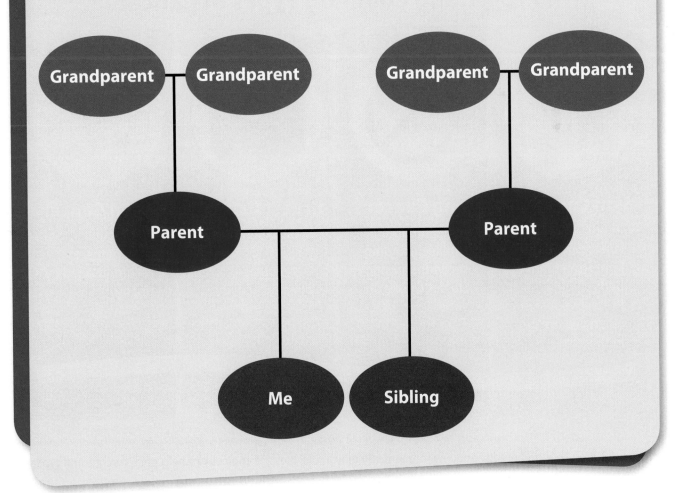

Heart Disease

Heart disease occurs as a result of damage to structures such as the blood vessels. The best method of prevention is making lifestyle choices that protect your blood vessels and heart. One important lifestyle choice is eating a healthy diet. Including more fruits and vegetables and fewer processed foods in your diet can improve heart health. Engaging in regular physical activity can also help you avoid heart disease. Getting regular physical activity will keep your heart in shape and working properly.

Maintaining a healthy weight also reduces the risk of heart disease. Eating a healthy diet and being physically active can help you manage your weight. In addition, avoiding tobacco and alcohol increases heart health. Making these healthy lifestyle choices can reduce your risk of developing heart disease.

Cancer

Maintaining a healthy lifestyle is also important for preventing cancer. To reduce your risk for cancer, be sure to maintain a healthy weight and eat a healthy diet. Physical activity is also important. In addition, each of the common types of cancer can be prevented in specific ways (**Figure 12.26**).

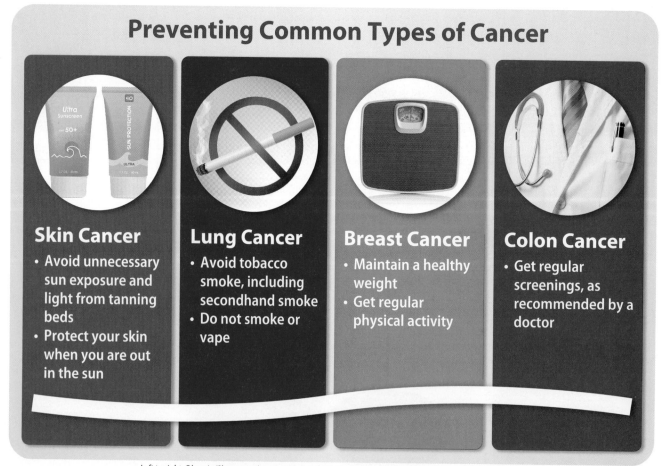

Preventing Common Types of Cancer

Skin Cancer
- Avoid unnecessary sun exposure and light from tanning beds
- Protect your skin when you are out in the sun

Lung Cancer
- Avoid tobacco smoke, including secondhand smoke
- Do not smoke or vape

Breast Cancer
- Maintain a healthy weight
- Get regular physical activity

Colon Cancer
- Get regular screenings, as recommended by a doctor

Figure 12.26 Though heredity and environment still play a role, lifestyle choices can help prevent common types of cancer.

Love Your Heart

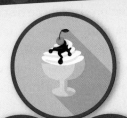

EAT LESS SUGARY AND SALTY FOODS

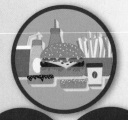

LIMIT INTAKE OF FATTY FOODS

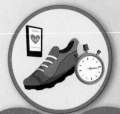

ENGAGE IN CARDIO ACTIVITIES FOR AT LEAST 30 MINUTES FIVE DAYS PER WEEK

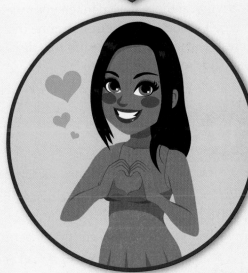

FOCUS ON MUSCLE STRENGTHENING ACTIVITIES TWO DAYS PER WEEK

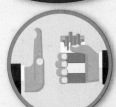

AVOID SMOKING, VAPING, AND OTHER USES OF TOBACCO

TRY EATING SOME MEALS WITHOUT MEAT

Girl: Kakigori Studio/Shutterstock.com; Icons, clockwise from top: PureSolution/Shutterstock.com; Elegant Solution/Shutterstock.com; Macrovector/Shutterstock.com; hvostik/Shutterstock.com; Elegant Solution/Shutterstock.com; Vadim Ermak/Shutterstock.com

Chronic Respiratory Diseases

Chronic respiratory diseases include bronchitis, emphysema, and asthma. The main causes of bronchitis and emphysema include tobacco smoke and pollutants in the home or workplace. You can reduce your risk of developing bronchitis or emphysema by avoiding these substances. In addition, early detection of bronchitis and emphysema can prevent these diseases from getting worse and leading to COPD. Once a respiratory disease is detected, a person who smokes or vapes should stop immediately and reduce exposure to substances that cause COPD.

People cannot prevent the development of asthma. People can manage the symptoms of asthma, however. For example, people can manage asthma by avoiding substances or situations that trigger asthma attacks. In addition, medicine can reduce asthma attacks and improve a person's breathing.

Diabetes

Risk factors for type 2 diabetes include having a physically inactive lifestyle and being overweight or obese. The best way to prevent type 2 diabetes is to avoid these risk factors. Maintaining a healthy weight can help reduce your risk of this disease. Eating a healthy diet and getting regular physical activity can help you manage your weight.

Since type 1 diabetes is an autoimmune disease, it cannot be prevented through lifestyle choices. People with this disease can manage it, however, by following doctor recommendations.

Lesson 12.3 Review

1. What are four ways to prevent communicable diseases?
2. Covering your nose and mouth with a tissue when coughing or sneezing is an example of _____ _____.
3. What are three food sanitation practices that help keep food safe to eat?
4. A(n) _____ is a substance that contains a dead or nontoxic part of a pathogen that is injected into a person to train the immune system.
5. **Critical thinking.** Name three ways to help prevent noncommunicable diseases and explain why they are helpful.

Hands-On Activity

Disease prevention is highly linked to the choices a person makes. Review the lesson and make a list identifying which prevention choices you make appropriately and which you need to work on. Why are some behaviors easy for you to do while others are not? How can you realistically improve your disease prevention behaviors? What support or help do you need from others to do this? Who can provide that support? On a separate sheet of paper, write a summary explaining your answers. Then, create a SMART goal you would like to achieve to help improve your overall health and well-being. Track your goal progress and adjust your goal as needed.

Summary

Lesson 12.1 Communicable Diseases

- Communicable diseases are diseases that can spread among living things and objects. These are diseases you can "catch" from others.
- Pathogens are microorganisms that cause communicable diseases. They are only visible with a microscope. Bacteria, viruses, fungi, and protozoa are pathogens that cause communicable diseases.
- Pathogens that cause communicable diseases travel by various methods of transmission from one organism or object to another. Methods of transmission may be direct or indirect.
- Communicable diseases include influenza, mononucleosis, tonsillitis, and conjunctivitis.
- Treatment with antibiotics is effective against most pathogenic bacteria, but is not effective against viruses, fungi, and protozoa.
- Certain antibiotics are ineffective against antibiotic-resistant bacteria, which are a serious public health concern. To decrease the chances of contributing to this, take antibiotics exactly as instructed by a doctor.

Lesson 12.2 Noncommunicable Diseases

- Noncommunicable diseases, or noninfectious diseases, do not spread among living things and objects. They are often long-term diseases with symptoms that come and go.
- Noncommunicable diseases are usually caused by a combination of heredity, lifestyle choices, and environment. The exact causes depend on the disease.
- Noncommunicable diseases include heart disease, cancer, chronic respiratory diseases, diabetes, and arthritis.
- Understanding the risks of noncommunicable diseases helps you make lifestyle choices to promote optimal health.

Lesson 12.3 Preventing Diseases

- Preventing communicable diseases involves taking actions to ensure microorganisms do not spread and make people sick.
- Prevention methods for communicable diseases include frequently washing hands, using respiratory etiquette, and practicing food sanitation.
- Vaccines prevent communicable diseases by stimulating the immune response. The immune response is like a rehearsal for an encounter with the real pathogen.
- Lifestyle choices such as a healthy diet and regular physical activity help prevent noncommunicable diseases.
- Additional methods of treating noncommunicable diseases include medicine and following doctor recommendations. These are helpful for treating asthma and diabetes.

Check Your Knowledge

Record your answers to each of the following questions on a separate sheet of paper.

1. Describe the difference between communicable and noncommunicable diseases.

2. What communicable disease is also known as *pinkeye*?
   A. Influenza.
   B. Conjunctivitis.
   C. Mononucleosis.
   D. Tonsilitis.

3. What does *method of transmission* mean?

4. Substances that target and kill pathogenic bacteria are called _____.

5. How can you avoid contributing to antibiotic resistance?

6. **True or false.** All noncommunicable diseases develop due to lifestyle choices.

7. Which of the following actions is *not* a method to help prevent heart disease?
   A. Eat a healthy diet that includes many fruits and vegetables.
   B. Engage in physical activity.
   C. Use tobacco and alcohol.
   D. Maintain a healthy weight.

8. Which noncommunicable disease is characterized by the uncontrolled growth of abnormal cells?

9. Which type of diabetes is an autoimmune disease?

10. **True or false.** Improper hand washing and heredity are risk factors for noncommunicable diseases.

11. **True or false.** Refrigerating and freezing certain foods is an example of a food sanitation practice.

12. What is the practice of covering your mouth and nose with a tissue while coughing or sneezing, or sneezing into your sleeve?

13. **True or false.** Making healthy lifestyle choices early in life can help you prevent noncommunicable diseases.

Use Your Vocabulary ↗

antibiotics	food sanitation	pathogens
arthritis	heart attack	respiratory etiquette
autoimmune disease	influenza	stroke
cancer	method of transmission	tonsillitis
communicable disease	mononucleosis	tumor
conjunctivitis	noncommunicable	vaccine
diabetes mellitus	diseases	

14. On a separate sheet of paper, list words that relate to each of the terms above. Then, work with a partner to explain how these words are related.

15. Write down terms from this chapter that use the word part *anti-*. Explain what *anti-* means and how this affects the definitions of these words. Then, write any other health-related words you can think of that also use this word part. You can look in the text glossary for inspiration.

Think Critically

16. **Cause and effect.** What dangers to self and others does a person create by coming to school sick with a communicable disease?

17. **Identify.** What agencies and resources are available in your community for getting healthcare for communicable diseases? How do you know if you need to see the doctor for a communicable disease?

18. **Analyze.** Why are behaviors that help prevent communicable diseases from spreading critical for personal and community health?

19. **Draw conclusions.** What prevention behaviors can help prevent more than one noncommunicable disease? Which behaviors do you believe are the most important for maintaining health? Why?

DEVELOP Your Skills

20. **Teamwork and advocacy skills.** Practicing health-enhancing behaviors and avoiding health risks are important, especially when it comes to preventing illnesses. In small groups, choose to explore a disease of interest to you. Then, as a group, write a script for a role-play scenario in which a person, a group of friends, or a family makes a responsible decision to prevent that disease. Include refusal skills, other healthy behaviors, and important or useful information about the disease in your role play. After reviewing your role play with your teacher, present it to your class to encourage your classmates to act healthfully.

21. **Communication and advocacy skills.** Working in a small group, create a presentation about how to use healthy behaviors to prevent or reduce the risk of one noncommunicable disease discussed in the chapter. Decide with your group the most important information people need to know. Use a school-approved software application to create a digital poster or digital public service announcement. Present your announcement to the class.

22. **Literacy and accessing information skills.** Listen to a podcast or watch a video about a middle-school student facing one of the diseases discussed in the chapter. Complete a report that assesses the accuracy of the information about the disease. Also, include the take-home message, theme, or moral of the podcast or video, and a recommendation for listening. Share your report with a classmate.

23. **Goal-setting skills.** To improve your personal hand-washing behavior, set a SMART goal for yourself. Create a plan of small steps to achieve this goal. Implement your plan and keep track of your progress in a journal. Write a reflection on the process after achieving your goal. How realistic was your goal? What strategies helped you?

24. **Communication and accessing information skills.** Imagine you are a writer for a middle-school newspaper or website. Write an editorial targeted at middle-school students. Choose a topic based on what you have read in the chapter. Use appropriate language to communicate your message clearly and be sure the information you provide is accurate. Use other valid and reliable sources to help formulate your writing. Be sure to cite your sources. Make any corrections for grammar, spelling, and punctuation.

Chapter 13

Promoting Safety and Preventing Injuries

Essential Question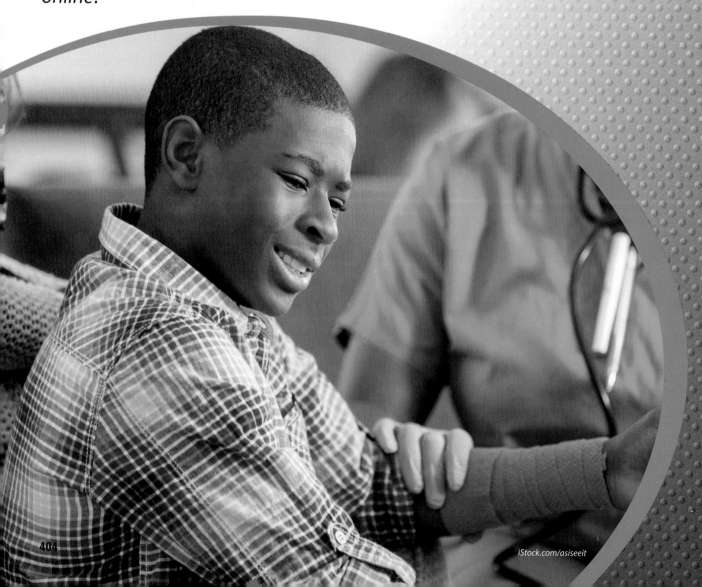

How can you protect yourself at home, in the community, and online?

Lesson 13.1 Promoting Safety in the Home

Lesson 13.2 Promoting Safety in the Community and Online

Lesson 13.3 Knowing Basic First Aid

iStock.com/asiseeit

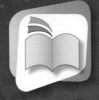

Reading Activity

Before you read the chapter, write all of the key terms for the chapter on a piece of paper and what you think each term means. As you read the chapter, compare your definitions to the definitions in the text. Change and highlight any of your definitions that are incorrect. Make flash cards for the terms you highlighted.

How Healthy Are You?

In this chapter, you will be learning about staying safe and preventing accidents and injuries. Before you begin reading, take the following quiz to assess your current safety and injury prevention habits.

Healthy Choices	Yes	No
Do you know the phone number for the Poison Control Center?		
Do you and your family have an established emergency evacuation plan in case of a fire?		
Do you and your family have a first-aid kit and other emergency supplies stored in your home and in any vehicles?		
Do you practice caution with strangers and get away from any stranger who makes you uncomfortable?		
Do you use the privacy settings on any social media accounts you have to protect your personal information?		
Do you take precautions as a pedestrian to make yourself visible and safe from getting hit by a car?		
Do you always wear a helmet when riding a bike and follow all traffic rules?		
Do you know what to do in the case of cuts, scrapes, severe bleeding, bites, stings, electrical shocks, and burns?		
Would you immediately call 911 if someone's breathing (including choking) or heart stopped?		

Count your "Yes" and "No" responses. The more "Yes" responses you have, the more healthy safety and injury prevention habits you exhibit. Now, take a closer look at the questions with which you responded "No." How can you make these habits part of your daily life? Identify a SMART goal you would like to achieve to help improve your overall health and well-being. Refer to Figure 1.11 to help you set up your SMART goal. If you do not understand the instructions, ask for clarification from your teacher.

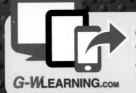

Click on the activity icon or visit www.g-wlearning.com/health to access online vocabulary activities using key terms from the chapter.

Promoting Safety in the Home

Key Terms

precautions actions you take to prevent something bad from happening

poisonous able to cause illness or death upon entering the body

fire triangle model to help you remember the elements that are needed for a fire to occur; elements include fuel, heat, and oxygen

flammable easily set on fire

extinguish put out

escape plan strategy that outlines safe routes and procedures for leaving the home in the event a fire occurs

emergency preparedness knowing how to respond to a specific type of emergency

natural disasters events or forces of nature that usually cause great damage

Learning Outcomes

After studying this lesson, you will be able to

- **give examples** of ways to prevent falls.
- **explain** how to prevent illness or injury from potentially hazardous products in the home.
- **describe** how the presence of weapons in the home increases the risk of serious injuries.
- **create** an escape plan for leaving your home in case of a fire.
- **develop** an emergency preparedness plan for your family.
- **identify** ways to remain safe when staying home alone.

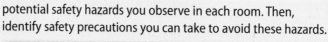

Graphic Organizer

Safety at Home

Before listening to your teacher present this lesson, draw or create a floor plan of the place you live to visually understand safety conditions in your home. An example floor plan is shown. Label each room and leave enough space to take notes. Throughout this lesson, list potential safety hazards you observe in each room. Then, identify safety precautions you can take to avoid these hazards.

Black Jack/Shutterstock.com

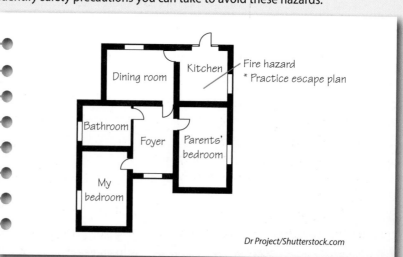

Dr Project/Shutterstock.com

Throughout her day, 13-year-old Jada may encounter unsafe situations. It is important for Jada to understand these potential situations and learn practices she can use to ensure her personal safety. For example, Jada and her family are very careful to avoid overloading electrical outlets. They regularly check smoke detectors and fire extinguishers to make sure they are working properly. They even have an escape plan in the event a fire occurs. Jada's family also stores various supplies such as flashlights and a first-aid kit in case of emergencies.

The safety practices Jada and her family take to prevent something bad from happening are known as **precautions**. Jada and her family take precautions to remain safe in their home. In this lesson, you will learn about simple safety precautions you and your family can take to protect yourselves from unsafe situations in the home.

Fall Prevention

Most falls people experience happen at home while doing regular daily activities. Some falls may be a result of hazards in the environment. Other falls may occur because someone takes risks, is not paying attention, or has a physical or medical condition. A simple fall can result in a broken bone, a head injury, or another medical condition.

One way to prevent falls is to reduce the risk in your home (**Figure 13.1**). You can also reduce your risk by avoiding dangerous activities and paying attention to your environment, both at home and in the community. Many falls occur because people text or use social media while walking. Distracted walking can also lead to a motor vehicle accident. Some communities issue tickets to people who text and walk.

Prevent Falls in the Home

- Clear the floor and stairs of clutter.
- Keep electrical cords and cables away from walkways.
- Cover slippery floors with nonslip rugs.
- Install handrails for stairs, in bathtubs, and near toilets for older adults.
- Use step stools or ladders to reach high cabinets or shelves.
- Ensure good lighting by replacing burned light bulbs and using night-lights.
- Repair or replace worn carpet edges and seams.

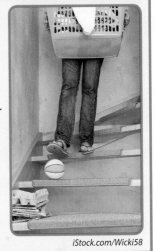

iStock.com/Wicki58

Figure 13.1 Activities and situations you encounter every day can cause falls. *What fall hazards are present in this photo?*

Poisoning Prevention

Many chemicals and natural substances are poisonous and can be hazardous if used incorrectly. A **poisonous** substance can cause illness or death upon entering the body. Poisonous substances around the home may include cleaning products, garden and yard products, automotive chemicals, gasoline, and carbon monoxide. *Carbon monoxide* is a toxic, odorless, invisible gas produced during the burning of gasoline, natural gas, oil, kerosene, charcoal, and other fuels. Examples of natural poisonous substances include some mushrooms and berries and mold. Understanding which substances are potentially hazardous can help prevent poisonings (**Figure 13.2**).

Figure 13.2

Some examples of poisons are mold, some mushrooms, cleaning supplies, fertilizers and pesticides, and chemicals such as gasoline and antifreeze. *Where might you find these poisons in a home?*

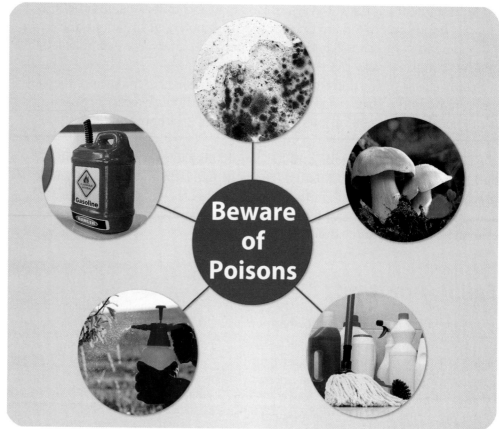

To prevent illness or injury from potentially hazardous products, read and follow label directions for safe use. Store all chemicals in original containers in a locked area that children and pets cannot access. When using a chemical, wear protective equipment required by the label directions. Unless you are certain about the safety of a plant or other natural substance, do not eat it. Dispose of chemicals as described on the label. If poisoning does occur, call the Poison Control Center (800-222-1222) immediately.

Weapons Safety

Your parent or guardian may keep a gun or other weapon in the home for hunting or personal safety. Weapons, however, can pose serious dangers to children and teens who find them. Accidents involving weapons can seriously injure or kill someone.

To help prevent accidents in homes that contain weapons, adults should keep guns and other weapons locked in a safe place that is out of reach of children. When storing a gun, adults should remove the ammunition (bullets) and keep it in another locked place away from the gun.

If you happen to see a weapon, leave the area without touching it. Find a trusted adult to tell right away. It is very important to report any weapon you find, as well as any person using or playing with the weapon. Also tell an adult if you hear anyone talking about using a weapon or see photos or messages about using a weapon online. These safety rules apply wherever you are (**Figure 13.3**).

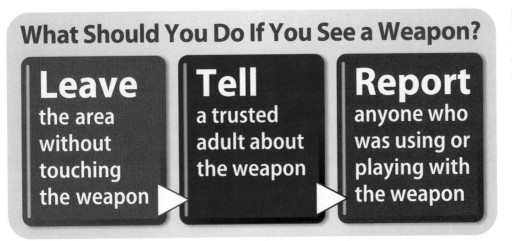

What Should You Do If You See a Weapon?

Leave the area without touching the weapon

Tell a trusted adult about the weapon

Report anyone who was using or playing with the weapon

Figure 13.3
If you see a weapon, you should follow these steps to ensure your safety and the safety of others.

Fire Prevention and Safety

A fire in the home is a dangerous emergency that can be deadly. Fortunately, there are steps you can take to help prevent a fire. If a fire does break out, you and your family need to know how to exit the home safely. The following steps can help you prevent fires and remain safe if one does occur:

- **Step 1.** Know how a fire starts by understanding the fire triangle.
- **Step 2.** Conduct a fire safety inspection within the home and address any concerns.
- **Step 3.** Have an escape plan in place and practice it so everyone knows what to do.

Understand the Fire Triangle

Before you can learn how to prevent a fire, you must know how a fire starts. There are three elements needed to start a fire. These elements include fuel, heat, and oxygen. The **fire triangle**, also known as the *combustion triangle*, is a model that can help you remember these elements (**Figure 13.4**). When fuel, heat, and oxygen are present in the right amounts, a chemical reaction occurs that can start a fire.

The fuel in the fire triangle refers to the material that is burning. Materials that are easily set on fire are **flammable**. Examples of flammable materials include wood, oils, paper, fabrics, and some liquids such as gasoline. When a heat source, such as a match, comes in contact with flammable materials, a fire starts. To stay burning, the fire needs oxygen.

To **extinguish** (put out) the fire, you need to remove one of the elements in the fire triangle. For example, putting a fire blanket over the flames will remove the oxygen from the fire and cause the fire to stop burning. When firefighters use water to put out the fire, they are removing the heat, which cools down the fire and extinguishes it.

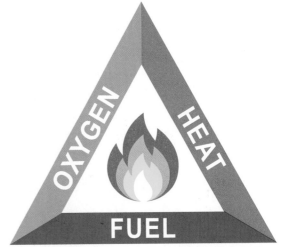

BALRedaan/Shutterstock.com

Figure 13.4 The fire triangle consists of the three elements needed to start a fire: fuel, heat, and oxygen. Knowing how to use a fire extinguisher can help you put out a fire.

Conduct a Fire Safety Inspection

Now that you understand how fires start, you can inspect your home using the fire safety inspection checklist in **Figure 13.5**. Using a checklist like that can help you make sure the environment is safe and no fire hazards are present. Properly installed smoke detectors on every level of the home, including the attic and basement, can reduce your risk of injury and death from fire. Smoke detectors should be installed outside all sleeping areas, in the kitchen, and near the furnace. Families should test smoke detectors monthly and replace the batteries at least yearly to make sure they are working properly.

Everyone in the family who is old enough should know the location of fire extinguishers in the home and learn how to use them. Fire extinguishers can control small fires and prevent them from causing damage or injury. A fire extinguisher should be available near the furnace, in the garage, and in the kitchen. There are different types of fire extinguishers, so be sure to check fire extinguisher labels carefully. Fire departments often provide training on how to properly use fire extinguishers.

Have an Escape Plan

A fire may break out in your home despite your best prevention efforts. This is why families should have an escape plan in place. An **escape plan** outlines safe routes and procedures for leaving the home in the event a fire occurs.

Because you never know where the fire may start, an escape plan should show two ways to exit each room of the home. If one exit becomes blocked or is too dangerous to pass through, you still have another way out.

Figure 13.5
Use this checklist to check for potential fire hazards in your home. Then, work with your parents or guardian to address any areas of concern that you note during your inspection.

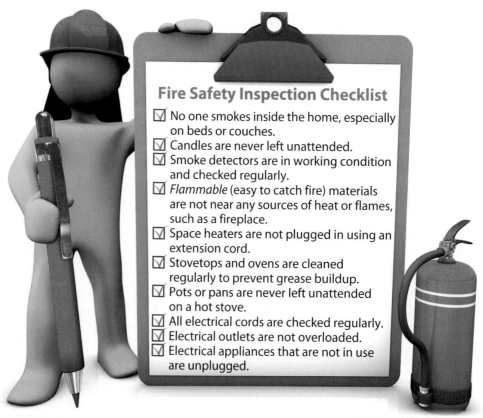

Fire Safety Inspection Checklist

☑ No one smokes inside the home, especially on beds or couches.
☑ Candles are never left unattended.
☑ Smoke detectors are in working condition and checked regularly.
☑ *Flammable* (easy to catch fire) materials are not near any sources of heat or flames, such as a fireplace.
☑ Space heaters are not plugged in using an extension cord.
☑ Stovetops and ovens are cleaned regularly to prevent grease buildup.
☑ Pots or pans are never left unattended on a hot stove.
☑ All electrical cords are checked regularly.
☑ Electrical outlets are not overloaded.
☑ Electrical appliances that are not in use are unplugged.

style-photography/Shutterstock.com

Part of the plan should identify who will assist babies and young children so everyone gets out safely. The plan should also include a place outside for all family members to meet once they are safely out of the home (Figure 13.6).

Once your family has an escape plan, arrange to practice the plan before a fire occurs. This way all family members can learn the plan without the stress of an actual emergency. The more you and your family practice, the more you increase your chances of everyone getting out of the home safely.

As your family practices the escape plan, make sure everyone knows how to respond to the sound of the smoke alarm. You may want to have a family member time how long it takes everyone to exit the home. As you leave the home, there are certain procedures you should follow to stay safe. These emergency evacuation procedures include the following:

- During a fire, feel doors with the back of your hand to determine if they are hot before opening them. If the door is hot, escape through a window. If you are trapped in a room, keep the door closed and signal or call for help.
- Check that all bedrooms in your home have a window that opens. Windows should be easy to unlock and open quickly.
- If you can, alert people in your home about the fire. Get out of the building and call 911 from a neighbor's home or a cell phone.
- Crawl near the floor to escape dangerous smoke, toxic fumes, and heat, which will rise toward the ceiling.
- If your clothing catches fire, stop, drop, and roll to put out the flames (Figure 13.7).
- Once outside, never reenter a burning building.

What Is in an Escape Plan?

EXIT

What are two ways to exit each room?

Who will assist babies and young children?

Where will we meet outside?

Top to bottom: Lester Balajadia/Shutterstock.com; Anna Baburkina/Shutterstock.com; motorolka/Shutterstock.com

Figure 13.6 An escape plan should answer the three questions shown here. *Why is it important to identify two ways to exit each room?*

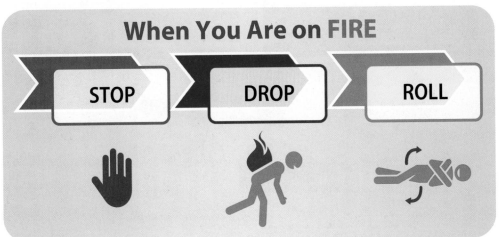

When You Are on FIRE

STOP **DROP** **ROLL**

Figure 13.7 Stop, drop, and roll if your clothing catches fire. Rolling will help smother the flames.

iStock.com/elenabs

Emergency Preparedness

In addition to a house fire, families should prepare for other types of disasters. **Emergency preparedness** involves knowing how to respond to a specific type of emergency.

Depending on where you live, you may experience one or more types of natural disasters. **Natural disasters** are events or forces of nature that usually cause great damage. Examples of natural disasters may include tornadoes, floods, hurricanes, earthquakes, and winter storms (**Figure 13.8**). Other emergencies may include power failure, landslide, wildfire, violent attacks, and terrorism. With some simple preparation and the appropriate supplies, you and your family can be ready to deal with natural disasters and other emergencies.

Most emergencies you might experience include similar challenges, such as exposure to the elements, loss of power, lack of sanitation, and lack of access to food or water. Planning for these is part of *emergency preparation.* In emergencies, people also need to communicate and receive emergency information. Doing so improves your chances of staying safe during a disaster.

Figure 13.8
Natural disasters can cause emergency situations and result in injuries, loss of power, exposure to the weather, and lack of food or water. *What natural disasters pose a risk to your community?*

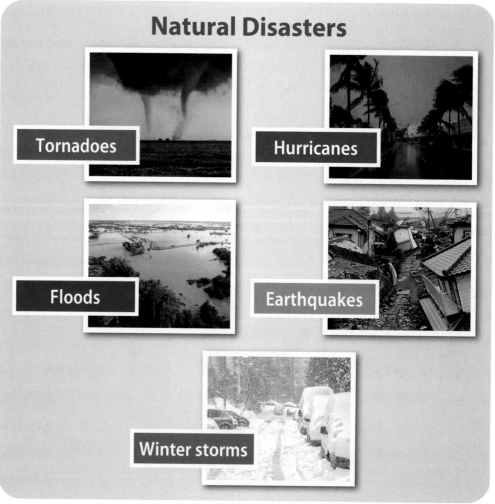

Natural Disasters

Tornadoes

Hurricanes

Floods

Earthquakes

Winter storms

Top row: Eugene R Thieszen/Shutterstock.com; Miami2you/Shutterstock.com; Middle row: wachira tasee/Shutterstock.com; austinding/Shutterstock.com; Bottom: Tainar/Shutterstock.com

Are You Prepared?

Tornadoes
- Take shelter in a safe, interior room with no windows on the lowest level of your home or below ground.
- Do not open windows.
- If outdoors, take cover in a vehicle or seek shelter in the nearest building.
- Do not hide under a bridge or overpass. You are safer in a low, flat area.

Hurricanes
- Build and store an emergency kit that can sustain you and your family for 3–5 days.
- Have an emergency plan in the case of evacuations.
- As a storm approaches, promptly follow instructions from public safety officials.

Winter Storms
- Stock up on food and water before the storm begins.
- Make sure you have a fully stocked first-aid kit.
- Stay indoors.

Earthquakes
- Practice "Drop, Cover, and Hold On."
- Stay indoors until the shaking stops.
- Cover your head.
- If outdoors, stay away from buildings, tall trees, and power lines.
- Move around as little as possible. Most earthquake injuries are from people moving around or falling.

Floods
- Move immediately to or stay on higher ground.
- Evacuate if directed.
- Avoid walking or driving through flood waters.

Keeping emergency supplies on hand can help you stay safe during many kinds of emergencies (**Figure 13.9**). Store emergency supplies in an easily accessible area of your home or car, and make sure everyone in your family knows where to find them.

After assembling emergency supplies, write an emergency plan. Different emergencies require different actions. Regardless of the type of emergency, an emergency plan should answer the following questions:

- Where will you take shelter during this emergency? For example, plan to go to a basement or a sturdy inner room, such as a bathroom, during a tornado. If you live in an area affected by hurricanes, know evacuation routes and shelters.
- How will you communicate with your family? Do you know how to reach a parent or guardian at work? Can you designate a contact person who lives outside of the area to relay information to all family members? How and where will you meet if family members are separated?
- Whom will you contact for emergency assistance, and how will you contact them? For example, know how to contact the police, fire department, and paramedics in an emergency.
- What supplies and equipment will you need to get through the emergency? Where will the supplies be located? What do you need to do to make sure these supplies are available?
- How will you learn when the danger has passed?

Figure 13.9
Emergency supplies may include a multi-tool or pocketknife, flashlights, masks, lanterns, matches, a first-aid kit, candles, nonperishable food, bottled water, a battery-powered radio, batteries, and blankets. *What other supplies could be helpful in an emergency?*

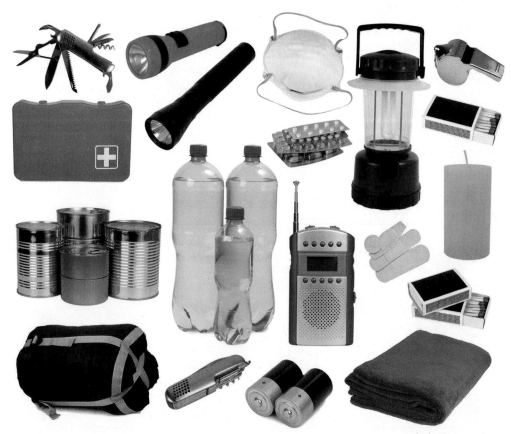

photka/Shutterstock.com

Safety When Home Alone

A major milestone occurs when parents or guardians decide that the young person is responsible enough to stay home alone for a short period of time. Some cities and states have laws indicating that children cannot be legally left home alone until they are at least 11 years old. Laws vary from state to state, however, and some responsible children may be able to stay home alone for short periods at an earlier age.

BUILDING Your Skills

Planning for an Emergency

Dangerous weather or a fire can cause an emergency quickly and unexpectedly. Having an emergency plan can help minimize the chaos and panic that accompany emergency situations and increase the chance of survival. An effective emergency plan should do the following:

- Identify a dangerous situation.
- List the needed emergency supplies and where they are located.
- Provide a detailed plan for responding to the emergency. The plan should answer questions such as the following: Where will you take shelter? With whom will you communicate (for example, family, friends, and emergency services)? How will you communicate? How will you know when the emergency has ended?

Write Your Family's Emergency Plan

Complete the first few steps of this activity with members of your family. After creating an emergency plan, share it with a partner, give feedback, and present it to the class. To create a family emergency plan, use the following steps:

1. With your family, consider the likelihood of the following dangerous situations: floods, tornadoes, hurricanes, winter storms, power failures, landslides, house fires, wildfires, earthquakes, and violent attacks. Choose two situations.

2. Refer to the information in this lesson and work with your family to create emergency plans for the two situations. Illustrate the emergency plans with pictures of emergency supplies and plan details.

3. Bring your emergency plan to class and share it with a partner. You should also review your partner's emergency plan. Exchange feedback and make changes or additions to your plans as needed.

4. Present your plans to the class.

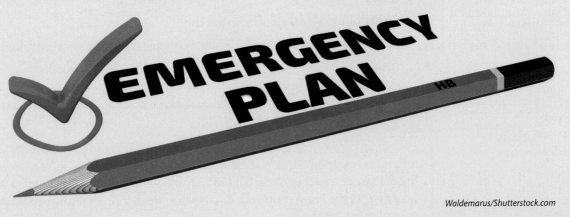

Waldemarus/Shutterstock.com

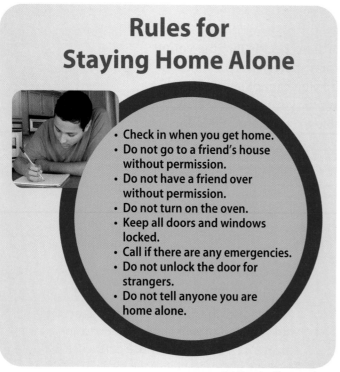

Rules for Staying Home Alone

- Check in when you get home.
- Do not go to a friend's house without permission.
- Do not have a friend over without permission.
- Do not turn on the oven.
- Keep all doors and windows locked.
- Call if there are any emergencies.
- Do not unlock the door for strangers.
- Do not tell anyone you are home alone.

Rob Marmion/Shutterstock.com

Figure 13.10 Some examples of rules for staying home alone are shown here. Marco's parents set these rules to keep Marco safe.

Your parents or guardian will probably set rules for you to follow when staying home alone (**Figure 13.10**). It is important that you follow these rules. The rules your parents or guardian set are meant to keep you safe and to prevent accidents from occurring. If you are staying home alone after school, your parent or guardian may expect you to call or text to check in as soon as you safely arrive home. Other rules may involve whether you can leave to go to a friend's house or whether you can have friends come over to visit. There may also be rules about whether you can do any cooking.

When you stay home alone, you need to know about fire safety, emergency preparedness, and first aid. You also need to know whom you can call if you need help. Other precautions you can take when staying home alone include making sure that all doors and windows are locked. Never unlock the door for strangers, including delivery people. Do not tell anyone on the phone or online (including social media), that you are home alone. Instead, say that your parent or guardian is home, but is busy. You will learn about other safety precautions in the next lesson.

Lesson 13.1 Review

1. Safety practices that you use to prevent something bad from happening are called _____.
2. Which of the following is a fall risk?
   - **A.** Good lighting.
   - **B.** Texting and walking.
   - **C.** Handrails.
   - **D.** Dry floor.
3. What should you do if a poisoning occurs?
4. **True or false.** When you are home alone, you should unlock the door for delivery people.
5. **Critical thinking.** How does the media portray dangerous situations, such as fire or explosives? Are these portrayals realistic or not? Explain.

Hands-On Activity

For this activity, sit down with your family and discuss the fire-prevention measures you and your family members already take. As a family, read aloud the fire inspection checklist in Figure 13.5 and review the family escape plan. Take five photos illustrating your family's fire-prevention measures and share your photos with the class.

Promoting Safety in the Community and Online

Learning Outcomes

After studying this lesson, you will be able to

- **describe** safety precautions you can take to stay safe at school.
- **give examples** of ways you can stay safe in public places.
- **demonstrate** how to protect your privacy and safety online.
- **explain** precautions you can take to stay safe on the road.
- **identify** ways to stay safe while participating in outdoor activities.

Key Terms

strangers people whom you do not know

digital footprint everything you share, access, or have shared about you online

digital citizenship taking responsible, healthy actions as part of the digital community

identity theft using people's personal information to pretend to be them, often for financial gain

Internet predators people who use personal information to find and harm people or violate their privacy

hackers people who illegally access data on digital devices

sext to send sexual content as digital text, a picture, or a video

pedestrians people on foot or using small wheels, such as bicycles, skateboards, or wheelchairs

Graphic Organizer

A Safe Day

In a table like the one shown, list your activities for each day. Include activities such as going to school, spending time on social media, and swimming. As you read this lesson, identify the risks associated with your daily activities. List precautions pertaining to each activity.

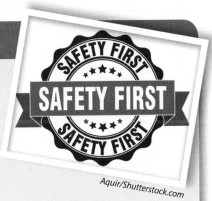

Aquir/Shutterstock.com

Day	Activities	Precautions
Monday	School Video-call with Beverley	Follow P.E. rules Ask permission to share our photo online
Tuesday		
Wednesday		
Thursday		
Friday		
Saturday		
Sunday		

Although your community is likely a safe place, it may also contain potential dangers. You may face hazards in familiar places, such as your school, or in unfamiliar public places. When doing outdoor activities, you need to know how to keep yourself safe. Being part of an online community also has risks you need to be aware of so you can protect yourself (**Figure 13.11**).

Remember in the first lesson how Jada's family takes precautions against emergencies. Jada extends these precautions into her community as well. She always wears her helmet when riding her bike and pays attention when crossing any street. Jada also spends a lot of time online. She uses the security and privacy settings on all of her profiles and she does not talk online to people she does not know.

When you encounter hazards within your community, you need to know how to respond. Luckily, in this lesson you will learn about certain precautions you can take to stay safe.

Staying Safe at School

Your school may feel like a very safe place, and it probably is safe most of the time. There are times, however, when you might encounter hazards, or dangers, at your school. Someone may try to start a fight with you. Another student may bring a weapon into the school. You may experience an injury during sports practice or physical education (P.E.) class.

Figure 13.11
It is important to engage in your community at school, in public, outdoors, and online. Keep in mind, however, that all of these settings have certain dangers. To keep yourself safe, you should know about these dangers and act safely.

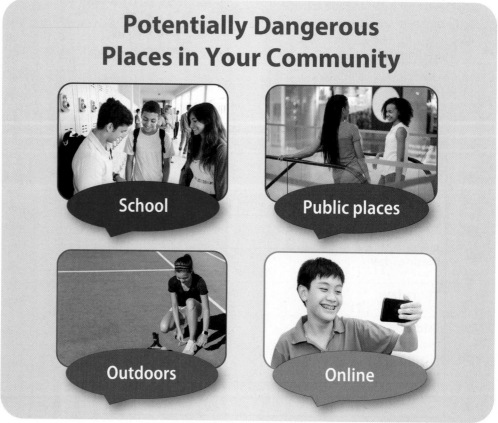

Potentially Dangerous Places in Your Community

School

Public places

Outdoors

Online

Top left to right: Monkey Business Images/Shutterstock.com; Mangostar/Shutterstock.com; Bottom left to right: Maridav/Shutterstock.com; Studio concept/Shutterstock.com

Schools have safety rules and procedures in place to protect you from school-related hazards. You have a responsibility to follow these safety rules and procedures whenever you are on school property. You also have a responsibility to alert school staff to unsafe conditions and emergencies that may exist, such as the presence of weapons. If you are uncomfortable about anything you see at school or during extracurricular activities, tell a teacher, counselor, dean, or school security officer (**Figure 13.12**). By alerting the appropriate staff to potential risks, you may be able to reduce the risk of an accident or injury occurring.

During sporting events and P.E. classes, follow rules to help protect your safety and the safety of other students. To reduce the risk of sports-related injuries, use safety equipment, such as helmets and kneepads, whenever necessary. Always be respectful of your fellow students and use gym equipment appropriately.

School personnel and family members can also play a role in keeping schools safe. Principals and school administrators set the rules you should follow at school. Teachers and family can reinforce these rules. Ultimately, however, you are responsible for keeping yourself and others safe at school.

Staying Safe in Public Places and Social Situations

As you get older, you may enjoy spending time with your friends in public places rather than staying at home. Your family may drop you off at the mall or the park to hang out with your friends. These are examples of public places, which include anywhere that is not your home or a friend's home. Spending time in social situations and public places like the mall can be fun, but dangers also exist.

When you are in public places, you are often around people you do not know. These people are **strangers**. Someone who is a stranger could be a danger to you. The rules in **Figure 13.13** can help you stay safe in public places and social situations.

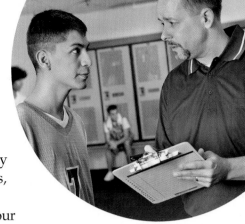

iStock.com/asiseeit

Figure 13.12
If you encounter a dangerous or uncomfortable situation at school, be sure to tell a trusted adult at the school. These adults have the responsibility to act on situations that put students at risk. *Should you tell trusted adults at school about unsafe situations during extracurricular activities? Why or why not?*

Figure 13.13
In public places, you will encounter many different types of people, including strangers who may be dangerous. It is important to take precautions to protect yourself before going out in public.

Staying Safe in Public Places

- Tell your parents or guardian where you are going, how you will get there, and when you will be home.
- Take identification and only enough money for your needs. Carry a charged cell phone to call for a ride or help.
- Travel in well-lit areas and with other people.
- Do not go anywhere with someone you do not know.
- If a stranger makes you or your friends uncomfortable, get away from the person and go tell a trusted adult.
- If a thief confronts you and wants your purse or phone, hand the items over without fighting.
- Leave situations where alcohol or drugs are present. Do not enter a vehicle with a driver who has been using drugs or alcohol.
- Do not accept food or drinks from other people in social situations. Get your own food and drinks and watch them to make sure others do not put anything else in them.

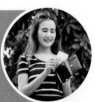
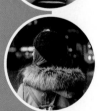
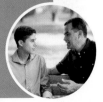

Top to bottom: iStock.com/Jillwt; iStock.com/finwal; iStock.com/Aldo Murillo

Staying Safe on the Internet

Using the Internet has many benefits. Communicating online takes seconds, and online communities can support and motivate people. People can use the Internet to find reliable information.

When you share a picture, post a message, or communicate with a friend online, these actions are recorded. Others can see what you shared. Your friend can look back at old messages at any time. Even if you delete a picture or post, people can still find it. All of these actions, even those you took a long time ago, make up your **digital footprint**.

Positive Online Behavior

Acting respectfully online is an important part of safety and your digital footprint. By engaging in positive online behaviors, you are practicing **digital citizenship**, or responsible, healthy actions as part of the digital community. Positive online behavior means acting respectfully and honestly by treating others well and not pretending to be someone else.

Another part of positive online behavior is following rules. You have probably seen some rules when joining a website. The website may have asked you to verify your age or agree to a set of rules about acceptable and unacceptable behavior. Pay attention to rules and do not try to get around them. Do not try to fake your age and do not violate rules by sharing content others created or posting violent material.

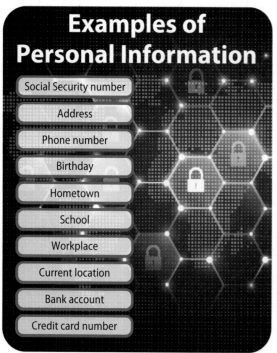

Examples of Personal Information

- Social Security number
- Address
- Phone number
- Birthday
- Hometown
- School
- Workplace
- Current location
- Bank account
- Credit card number

Pasko Maksim/Shutterstock.com

Figure 13.14 Keeping your personal information private keeps you safe.

Privacy

As you make friends and communicate online, you will probably share a lot of information about yourself. You will want to tell friends about your interests, activities, and plans.

Some personal information can make it possible for people to identify you or know where you are (**Figure 13.14**). This can lead to **identity theft** (when people use your personal information to pretend to be you). It can also put you in great danger from **Internet predators**, who use personal information to find and harm people or violate their privacy.

To protect yourself, use privacy settings, keep passwords private, and do not click on links or download apps from suspicious sources. Suspicious links and apps can expose your information to **hackers**, who illegally access data on digital devices.

Do not post any personal information online. If you want to post this kind of information, talk with a parent or guardian first. Avoid posting photos of your school, home, or other locations that could help someone find you. Avoid tagging yourself at certain locations or saying you will be at certain public events. In addition, always ask permission before sharing photos of another person.

When talking with people you met online, *never* share personal information or photographs or agree to video-call or meet. A video-call can help an Internet predator identify you. Meeting in person can put you at risk. If someone you met online asks for your personal information or asks to video-call or meet with you, leave the conversation and tell a trusted adult what happened.

Thinking Before You Post

When communicating online, consider whether you want everyone to see what you are saying now and in the future. Posts that promote bullying or illegal activity may become an issue when you apply for schools or jobs. Posts with sexual content can be shared with anyone and remain on the Internet for a long time. Before you post online, think about whether you will regret it later (**Figure 13.15**). If you are unsure, read your draft out loud or show the photo or video you are sharing to a trusted friend or adult. If you receive any message or see any content that makes you uncomfortable, tell a trusted adult immediately.

As young people learn more about themselves, they may be tempted to **sext**, or send sexual content in the form of actual text, pictures, or videos. Sexting has many potentially serious consequences.

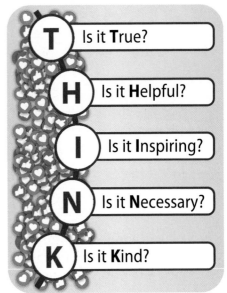

T — Is it **True**?

H — Is it **Helpful**?

I — Is it **Inspiring**?

N — Is it **Necessary**?

K — Is it **Kind**?

Alex Gontar/Shutterstock.com

Figure 13.15
Asking these questions before you post online can help you interact positively, respectfully, and honestly with others.

CASE STUDY

Brianna's Online Relationship

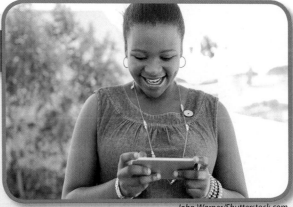

John Warner/Shutterstock.com

Now that Brianna is 13 years old, her parents are giving her more and more freedom. This year, Brianna's parents let her begin using social media, and according to Brianna, life is *finally* getting interesting. Brianna likes to send her friends funny pictures and follow their lives.

Last week, Brianna met a boy named James on social media. James lives in her city and messages her throughout the day. Brianna likes James and feels like he really understands her. She has told her friends about James, but has not told them everything because James wants to keep their relationship private. Brianna wants to tell her parents, but feels nervous.

Brianna decides that she will tell her parents after she meets James. After all, she may not like him when they meet. Brianna makes plans to meet James at the mall and tells her friend Addison about her plan. Addison tells Brianna that James sounds a bit weird, but Addison does not really know James. Brianna feels nervous just thinking about the day she and James will meet.

Thinking Critically

1. List the benefits and risks of Brianna meeting James in person.

2. If you were Addison, what advice would you give Brianna about talking with and meeting James? What should you do to help keep Brianna safe?

3. Are there any red flags that Brianna and James may not have a healthy relationship? If so, what are they?

4. If Brianna is going to meet James in person, how should she do so safely?

Staying Safe on Social Media

If someone sends you a photo that makes you uncomfortable or could embarrass, endanger, or harm another person, do not share it and let the person know.

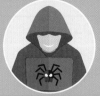

Do not open or click on suspicious e-mails, messages, or links. They can contain viruses that affect digital devices or allow hackers to illegally access personal data.

Only download applications and software from reliable, credible websites. Ask a trusted adult if you are unsure if a website is secure.

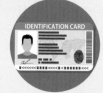

Be careful what personal information or revealing information you share online. You never know who will see it.

Adjust your privacy settings so only people you know and trust can see your posts.

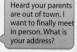

Never give your address or personal information to someone you have never met in real life. People may or may not be exactly who they say they are.

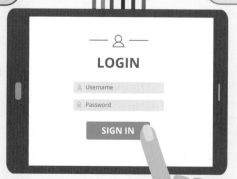

Group of teens: Lorelyn Medina/Shutterstock.com; Hacker: Fireofheart/Shutterstock.com; Download icon: Nobelus/Shutterstock.com; Identification card: BlueberryPie/Shutterstock.com; Lock icon: T-Kot/Shutterstock.com; Hand and tablet: Olga Lebedeva/Shutterstock.com

Legally, it can be seen as harassment and lead to serious consequences. Once sexual photos have been sent, they can be posted online or shared with others. If someone sends you a sext, do not share it with others. Immediately delete the sext and tell a trusted adult. If someone asks for a sext, use refusal skills to say *no*. Remember, if someone really cares about you, that person will not pressure you.

Staying Safe on the Road

Did you know that motor vehicle crashes are the leading cause of death among young people? In fact, motor vehicle crashes account for about 70 percent of the deaths associated with unintentional injuries. Many of these deaths occur among pedestrians involved in the accidents. **Pedestrians** are people on foot or using small wheels, such as bicycles, skateboards, or wheelchairs (**Figure 13.16**). To protect yourself and remain safe, there are certain precautions you can take as a pedestrian. You can also take precautions to stay safe while riding in a car or school bus.

Pedestrian Safety

On the road, pedestrians have the "right of way." This is the legal right of a pedestrian to move before a vehicle moves, in certain situations. For example, if a vehicle comes to a stop sign, and pedestrians are waiting at the corner, the pedestrians have the right of way to cross the street first. The driver must respect that right and allow the pedestrians to cross.

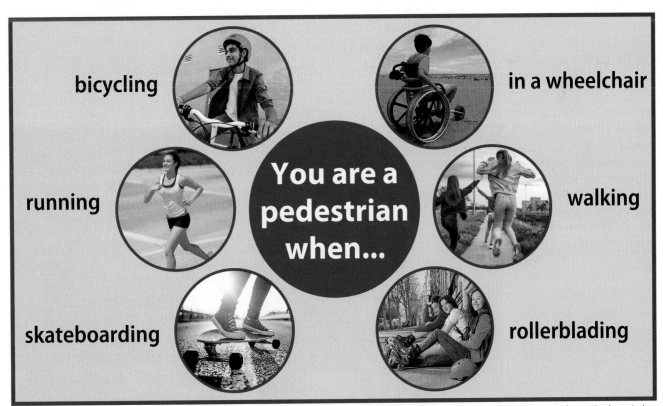

Clockwise from top left: iStock.com/kate_sept200; ChiccoDodiFC/Shutterstock.com; iStock.com/golero; Sergey Novikov/Shutterstock.com; kaca kaca/Shutterstock.com; iStock.com/nycshooter;

Figure 13.16 Whenever you go for a walk or a bike ride in your community, you are a pedestrian.

As a pedestrian, however, you also have responsibilities. These include the following:

- Always assume that drivers cannot see you. Drivers should stop for pedestrians, but that does not mean they always do.
- Walk where drivers would expect you to walk, which is on sidewalks, if possible.
- If walking on the road, always walk facing traffic, not in the direction of traffic.
- Make eye contact with drivers at intersections to make sure they see you.
- Obey all traffic signals and use specific crosswalk areas at intersections, where it is safer for you to cross.
- Pay attention to your surroundings (**Figure 13.17**). Distracted walking contributes to many pedestrian deaths each year.
- Wear proper safety equipment, such as a helmet, when skateboarding or rollerblading.
- If you must walk at night, wear bright clothing or carry a flashlight.

Riding a bicycle is an inexpensive form of transportation and a fun way to get physical activity. Use the following guidelines to remain safe while riding a bicycle:

- Always wear a properly fitted helmet.
- Know and obey all traffic rules.
- Ride on the right side of the road and with traffic, never facing traffic.
- Ride with friends in a single file.
- Signal your turns at intersections so drivers can anticipate your movements. With your left arm, point left to indicate a left turn and bend your forearm up to indicate a right turn.
- Always stop at red lights.
- Wear bright clothing during the day and reflective clothing at night.
- Use front and rear lights if riding after dark.

Figure 13.17
Paying attention to your surroundings will help keep you safe as a pedestrian. *Why should you make eye contact with drivers at intersections?*

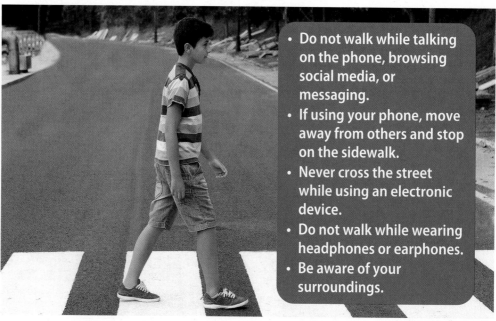

- Do not walk while talking on the phone, browsing social media, or messaging.
- If using your phone, move away from others and stop on the sidewalk.
- Never cross the street while using an electronic device.
- Do not walk while wearing headphones or earphones.
- Be aware of your surroundings.

Gelpi/Shutterstock.com

Vehicle Safety

Although you cannot drive yet, you probably spend a lot of time as a passenger in a car. The most important safety precaution you can take in the car is to wear a seat belt (**Figure 13.18**).

Another safety precaution you can take is to avoid distracting the driver. Any distractions in the car, such as noisy passengers, can make it difficult for the driver to concentrate. This increases the risk of an accident. Using a phone while driving is another distraction that can cause accidents. If you see the driver using the phone, ask the person to stop and pay attention to the road to stay safe.

Perhaps you take the school bus each morning and afternoon. If so, there are specific precautions to take when riding the school bus. Only get on the bus once the bus has stopped and the driver says it is safe. Always listen to instructions from the bus driver. Wear your seat belt if the bus has seat belts, and avoid distracting the bus driver.

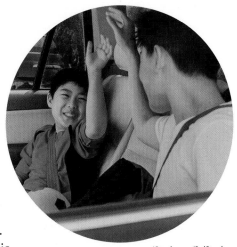

iStock.com/SolStock

Figure 13.18
When used properly, seat belts can reduce crash-related injuries and deaths by half.

Staying Safe in the Water

In the summer when the weather is hot, people often like to engage in water-related activities such as swimming in the local public swimming pool. Sailing, water-skiing, and spending time at the beach are also fun water-related activities (**Figure 13.19**). This means that water-related accidents can occur.

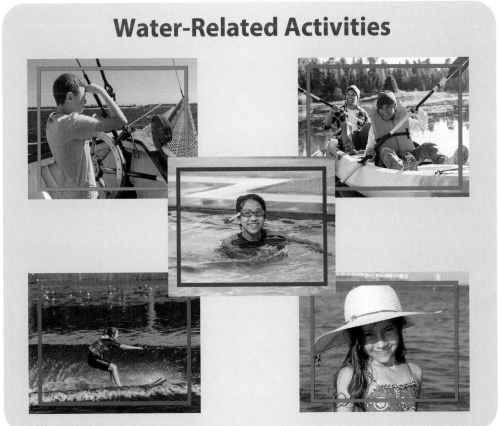

Water-Related Activities

Clockwise from top: iStock.com/arkanex; Monkey Business Images/Shutterstock.com; Katya Shut/Shutterstock.com; ChrisVanLennepPhoto/Shutterstock.com; photonewman/Shutterstock.com

Figure 13.19
Water-related activities are fun, but pose safety risks.

You can prevent accidents by learning and practicing the following water-safety tips:

- Never leave children alone in or near water of any kind—including ponds, lakes, swimming pools, and beaches—even when lifeguards are on duty. This also means never leaving children alone in bathtubs. A drowning can occur in minutes when someone stops paying attention or turns away.
- Teach children how to swim.
- Wear a life jacket when swimming.
- Never swim alone or in unsupervised areas.
- Do not dive in shallow water.
- Check the weather and avoid getting in the water if a storm is coming.
- Do not swim in a river after a storm because currents may be stronger.
- Check the water temperature and avoid swimming in really cold water.
- If you believe someone is drowning, call 911 or tell someone to call right away. The American Red Cross recommends that untrained rescuers avoid entering the water. Drowning people panic and may push you down. They can even drown you. Instead, rescuers should reach for the drowning person or throw a flotation device, life jacket, rope, or any object that will float.

Lesson 13.2 Review

1. You should tell your _____ if you see something that is unsafe or that makes you uncomfortable at school.

    A. friend   **C.** teacher

    B. sibling   **D.** classmates

2. Why is it unsafe to share personal information online?

3. When you are riding a bicycle, should you ride with traffic or facing traffic?

4. What should you do if you believe someone is drowning?

5. **Critical thinking.** Give some examples of messages, photos, or videos that would be inappropriate to share online. Explain why these examples are inappropriate and discuss the consequences of sharing them.

Hands-On Activity

Review the guidelines in this lesson for staying safe in a public place. Then, create a table like the one shown. Over the next three days, pay attention to safety mistakes you and others make in public. Identify at least five safety mistakes and list precautions to prevent them. Share your findings with the class. If you know the person who made the mistake, share the recommended precaution with that person.

Safety Mistake	Who Did It?	What Was the Risk?	Precautions

Knowing Basic First Aid

Learning Outcomes

After studying this lesson, you will be able to

- **identify** items needed in a first-aid kit.
- **describe** the three steps you should take after determining that you can help someone in need of first aid.
- **summarize** ways to provide treatment for various common injuries.
- **explain** what a medical emergency is and how you should respond to one.

Graphic Organizer

First-Aid Guidelines

Skim this lesson and find pictures or illustrations online of the injuries and emergencies described in this lesson. Arrange the images like in the example shown. As you read this lesson, take notes underneath each image to help comprehend the topics.

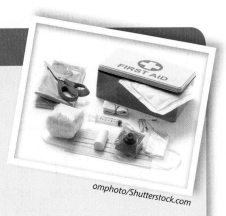

omphoto/Shutterstock.com

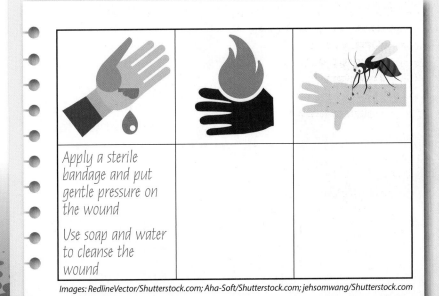

Apply a sterile bandage and put gentle pressure on the wound		
Use soap and water to cleanse the wound		

Images: RedlineVector/Shutterstock.com; Aha-Soft/Shutterstock.com; jehsomwang/Shutterstock.com

Key Terms

first aid treatment given in the first moments of an accident or injury—usually before medical professionals arrive on the scene

first-aid kit container that includes the supplies needed to treat most types of minor injuries

standard precautions infection control practices that apply when giving first aid to any person under any circumstances

anaphylaxis allergic response in which fluid fills the lungs and air passages narrow, restricting breathing

medical emergency urgent, life-threatening situation

cardiopulmonary resuscitation (CPR) emergency procedure that uses chest compressions to restore heartbeat; may also involve mouth-to-mouth breathing

automated external defibrillator (AED) rescue device that delivers a controlled, precise shock to the heart

Despite your best efforts to stay safe, accidents and injuries can still occur. When an accident or injury does happen, a person with first-aid skills can help the injured person. **First aid** is treatment given in the first moments of an accident or injury—usually before medical professionals arrive on the scene. First-aid skills allow you to provide treatment for a person while you are waiting for emergency medical professionals to arrive. The first aid given right after an injury occurs could actually help save a life.

Jada from the previous lessons takes first aid very seriously. She knows that professional organizations such as the American Red Cross and the American Heart Association offer basic first-aid certification classes. She takes these classes to learn how to administer first aid properly (**Figure 13.20**). Even before she took one of these classes, there were basic first-aid skills she had learned. This lesson will discuss some of those basic first-aid skills.

Keep a First-Aid Kit on Hand

To administer first aid, you need to have certain supplies on hand. A **first-aid kit** contains the supplies needed to treat many types of minor injuries. You can put together your own kit or purchase a ready-made kit at most drugstores or from the American Red Cross. The American Red Cross suggests keeping a first-aid kit in the home and in vehicles. When spending time doing outdoor activities, such as hiking or camping, it is a good idea to carry a first-aid kit with you. Keep the first-aid kit out of reach and out of sight of small children, and away from family pets. **Figure 13.21** shows supplies often included in a first-aid kit.

Figure 13.20
First-aid classes teach students the basics of delivering first aid.

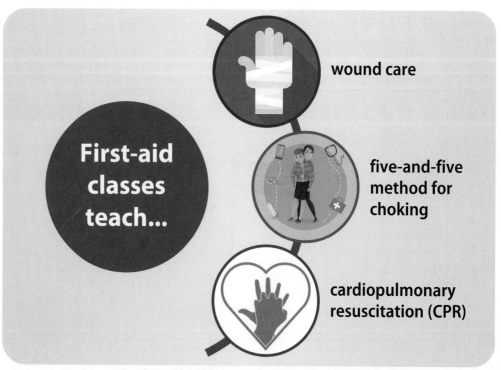

First-aid classes teach...

wound care

five-and-five method for choking

cardiopulmonary resuscitation (CPR)

Top to bottom: lukpedclub/Shutterstock.com; Macrovector/Shutterstock.com; Dzm1try/Shutterstock.com

First-Aid Kit Essentials

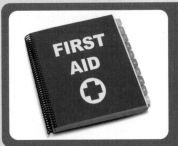

Resources
- First-aid manual
- Phone numbers for the Poison Control Center, family doctor, police department, and fire department

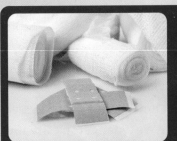

Supplies for Treating Wounds
- Gauze pads and assorted bandages
- Medical tape
- Cotton balls and cotton swabs
- Scissors

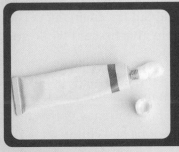

Supplies for Preventing Infections
- Antibiotic ointment (cream)
- Antiseptic wipes
- Hand sanitizer
- Disposable latex or synthetic gloves

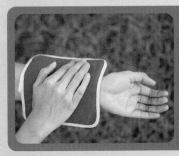

Supplies for Treating Various Injuries
- Elastic wrap
- Instant cold packs
- Tweezers
- Sterile eyedrops or eyewash solution
- Oral thermometer (nonmercury/nonglass)

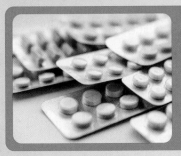

Over-the-Counter Medications
- Pain relievers such as ibuprofen or acetaminophen
- Hydrocortisone cream
- Antihistamine medications

Top to bottom: Mega Pixel/Shutterstock.com; Henrik Dolle/Shutterstock.com; nokwalai/Shutterstock.com; Chutima Chaochaiya/Shutterstock.com; DedMityay/Shutterstock.com

Figure 13.21
A first-aid kit should include the essentials shown here and any additional supplies you need for yourself or your family. *Where in your home should you keep a first-aid kit?*

Determine If You Can Help

Before administering any first aid, you need to check the scene to determine if you can safely help the injured person. If you cannot safely get to the person because of that person's location, or because of hazardous conditions, call 911 immediately. Do not risk becoming injured yourself. If you can remain safe and provide help, then stay calm and perform the following three steps:

1. **Check the injured person's condition.** Do a very quick assessment of the situation. Is the person awake and responsive, or is the person unresponsive? Does the injury appear to be life threatening? Signs of a life-threatening injury may include the following:

    - severe bleeding
    - labored or no breathing
    - *shock*—a life-threatening condition in which the vital organs do not receive enough blood and oxygen
    - unconsciousness—the person passes out and cannot be awakened

    Do not move the person unless you must leave a dangerous situation.

2. **Call 911.** As soon as you can, call 911 or your local emergency services, or tell someone else to call while you perform first aid (**Figure 13.22**). If you are at school, tell a teacher or coach about the emergency. These trusted adults may be able to call 911 or help give first aid while you call 911.

3. **Give first aid.** If possible, ask the injured person whether that person wants to receive first aid. This is called *obtaining consent*, and it is typically done for legal reasons. Under the law, you may perform first aid without consent if the person is unconscious or a child.

Figure 13.22
Communicating appropriately with 911 dispatchers can help them understand the situation better and get aid to you faster. *What should you tell a 911 dispatcher about the injured person?*

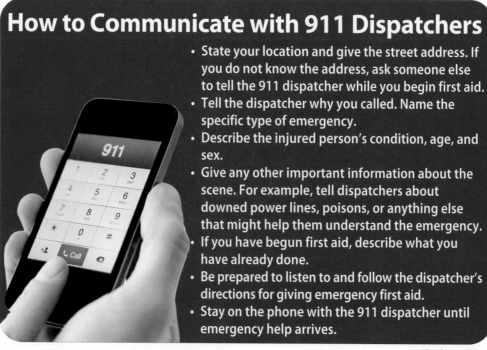

How to Communicate with 911 Dispatchers

- State your location and give the street address. If you do not know the address, ask someone else to tell the 911 dispatcher while you begin first aid.
- Tell the dispatcher why you called. Name the specific type of emergency.
- Describe the injured person's condition, age, and sex.
- Give any other important information about the scene. For example, tell dispatchers about downed power lines, poisons, or anything else that might help them understand the emergency.
- If you have begun first aid, describe what you have already done.
- Be prepared to listen to and follow the dispatcher's directions for giving emergency first aid.
- Stay on the phone with the 911 dispatcher until emergency help arrives.

iStock.com/TommL

Provide Treatment for Common Injuries

By learning and practicing first-aid skills, you will be able to remain calm, think clearly, and act rationally during the stress of helping an injured person. By studying Chapter 8, you have already learned how to treat sprains and know what to do if a bone becomes fractured or dislocated. In the following sections, you will learn about standard precautions and basic first-aid treatments for some other common injuries.

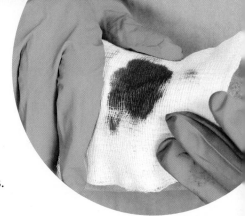

Joe Belanger/Shutterstock.com

Figure 13.23
Bodily fluids such as blood can contain pathogens. You cannot know if someone you are helping has a communicable disease.

Standard Precautions

A person giving first aid is often at risk for infection. This is because first-aid procedures often bring a person in contact with bodily fluids (**Figure 13.23**). People who perform first aid should follow standard precautions to protect themselves from infection.

Standard precautions are infection control practices based on universal precautions. Standard precautions were developed by the Centers for Disease Control and Prevention (CDC). Like universal precautions, standard precautions protect from bloodborne infections, such as HIV. Standard precautions, however, also protect from infections transmitted by respiratory droplets.

Standard precautions apply when giving first aid to any person under any circumstances. An example of a standard precaution is to wear protective gloves when there is a risk of contact with blood or bodily fluids that may contain blood. Washing hands with soap and water after giving first aid is another example of a standard precaution.

Cuts, Scrapes, and Puncture Wounds

A person who gets a minor cut or scrape often does not need to receive professional medical treatment. Some bleeding may occur, but the bleeding will often stop on its own. If the bleeding does not stop, follow the steps in **Figure 13.24**.

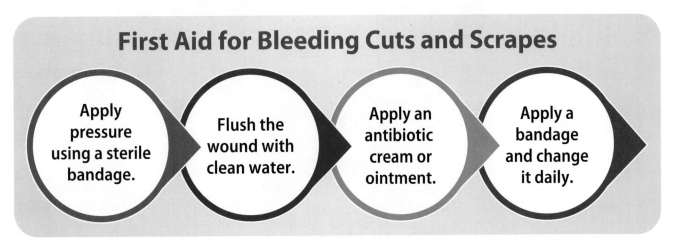

First Aid for Bleeding Cuts and Scrapes

Apply pressure using a sterile bandage. → **Flush the wound with clean water.** → **Apply an antibiotic cream or ointment.** → **Apply a bandage and change it daily.**

Figure 13.24 These steps can help you care for a cut or scrape that does not stop bleeding. If the cut is deep enough that it does not easily press together, however, you should seek medical attention. You should also seek medical attention if the bleeding does not stop after these steps. *Should you apply antibiotic ointment before or after flushing the wound?*

Deep cuts usually require stitches provided by a medical professional. A cut is considered deep if the edges of the cut do not easily press together when you apply gentle pressure. Some cuts are so deep that they expose the dermis or fatty tissue. People with deep cuts, scrapes, and puncture wounds may also need a vaccine to prevent *tetanus*, a serious bacterial infection associated with these types of wounds.

Puncture wounds—such as penetrating wounds from nails, thorns, or other sharp objects—usually bleed a small amount and appear to close up right away. The object that caused the puncture, however, can introduce bacteria deep into the tissues where it can become trapped and cause infections.

Severe Bleeding

The most important part of first aid for severe bleeding is the application of pressure to the wound. Other steps slow blood loss by careful positioning of the body. Following are steps to take when providing first aid to someone experiencing severe bleeding:

1. Apply pressure to wound using a sterile bandage, if possible.
2. Position the wound higher than the heart.
3. Continue applying pressure and cover the wound with gauze and bandages.
4. Keep the injured person calm.
5. Treat the injured person for shock (**Figure 13.25**).

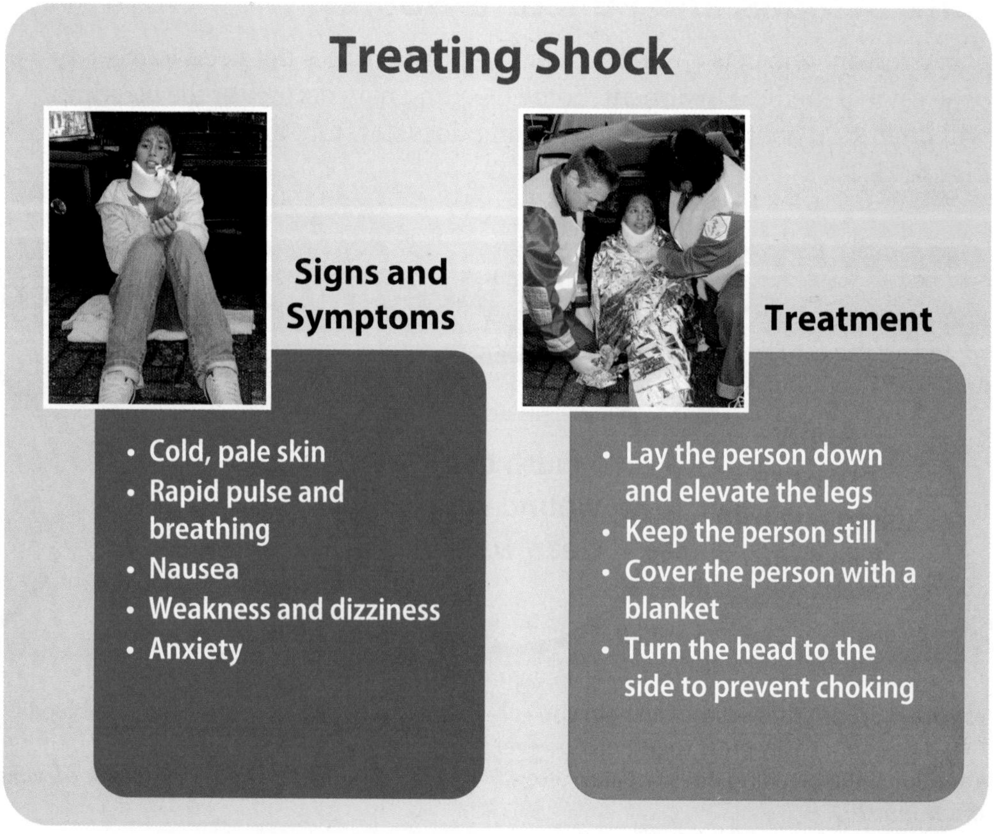
Treating Shock
Signs and Symptoms
• Cold, pale skin
• Rapid pulse and breathing
• Nausea
• Weakness and dizziness
• Anxiety
Treatment
• Lay the person down and elevate the legs
• Keep the person still
• Cover the person with a blanket
• Turn the head to the side to prevent choking

Anneka/Shutterstock.com

Figure 13.25
Shock is a life-threatening condition that can result from severe bleeding or trauma. Treating a person for shock can help the person stay calm and warm.

Bites and Stings

People may experience bites from domestic animals, such as dogs or cats. Wild animals, such as raccoons or snakes, may also bite people. Common biting and stinging insects include bees, wasps, mosquitoes, and some types of ants.

All animal bites require a doctor's attention. Bite wounds that break or puncture the skin carry the risk of infection. For example, the *rabies virus* infects the nerves, brain, and spinal cord. The disease is fatal if not treated immediately, before the virus reaches the brain and symptoms begin. Until you see the doctor, you can wash the bite wound with soap and water, cover it with a clean bandage, and elevate the affected area.

Mild reactions to insect bites are common, and often include swelling or itching at the site of the bite. Treat these reactions with cool cloths, calamine lotion, or over-the-counter hydrocortisone cream if the itching is severe.

More severe reactions are typically associated with stings from bees, wasps, yellow jackets, and fire ants. The venom of these insects triggers pain, swelling, and redness. Some people develop *hives*—a swollen, fluid-filled skin rash (**Figure 13.26**). Treat these stings with cold compresses or ice, pain reliever, elevation of the stung area, and rest. Use tweezers to remove any stingers stuck in the skin, wash the area, and apply hydrocortisone cream to relieve swelling and itching.

A few people experience an extremely severe, life-threatening allergic reaction to insect stings, called *anaphylaxis*. **Anaphylaxis** is an allergic response in which fluid fills the lungs and air passages narrow, restricting breathing. This type of reaction requires immediate emergency care or the person could die. People who have such severe allergic reactions often have medication such as the EpiPen® (**Figure 13.27**).

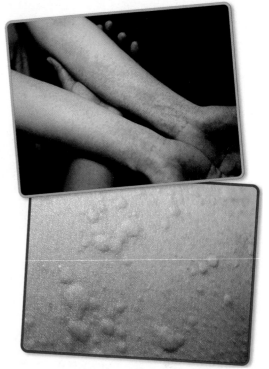

Chatchai.wa/Shutterstock.com; lpen/Shutterstock.com

Figure 13.26 Hives can break out in response to venom or as an allergic reaction.

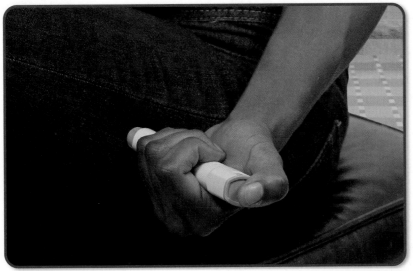

EpiPen® in use: Bob Byron/Shutterstock.com; Goodheart-Willcox Publisher

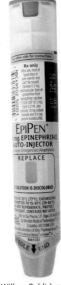

Figure 13.27 EpiPens® help treat allergic reactions and are important in emergency situations. *Why is anaphylaxis an emergency situation?*

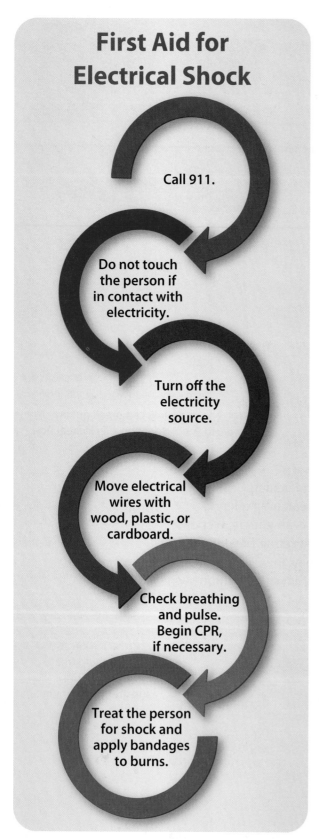

First Aid for Electrical Shock

Call 911.

Do not touch the person if in contact with electricity.

Turn off the electricity source.

Move electrical wires with wood, plastic, or cardboard.

Check breathing and pulse. Begin CPR, if necessary.

Treat the person for shock and apply bandages to burns.

Figure 13.28 These steps can help you care for someone after electrical shock. *When should you call 911 if someone experiences electrical shock?*

Electrical Shock

Electrical shock occurs when the body is in contact with an electrical current. The shock could come from fallen power lines or damaged or frayed cords or wiring. People also get shocked when standing in flooded streets or basements. In these situations, the water conducts electricity to the body from electrical wires, outlets, or downed power lines.

An electrical shock may cause burns, internal injuries, cardiac arrest, or even death. Use the first-aid steps in **Figure 13.28** to treat electrical shock while waiting for emergency medical help to arrive.

Burns

Burns are common injuries that range from mild to life threatening. Causes of a burn can include exposure to any source of heat and energy such as fire, burning or smoldering materials, steam, hot surfaces, or extremely hot gases and liquids. Chemicals, electric current, and the sun are also possible causes of burns.

All types of burns can seriously damage skin. Dangerous complications from burns include infection, shock, dehydration, pain, and immobility of the affected body part. First aid is essential for all burns. To give appropriate first aid, you need to identify whether the burn is a first-, second-, or third-degree burn (**Figure 13.29**).

Respond to Medical Emergencies

A **medical emergency** is an urgent, life-threatening situation. Examples of medical emergencies may include a person choking or requiring cardiopulmonary resuscitation (CPR). When medical emergencies such as these arise, call 911 right away. Then, follow emergency first-aid treatment. These medical emergencies require an immediate first-aid response. Otherwise, the injured person could die.

Types of Burns

First-Degree Burns	Second-Degree Burns	Third-Degree Burns
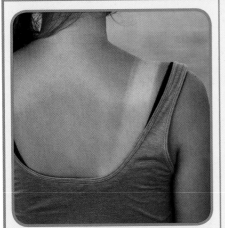	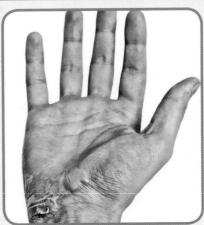	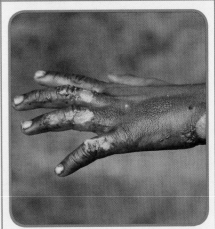
yurakrasil/Shutterstock.com	*nikkytok/Shutterstock.com*	*Naiyyer/Shutterstock.com*
• Damage only the outer layer of skin • Cause redness, swelling, and pain • Treatment includes holding the burned skin under cool water, covering the burn, and taking pain reliever	• Affect the second layer of skin • Cause blisters, redness, and swelling • Burns affecting less than 3 inches can be treated like first-degree burns • Burns affecting more than 3 inches are medical emergencies and should be treated like third-degree burns	• Affect all layers of skin and underlying tissue • Are medical emergencies • To respond, call 911 immediately and check the person's breathing and pulse, elevate the burned body part, cover the burn, and treat for shock until help arrives • Do not remove burned clothing or immerse burns in cool water

Figure 13.29 First-, second-, and third-degree burns require different care. *Which type of burn affects only the outer layer of skin?*

Choking

Choking is a medical emergency in which an object, such as a piece of food, blocks the airway. This means that a choking person cannot breathe. Choking may occur when people chew their food too quickly or when young children put objects in their mouths.

Many people instinctively grab their throats with both hands when they are choking, but there are other signs as well. If you know these signs, you can quickly recognize when someone is choking and provide help. The following are signs of choking:

- hand signals or pointing to throat
- wheezing
- inability to breathe normally
- inability to talk or make noise
- inability to cough or expel air forcefully
- passing out
- blue skin, lips, and nails

The American Red Cross recommends the *five-and-five method* for helping a person who is choking (**Figure 13.30**). This method involves a series of back blows alternating with abdominal thrusts, which force air out of the choking person's lungs. This should help push the stuck object out of the airway. Abdominal thrusts are also called the *Heimlich maneuver*.

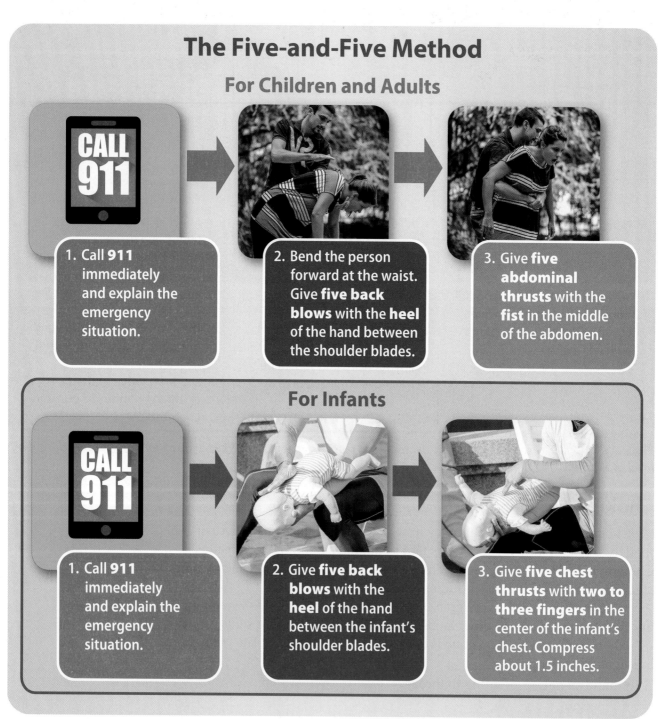

The Five-and-Five Method

For Children and Adults

CALL 911

1. Call **911** immediately and explain the emergency situation.

2. Bend the person forward at the waist. Give **five back blows** with the **heel** of the hand between the shoulder blades.

3. Give **five abdominal thrusts** with the **fist** in the middle of the abdomen.

For Infants

CALL 911

1. Call **911** immediately and explain the emergency situation.

2. Give **five back blows** with the **heel** of the hand between the infant's shoulder blades.

3. Give **five chest thrusts** with **two to three fingers** in the center of the infant's chest. Compress about 1.5 inches.

Top left to right: gst/Shutterstock.com; pixelaway/Shutterstock.com; Bottom: narin phapnam/Shutterstock.com

Figure 13.30 If a person is choking, use the five-and-five method to give aid. After you call 911, perform step 2 and step 3 and continue them, if necessary, until help arrives or until the person stops choking. ***Which part of your hand should you use to give back blows?***

Cardiopulmonary Resuscitation (CPR)

Your heart beats and your lungs breathe in air to keep you alive. Medical emergencies in which a person's heart stops beating or someone stops breathing are life threatening. In these situations, first aid and medical care must begin as soon as possible to restore breathing and heartbeat. The main technique used to restore breathing and heartbeat is cardiopulmonary resuscitation, or *CPR*.

Cardiopulmonary resuscitation (CPR) is an emergency procedure that uses chest compressions to restore heartbeat. Full CPR involves mouth-to-mouth breathing, or *rescue breaths*. *Hands-Only™ CPR* only involves chest compressions. The American Heart Association (AHA) and the American Red Cross recommend that rescuers use Hands-Only™ CPR for adults in most cases. This is because rescue breaths require training, and almost anyone can perform chest compressions without training. Hands-Only™ CPR delivers blood circulation to people who experience cardiac arrest. Cardiac arrest describes a condition in which the heart stops beating. **Figure 13.31** describes how to perform Hands-Only™ CPR for adults.

Do not slow down or stop performing CPR until emergency services arrive, or an **automated external defibrillator (AED)** is available and ready for use. This rescue device delivers a controlled, precise shock to the heart and gives automated instructions (**Figure 13.32**). An AED can restore a person's heartbeat after cardiac arrest. Hands-Only™ CPR and AEDs can be used even by people with little or no training.

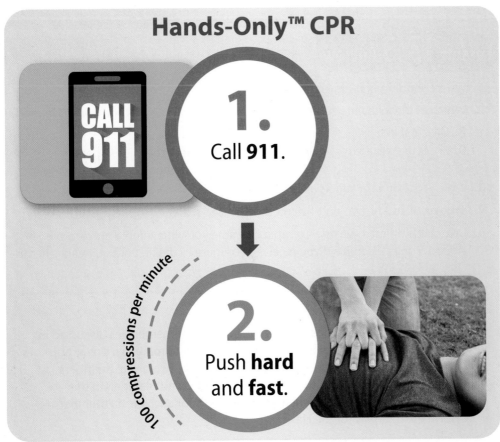

Hands-Only™ CPR

CALL 911

1. Call **911**.

100 compressions per minute

2. Push **hard** and **fast**.

Figure 13.31
Hands-Only™ CPR is used to help adults who are not breathing and whose hearts are not beating. To deliver 100 compressions per minute, you can push to the song "Stayin' Alive" by the Bee Gees.

Top to bottom: gst/Shutterstock.com; Sajee Rod/Shutterstock.com

Figure 13.32
An AED can be found in most public places. AEDs usually give automated instructions for their use. The steps for using an AED are listed here.

Using an Automated External Defibrillator (AED)

After calling 911, adults trained in using an AED can use the following steps if an infant, child, or adult is unconscious and not breathing. If the person is an infant or child, obtain parental consent, if possible.

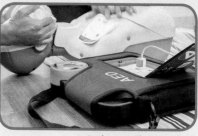

narin phapnam/Shutterstock.com

- **Step 1.** Turn on AED.
- **Step 2.** Wipe bare chest dry.
- **Step 3.** Attach pads.

For infants and children younger than eight years of age

Use *pediatric pads,* if possible. Place one pad on the upper-right side of the chest and the other pad on the left side of the chest. If the pads touch (because the infant or child is too small), place one pad in the middle of the chest and one pad in the middle of the back.

For children older than eight years of age and adults

Place one pad on the upper-right side of the chest and the other pad on the left side of the chest.

- **Step 4.** If necessary, plug in connector.
- **Step 5.** Tell everyone to stand clear.
- **Step 6.** Deliver shock.
- **Step 7.** Perform about five cycles of CPR.

Lesson **13.3** Review

1. Where should a first-aid kit be kept?
2. Which of the following should you do first when you see that someone is injured?
   - **A.** Give first aid.
   - **B.** Check the scene to make sure it is safe.
   - **C.** Call 911.
   - **D.** Check the injured person's condition.
3. Which type of burn affects all layers of the skin?
4. **True or false.** The five-and-five method is used to help people who are choking.
5. **Critical thinking.** Give one example of a time you were injured and received first aid. How does the first aid you received compare to the first-aid guidelines in this chapter?

Hands-On Activity

In groups of three, choose one of the injuries or emergencies discussed in this lesson and create a real-life scenario involving it to role-play. One group member should be the injured person, and the other two group members should respond correctly to the situation. Use items and materials in the classroom as first-aid equipment and write scripts for each group member. Perform the role-play for the class.

Summary

Lesson 13.1 Promoting Safety in the Home

- Falls are dangerous accidents. You can help prevent them by being aware and reducing fall risks in the environment.
- Poisonous substances include chemicals found outside and in the home, gasoline, and carbon monoxide. If a poisoning occurs, you should call the Poison Control Center immediately.
- All weapons should be kept in a locked safe place away from children. Ammunition should be stored separate from a gun.
- Knowing how fires start and being aware of fire hazards can help prevent fires. Your family should establish an escape plan in case a fire does occur.
- Emergency preparedness involves knowing how to respond to an emergency. You can prepare by gathering emergency supplies and making an emergency plan.
- Always follow your parents' or guardian's rules when home alone and do not open the door for strangers.

Lesson 13.2 Promoting Safety in the Community and Online

- Always follow safety rules at school. If you encounter unsafe or uncomfortable situations at school, you should tell a teacher, counselor, dean, or school security officer.
- In public places and social situations, pay attention to your surroundings and never go with or accept gifts from strangers.
- To remain safe online, never share your personal information or inappropriate content. Think before you post and use privacy settings. If you receive a message or photo online that makes you uncomfortable, tell a trusted adult.
- When walking on the road, walk facing traffic. When riding a bike on the road, ride with traffic. When in a vehicle, never distract the driver.
- To be safe in the water, swim only in supervised areas and do not dive in shallow water. If you see someone drowning, call 911 immediately.

Lesson 13.3 Knowing Basic First Aid

- Before giving first aid, always check the scene and check the injured person's condition. If the injury is life threatening, call 911. Follow standard precautions to prevent infection.
- Cuts, scrapes, and puncture wounds need to be cleaned and bandaged. If wounds are deep, they may require professional treatment or a vaccine. If wounds bleed severely, applying pressure and dressing the wound can help. All animal bites and some insect bites and stings require a doctor's attention. Electrical shock is always an emergency, as are third-degree burns. First- and second-degree burns that are minor can be treated with cool water, bandages, and pain reliever.
- You can use the five-and-five method when a person is choking. If a person's heart and breathing stop, performing Hands-Only™ CPR can save the person's life.

Check Your Knowledge

Record your answers to each of the following questions on a separate sheet of paper.

1. If you find a weapon in an unsecured area, what should you do?
2. **True or false.** During a fire, you should crawl on the floor to escape smoke.
3. What is emergency preparedness?
4. **True or false.** If a thief demands your phone, you should refuse to hand it over.
5. **True or false.** Deleting a photo online completely removes it from the Internet.
6. How should you signal that you are turning left when riding a bike?
   - **A.** Bending your forearm.
   - **B.** Pointing left.
   - **C.** Waving your left arm.
   - **D.** Veering left.
7. Which of the following is a good water-safety practice?
   - **A.** Diving in shallow water.
   - **B.** Wearing a life jacket.
   - **C.** Swimming in an unsupervised area.
   - **D.** Swimming in cold water.
8. Which of the following is a sign of a life-threatening injury?
   - **A.** Shock.
   - **B.** Minor bleeding.
   - **C.** Swelling.
   - **D.** Bruising.
9. How should you provide first aid to someone experiencing severe bleeding?
10. What happens during anaphylaxis?
11. When should you call 911 if you find someone who is *not* breathing and whose heart is *not* beating?
    - **A.** After giving five abdominal thrusts.
    - **B.** Immediately.
    - **C.** After giving one cycle of CPR.
    - **D.** After finding an AED.
12. What is Hands-Only™ CPR?

Use Your Vocabulary ↗

anaphylaxis
automated external
    defibrillator (AED)
cardiopulmonary
    resuscitation (CPR)
digital citizenship
digital footprint
emergency
    preparedness

escape plan
extinguish
fire triangle
first aid
first-aid kit
flammable
hackers
identity theft
Internet predators

medical emergency
natural disasters
pedestrians
poisonous
precautions
sext
standard precautions
strangers

13. Draw a cartoon for one of the terms above. Use the cartoon to express the meaning of the term. Share your cartoon with the class. Explain how the cartoon shows the meaning of the term.
14. Write a brief scene in which 5–10 terms from the chapter are used by medical professionals in a real-life context. Then rewrite the dialogue using simpler sentences and transitions, as though an adult were describing the same scene to a child. Read both scenes to the class and ask for feedback on whether the two scenes were appropriate for their different audiences.

Think Critically

15. **Cause and effect.** What are the consequences of being unprepared for an emergency? Give examples of consequences for at least three emergency situations.

16. **Draw conclusions.** In a small group, discuss whether a middle school student is old enough and responsible enough to stay home alone.

17. **Compare and contrast.** Compare and contrast a safe and unsafe school environment. Give examples of how the school environment can positively or negatively impact a middle school student's physical and emotional health.

18. **Identify.** What are some ways that middle school students can have fun on social media without putting their personal safety at risk?

DEVELOP Your Skills

19. **Healthy behaviors and communication skills.** Talk with your parents or guardian about expectations and rules for staying home alone. Create a *Guide to Staying Home Alone* that lists at least five safety rules for staying home alone. Use pictures or graphics to illustrate each rule and display your guide in a visible place in your home.

20. **Refusal and communication skills.** Imagine that you are flirting with someone you met on social media. You have been talking with this person for three weeks and enjoy your online relationship. One day, this person sends the following message to you. How would you respond to protect your personal safety?

> You are amazing. Tell me more about yourself. I want to know everything about you.

21. **Decision-making skills.** Imagine that you are seeing a movie with two friends. The movie is not very good, so you and your friends decide to walk to the mall 10 blocks away. To save time, your friends plan to walk behind buildings and on side streets. When you reach the lobby of the theater, however, you notice how dark it is outside. List the pros and cons of each decision you could make and write a summary describing the pros and cons, safety risks and precautions, and what you would do.

22. **Advocacy skills.** Think about the personal safety threats that endanger students in your school and create a personal safety flyer highlighting one safety threat. Include at least five safety tips related to the threat and at least two pictures to support your content. If you have permission, hang your flyer on a wall in your school.

23. **Teamwork and technology skills.** In a team of three, review Lesson 13.3 on basic first aid. Choose three common injuries and/or medical emergencies. With your team, create three short video clips reenacting the injury or medical emergency and demonstrating effective response and first aid. While demonstrating effective response and first aid, verbally communicate these steps in the video. Also include information about where students can receive valid information and training in this type of first aid. Present your videos to the class and adapt your vocabulary as needed to respond to questions and clarify information.

Chapter 14

Protecting Environmental Health

Essential Question

How is your health influenced by the environment in which you live?

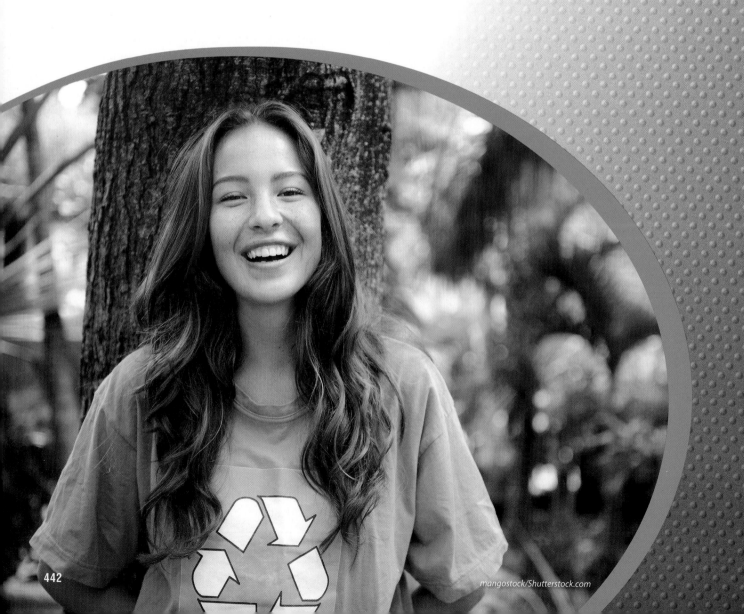

mangostock/Shutterstock.com

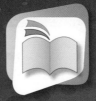

Reading Activity

Write the Learning Outcomes for this chapter on a piece of paper. Then, beneath each outcome, rewrite it as a question. While reading the chapter, take notes about information relating to these outcomes. After reading, refer to your notes and write two or three sentences answering each outcome's question.

How Healthy Are You?

In this chapter, you will be learning about environmental health. Before you begin reading, take the following quiz to assess your current environmental health habits.

Healthy Choices	Yes	No
Do you know how to properly dispose of products that contain chemicals and pollutants?		
Do you know what to do if you or someone you know has been in contact with a harmful substance?		
Do you know what the symbols on packages of chemicals mean? Do you make sure to read warning labels carefully before using or storing chemicals?		
Do you limit your exposure to high levels of noise, such as through headphones?		
Do you use a reusable bottle instead of disposable plastic bottles?		
Do you reduce the amount of energy you use by turning off the lights when you leave a room or by turning off the water while you brush your teeth?		
Do you recycle items made from paper, aluminum, glass, or plastic?		
Do you safely dispose of hazardous materials such as aerosol cans, batteries, or medical waste?		
Do you use energy-efficient, green, and biodegradable products as much as possible?		
Do you do your best to reuse materials or make green choices away from home and on the road, as well as in your home?		

Count your "Yes" and "No" responses. The more "Yes" responses you have, the more healthy environmental habits you exhibit. Now, take a closer look at the questions with which you responded "No." How can you make these healthy habits part of your daily life? Identify a SMART goal you would like to achieve to help improve your overall health and well-being. Refer to Figure 1.11 to help you set up your SMART goal. If you do not understand the instructions, ask for clarification from your teacher.

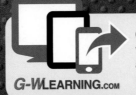

Click on the activity icon or visit www.g-wlearning.com/health to access online vocabulary activities using key terms from the chapter.

Common Hazards in the Environment

Learning Outcomes

After studying this lesson, you will be able to

- **describe** different types of air pollution and their effects.
- **assess** causes of water pollution and ways to keep water safe.
- **identify** types of chemicals that are harmful to health and the environment.
- **explain** how to handle chemicals safely.
- **recognize** the health dangers of noise pollution and how to avoid them.

Graphic Organizer

Pollution Basics

Find or take photos that illustrate the following types of pollution: air pollution, water pollution, chemicals, and noise pollution. Under each photo, draw two circles labeled *Sources* and *Effects*. An example is shown. As you read this lesson, identify the sources and effects of the different types of pollution. Write them next to the appropriate circles.

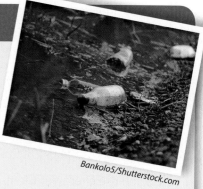

Bankolo5/Shutterstock.com

Sources — Effects
Sources — Effects
Sources — Effects
Sources — Effects

Left to right, top to bottom: cubicidea/Shutterstock.com; Mjosedesign/Shutterstock.com; Makc/Shutterstock.com; grmarc/Shutterstock.com

Ten-year-old Diego lives in a city with his family, and he has experienced more than a few hazards in his home environment. He can visibly see and smell the smog from cars. Even indoors, Diego inhales tobacco smoke and dust. Diego has asthma and has had a hard time breathing lately, even when he is not having an asthma attack. To improve Diego's health and wellness, Diego's parents have started to discuss moving to an area with cleaner air and less pollution. Air pollution is one of a few hazards in your environment that will be covered in this lesson.

The Environment

When you think about health, you probably think about the actions you take to stay healthy. How and when you get physical activity, the food you eat, and how much sleep you get all have important effects on your health. Your health is also influenced by the environment in which you live, however.

Humans all live on planet Earth and depend on the planet's resources, such as water, animals, trees, air, other plants, and fossil fuels. How people use these resources affects the environment, which then influences people's health (**Figure 14.1**).

Humans and the Environment Affect Each Other

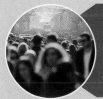
Population
As the human population grows, people use more resources and produce more waste. This can lead to shortages in food and water.

Waste Management
Communities may store waste in landfills, which have limited storage. Suitable land for landfills becomes hard to find.

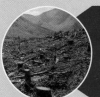
Deforestation
People use wood for power, construction, and other purposes. Consuming wood can lead to deforestation, which reduces the benefit trees have on the environment.

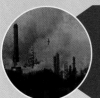
Greenhouse Gases
Activities that release greenhouse gases like carbon dioxide and methane contribute to rising temperatures, which worsen weather conditions.

Figure 14.1
These are a few examples of how humans and the environment affect each other.

Top to bottom: dotshock/Shutterstock.com; vchal/Shutterstock.com; Marten_House/Shutterstock.com; Susan Santa Maria/Shutterstock.com

Unfortunately, people do not always treat their environment with the care it deserves. Human activities can harm the environment and negatively affect people's health. This harm can lead to hazards like air pollution, water pollution, and chemical pollution.

The field of *environmental health* examines how factors in the natural environment, such as air, water, and soil, impact your health. Environmental factors also include spaces made by people, such as homes, apartments, schools, and offices.

Air Pollution

Humans survive by breathing in air. Air contains oxygen, which people need to survive. Air also contains other gases, including nitrogen, argon, and carbon dioxide. Sometimes, air contains other substances, known as **pollutants**, which contaminate the environment and can harm people.

Outdoor Air Pollution

The air outside is influenced by natural forces in the environment. For example, a wildfire releases smoke and carbon monoxide into the air. A volcanic eruption releases carbon dioxide, sulfur dioxide, and other chemicals, as well as ash (**Figure 14.2**). Wind currents can carry these pollutants for thousands of miles.

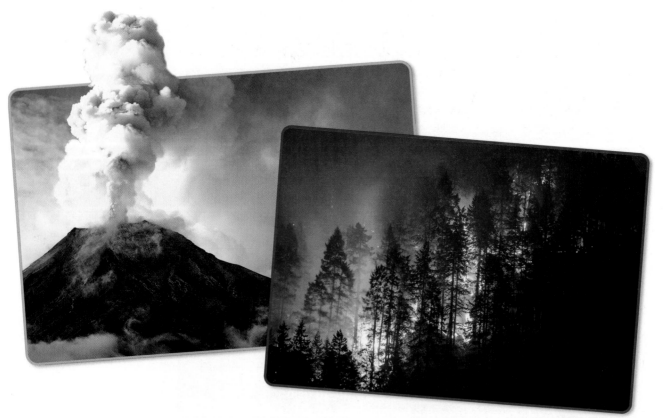

Kali Guerra/Shutterstock.com; Christian Roberts-Olsen/Shutterstock.com

Figure 14.2 Volcanic eruptions and wildfires release pollutants into the air. Wind can carry these pollutants for miles. *What pollutants does a volcanic eruption release?*

The air outside is also affected by human activity. You might have seen pictures of smog hanging over a big city. **Smog** is a fog that has mixed with smoke and chemical fumes (**Figure 14.3**). Car exhaust is a major cause of smog in cities. The burning of coal, oil, and gas to power cars and produce electricity also pollutes the air. Even tractors on farms create dust clouds when plowing the fields.

When polluting gases are released into the air, they mix with water, oxygen, and other chemicals to form acids. These acids then fall to the ground as rain, snow, hail, fog, or even dust. Any form of precipitation that includes particles containing acid is known as **acid rain**.

Another source of air pollution is *particulate matter*, which is made up of tiny particles and drops of liquid. These tiny particles and liquids that float in the air can include chemicals, metals, and dust. Some particulate matter is natural. One example is pollen from flowers and trees carried on the wind. Particulate matter can also be created by human actions, such as cooking on a grill or burning fuel in a power plant.

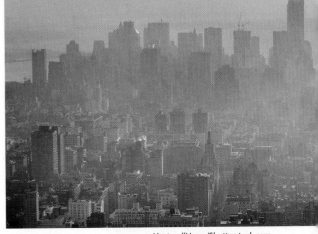

Venturelli Luca/Shutterstock.com

Figure 14.3 Smog sometimes hangs over densely populated areas such as cities. *What are the components of smog?*

Indoor Air Pollution

Indoor air can also contain pollutants. Indoor pollution can be caused by many different factors (**Figure 14.4**). Some of these pollutants can be seen or smelled. For example, you can see smoke from cigarettes and smell some cleaning products.

Mold can be seen growing in wet places and can cause respiratory diseases and infections. The natural mineral asbestos can release cancer-causing fibers. Scented products such as candles and perfumes release chemicals that can irritate the eyes, nose, and throat.

Other types of pollutants have no odor and are so small that you cannot see them. For example, very tiny bugs, called *dust mites*, are one of the most common causes of indoor air pollution. Dust mites live in mattresses, upholstered furniture, rugs, or curtains. Their bodies and waste matter can trigger allergic reactions and asthma in humans.

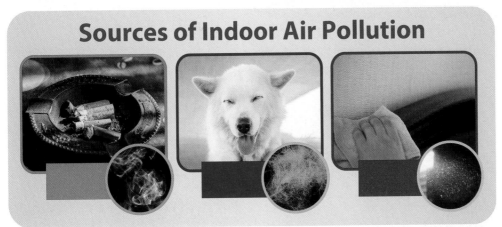

Sources of Indoor Air Pollution

Left to right: Greentellect Studio/Shutterstock.com; bstecko/Shutterstock.com; narin phapnam/Shutterstock.com; February_Love/Shutterstock.com; Evg Zhul/Shutterstock.com; struvictory/Shutterstock.com

Figure 14.4 Tobacco smoke, pet dander, and dust are three substances that can pollute the air indoors. Paint and cleaning products are other sources of indoor air pollution.

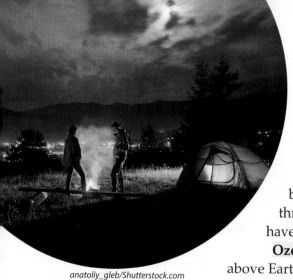

Figure 14.5
Particulate matter, such as the particles found in smoke from a campfire, can irritate the eyes, nose, and throat.

Effects of Air Pollution

Breathing in pollutants can cause health conditions. In some cases, it can cause very serious conditions, such as cancer and heart disease. Air pollution can also make current health conditions worse. For example, smog can make it very difficult for people with respiratory disease to breathe.

Particulate matter can get into people's lungs and bloodstream. Larger particles can irritate the eyes, nose, and throat. You have probably experienced this type of irritation if you have sat close to a charcoal grill or beside a campfire (**Figure 14.5**).

Ozone is a gas made up of oxygen that naturally exists high above Earth's atmosphere. It helps protect people from the damaging ultraviolet (UV) rays produced by the sun. Some kinds of air pollution caused by humans can damage this ozone layer, which increases the amount of UV rays reaching Earth. UV rays can cause skin cancer. Too much UV radiation may also damage plants, including crops grown for food. Ozone poses other dangers, too. Ozone close to the ground can cause respiratory conditions and environmental harm. Ground-level ozone is usually caused by chemical reactions between different pollutants in the air.

Air pollution also has an effect on Earth's climate. Earth's atmosphere is made up of different gases, including nitrogen, oxygen, and carbon dioxide. These *greenhouse gases* trap the energy produced by the sun, which warms Earth. As a result, Earth maintains a balanced and stable temperature over time.

When these gases build up in the atmosphere, however, they trap more heat near the surface of Earth. The effects of this buildup can change climates around the world. Many scientists have concluded that the buildup of gases released by burning fuels to produce energy has resulted in climate change. Climate change can lead to shifts in weather patterns. These changes can lead to more major disasters, such as hurricanes, heat waves, droughts, and floods. Scientists also warn that rising temperatures will melt ice on Earth's surface. This melting ice can raise sea levels and threaten flooding in coastal areas (**Figure 14.6**).

Figure 14.6
The buildup of gases in Earth's atmosphere may lead to rising temperatures, which could melt ice on the planet's surface.

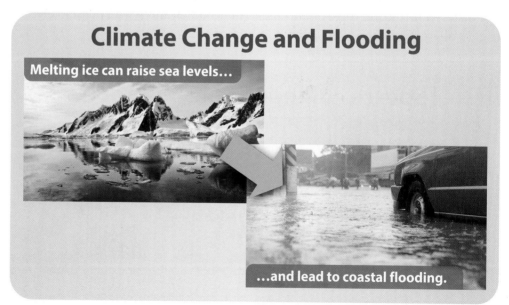

Climate Change and Flooding

Melting ice can raise sea levels...

...and lead to coastal flooding.

Water Pollution

Humans need water to drink in order to survive. More than two-thirds of Earth's surface is covered by water, but most of this water is in the ocean. People cannot use salty ocean water for drinking. They need freshwater for drinking.

Only about three percent of the water on Earth is freshwater. Most of this freshwater is frozen in the polar ice caps and glaciers. This leaves only about one percent of the water on Earth available to use as drinking water. Usable sources of freshwater are found in lakes, rivers, and reservoirs. There is also freshwater inside Earth. These combined sources provide the freshwater needed for farms, homes, businesses, factories, and communities. Unfortunately, if this water becomes polluted, it is no longer safe for humans to drink.

A number of factors can pollute the water. Water can be polluted by human-made products, such as chemicals and pollutants, but also by natural disasters.

Human Causes of Water Pollution

The products that people use in their daily lives can end up in the water supply. When rain or melted snow is not absorbed on Earth's surface, it becomes runoff, travels over the ground, and picks up loose soil and pollutants (**Figure 14.7**). These pollutants can include the following:

- pesticides and fertilizers from lawns and fields
- oil, grease, and chemicals from cars, trucks, and other vehicles
- metals and chemicals from factories and construction sites
- animal waste from agriculture

Runoff travels to bodies of water, such as ponds, lakes, streams, and rivers. People can then use it for washing food, bathing, or drinking. Exposure to chemicals and pollutants through these activities can make people sick (**Figure 14.8**).

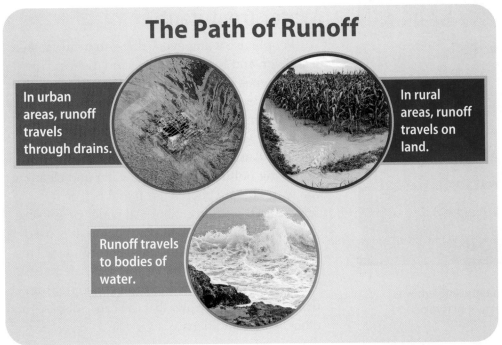

The Path of Runoff

In urban areas, runoff travels through drains.

In rural areas, runoff travels on land.

Runoff travels to bodies of water.

Figure 14.7
Rain or melted snow that is not absorbed on Earth's surface becomes runoff. In urban areas, runoff travels through drains. In rural areas, runoff travels on land. In both situations, runoff can pick up pollutants before reaching bodies of water.

Left to right: PowerUp/Shutterstock.com; michael sheehan/Shutterstock.com; NokHoOkNoi/Shutterstock.com

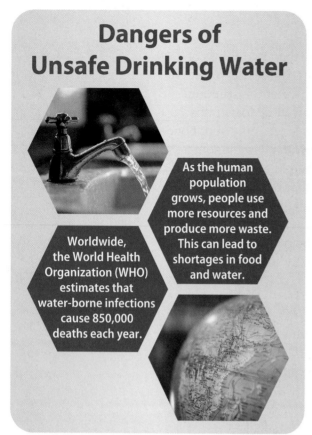

Dangers of Unsafe Drinking Water

As the human population grows, people use more resources and produce more waste. This can lead to shortages in food and water.

Worldwide, the World Health Organization (WHO) estimates that water-borne infections cause 850,000 deaths each year.

Top to bottom: BeautifulPicture/Shutterstock.com; Aris Suwanmalee/Shutterstock.com

Figure 14.8 In many parts of the world, safe drinking water is hard to find. Drinking unsafe water can have serious health consequences.

Water pollution can also occur when people do not properly dispose of products containing chemicals and pollutants. These products include paint cans, some batteries, and medicines. There are special rules for disposing of these products to help prevent water pollution. Sometimes, however, people do not know these rules or do not follow them.

Natural Causes of Water Pollution

Major natural disasters, such as hurricanes, typhoons, and earthquakes, can cause water pollution. During hurricanes and floods, pollutants that are usually stored in landfills or other disposal areas are swept into waterways. Examples are raw sewage, fertilizers, chemicals, and oil. Earthquakes can trigger tsunamis, or tidal waves, which flood an area with saltwater. This water can destroy farmland and crops.

Tiny organisms, such as bacteria, viruses, and parasites, can live in the water supply. Even though you cannot see these organisms, drinking water that contains them can make people sick. In the case of a disaster, the water supply of a whole town or area can be dirtied. In some cases, people can even die from drinking this water.

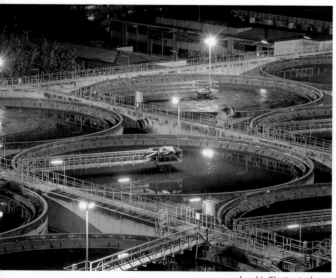

arhendrix/Shutterstock.com

Figure 14.9 A water treatment plant removes pollutants from water and cleans it before people drink it.

Water Treatment

People use water every day—to drink, to take a shower, and to wash clothes and dishes. This water comes from natural bodies of water, such as streams, ponds, and rivers.

Drinking water in the United States is treated in a water treatment plant. This process takes between 8 and 16 hours. The process involves removing pollutants from the water and cleaning the water before people use it and before it returns to the environment. All water people use goes through a treatment plant before it is used in homes, farms, or industries (**Figure 14.9**). This water is also tested to make sure it is safe to use. This process is designed to protect people from drinking polluted water that can cause diseases and other health conditions.

Chemicals

Chemicals are substances that have specific properties or characteristics. Some chemicals are found in nature. For example, vitamin C (ascorbic acid) is a chemical naturally found in some fruits. Other chemicals are made by people. For example, aspirin (acetylsalicylic acid) is a chemical made by people from substances found in tree bark. People use chemicals every day, in many different ways. You are exposed to chemicals through items you eat and drink, but also through the air you breathe and even through the objects you touch.

Types of Chemicals

Many chemicals are safe for people to use, at least in reasonable amounts. Minerals, such as iron, are naturally occurring chemicals that your body needs to stay healthy. Some kinds of chemicals, however, are *toxic*. This means people can get sick from coming into contact with these chemicals by touching them, eating or drinking something that contains them, or inhaling them (**Figure 14.10**). It is important to know what these chemicals are and where they are found so you can be safe. These chemicals include the following:

- **Mercury.** Mercury is found in fish and household products such as batteries, paint, glass thermometers, and compact fluorescent light bulbs. Eating fish with high levels of mercury and disposing of mercury-containing products inappropriately can have harmful effects. Natural events, such as forest fires, and the burning of fossil fuels can also release mercury into the air.
- **Lead.** Lead was used in household products such as paint, gasoline, and pesticides before 1978. It was used in water pipes before 1986. Exposure to lead-based products and water containing lead can harm people's health. Trained people can test homes for lead and recommend steps to take to remove it.

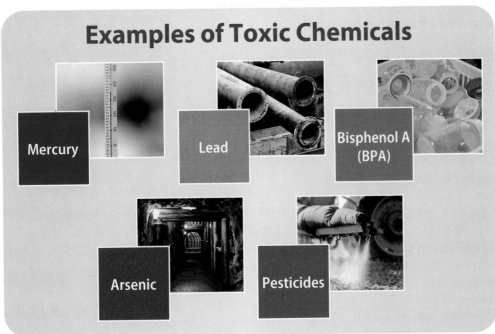

Examples of Toxic Chemicals

Mercury

Lead

Bisphenol A (BPA)

Arsenic

Pesticides

Figure 14.10
Chemicals are in everything, and not all chemicals are bad for health. Some chemicals, however, are toxic. *What does it mean for a chemical to be toxic?*

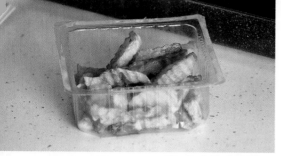

Africa Studio/Shutterstock.com

Figure 14.11 Plastic containers release chemicals into whatever substance they are holding, including food and drinks. Therefore, when people eat or drink items from a plastic container, they ingest the chemicals found in the plastic. Thus, toxic chemicals in plastics can cause great harm. *What is the name of the chemical found in many plastics?*

- **Bisphenol A (BPA).** BPA is a chemical found in many plastics. Scientific research shows that BPA may pose health risks (**Figure 14.11**). Many plastic products, such as water bottles and food containers, are now labeled *BPA-free* if this chemical is not used in the product.
- **Arsenic.** Arsenic naturally occurs in rocks, soil, water, and air. It can lead to water pollution when rain or melted snow runs over the ground. Arsenic can also be released from mining and is used in some products that protect wood against termites. Exposure to arsenic can cause serious health conditions.
- **Pesticides.** Pesticides are chemicals that control, or kill, weeds, bugs, and rodents. Pesticides can cause harm if they are ingested with food. Water can also carry pesticides from lawns, gardens, and farms into nearby bodies of water.

Whether a chemical is harmful to your health depends on a number of factors. These factors include how you are exposed to the chemical, how long you are exposed to it, and the amount of the chemical to which you are exposed.

CASE STUDY

Seiji's Paint Job

For months, Seiji has been telling his parents he wants to paint his bedroom. Seiji's bedroom has the same light-blue wallpaper it had when he and his parents moved into the old apartment. Seiji liked the wallpaper when he was younger, but now he wants the bedroom to be darker. Last week, Seiji's parents finally agreed to let him remove the wallpaper and paint the bedroom.

Seiji and his father work together to remove the wallpaper from Seiji's bedroom, and Seiji enjoys working with his father. The wallpaper-removal process produces a lot of dust, and underneath the wallpaper, Seiji and his father discover peeling, yellow paint. Seiji and his father do not feel well that evening, but they decide to wait until the morning to see if they feel better.

The next morning, both Seiji and his father have headaches and feel tired. Seiji's father says they should not continue working on the bedroom until professionals come to test the bedroom for lead paint. Seiji is glad his father cares about his health, but is disappointed he and his father will not finish painting over the weekend. When Seiji tells

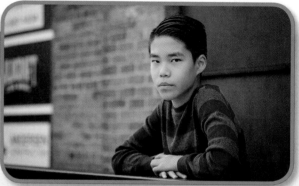

Torgado/Shutterstock.com

his teacher about the paint job, his teacher tells him that lead exposure can have very harmful effects. That makes Seiji feel a little better about the delay.

Thinking Critically

1. Why do you think Seiji's father suspected that the peeling paint underneath the bedroom's wallpaper might contain lead?

2. Should Seiji spend time in his bedroom before the professionals come to test the paint? Why or why not?

3. If Seiji told you he was disappointed his father delayed their painting project, what would you say to him? How would you explain to Seiji that his father is looking out for his safety?

Certain groups of people, such as babies, have an increased risk of harm due to chemical exposure (**Figure 14.12**). Exposure to toxic chemicals can lead to nausea and vomiting, skin or eye conditions, and cancer. Exposure to some chemicals, such as pesticides (which are poisons), can cause death.

If you are worried that you have been exposed to a dangerous chemical, talk with your doctor, school nurse, or another trusted adult. You can also call the Poison Control Center at (800) 222-1222. This resource is very helpful if you think you or someone you know has been in contact with a harmful substance.

Safe Chemical Use

To prevent harm from toxic chemicals, use household chemicals, such as paint and cleaning supplies, properly. Make sure to read warning labels carefully before using any kind of chemical. Other strategies for protecting yourself—and the environment—from chemicals include the following:

- Read warning labels and learn the symbols placed on the packages of chemicals (**Figure 14.13**). These symbols explain how the chemicals may impact a person's health and whether they can hurt the environment.
- Be very careful about mixing different chemicals together. For example, mixing bleach and products containing ammonia produces a highly toxic gas.

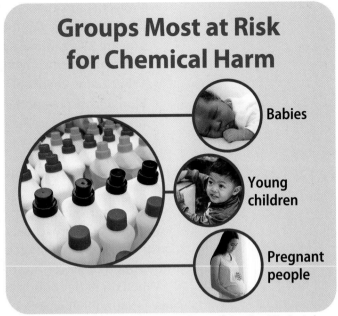

Groups Most at Risk for Chemical Harm

Babies

Young children

Pregnant people

Chemicals: Sfocato/Shutterstock.com; Top to bottom: Tatiana Katsai/Shutterstock.com; Titikul_B/Shutterstock.com; Africa Studio/Shutterstock.com

Figure 14.12 Exposure to chemicals is particularly dangerous for babies and young children. This is because babies' and young children's bodies are still growing. People who are pregnant need to avoid exposure to chemicals, which can cause health issues for the fetus.

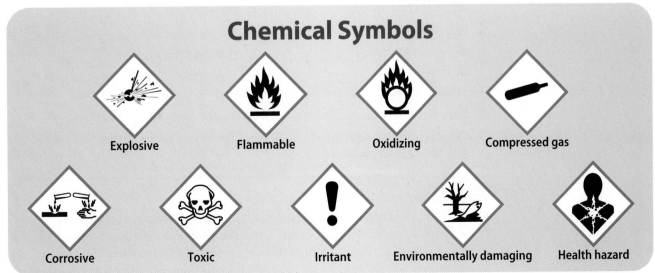

Chemical Symbols

Explosive

Flammable

Oxidizing

Compressed gas

Corrosive

Toxic

Irritant

Environmentally damaging

Health hazard

Rainer Lesniewski/Shutterstock.com

Figure 14.13 By recognizing the chemical symbols on packaging, you can understand the warnings about health risks associated with chemicals in different products. ***Look at the packaging of a cleaning product you use regularly. What chemical symbols are on the packaging?***

- Protect your skin and eyes from chemical exposure. Wear gloves and other protective equipment, depending on the type of chemical product you are using. Make sure to wash your hands carefully with soap and water after using chemical products.
- When using chemical products, work outside or leave windows open.
- Store and dispose of chemical products properly. Keep them away from items used in cooking and eating. Do not move chemicals into new containers.

Noise Pollution

You are surrounded by sounds. People listen to music, television shows, and radio broadcasts. Cars, trucks, trains, and planes make sounds. Construction equipment generates sound, too. Some sounds are natural, such as the sound of waves hitting the shore or birds calling to one another.

When do these sounds become a concern? When do sounds become noise? *Noise* is sound that a person does not want to hear or is bothered by. Noise can be more than simply bothersome. It can negatively affect a person's health.

High levels of noise over a period of time can lead to a loss of hearing. That is one reason that doctors warn about listening to music over earphones at high volume levels. Some studies have found that one in five teens suffers from some hearing loss. Other health effects of noise include stress, high blood pressure, difficulty sleeping, and lower productivity.

Experts recommend setting the volume at no more than about 60 percent of full volume when listening to a device through earphones. Wearing earplugs when operating loud equipment such as power mowers also helps.

Lesson 14.1 Review

1. What does the field of environmental health examine?
2. Which of the following is a potential effect of air pollution?
   - **A.** Easier breathing.
   - **B.** Hearing loss.
   - **C.** Water treatment.
   - **D.** Heart disease.
3. **True or false.** You can see bacteria and viruses in contaminated water.
4. **True or false.** High noise levels can lead to stress and difficulty sleeping.
5. **Critical thinking.** Should you microwave food in a plastic container that is *not* BPA-free? Explain why or why not.

Hands-On Activity

Using valid and reliable resources, find a true story about a community impacted by pollution. Then, create a realistic illustration, shadow box, cartoon strip, digital slide show, or other artistic representation describing how the community was affected. Be sure to emphasize the impact that pollution had on people's health and well-being. Present your visual to the class and share the true story behind it. Use effective communication skills and include a call to action.

Pollution Prevention and Greener Living

Learning Outcomes

After studying this lesson, you will be able to

- **give examples** of federal and state laws that protect the environment.
- **describe** what the environmental protection hierarchy is and how to use it.
- **determine** strategies you can use to reduce energy consumption and conserve natural resources at home.
- **identify** ways to be green at school.
- **explain** green choices people can make when traveling.

Graphic Organizer

Living Greener Every Day

Think about the places you visit every day—for example, your school, your home, or the park. List these places on a piece of paper as shown. As you listen to the presentation of this lesson, take notes about environmental laws that affect each location and about strategies you can use to preserve the environment in each place you visit. An example is provided for you.

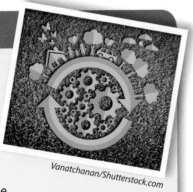

Vanatchanan/Shutterstock.com

Home	School	Public Transit Station	Alley's House
Laws Safe Drinking Water Act (makes water safe)			
Strategies Turn off the lights before going to school			

Key Terms

Air Quality Index (AQI) number that communicates to the public the level of pollutants in the air

brownfield site land, such as an old factory or gas station, that contains hazardous waste

fossil fuels natural forms of energy, such as oil, natural gas, and gas, that were formed a very long time ago, when dinosaurs lived on Earth

renewable energy type of energy that cannot be used up, such as wind, water, or solar power

recycling process in which used materials are turned into new products

sustainability actions that maintain the natural resources in the environment

green products goods that have a less harmful impact on the environment than traditional products

biodegradable able to break down without causing harm when thrown out

composting process of gathering food scraps and organic waste into a bin and letting it decompose and then adding it to soil to help plants grow

R emember Diego from the first lesson. Because of the direct impact pollution has had on his life, Diego wants to live as green as he can. Diego carries a reusable water bottle instead of disposable cans or bottles, turns off any lights he is not using, and reuses items whenever possible. To avoid wasted food, Diego is careful at restaurants to order only the amount of food he can eat and to take home any leftovers to eat later. He also set up a carpool with a few of his friends at school to help minimize car exhaust pollution. You will learn about these and more ways to prevent pollution and live greener in this lesson.

Society's Actions to Protect the Environment

Federal and state governments have passed laws to promote a safe environment. The *Environmental Protection Agency (EPA)* is the federal government agency that sets rules and regulations to protect people's health and the environment in the United States (**Figure 14.14**). These rules put into practice laws passed by Congress. They are based on scientific research.

States have their own laws aimed at protecting the environment. Each state has departments with power to enforce those laws.

Clean Air Act

The *Clean Air Act* is a federal law that regulates air pollution levels to protect people's health. This law sets specific limits on the amounts and types of pollution that power plants can release into the air. It also regulates the amounts and types of pollution produced by motor vehicles. This law has had a major impact on reducing air pollution.

Figure 14.14
When federal and state governments pass environmental safety laws, the EPA regulates and enforces these laws.

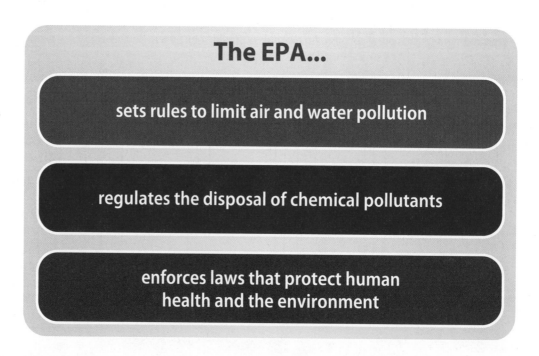

The EPA...

sets rules to limit air and water pollution

regulates the disposal of chemical pollutants

enforces laws that protect human health and the environment

The EPA works with state and local agencies to create a measure of air pollution. This measure is called the **Air Quality Index (AQI)**. The AQI tells you about five major air pollutants (**Figure 14.15**). Large cities are required to report the AQI every day. Many smaller communities do as well. This index is available on the Internet or through a free e-mail or app.

People can use the AQI to protect themselves. If air pollution is high in an area one day, people can spend more time inside. This is especially important for people with allergies or asthma. If air pollution levels are high, stay indoors during the afternoon. This is when ozone levels are typically the highest.

Safe Drinking Water Act

The *Safe Drinking Water Act* requires that drinking water is tested for more than 90 different pollutants. This testing includes metals, such as lead. It also includes pollutants that could spread diseases, such as *E. coli* and salmonella. Water systems are continually tested to make sure they meet safe standards.

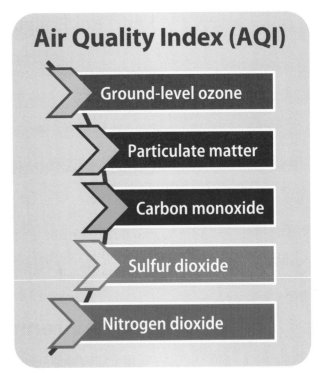

Air Quality Index (AQI)

- Ground-level ozone
- Particulate matter
- Carbon monoxide
- Sulfur dioxide
- Nitrogen dioxide

Figure 14.15 The five major air pollutants identified in the AQI are ground-level ozone, particulate matter, carbon monoxide, sulfur dioxide, and nitrogen dioxide. *Which law has had a major impact in reducing air pollution?*

Resource Conservation and Recovery Act

The *Resource Conservation and Recovery Act* provides rules and regulations about managing hazardous waste. For example, some chemicals can cause harm if they are simply dumped in the trash. Some trash contains dangerous chemicals. If those chemicals are not in a special container, they can leak into the ground or water (**Figure 14.16**). There are now specific rules about disposing of such waste.

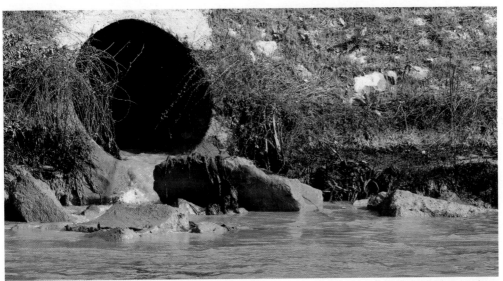

Figure 14.16 Hazardous waste in people's garbage can contaminate the water people use for cleaning, cooking, and drinking. *Which law provides rules and regulations about managing hazardous waste?*

Land Revitalization Program

Sometimes land contains hazardous waste that can hurt people's health. These areas that contain hazardous waste are called *brownfield sites*. A **brownfield site** may be the site of an old factory or gas station. The EPA's Land Revitalization Program cleans up potentially contaminated land so that it is safe to use. This process removes any polluting substances and creates more usable land.

Celebrate Earth Day

People around the world celebrate Earth Day on April 22 each year. Earth Day events are held to demonstrate support for protecting the environment and taking care of the planet. Join an Earth Day celebration in your school or community—or start your own. You can find lots of ideas for activities to do in support of Earth Day online.

The Environmental Protection Hierarchy

The EPA has created a graphic called the *environmental protection hierarchy*. It shows five different ways of protecting the environment. The higher up in the hierarchy, the better the approach (**Figure 14.17**).

Source Reduction

The best strategy for protecting the environment is to *reduce* trash and pollution. This eliminates the *source*, or cause, of pollution. For example, many people buy bottled water and then throw out the plastic container. Instead, they could buy a reusable bottle and refill it. This approach would

Figure 14.17
Ways to protect the environment include a reduction of trash and pollution, recycling and reusing items and materials, treatment of waste to make it less dangerous, and disposal of hazardous materials. *What is the most preferred way to protect the environment?*

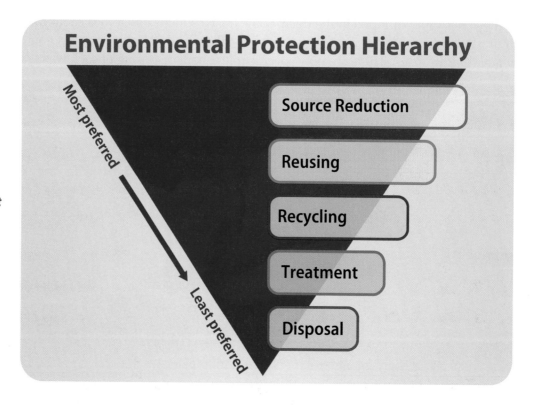

Environmental Protection Hierarchy

Most preferred

Least preferred

- Source Reduction
- Reusing
- Recycling
- Treatment
- Disposal

reduce the amount of plastic thrown away. Very simple strategies, such as turning off the lights when leaving a room and turning off the water when brushing teeth, reduce the amount of energy used.

Reducing the use of oil, gas, and coal is another way to help the environment. These energy sources are called **fossil fuels** and were formed a very long time ago, when dinosaurs lived on Earth. Burning these fuels releases gases and particulate matter into the air. Many scientists also believe that they contribute to climate change. Driving electric or hybrid cars, for example, can reduce the amount of exhaust from fossil fuels.

Alternative sources of electric energy such as solar power, wind power, and water power help as well. These sources of energy come from resources that do not run out, such as wind, water, and sunlight. These types of energy are called **renewable energy** (**Figure 14.18**). People can use as much energy as possible from these sources and never run out. Another advantage about this type of energy is that it does not cause pollution. That is why this type of energy is sometimes called *clean energy*. The more people can use renewable energy sources, the more they protect the environment.

Another way of reducing waste is to take care of your belongings, such as clothes and electronics, so they last longer. Buy used clothes or books instead of new ones. Shop at thrift stores, garage sales, and flea markets to save money and protect the environment at the same time. All of these strategies reduce the need to manufacture new products, which takes energy.

Reusing and Recycling

The next best approach to reducing pollution is to reuse and recycle items you use, instead of just throwing them away. Reusing products means they do not have to be thrown away or recycled. For example, instead of using a new plastic bag and throwing it away every time you go shopping, carry a reusable bag.

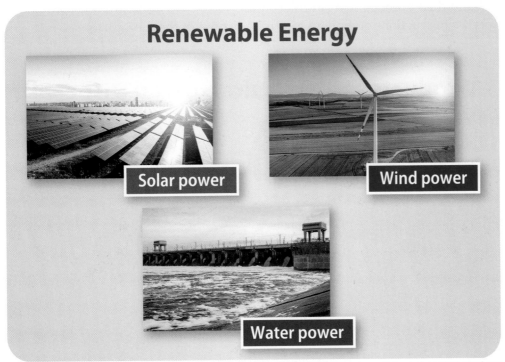

Renewable Energy

Solar power

Wind power

Water power

Figure 14.18
Sunlight, wind, and water are natural sources of energy that cannot run out. They also do not cause pollution.

Left to right, top to bottom: Wang An Qi/Shutterstock.com; Stockr/Shutterstock.com; Getmaneclnna/Shutterstock.com

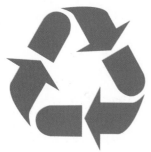

Figure 14.19
The symbol shown here can help you identify recycling receptacles when you are disposing of paper, plastic, glass, and aluminum items. *What happens in the process of recycling?*

Buy rechargeable batteries, which you can reuse. When you are done using something, donate it so someone else can use it, too. For example, you could donate clothes you have outgrown to a local homeless shelter, thrift store, or charitable organization.

Recycling is a process in which used materials are turned into new products. This reduces the amount of trash sent to landfills. Recycling conserves natural resources and saves energy. Recycling also helps limit the burning of fossil fuels, which contributes to climate change. Many items people use every day are recyclable. For example, newspapers and magazines, aluminum cans, glass bottles, and plastic containers are all recyclable (**Figure 14.19**).

Certain types of products need to be recycled in particular ways to protect the environment. These include electronics, such as televisions and computers, and appliances, such as microwaves and refrigerators. These products can contain dangerous substances. It is important to recycle these products properly so that these substances do not pollute landfills. Many towns have special days these products can be dropped off for recycling. Some stores also collect these products for recycling.

Treatment

The next step in the hierarchy is *treating* substances that may be dangerous. This approach uses processes that make the substance less dangerous. For example, sewage is treated in water treatment plants to avoid the harmful effects of human waste entering the environment.

Disposal

Some products contain hazardous materials, and therefore are not able to be treated or recycled. These products need to be disposed of very carefully to avoid harming the environment. They cannot simply be placed in a trash can and then dumped in a landfill (**Figure 14.20**). Most communities provide specific instructions on how to carefully dispose of these products.

Figure 14.20
Products such as some batteries, tires, full or partially full aerosol cans, household chemicals, and medical waste require special disposal because they can harm the environment if dumped in a landfill.

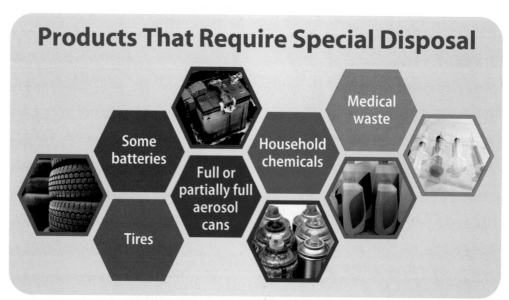

Greener Living

"Green" living means living in a way that protects the environment. It involves limiting or preventing actions that pollute and conserving resources. One goal of green living is to make choices that create **sustainability**, or actions that maintain the natural resources in the environment.

BUILDING Your Skills

Advocating for the Environment

One way to protect the environment is to advocate for it. An *advocate* is a person who stands up for what that person believes is right. To be an advocate, a person must

- be passionate about a cause
- use power of persuasion to prove the importance of the cause
- inspire a behavior change among others

There are many ways to advocate for a cause, and one way is to create a campaign. You may have encountered campaigns before. For example, you have probably seen billboards, commercials, and T-shirts advertising a cause. You may have participated in awareness walks or worn a certain color ribbon for a meaningful day. All of these strategies aim to inspire awareness and action in certain people. You can create a campaign about a cause you care about, too.

Start a Campaign

The environment needs your help, so start a campaign to advocate for its health. First, form a small group to be your team. In your group, discuss environmental issues in your community (school, neighborhood, or town). Find an issue that your group is passionate about improving.

Once you have chosen an issue, research it. Become an expert on your chosen environmental topic. Remember that research should come from many sources, including books, online databases, and people. Research should also be valid and reliable, so use trustworthy sources.

Next, create a campaign to promote your cause. Your campaign might be an event, a series of advertisements or messages, or a movement promoting change. Whatever the nature of your campaign, make sure your campaign is innovative, or new, and promotes your cause. While creating your campaign, keep in mind the multiple age levels in your community. Your campaign should appeal to all ages, from young children to older adults. Consider what each age group can do to help solve your issue and make sure each person knows what you are asking. Write down the details of your campaign and plan so you understand how to put the campaign into action. Then, with the help of your teacher, get your campaign out into the community.

As your campaign runs its course, be sure to "practice what you preach," or live out the cause you are promoting. After a while, observe the campaign's effect on your community and consider the following questions:

- What worked in your campaign? What did not work?
- Did people make changes in their behavior because of your campaign?
- Has the community environment improved because of your campaign? Is it too soon to tell? When will you know?
- What did you learn about yourself, about advocacy, and about your community during this campaign? Did you "practice what you preached"?

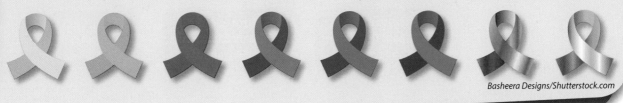

Basheera Designs/Shutterstock.com

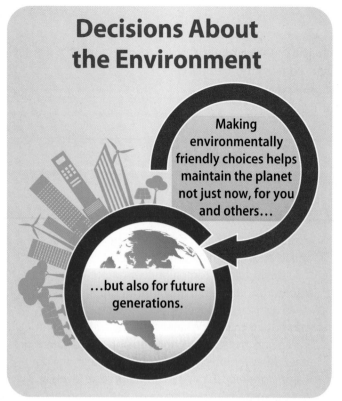

Decisions About the Environment

Making environmentally friendly choices helps maintain the planet not just now, for you and others...

...but also for future generations.

khonkangrua/Shutterstock.com

Figure 14.21 Every day, you make decisions that affect the environment and shape your health. These decisions do not just affect you. They also impact others, today and in the future.

When people make responsible choices about using and consuming products, they help protect Earth so that these natural resources can last for many, many years (**Figure 14.21**). For example, sustainable gardening is a way of growing plants that reduces any negative impact on the environment. It includes actions such as avoiding the use of chemicals that can pollute the soil and capturing rain to water plants.

People can take many different actions in their homes, schools, workplaces, and communities to help protect society and the environment.

Use Less Energy

Making small changes in your behavior can help reduce energy consumption and conserve natural resources. Following are some simple strategies for using less energy at home:

- Shut the refrigerator door as soon as you select what you need.
- Use light bulbs that run on less energy (**Figure 14.22**).
- Turn off lights when leaving a room.
- Use as little electricity as possible to heat and cool your home. Set the thermostat a bit higher in the summer and a bit lower in the winter to reduce the amount of energy used.

Figure 14.22
Energy-efficient light bulbs use less energy, which helps them last longer. By using less energy, these bulbs also produce less waste. *What is one way to tell if a product is energy efficient?*

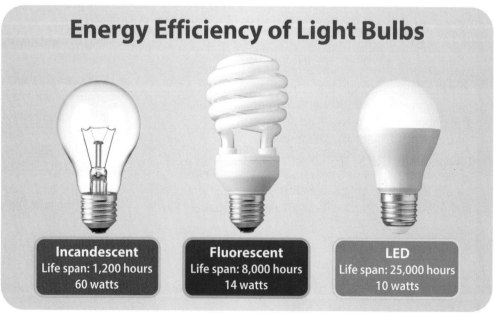

Energy Efficiency of Light Bulbs

Incandescent
Life span: 1,200 hours
60 watts

Fluorescent
Life span: 8,000 hours
14 watts

LED
Life span: 25,000 hours
10 watts

Somchai Som/Shutterstock.com

- Keep outside doors and windows shut when heating or cooling your home.
- Buy energy-efficient products. You can look for the *Energy Star* symbol to choose products that have energy efficiency. This symbol appears on products that use smaller amounts of energy. These products save people money over time because they require less energy to run. They also reduce energy use, which saves energy and reduces pollution. The symbol is given to various products that use electricity, including computers and fans. It is also given to new buildings that meet standards for lower energy use.

Buy Green Products

Another approach to green living is to make wise purchases. **Green products** are goods that have a less harmful impact on the environment than traditional products. Green products could include any of the following features:

- made of recycled materials
- obtained from local stores or farms, meaning less energy was needed to transport them (**Figure 14.23**)
- made without harmful chemicals
- **biodegradable**, or able to break down without causing harm when thrown out

Reduce Food Waste

Another way to live greener is to reduce the amount of wasted food. Every year, Americans throw away more than 38 million tons of food. This includes food that has spoiled, but it also includes leftovers people just do not finish. Most of this food ends up in landfills. Being more mindful about your food choices can help reduce food waste and save money. You can reduce food waste in the following ways:

- Only buy as much food as you expect to eat.
- Store food carefully so that it stays fresh longer.
- Have a "leftovers night" each week.
- When eating out, take home food you do not finish to avoid it being thrown away.

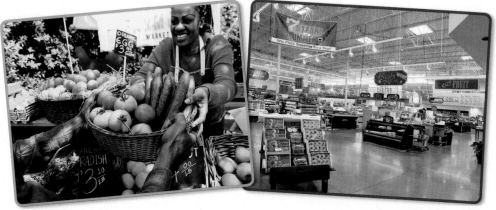

Figure 14.23
Locally grown food has had less exposure to potential contaminants in transport and is more likely to be fresh and full of nutrients than food shipped from far away.

Rawpixel.com/Shutterstock.com; B Brown/Shutterstock.com

Steps Toward a Greener Planet

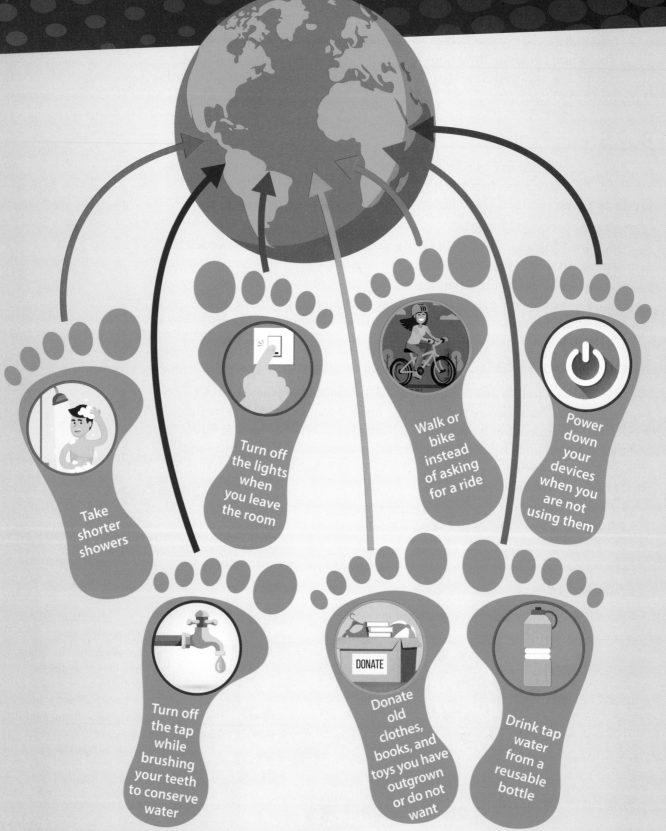

Earth: peiyang/Shutterstock.com; Footprints: Arcady/Shutterstock.com; Top to bottom, left to right: Boonyen/Shutterstock.com; Wor Sang Jun/Shutterstock.com; bioraven/Shutterstock.com; Jane Kelly/Shutterstock.com; Marnikus/Shutterstock.com; Maike Hildebrandt/Shutterstock.com; Creative Stall/Shutterstock.com

Plant a Tree

Planting a tree is a pretty simple way to protect the environment (**Figure 14.24**). Trees beautify surroundings and provide shade. The shade trees provide can make a home cooler and reduce the demand for air-conditioning. Trees also absorb carbon dioxide and other gases (including carbon monoxide and sulfur dioxide) from the air, and release oxygen into the air. This helps air quality. Trees also help the environment by holding water in the soil, preventing it from running off.

Be Green Away from Home

There are many ways people can be green at school or work. Reusing materials is one approach. Instead of buying new notebooks, pens, and other supplies each new school year, reuse supplies from the previous year. If buying new items, look for those made from recycled products. Office workers can use paper that is no longer needed as note paper.

People can make green choices in the school or workplace cafeteria. Following are some easy ways to make environmentally friendly choices:

- If you bring lunch from home, use reusable containers instead of disposable ones.
- Bring drinks in a thermos or safe reusable water bottle.
- If you bring cans or bottles to school or work, recycle them.
- If you buy lunch, take only what you need. Extra napkins and ketchup packages simply add extra waste.

Some schools have a composting program to help reduce the amount of food waste. **Composting** involves gathering food scraps and organic waste into a bin and letting it decompose and then adding it to soil to help plants grow (**Figure 14.25**). If your school has this type of program, make sure to dispose of your food scraps properly so they are composted and not just thrown away.

Benefits of Trees

Beautify surroundings
Provide shade
Absorb carbon dioxide
Release oxygen
Prevent runoff

John_T/Shutterstock.com

Figure 14.24 Planting trees is an easy, cheap activity that can have many benefits to the environment.

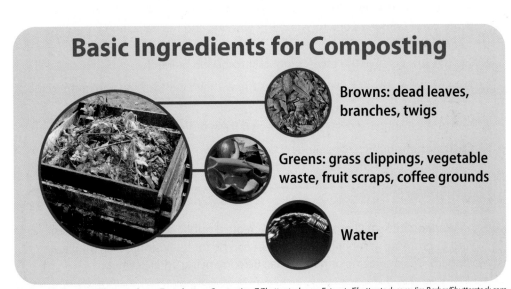

Basic Ingredients for Composting

Browns: dead leaves, branches, twigs

Greens: grass clippings, vegetable waste, fruit scraps, coffee grounds

Water

Figure 14.25
To create a compost pile, alternate layers of browns and greens in equal amounts. Add water to dry materials as they are placed in the bin to keep them moist. *What type of waste does composting help reduce?*

Compost pile: Evan Lorne/Shutterstock.com; Top to bottom: ConstantinosZ/Shutterstock.com; Fotocute/Shutterstock.com; Jim Barber/Shutterstock.com

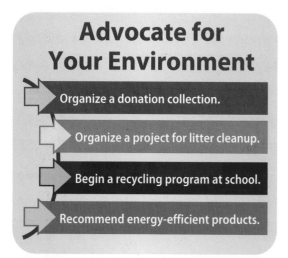

Advocate for Your Environment

Organize a donation collection.

Organize a project for litter cleanup.

Begin a recycling program at school.

Recommend energy-efficient products.

Figure 14.26
Educating others and advocating for the environment can help you promote environmental health.

If your school does not have this type of program, maybe you could work with friends to start one.

Many people do not understand how their choices impact the environment, and how even small changes can help protect the planet. Educating people in your school or community about the benefits of reducing energy consumption can help protect the environment and improve overall health in your community (**Figure 14.26**).

Be Green on the Road

You can reduce energy consumed and pollution by making greener choices when you travel. For example, walking or biking to school is a greener choice than riding in a car. For longer distances, try to use public transportation, such as a subway, train, or bus. These forms of transportation take many people and use much less energy than if people drove their own car.

Drivers can also make greener choices to help protect the environment. One way drivers can help the environment is to buy energy-efficient cars. Cars can differ a lot in how much gas they use. Cars with a high miles-per-gallon (MPG) use less gas than those with a low MPG. A high-MPG car costs less to drive and reduces pollution. Although most cars run on gasoline, some newer cars use different forms of energy that are better for the environment. Electric cars do not use any gas and do not produce exhaust. Of course, they do use some energy—the electricity needed to recharge their batteries. Hybrid cars are powered with both gasoline and electricity. Driving these cars may save money because less money is spent buying gas.

Lesson 14.2 Review

1. Which Act requires large cities to report the AQI every day?
   - **A.** *Safe Drinking Water Act.*
   - **B.** *Resource Conservation and Recovery Act.*
   - **C.** *Clean Air Act.*
   - **D.** Land Revitalization Program.

2. List the strategies of the environmental protection hierarchy.

3. **True or false.** Biodegradable products break down without causing harm to the environment.

4. How does storing food carefully to keep it fresh reduce waste?

5. **Critical thinking.** Research and report your community's guidelines for disposing of different kinds of batteries.

Hands-On Activity

Working in a small group, plan and create a public service announcement (PSA) to promote greener living. The PSA can be for television, social media, a billboard, or a magazine or newspaper. Be convincing and succinct.

Summary

Lesson 14.1 Common Hazards in the Environment

- Humans and the environment influence each other. The study of how factors in the natural environment impact your health is called *environmental health*. As a healthy environment can lead to better health, so can an unhealthy environment lead to poor health.

- Pollutants are substances that contaminate the environment and can harm people. Air pollution refers to the contamination of the air you breathe. Smog, acid rain, and particulate matter are examples of outdoor air pollution. Examples of indoor air pollution include tobacco smoke, paint, mold, and dust. Air pollution can cause health conditions in humans and is also believed to contribute to climate change.

- Polluted water poses major risks to human health. Sometimes, water pollution occurs because of human activity. For example, pesticides and chemicals that humans use can contaminate water. Water pollution can also be natural. Bacteria, viruses, and parasites can contaminate water and make people sick. To prevent water contamination, drinking water in the United States is treated according to a water treatment plan.

- Chemicals can also pollute the environment. Some chemicals are natural, while others are made by people. In large amounts, chemicals can harm health. For example, exposure to lead can have negative effects. Chemicals found in plastic can cause sickness. Identifying, storing, and disposing of chemicals safely can help prevent contamination.

- Noise pollution refers to noises you do not want to hear. High levels of noise can cause hearing loss and lead to stress. Listening to music at a moderate volume and wearing earplugs can help reduce noise pollution.

Lesson 14.2 Pollution Prevention and Greener Living

- The Environmental Protection Agency (EPA) sets regulations to help protect the environment. EPA initiatives include the *Clean Air Act*, *Safe Drinking Water Act*, *Resource Conservation and Recovery Act*, Land Revitalization Program, and Earth Day.

- The environmental protection hierarchy illustrates different ways of protecting the environment. The hierarchy's strategies are *reducing* trash and pollution, *reusing* and *recycling* items, *treating* dangerous substances, and *disposing* of hazardous materials carefully.

- Green living is living in a way that protects the environment. You can use many strategies to live more greenly. These include using less energy, buying green products, reducing food waste, and planting trees.

- You can make green choices away from home by reusing materials and educating others. You can make green choices on the road by using public transportation and energy-efficient cars.

Check Your Knowledge

Record your answers to each of the following questions on a separate sheet of paper.

1. **True or false.** Car exhaust is a major contributor to smog in cities.

2. How does runoff lead to the pollution of a water supply?

3. **True or false.** In the United States, drinking water travels from the water supply to your home without treatment.

4. Which of the following chemicals can be found in batteries, paint, and glass thermometers?
   - **A.** Mercury.
   - **B.** Arsenic.
   - **C.** Lead.
   - **D.** Aspirin.

5. Is it safe to move chemicals into different containers? Why or why not?

6. Which of the following is a health effect of noise pollution?
   - **A.** Low stress.
   - **B.** Deep sleeping.
   - **C.** High blood pressure.
   - **D.** High productivity at work.

7. Which EPA initiative cleans up brownfield sites so they are safe to use?

8. **True or false.** Burning fossil fuels releases gases and particulate matter into the air.

9. What is an example of a household product that requires special disposal?

10. **True or false.** Green products must be obtained from international sources.

11. How does planting a tree help the environment?

12. Which of the following is a good strategy for being green away from home?
    - **A.** Bring extra napkins for lunch.
    - **B.** Use disposable containers.
    - **C.** Drink out of plastic water bottles.
    - **D.** Recycle cans and bottles.

13. **True or false.** Using public transportation to get to school is a greener choice than riding in a car.

Use Your Vocabulary ⤴

acid rain	fossil fuels	renewable energy
Air Quality Index (AQI)	green products	smog
biodegradable	ozone	sustainability
brownfield site	pollutants	
composting	recycling	

14. In Lesson 14.2, you learned that biodegradable items can break down without causing harm to the environment when thrown away. The word *biodegradable* comes from the word parts *bio-* (meaning "life"), *degrade* (meaning "to deteriorate"), and *-able* (meaning "capable of"). With a partner, make a list of other words that contain the word parts *bio-*, *degrade*, or *-able*. These words may be used in everyday language or are common in the health field. You may use a dictionary to locate words. Some examples may include *affordable* (can be paid for) or *biohazard* (dangerous organic material).

Think Critically

15. **Determine.** Explain how personal health and the health of a person's environment are connected.

16. **Cause and effect.** How have the use of technology and technological advances helped and harmed the environment?

17. **Make inferences.** Even though people are making changes to protect the environment, pollution still exists. As long as pollution is an issue, what behavior changes can you make to protect your personal health?

18. **Predict.** What effect could climate change have on human health now and in the future?

19. **Identify.** Think about reasons people do not make choices for greener living. List these reasons and share them with a partner. For each reason not to make greener choices, write a sentence in favor of making greener choices.

DEVELOP Your Skills

20. **Access information.** Working with a partner, research five local, state, national, and international agencies that promote environmental health and protection. Make a resource list that includes the name of each agency, the agency's mission or purpose, and the agency's contact information (for example, website address). Share your list with your classmates and create a class list to take home.

21. **Goal-setting skills.** Review this chapter's information about green living and brainstorm other ways middle school students can have a positive impact on the environment and human health. Identify one realistic action you can either add to or remove from your daily routine to improve environmental health. Write this action as a SMART goal and track your progress toward achieving it over one month. At the end of the month, review your actions, your feelings, and any impact on your environment.

22. **Leadership, decision-making, advocacy, and communication skills.** Identify one change you can make in your home or school that will promote environmental and human health. Will you need to purchase or subscribe to anything to make the change happen? What routines will need to change, and whom will they impact? Talk with your family or teacher about putting this change into action and then try it out.

23. **Literacy, communication, and technology skills.** Watch a video or listen to a podcast that shares news about environmental health. Take notes as you watch or listen to the news story and identify the most important ideas. Then, share the video or podcast with your classmates and use a meme, hashtag, or other online feature to highlight the most important ideas in the story.

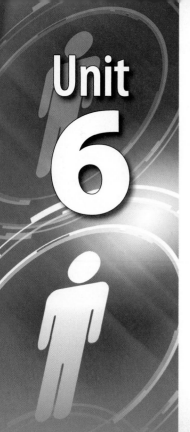

Unit 6

Social Health and Wellness

Chapter 15   Promoting Healthy Relationships

Chapter 16   Preventing and Responding to Violence

Warm-Up Activity

Questions About Relationships

This unit will discuss what relationships are and what makes them healthy or unhealthy. Without talking with anyone else, answer the following questions on six separate sticky notes:

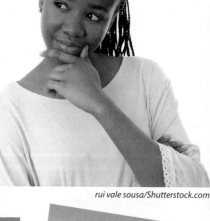

rui vale sousa/Shutterstock.com

1. What is a relationship?

2. What qualities are found in healthy relationships?

3. How can you strengthen a relationship?

4. How do you know when a relationship should end?

5. What makes a relationship unhealthy?

6. What makes a relationship abusive?

Squares: Brumarina/Shutterstock.com

When you are done answering these questions, post your answers on the wall. Everyone in the class should post their answers, and answers should be grouped by question. Then, pair up into small groups. Each group will be given one question and all of its associated answers. Working collaboratively, read all the provided answers and write one statement that summarizes the class' responses.

After reading the chapters in this unit, read these summary statements again and review how accurate they were. Enhance your statements to be more correct and complete.

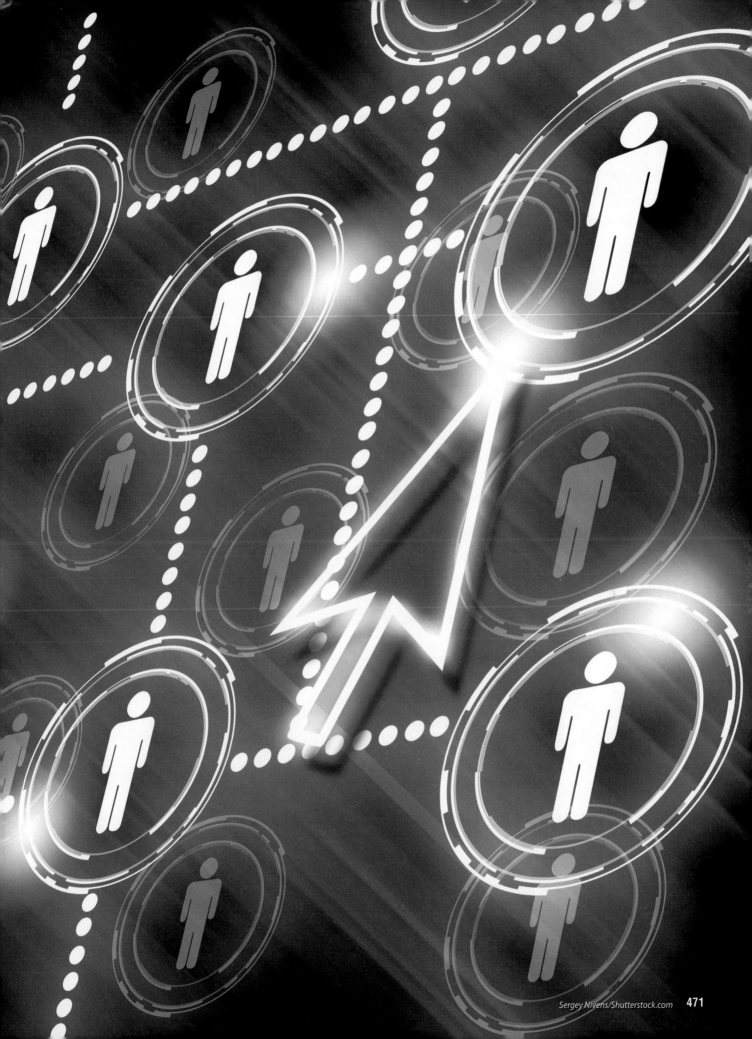

Promoting Healthy Relationships

 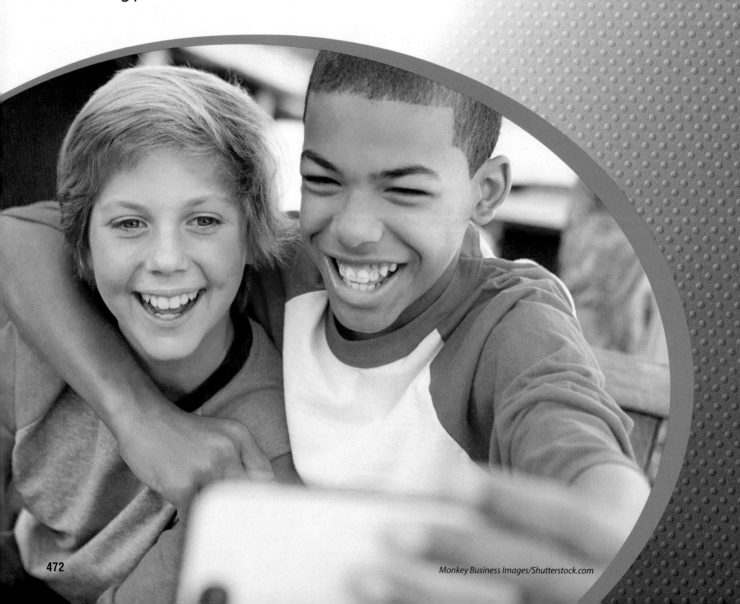

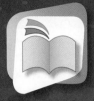

Reading Activity

In groups of three, review healthy and types of relationships. Arrange a study session to read the chapter aloud. Take care to speak clearly. Stop at the end of each lesson and work together to identify the main points. After reading this chapter, draw connections between the types of relationships as a group.

How Healthy Are You?

In this chapter, you will be learning about healthy relationships. Before you begin reading, take the following quiz to assess your current healthy relationship habits.

Healthy Choices	Yes	No
Do you have a social support system of people you can count on to help you in times of crises?		
Are you a patient and attentive listener?		
Can you clearly express to someone your wants, needs, opinions, and feelings?		
Are you able to prevent or resolve conflicts with family members?		
Do you and your friends avoid excluding other people from your group?		
Do you avoid interrupting, judging, or criticizing others when they are talking?		
Do you try not to rely too much on virtual interactions with your friends, choosing face-to-face interactions instead?		
Do you know the difference between casual dating and group dating?		
Are your relationships with others based on characteristics of honesty, trust, mutual respect, care, and commitment?		

Count your "Yes" and "No" responses. The more "Yes" responses you have, the more healthy relationship habits you exhibit. Now, take a closer look at the questions with which you responded "No." How can you make these healthy habits part of your daily life? Identify a SMART goal you would like to achieve to help improve your overall health and well-being. Refer to Figure 1.11 to help you set up your SMART goal. If you do not understand the instructions, ask for clarification from your teacher.

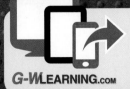

Click on the activity icon or visit www.g-wlearning.com/health to access online vocabulary activities using key terms from the chapter.

Lesson 15.1

What Is a Healthy Relationship?

Key Terms 📤

relationships connections that people form and maintain with others

affirmative consent direct, verbal, freely given agreement that occurs when someone clearly says yes

interpersonal skills skills that help people communicate and relate in positive ways with others

communication process exchange of messages and responses between two or more people

feedback constructive response to a message to communicate that it was received and understood

verbal communication use of words to send a spoken or written message

nonverbal communication communicating through facial expressions, body language, gestures, tone and volume of voice, and other signals that do not involve the use of words

active listening act of concentrating on person talking with the goal of understanding the message and the speaker's feelings about it

peer mediation process in which specially trained students work with other students to resolve conflicts

Learning Outcomes

After studying this lesson, you will be able to

- **discuss** the importance of relationships for physical, emotional, and social health.
- **identify** characteristics that can help you build and maintain healthy relationships with others and enhance your own health.
- **demonstrate** techniques to communicate clearly and effectively, both verbally and nonverbally, with others.
- **demonstrate** effective negotiating skills to resolve a conflict.
- **describe** the purpose of peer mediation.

Graphic Organizer

Alex Staroseltsev/Shutterstock.com

Visualizing Relationships

Before reading this lesson, skim the main headings and write each one in a different color on a separate piece of paper. As you silently read the lesson and then listen to your teacher, take notes in the color you chose for each main heading as shown. After you finish taking notes, draw a small illustration or visual next to each section that will help you remember what you learned.

The Importance of Relationships
Family relationships meet basic human needs

Communication Skills

Healthy Versus Unhealthy Relationships

Conflict Resolution Skills

Jemastock/Shutterstock.com

474

Relationships are an important part of every person's life, and as you grow up, you will form and maintain new types of relationships. For example, Kai is in eighth grade and is a very social person. For as long as he can remember, he has been close with his parents. He enjoys playing sports and video games with his younger brother. Since he started middle school, Kai has made many new friends. This year, he even likes a classmate. Some of Kai's peers have stopped talking to their friends and lost friendships because of conflict. Kai does not want this to happen to him and his friends. Kai understands that his relationships are important to his health and well-being.

The Importance of Relationships

People live in social groups and have many relationships with other people. **Relationships** are the connections you form and maintain with other people. Most people live in families and have friends. Young people have relationships with other students, teachers, and adults. Adults have relationships with coworkers and members of groups to which they belong. All of these relationships help contribute to a person's health and well-being (**Figure 15.1**).

Some relationships meet basic human needs. Most of these relationships are in families, which are responsible for meeting the needs of members. Other relationships, however, also play a crucial role in your overall health.

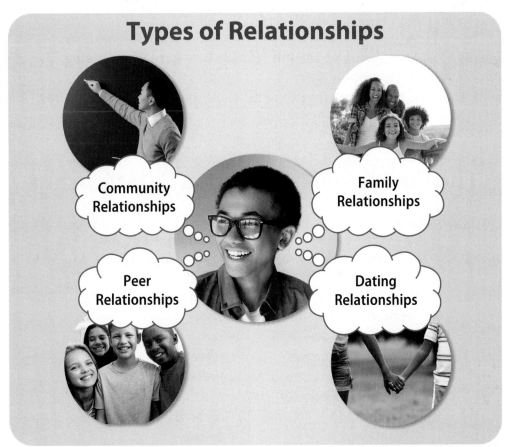

Types of Relationships

Community Relationships

Family Relationships

Peer Relationships

Dating Relationships

Figure 15.1
All of your relationships impact your well-being. As you grow up, you will have more types of relationships and will get to know more diverse people. *Which type of relationship is responsible for meeting the needs of members?*

Center: LightField Studios/Shutterstock.com; Clockwise from top left: Africa Studio/Shutterstock.com; Monkey Business Images/Shutterstock.com; Diego Cervo/Shutterstock.com; Monkey Business Images/Shutterstock.com

Researchers have found that people with good social support are less likely to get sick than people who lack social support. People with good social support also tend to recover from illnesses faster and even live longer. Relationships filled with tension and conflict can have the opposite effects on health.

Relationships also meet the need to belong to a group and to feel connected with and loved by other people. Relationships impact you emotionally. A smile or a compliment from a friend or a classmate can lift your spirits. An argument with a sibling can make you feel angry or sad. Relationships allow you to learn more about yourself, receive and provide emotional support, and gain skills for communicating and resolving conflicts.

Different relationships satisfy different needs. When you were younger, most of your relationships were probably in your family. As you grow up, your social world is expanding to include other relationships, such as those with peers, teachers, and even dating partners.

Healthy Versus Unhealthy Relationships

The impact of relationships depends on the health of the relationships (**Figure 15.2**). For example, in healthy relationships, people receive support from family and friends when they go through times of crises. This support helps give people the strength they need to recover from the challenges they face. People in unhealthy relationships often do not receive the support they need. In turn, this can result in experiencing more physical, mental, and emotional issues than people in healthy relationships. Healthy relationships can improve all aspects of health.

As you form new relationships, you can ensure your own health by building *healthy relationships*. Healthy relationships have the following important characteristics:

- **Honesty.** Honesty means telling the truth about what you have done, what you want, and how you feel.

Figure 15.2
A person with healthy relationships will experience more positive emotions and fewer negative emotions than a person with unhealthy relationships.

The Emotional Impact of a Relationship

In a **healthy** relationship, you will feel

- secure
- loved
- safe
- free to be yourself
- valued
- acknowledged
- understood
- confident

In an **unhealthy** relationship, you will feel

- anxious
- angry
- sad
- resentful
- pressured
- used
- ignored
- unsafe

- **Trust.** Trust is believing that another person is not going to do or say something to hurt you.
- **Mutual respect.** Respect is knowing that each person has worth as a human being and has a right to have one's feelings and desires recognized. Respect should be *mutual*, or go both ways.
- **Care and commitment.** You demonstrate care and commitment when you show concern for another person and work to make the relationship better.
- **Emotional control.** Controlling your emotions is an important part of building a healthy relationship. For example, controlling your anger can help you work through conflict in a positive way.
- **Understanding.** When you show understanding, you acknowledge and relate to the feelings and thoughts of another person.
- **Safety.** Each person feels safe, cares for each other's well-being, and respects personal *boundaries*, or rules about behavior. Part of respecting boundaries is giving and receiving affirmative consent. **Affirmative consent** is a direct, verbal, freely given agreement that occurs when someone clearly says "yes." For example, if a friend says no to hanging out after school, you do not show up to your friend's house uninvited. Do not force your friend to hang out and respect your friend's decision.
- **Good interpersonal skills. Interpersonal skills** are skills that help people communicate and resolve conflicts in positive ways. You can build healthy relationships by using interpersonal skills.

Paying attention to these characteristics can help you build and maintain healthy relationships. If a relationship does not have these characteristics, it is unhealthy and needs to change (**Figure 15.3**).

If a person in the relationship is not willing to invest in making the relationship better, the relationship may need to end. If you know a relationship is unhealthy, you can take action to change or leave the relationship and get help from a trusted adult or community resource. To build healthy relationships, you need to have good communication skills and conflict resolution skills.

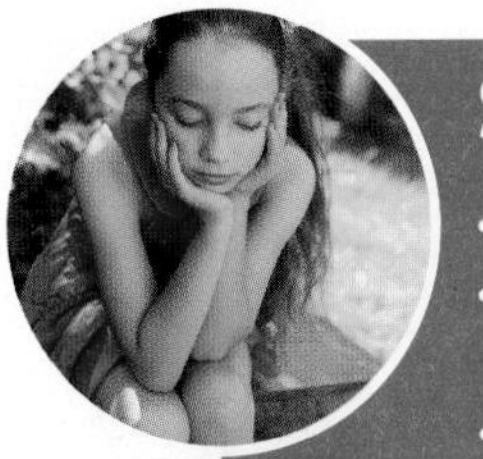

Signs of an Unhealthy Relationship

- You feel used, ignored, and unappreciated.
- One person is more interested in maintaining the relationship than the other person.
- You are subjected to angry outbursts.
- You feel you cannot say or do anything right.
- You and the other person are constantly fighting.
- You are made fun of or threatened.
- The other person is extremely jealous of you.
- The other person tells you to stay away from friends or family.
- The other person raises a hand as if to hit you.
- The other person has been violent toward you.
- You are being pressured to engage in activities that make you uncomfortable.
- The other person encourages unhealthy behaviors.
- The other person does not respect your boundaries and consent.

Figure 15.3
Some people may have trouble seeing the signs of an unhealthy relationship. This is especially true for people raised in environments without respect, kindness, or trust.

Katya Shut/Shutterstock.com

Communication Skills

Effective communication is perhaps the most important part of a healthy relationship. The **communication process** involves the exchange of messages and responses between two or more people. Effective communication happens when the receiver understands the message and sends **feedback**—a constructive response—to communicate to the sender that the message was received and understood (**Figure 15.4**). The communication process continues with the further exchange of messages. Two types of communication are used to send messages: verbal and nonverbal communication.

Verbal Communication

Verbal communication involves the use of words to send a spoken or written message. You use verbal communication all the time—through everyday conversation, text messages, phone calls, e-mails, social media posts, letters, and notes. For example, telling or texting a parent or guardian you will be home at a certain time is a form of verbal communication. Talking with a friend through video calls or online messages is another.

Nonverbal Communication

In many situations, communication involves more than just words. **Nonverbal communication** involves communicating through facial expressions, body language, gestures, tone and volume of voice, and other signals that do not involve the use of words. Your nonverbal communication shows people whether you are paying attention and are interested in the conversation. These signals are an especially important part of showing respect for the person communicating with you.

Figure 15.4
The communication process involves sending a message, such as a thought, idea, feeling, or information, to another person, called the *receiver*. *What is the term for a constructive response to a communicated message?*

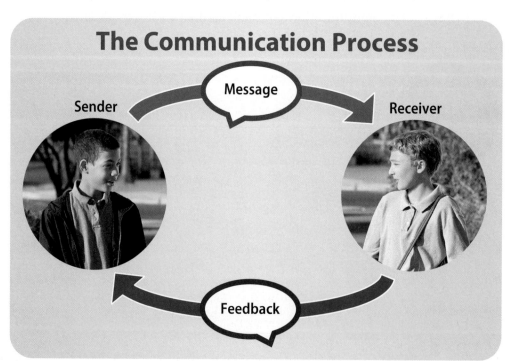

The Communication Process

Sender — Message → Receiver

Feedback

CREATISTA/Shutterstock.com

Nonverbal communication includes the following:

- eye contact or lack of eye contact
- facial expressions, such as smiling, frowning, or eye rolling
- gestures, such as nodding, shaking the head, or moving the hands
- posture, such as leaning forward, facing away, or slumping in a chair
- tone of voice, such as encouragement, doubt, or sarcasm
- volume of voice, such as loudness showing anger or excitement, or softness showing reluctance to speak
- pitch of voice, such as high-pitched excitement or low-pitched lack of interest

Nonverbal communication is only possible if you can see or hear the other person. For example, if you are talking with someone at school, you can see the other person's facial expressions. If you are talking over the phone, you can hear the other person's tone of voice.

Forms of communication where you cannot see or hear the other person, such as online messages, can present challenges. The possibility of miscommunication and conflict increases. Online communication has evolved to include some forms of nonverbal communication, such as emoticons, audio messages, pictures, and fonts such as capitalizing words. These cues help express tone, facial expressions, and gestures (**Figure 15.5**).

Ways to Communicate Effectively

In healthy relationships, people communicate their thoughts, values, feelings, and consent. They know the other person in the relationship will listen to and support them. You can use the techniques in the next sections to communicate care, consideration, and respect for yourself and others. These techniques help ensure that people communicate clearly and effectively.

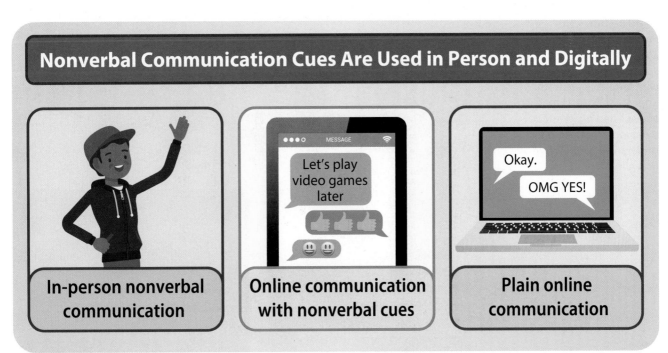

Nonverbal Communication Cues Are Used in Person and Digitally

In-person nonverbal communication

Online communication with nonverbal cues

Let's play video games later

Okay.

OMG YES!

Plain online communication

Figure 15.5 Nonverbal cues influence the tone and meaning of a message, whether the communication happens online or in person.

Use Active Listening

Good communication requires good listening skills. When you listen and focus on what the other person is saying, you work to understand the speaker's point of view and show respect. **Active listening** is the act of concentrating on the person talking with the goal of understanding the message and the speaker's feelings. Active listening involves the key steps shown in **Figure 15.6**.

Active listening is a great way to avoid misunderstandings. If you carefully listen to what others say, others will be more likely to do the same for you.

Clearly Express Your Needs and Preferences

To communicate effectively, people need to clearly, fully state their wants, needs, opinions, and feelings. Expecting the other person to be a mind reader is a sign of poor communication. Some people assume that others should be able to notice their subtle hints and know how they are feeling. This is also a poor communication strategy. Instead, explain what you want the other person to understand.

Be Assertive

As you communicate with others, you may notice that people use different communication styles. There are three common communication styles, which include the following:

1. **Passive.** Passive communication does not clearly state needs, wants, and feelings. A passive communicator may seem to say "yes" to everything, speak very quietly, and let hurt feelings build up.

Figure 15.6
Paying attention and acknowledging the speaker's message with feedback are both important aspects to active listening. *What is a person attempting to understand with active listening?*

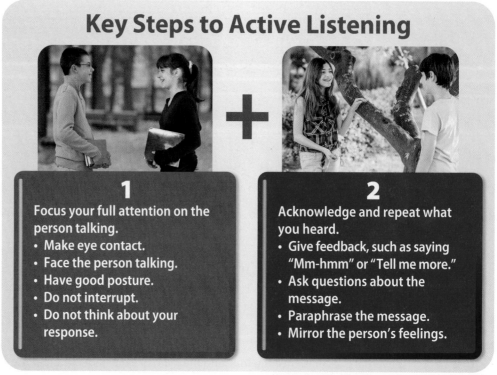

Key Steps to Active Listening

1
Focus your full attention on the person talking.
- Make eye contact.
- Face the person talking.
- Have good posture.
- Do not interrupt.
- Do not think about your response.

2
Acknowledge and repeat what you heard.
- Give feedback, such as saying "Mm-hmm" or "Tell me more."
- Ask questions about the message.
- Paraphrase the message.
- Mirror the person's feelings.

Left to right: iStock.com/Vesnaandjic; iStock.com/Angelafoto

2. **Aggressive.** Aggressive communication makes demands of another person and insults others. A person with this communication style expresses needs and feelings in a way that disrespects others.

3. **Assertive.** Assertive communication clearly expresses feelings, needs, and goals in a way that shows respect to the other person. This communication style values both people and seeks clarity.

BUILDING Your Skills

Be Assertive

You have probably encountered passive, aggressive, and assertive communication. For example, do you know people who say "yes" to everything? Have you seen people get what they want by being rude? Have you met people who seem to get what they need without demanding it?

Not all of these styles are equally effective. Passive and aggressive communication can hurt your health and relationships. Passive communicators often feel taken advantage of, and aggressive communicators often have difficulty making lasting relationships. The assertive communication style is the healthiest for relationships.

If being assertive does not come naturally to you, practice your assertive communication skills. The more you use assertive communication, the more comfortable you will feel being assertive. The following steps can help you improve your assertive communication skills:

- Have good posture. Stand or sit up straight with your shoulders back and down.
- Before starting the conversation, prepare yourself to act assertively. You could even write the word *assertive* on your hand as a reminder.
- Make eye contact. Do not stare at the other person, but make sure you can tell the color of the person's eyes. Glance at the person's eyes periodically during the conversation.
- Use a strong, but not overly loud voice and say what you mean.
- Remind yourself throughout the conversation to be assertive.
- Use I-statements instead of you-statements. For example, instead of saying, "You always steal my clothes," you could say, "I do not like

it when my clothes are borrowed without permission."
- Once the conversation is over, think about how it went. Consider what you could do in the future to be more assertive.
- Repeat. The next time an opportunity presents itself, be assertive again.

Practice Assertive Communication

With a partner, take turns role-playing how you would respond to the following scenarios using assertive communication. Continue practicing the role-plays until you feel comfortable using assertive communication.

Scenarios:

- You receive a grade on an assignment that you feel is much lower than you deserve. How would you discuss your grade with your teacher?
- Your best friend wants to see a movie that you really do not want to see. How would you respond to your friend?
- Your sibling comes into your bedroom unannounced, despite the door being closed and it bothers you. How would you ask your sibling for more privacy?

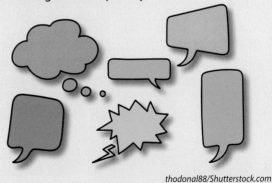

thodonal88/Shutterstock.com

The best communication style for building healthy relationships is assertive communication. This style allows you to express how you feel and make yourself known. If you do not express your feelings, goals, and consent, you are not letting other people truly know you. Assertive communication also helps you express yourself respectfully and in a way that is understanding of others. Communicating in a way that disrespects others can hurt healthy relationships. Communicating assertively, however, can help you build honest relationships based on trust and respect (**Figure 15.7**).

Use I-Statements

Effective communication uses I-statements to express feelings and desires. *I-statements* explain how the speaker feels without passing judgment on the receiver. An example of an I-statement is "I feel sad when I don't have anyone to talk to in class." This is more constructive than a you-statement, which makes assumptions about and blames the other person (for example, "You don't like me

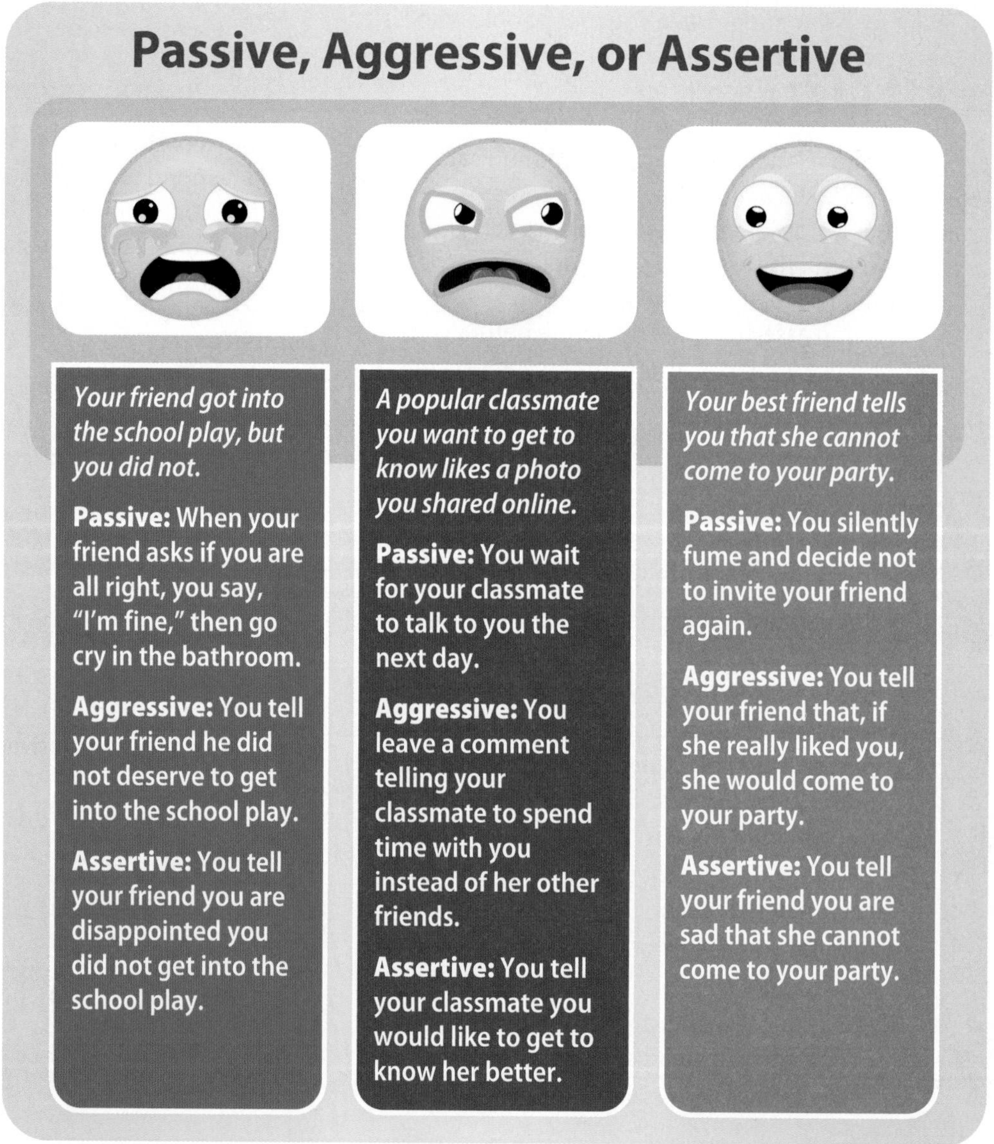

Figure 15.7
The way you communicate with others—passive, aggressive, or assertive—can impact whether or not you form healthy relationships with them. *Which communication style shows respect to the other person while clearly stating feelings and needs?*

Passive, Aggressive, or Assertive

Your friend got into the school play, but you did not.

Passive: When your friend asks if you are all right, you say, "I'm fine," then go cry in the bathroom.

Aggressive: You tell your friend he did not deserve to get into the school play.

Assertive: You tell your friend you are disappointed you did not get into the school play.

A popular classmate you want to get to know likes a photo you shared online.

Passive: You wait for your classmate to talk to you the next day.

Aggressive: You leave a comment telling your classmate to spend time with you instead of her other friends.

Assertive: You tell your classmate you would like to get to know her better.

Your best friend tells you that she cannot come to your party.

Passive: You silently fume and decide not to invite your friend again.

Aggressive: You tell your friend that, if she really liked you, she would come to your party.

Assertive: You tell your friend you are sad that she cannot come to your party.

Emojis: ChibVector/Shutterstock.com

anymore"). Using I-statements to tell other people how you feel can help them understand your point of view without making them feel attacked (**Figure 15.8**).

Watch Your Nonverbal Communication

Be aware of the nonverbal messages you are sending. What messages do your facial expressions and body language communicate to others? For example, suppose you are having a conversation with your sister. As she speaks, you look down at your phone and roll your eyes once in a while. These signals do not communicate active listening or respect for your sister. Making eye contact, nodding your head, and leaning forward would communicate that you value what she is saying.

Use Online Communication Wisely

Today, a lot of communication occurs online, such as text messages or social media. This type of communication has many advantages, some of which are instant feedback and long-distance communication. It also has some disadvantages. For example, it lacks some of the nonverbal communication present in face-to-face contact. People can also misjudge the tone or meaning of an online message. Following are strategies to help communicate online safely and effectively:

- **Be kind and respectful.** Treat people the way you would like to be treated. If someone is mean or rude, you can ignore the message, tell the person to stop, or block the person.
- **Solve conflicts offline.** Do not post or share conflicts with a person online. Agree to meet the person face-to-face to work through the conflict together.
- **Think before you share.** Think carefully before you share anything you would not want other people to see. Assume everyone will be able to see anything you post, even if you try to remove it.

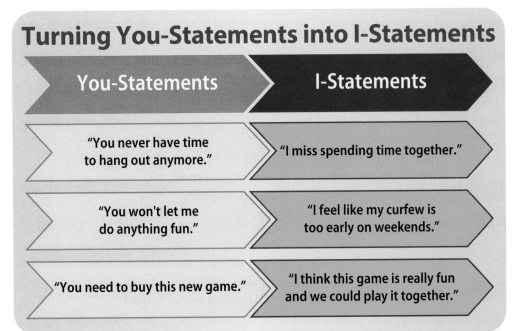

Turning You-Statements into I-Statements

You-Statements	I-Statements
"You never have time to hang out anymore."	"I miss spending time together."
"You won't let me do anything fun."	"I feel like my curfew is too early on weekends."
"You need to buy this new game."	"I think this game is really fun and we could play it together."

Figure 15.8
Using you-statements can make the other person feel blamed or judged, which can prevent positive communication. Instead, try to make I-statements.

Conflict Resolution Skills

Even with good communication, people can still have disagreements. These disagreements are called *conflicts* and are a normal part of life. Conflicts are present even in healthy relationships. **Figure 15.9** shows common sources of conflicts. What separates conflict in healthy relationships from conflict in unhealthy relationships is how conflict is resolved.

In disagreements of little importance, it may be best to simply accept differences between yourself and another person. There is no point arguing with a sibling who does not like a food you enjoy eating, for example. Other conflicts, such as you and your friend disagreeing about which movie to see, are easy to settle with no hurt feelings. Many conflicts, however, are more complicated and are too serious to ignore.

Conflicts that are not resolved can be quite hurtful. Unresolved conflicts can weaken feelings of trust and harm a person's mental and emotional health. Many people worry that addressing a conflict with another person can destroy a relationship or make conflict worse. In fact, working through and resolving a conflict can actually strengthen a relationship. The only way to settle a conflict is to address it. When people work together to resolve a conflict, they can end a hurtful situation and show their commitment to the relationship. When the conflict is settled, they can even feel closer to each other.

Common Sources of Conflict

Different Priorities
Your friend practices soccer instead of hanging out with you.

Different Values
You disagree with how your teacher treats a struggling classmate.

Different Goals
You want more independence, but your parents want to keep you safe.

Different Needs
You need alone time, but your sibling needs to talk after a fight with your parents.

Misunderstandings
You tell a classmate you had a bad weekend, and your friend thinks you are complaining about the time you spent together.

Left to right: Lapina/Shutterstock.com; Tyler Olson/Shutterstock.com; digitalskillet/Shutterstock.com; iStock.com/SolStock; Komkrit Noenpoempisut/Shutterstock.com

Figure 15.9 Conflicts can arise, even in healthy relationships, when people have different priorities, values, goals, needs, or understandings of a situation. *What effect can resolving a conflict have on a relationship?*

Negotiation

Settling a conflict requires negotiating skills. *Negotiating* is a process in which people work together (to think and talk) through a solution to a conflict. Figure 15.10 shows the six steps of the negotiation process.

Prepare

To prepare, agree with the other person on a time and place to discuss the conflict. Meet when you both have enough time to focus on the issue. Choose a meeting place away from other people and distractions. Before the meeting, get yourself ready. Think about what you want, what reasons you have, and what the other person may want. Consider what you are willing to give up to satisfy the other person's goals.

Keep Calm

Intense feelings such as frustration and anger can make a conflict worse. Feeling angry is normal, but acting aggressively in anger can hurt a relationship. Resolving conflict requires you to manage your emotions and share your feelings without letting them get out of control. If you feel anger building up, set that anger aside. Try taking several deep breaths or taking a break. Walk away and give yourself and the other person a chance to calm down.

State Your Position

When it is your turn to talk, state your position assertively. Speak honestly about your feelings, needs, and goals. Avoid behaving passively or aggressively. Behaving passively can cause you to avoid the conflict and let it continue to build. Aggressive behavior can offend the other person and put that person on the defensive. To state your position assertively, use I-statements instead of you-statements. Make sure your body language and other nonverbal cues match the position you are stating.

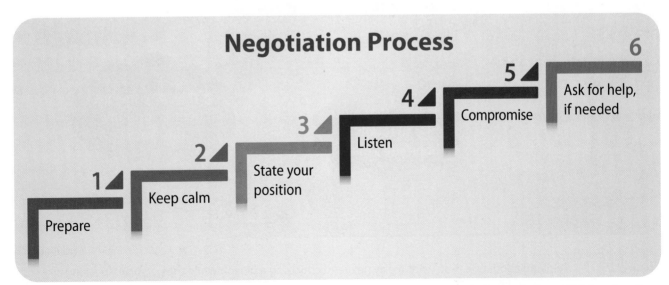

Figure 15.10 To work through a conflict, the people involved need to negotiate a solution to the issue. This involves time and effort.

Listen

Listen carefully to what the person is saying and try to understand that person's thoughts and feelings. Consider what good points the person is making and do not think about your response while the other person is talking (**Figure 15.11**). Also pay attention to the person's body language and tone of voice.

Compromise

In a *compromise*, both parties give up something they each want to reach a solution that is acceptable for everyone involved. For example, if you and your friends disagree about which movie to see, you could agree to see one movie this weekend and the other movie next weekend. Effective compromise is only possible if both sides are willing to be flexible.

Ask for Help

Sometimes a person is not ready to talk directly to the other person in a conflict. In that case, it might be best to talk to someone else first. Explaining the situation to a trusted adult or another friend can help you work out how you feel and what you want. It can give you a new perspective on the issue and clarify what to do next.

Mediation

In some cases, a conflict is too serious or difficult for the people directly involved to manage by themselves. In this situation, an outside individual can help the people or groups find a good solution.

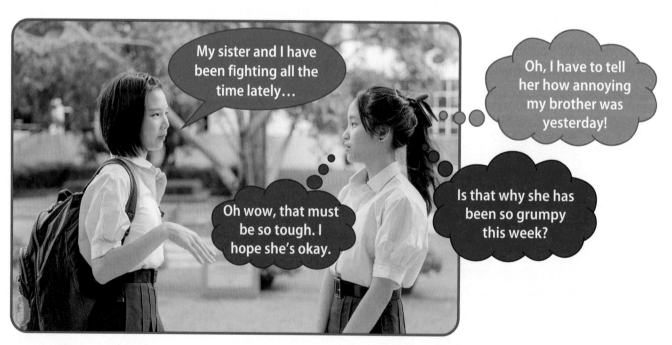

Crystal Home/Shutterstock.com

Figure 15.11 Thinking about what you want to say next and criticizing a person while the person is speaking are examples of poor listening skills.

As you learned in Chapter 1, *mediation* is a strategy for resolving difficult conflicts by involving a neutral third party, or *mediator*. A neutral person is someone who does not favor one side or another in a conflict.

Conflict resolution programs in many schools provide **peer mediation**, in which specially trained students work with other students to resolve conflicts (**Figure 15.12**). Peer mediators learn about conflicts and methods for resolving them. They work under the guidance of faculty advisors. When a conflict arises, the faculty member assigns a mediator to handle the situation. The mediator sets up a meeting to talk to the people involved in the conflict and to work through a solution.

At the meeting, the mediator invites everyone to state their view of the conflict. The mediator asks if those involved have thought of any possible solutions. If not, the mediator helps brainstorm possible solutions. The group discusses each alternative until everyone agrees on a solution.

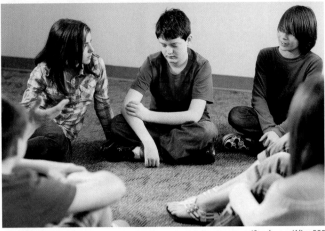

iStock.com/Alina555

Figure 15.12 In school peer mediation programs, students can help one another resolve conflicts in ways that maintain healthy relationships. *What is the term for a strategy for resolving difficult conflicts by involving a mediator?*

Lesson **15.1** Review

1. What are three characteristics of a healthy relationship?
2. Which of the following is an example of nonverbal communication?

   A. Letters.

   B. Posture.

   C. Text message.

   D. Phone call.
3. **True or false.** Active listening is thinking about your response while another person is talking.
4. What happens in a compromise?
5. **Critical thinking.** Explain why the assertive communication style is most effective for building healthy relationships.

Hands-On Activity

With a partner, review the information about I-statements in this lesson. Then, on a separate piece of paper, write five you-statements expressing negative emotions you have felt over the past year. Trade with your partner and rewrite your partner's you-statements into I-statements that would improve communication. Share the I-statements with your partner and discuss what each statement communicates.

Lesson 15.2

Family Relationships

Key Terms ☞

immediate family person's parents or guardians and siblings

extended family distant relatives, including aunts, uncles, cousins, and grandparents

socialize teaching children to behave in socially acceptable ways

traditions specific patterns of behavior passed down in a culture

rituals series of actions performed as part of a ceremony

sibling rivalry competitive feelings between siblings

Learning Outcomes

After studying this lesson, you will be able to

- **analyze** the functions of the family.
- **explain** the role of community in supporting families.
- **identify** strategies to promote healthy relationships with parents or guardians and siblings.
- **describe** various changes that occur within families and ways to adjust to them.

Graphic Organizer

Healthy and Unhealthy Families

On a separate piece of paper, draw two pictures—one illustrating a healthy family and the other illustrating an unhealthy family—as in the example shown. Then, as you read this lesson, organize your notes according to qualities that make families healthy and qualities that make families unhealthy. An example is provided for you.

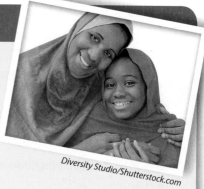

Diversity Studio/Shutterstock.com

Healthy Family   **Unhealthy Family**

Provide for members' physical needs
Meet mental and emotional needs

Healthy and unhealthy families: Melinda Varga/Shutterstock.com

The word family has several definitions. Legally, a *family* is two or more people related by marriage, blood, or adoption who live in the same home. A family may also include other relatives, partners, and diverse members. There are many different types of family structures (**Figure 15.13**). No matter the type of family, family relationships are important.

The very first relationship most people have are with their family members. As they grow up, many people spend lots of time with members of their **immediate family**, meaning their parents or guardians and siblings. **Extended family** members, such as aunts, uncles, cousins, and grandparents, can also play a significant role in a person's life. Together, many people consider these family relationships to be among their closest.

In this lesson, you will learn about different conflicts that can occur in family relationships and ways to prevent and resolve them. You will also learn about changes in family relationships and skills to help cope with these changes.

Functions of Family Relationships

Family relationships have several unique functions that make them different from other relationships. Unlike other types of relationships, relationships in families have the responsibility of providing for members' physical needs, fulfilling members' mental and emotional needs, and educating and socializing children.

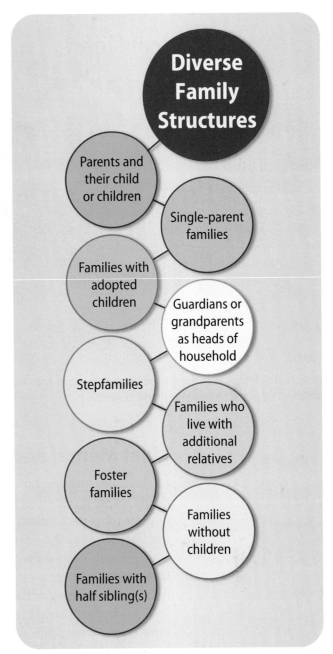

Figure 15.13 There are many different structures that make up a family. *Which family members are considered extended family?*

Provide for Physical Needs

Families typically provide for members' physical needs, such as needs for food. Families are also responsible for ensuring that members are healthy and safe (**Figure 15.14**). Your parents or guardians may take you to the doctor and dentist on a regular basis. They probably set rules—even rules you may not like—with the goal of keeping you safe and healthy.

As children grow older, they can take on tasks to help meet the family's physical needs. For example, doing some cleaning chores helps keep the home a healthy place to live. It also takes tasks away from parents or guardians who have to spend many hours a day working.

Physical Needs That the Family Meets

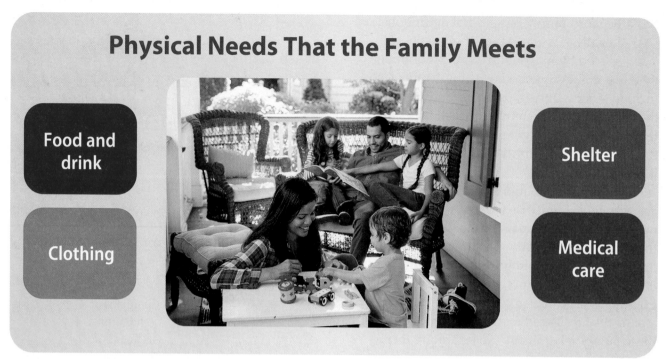

Monkey Business Images/Shutterstock.com

Figure 15.14 It is the responsibility of your family to make sure that you have enough to eat and drink, clothes to wear, a safe place to live, and medical care.

Meet Mental and Emotional Needs

Families also help meet members' mental and emotional needs, such as the needs for love, self-esteem, and emotional comfort. For example, your parents or guardians may attend your school performances and sporting events. Family members may celebrate your birthday and your achievements. The support and love you receive from your family members help you feel secure and good about yourself. Many people rely on their families for advice about how to solve issues or handle challenges.

Children can help meet the mental and emotional needs of adults in the family, too. When children show love for parents or guardians, grandparents, or other extended family members, those adults feel good. Children can provide words of support or encouragement when adults feel down.

Educate and Socialize Children

Families educate children by teaching them about the world and sending them to school. They also **socialize** children by teaching them to behave in socially acceptable ways (**Figure 15.15**). Children learn about culture, values, and **traditions** (specific patterns of behavior) through their families. They learn language from family members, as well as information about their families' culture and religion. All families have unique traditions, which may include celebrating special occasions, holding particular values and beliefs, and participating in certain religious **rituals**, or series of actions.

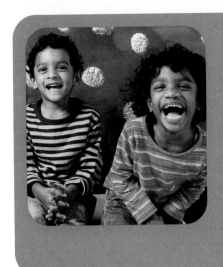

Through socialization, children learn about

- culture
- language
- social norms
- society
- relationships
- gender
- appropriate behavior

alexandre zveiger/Shutterstock.com

Figure 15.15
Families typically prepare their children for the outside world by teaching them lessons and sending them to school. *What are the specific patterns of behavior children learn through their families?*

Families and the Community

Families live in larger social groups, or *communities*. Because of this, neighbors and even strangers can have an impact on family relationships. For example, they can give support to family members in times of trouble by providing meals when a parent or guardian is ill. Neighbors can be friends to family members and join with them in enjoyable social events.

A community is more than just a neighborhood, however. Families live in towns or cities, and these locations have institutions and services that can help families, such as police and fire departments, hospitals, and government agencies. State laws require that children receive certain vaccines to promote public health and prevent the spread of diseases. School officials take steps to remove students who threaten classmates, helping families meet the goal of keeping members safe.

It is important to have healthy relationships within your community. You can build healthy relationships in your community by treating other people with respect, being open and honest about what you think and feel, and being reliable and trustworthy (**Figure 15.16**).

Relationships with Parents or Guardians

Family relationships are some of the most important relationships you will have in your life. These relationships, however, can be difficult at times. For example, many children experience some conflict in their relationships with parents, guardians, or other caregivers. These conflicts can get worse as children grow older. Identifying common issues in these relationships and using certain strategies can help strengthen the relationship between caregivers and young people.

Skills to Build Healthy Relationships in the Community

- Advocate for diversity
- Communicate effectively
  - Show respect
  - Demonstrate confidence
  - Be receptive to feedback
  - Acknowledge other people
  - Proofread communication
- Maintain healthy boundaries
- Be involved in your community
- Participate in clubs that involve other students and families

Figure 15.16 You can build healthy relationships in your community by communicating effectively and being involved in the community.

Common Issues in Relationships with Parents or Guardians

Many issues between parents or guardians and young people result from conflicting goals. For example, one major goal young people have is to form a unique identity apart from family. Adolescence is a time of self-exploration. During this time, young people naturally push for things such as freedom and independence (**Figure 15.17**).

At the same time, parents' or guardians' goals include keeping young people safe and healthy and teaching them how to function well in society. To do this, parents or guardians set rules that young people might find restrictive, or limiting. This is one reason why conflicts between parents or guardians and young people often escalate during adolescence.

Conflicts between parents or guardians and young people may also develop as a result of media influences such as television and movies. Young people may see messages about living in families that conflict with the traditions or customs of their own families. These differences can be a source of conflict.

Maintaining Healthy Relationships with Parents or Guardians

Maintaining healthy relationships with parents or guardians takes effort. Fortunately, the following strategies for having healthy relationships and resolving conflicts with parents or guardians can help:

- Share your plans ahead of time. Make sure to get approval before you commit to do something with a friend. Answer any questions your parents or guardians may have and revise the plan, if needed.
- Discuss family rules. If you disagree with a rule, calmly explain why you think the rule should change and give reasons for your suggested change (**Figure 15.18**). Your parents or guardian may agree to reconsider the rule.

Figure 15.17
During adolescence, young people want more independence, freedom, and responsibility, which can cause arguments with guardians or parents. *What type of identity do young people want to form during adolescence?*

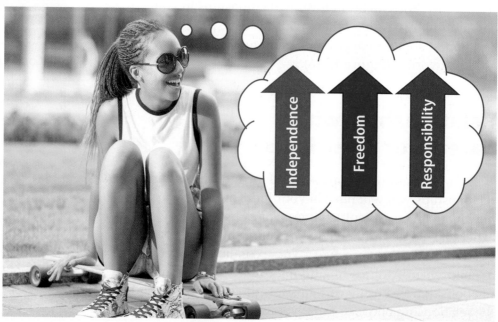

Dmitry Morgan/Shutterstock.com

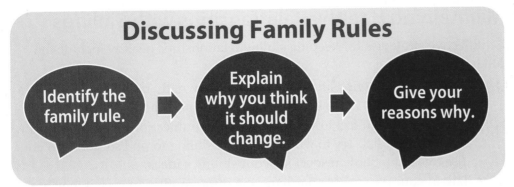

Discussing Family Rules

Identify the family rule. → Explain why you think it should change. → Give your reasons why.

Figure 15.18
If you think a family rule is unfair or unnecessary, the best response is to calmly discuss a possible change with your parent or guardian.

- Follow your family's rules, even if you disagree with them. Remember that parents and guardians may relax or lift these rules if you show responsible behavior and a willingness to obey limits. On the other hand, if you do not follow the rules, you may weaken your family's trust in you.
- Remain calm. When you have a disagreement, do not resort to yelling and do not walk away. Show your parents or guardians that you are capable of having a mature discussion and that you can be responsible.
- Spend time doing enjoyable activities with your family. You might suggest having a special family dinner one night a week or planning a trip. These types of activities can bring families together.

Adolescents who have healthy relationships with their parents and guardians can communicate their thoughts and feelings, learn to navigate challenges, and learn to make healthy decisions. Unfortunately, some adolescents may feel their relationship is unhealthy. If you have an unhealthy relationship with a parent or guardian, do what you can to improve the relationship. Talk to other adults you trust, such as a teacher, school counselor, or school nurse. You can also reach out to community resources.

Relationships with Siblings

Sibling relationships are often the earliest friendships people have. Many siblings often fight and argue, however. Keeping these relationships healthy can lead to greater satisfaction as you grow older.

Common Issues in Sibling Relationships

Even siblings who are biologically related or who grow up in the same household may not share interests. Siblings may have different personalities, find different activities interesting, or have different ways of handling major life events. These differences can create conflict, especially when siblings spend a lot of time together.

Another source of conflict among siblings is competition, which is called **sibling rivalry**. Siblings may compete for material or nonmaterial items. Examples of sibling rivalry include competing for a parent's or guardian's attention or fighting over use of the television. When teasing is involved, feelings of competition may increase. Sibling rivalry may lead to negative feelings, such as resentment, anger, or jealousy.

Maintaining Healthy Relationships with Siblings

Effective strategies for keeping sibling relationships healthy include the following:

- Get away from tense situations and cool down. By taking a break from a heated situation, you will avoid making the argument worse.
- Express how you feel to your sibling. Communication is the first step in resolving conflict. Try to work with your sibling to find solutions to your disagreement. Show respect for your sibling's ideas.
- Talk to your parents or guardians about the conflict and see if they have advice for finding a good solution.
- Compromise when issues arise. Try to work out a solution that both you and your sibling think is fair (**Figure 15.19**). Together, you can develop specific rules for handling ongoing sources of conflict.
- Identify a personal space for each person. For example, if you share a bedroom with a sibling, talk to your sibling about setting aside areas for each of you.
- Respect your sibling's space and privacy. Do not enter a sibling's room without knocking. If you share a room, respect your sibling's private space within that room.
- Find enjoyable ways of spending time with your sibling. This could include going for a bike ride or having a family game night.

Figure 15.19
When you disagree with a sibling, working out a solution that is fair to both parties can stop the disagreement before it causes a fight.

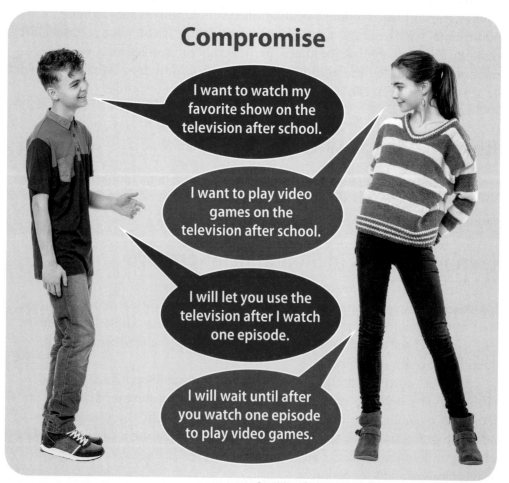

Boy: VaLiza/Shutterstock.com; Girl: Armin Staudt/Shutterstock.com

Changes in Family Relationships

All families encounter changes over time. For example, a member may have a physical or mental illness, lose a job, or move to a new community. Change can create stress in a family and disrupt family relationships. These changes are a normal, although difficult, part of family life.

Even positive changes—such as a job promotion or starting middle school—can create stress. This is because new events lead to changes in how family members interact every day. For example, suppose a parent or guardian gets a big promotion at work. This may mean that the parent or guardian must work longer hours or travel more. Other family members may need to take on additional chores at home.

Some of the most challenging changes families experience are those that affect family structure—the addition or loss of a family member. These changes include the birth or adoption of a new family member, separation or divorce, remarriage, and the death of a family member. Although these events can be difficult, healthy families can work through them together. Sometimes, families even grow closer when dealing with changes such as these. Using good communication skills and effective strategies for maintaining family relationships will help family members get through these challenging periods (**Figure 15.20**).

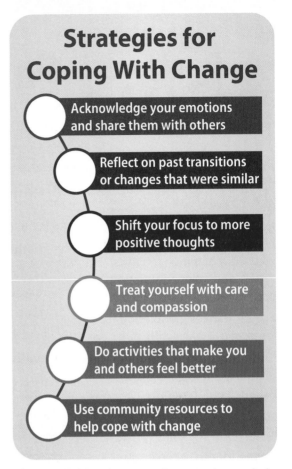

Strategies for Coping With Change

- Acknowledge your emotions and share them with others
- Reflect on past transitions or changes that were similar
- Shift your focus to more positive thoughts
- Treat yourself with care and compassion
- Do activities that make you and others feel better
- Use community resources to help cope with change

Figure 15.20 Using certain strategies can help family members cope with changes and maintain healthy relationships, even during challenging times.

Lesson 15.2 Review

1. Name three unique functions that make family relationships different from other relationships.
2. **True or false.** Neighbors and strangers can influence family relationships.
3. If you disagree with a family rule, what should you do?
4. What is sibling rivalry?
5. **Critical thinking.** Why do even positive changes in families cause stress?

Hands-On Activity

Over several days, become an observer of your family's interactions. Pay attention to any signs of the conflicts discussed in this lesson and note how your family resolves these conflicts. Write a summary of your observations and then draw conclusions about your family's relationships. Identify healthy and unhealthy characteristics in your family's interactions. For each unhealthy characteristic, describe what you can do to make your family relationships healthier.

Lesson 15.3

Peer Relationships

Key Terms

friendship relationship between two or more people who share common interests, values, and goals and support each other

acquaintances people you know and interact with, but may not consider friends

diversity inclusion of people with different backgrounds

stereotypes oversimplified ideas about a group of people

online friends people you meet through social media, websites, chat rooms, or gaming

clique small group of friends who deliberately exclude other people from joining or being a part of their group

Learning Outcomes

After studying this lesson, you will be able to

- **distinguish between** different types of friendships.
- **explain** how to promote tolerance and celebrate diversity in relationships.
- **devise** a plan to use strategies for building and maintaining healthy friendships.
- **evaluate** common issues in friendships.
- **differentiate between** positive and negative types of peer pressure.

Graphic Organizer

Friendship Inventory

Take an inventory of your friendships by listing your closest peer relationships in the middle column of a table like the one shown. As you read this lesson, identify each type of friendship and record the information after the person's name. In the left-hand column, write factors that could harm your friendships. In the right-hand column, write strategies for keeping your friendships healthy.

William Perugini/Shutterstock.com

Harmful Factors	Friendships	Strategies
Feelings of jealousy	Jade (best friend)	Make more time for friends
Pressure to tease Jade	Abdul (school friend)	Talk to Abdul in person more often
	Josiah (online friend)	
	Sheila (acquaintance)	

496

P eer relationships, or friendships, are some of the most important relationships in your life. Friendships are especially important during adolescence, when relationships with peers can become the center of your world. Consider Kai from the first lesson. Kai loves talking with his friends. He spends a lot of time online joking with his classmates on social media. He has a best friend named Jacqueline, and they like to play soccer and video games together. He avoids cliques because he would prefer to be friends and get along with everyone.

Types of Friendships

The most common type of peer relationship is friendship. **Friendship** is the relationship between two or more people who share common interests, values, and goals and support each other. The term *friendship* describes many different types of peer relationships (**Figure 15.21**). For example, you probably know the difference between your very closest friends and your more casual friends. Perhaps you have a single friend whom you consider your best friend. You may also have many **acquaintances**—people you know and interact with, but may not consider friends.

Living in a diverse culture, you are likely to meet people who see the world differently than you do. **Diversity** is present in a group of people with different backgrounds, including ages, sex, family traditions, ethnicities, and cultures.

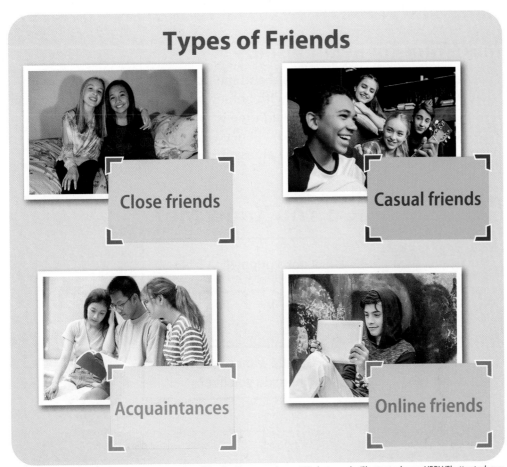

Types of Friends

Close friends

Casual friends

Acquaintances

Online friends

Left to right: May Hayward/Shutterstock.com; LightField Studios/Shutterstock.com; NiP photography/Shutterstock.com; HBRH/Shutterstock.com

Figure 15.21
There are many different types of peer relationships that can all be considered friendships. *What is it called when you have a friendship with someone who has a different background than you?*

In healthy relationships, people respect others for who they are. They celebrate differences and avoid stereotyping. **Stereotypes** are oversimplified ideas about a group of people. Diversity in a culture can broaden people's knowledge. Ideally, people challenge and learn from others, while respecting others' values.

In the past, most people had friends they went to school with or who lived in the neighborhood. Today, however, many people have friends who live farther away.

You may have **online friends**, or people you meet through social media, websites, chat rooms, or gaming. True friendships can sometimes develop between online friends, especially if friends share some real-life friends. You should be careful, however, about sharing information with people you have only met online (**Figure 15.22**). These people might not be representing themselves truthfully. If an online friend offers to meet you in person, talk about the situation with a trusted adult before agreeing to meet.

Strategies for Building Healthy Friendships

Healthy friendships provide emotional and social support, companionship, and help you learn more about yourself and others. Sometimes it can be hard to make and keep friends. Determining whether someone shares your core values and beliefs can take time, especially if you are still trying to figure out your values and beliefs. Even when arguments arise, however, there are ways to maintain healthy friendships over time.

Make Time for Relationships

It takes time and energy to build and maintain close relationships with friends. Even when you are busy with homework, sports, or other activities, try to find time to connect and spend time with acquaintances and friends. As you build new friendships, you will need time to get to know other people and understand how their values and beliefs align with yours.

Figure 15.22
You can form meaningful relationships online, but you should keep in mind that you cannot truly know who you are talking to. *What is the term for people you meet online and do not interact face-to-face?*

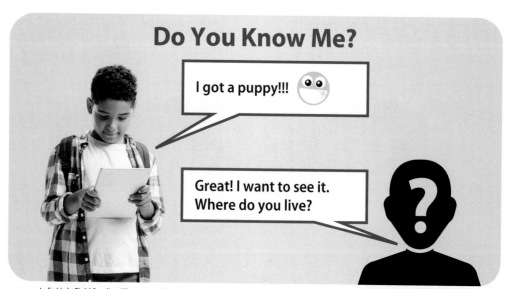

Left: LightField Studios/Shutterstock.com; Emoji: Dmytro Onopko/Shutterstock.com; Right: Best Vector Elements/Shutterstock.com

If you want to get to know someone, you could try spending time in a group, doing an activity together, or talking throughout the day. If finding free time is hard, plan ahead and set dates to get together with friends to set aside the needed time to build friendships.

Meet Friends Face-to-Face

Online communication is a great way to connect with friends and get to know people. It is also important to form and maintain friendships through face-to-face interactions. In-person communication is an important part of having a close relationship. While online communication makes it easier to stay in touch, do not rely on these types of interactions alone. Remember that online conversations lack important aspects of nonverbal communication. One of the best ways to keep a relationship healthy is to step away from the screen and make time to be physically present with someone (**Figure 15.23**).

Be a Good Friend

In healthy friendships, each person contributes equally to the relationship. You can be a good friend by listening carefully to what your friends are saying. Also, avoid interrupting or judging them when they are talking. Other strategies you can use to keep your friendships healthy include the following:

- Support and encourage your friends, and celebrate their successes.
- Avoid teasing or criticizing your friends.
- Do not gossip or spread rumors about your friends. Spreading gossip and rumors is hurtful and makes others feel bad.
- Work with your friends to solve disagreements and conflicts.
- Express your feelings openly during conflicts, and listen carefully to your friend's point of view.
- Apologize if you hurt your friend and try to find ways to make it better.

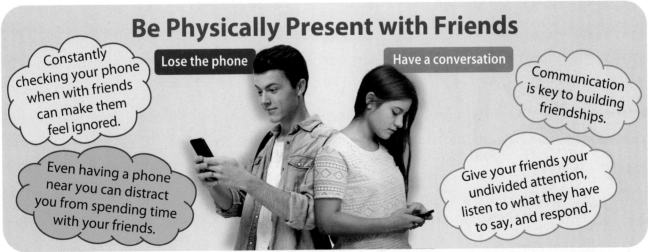

Be Physically Present with Friends

Constantly checking your phone when with friends can make them feel ignored.

Lose the phone

Even having a phone near you can distract you from spending time with your friends.

Have a conversation

Communication is key to building friendships.

Give your friends your undivided attention, listen to what they have to say, and respond.

Ljupco Smokovski/Shutterstock.com; antoniodiaz/Shutterstock.com

Figure 15.23 Having your phone in front of you while spending time with friends, whether you are on it or not, can prevent you from forming meaningful friendships. ***What type of interaction is important to form and maintain friendships?***

Damage Control: The Negative Effects of Gossip and Rumors

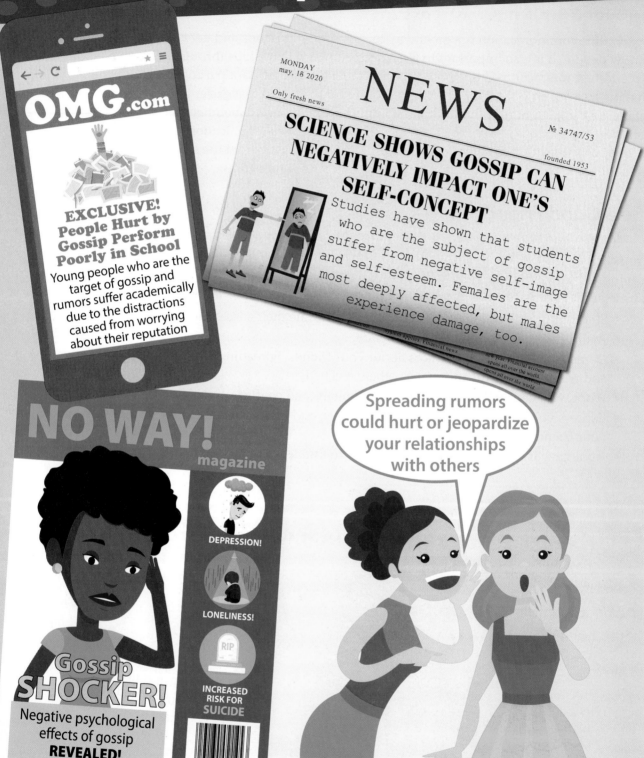

OMG.com

EXCLUSIVE!
People Hurt by Gossip Perform Poorly in School

Young people who are the target of gossip and rumors suffer academically due to the distractions caused from worrying about their reputation

MONDAY may, 18 2020

Only fresh news

NEWS

№ 34747/53

founded 1953

SCIENCE SHOWS GOSSIP CAN NEGATIVELY IMPACT ONE'S SELF-CONCEPT

Studies have shown that students who are the subject of gossip suffer from negative self-image and self-esteem. Females are the most deeply affected, but males experience damage, too.

NO WAY! magazine

DEPRESSION!

LONELINESS!

RIP

INCREASED RISK FOR SUICIDE

Gossip SHOCKER!
Negative psychological effects of gossip REVEALED!

0 10421 25071 3

Spreading rumors could hurt or jeopardize your relationships with others

Common Issues in Friendships

Although friendships can improve your life in many ways, they can also be a source of conflicts and issues. At times, even close friendships can be complicated and confusing. Cliques, jealousy, and changes over time are common issues in friendships.

Cliques

Many middle school students enjoy spending time with groups of friends. Sometimes, these groups of friends may exclude other people, which can lead to hurt feelings. A **clique** is a small group of friends who deliberately exclude other people from joining or being a part of their group.

People in a clique often feel pressured to act a certain way or adopt the attitudes and behaviors of group members (**Figure 15.24**). Sometimes, cliques can also pressure group members to do unhealthy actions. For example, a group may encourage vaping. In this way, cliques can reduce each person's individuality and compromise well-being, which is unhealthy.

You can learn to handle cliques by being true to yourself. If you are in a clique, think about if being part of the group feels good or not. Make sure to spend time with people who make you feel good about yourself and respect you for who you are. Do not limit yourself to only making friends with people in one group. You might miss out on some great friendships.

Jealousy

Jealousy may sometimes occur in a friendship. You may feel jealous of your friend's achievement in a particular area, such as schoolwork, athletics, or music. You may also feel jealous of other aspects of a friend's life, such as the friend's home, dating relationship, or family life. Feelings of jealousy are normal if they occur once in a while. Continuous jealous feelings, however, can harm a relationship over time.

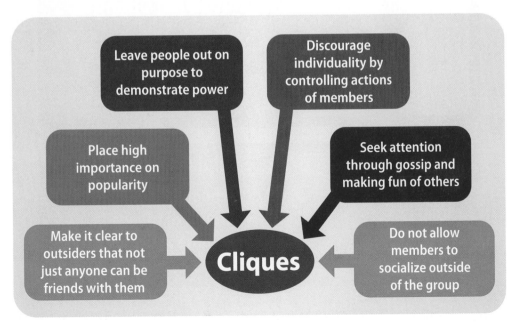

Figure 15.24
There are various signs that can help identify if a group of friends is a clique.

Honestly expressing your emotions, including jealousy, can prevent negative feelings from building up over time and weakening your friendship. If you value your friendship and want to keep it, try to move beyond feelings of jealousy.

Changes over Time

Friendships evolve as people change over time. Experiencing physical, emotional, and social changes can influence your friendships (**Figure 15.25**). This is particularly true if you and a friend change in different ways. You may no longer share the same interests with your childhood friends. You may need to stop spending time with a friend who makes unsafe or unhealthy decisions.

Sometimes, old friendships can be maintained, but change in some way. For example, you might see an old friend less frequently as your interests and peer groups change. If you want to maintain an old friendship, invest time and energy in that friendship. Make a point of connecting with your friend, either online or in person, so you can stay up-to-date on each other's lives. These check-ins will help you stay connected.

Figure 15.25
If one friend changes physically, emotionally, or socially at a different rate or in a different way than another friend, distance between the two people can result.

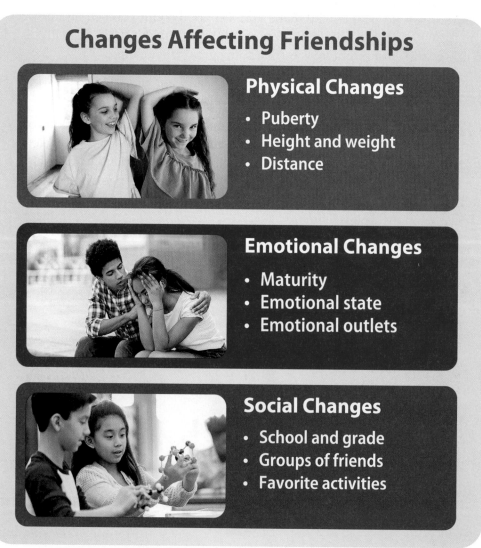

Changes Affecting Friendships

Physical Changes
- Puberty
- Height and weight
- Distance

Emotional Changes
- Maturity
- Emotional state
- Emotional outlets

Social Changes
- School and grade
- Groups of friends
- Favorite activities

Top to bottom: Monkey Business Images/Shutterstock.com; Prostock-studio/Shutterstock.com; iStock.com/SDI Productions

If you feel that you and a friend are drifting apart, tell your friend how you feel. If both of you are interested in maintaining the friendship, you can work together to find ways of remaining close.

Peer Pressure

Peer pressure is a common element present in friendships. *Peer pressure* is the influence a person feels from *peers*, or people of the same age range or status, to act or think in certain ways. Pressure from peers can be positive or negative.

Positive Peer Pressure

Although people often associate peer pressure with negative activities, it can have a positive influence (**Figure 15.26**). For example, you might feel pressured to participate in community service projects with a school group. A friend may encourage you to study harder to improve your grades. In these cases, pressure from peers can help broaden your perspective of the world, help your community, or help you succeed in school. Positive peer pressure is also respectful. It values your opinions, preferences, and individuality. For example, a friend should accept your answer if you decline an invite to see a movie.

Negative Peer Pressure

In some friendships, one person pressures another to do something that person is not comfortable doing. Friends might pressure each other to drink alcohol, skip class, or tease a classmate. Most people want to be liked and to fit in with a group. They may decide to go along with a certain behavior, even if they are uncomfortable with it. They may worry about being teased or excluded if they do not join in a group activity. Sometimes, youths worry that standing up for what they believe could cause them to lose a friendship.

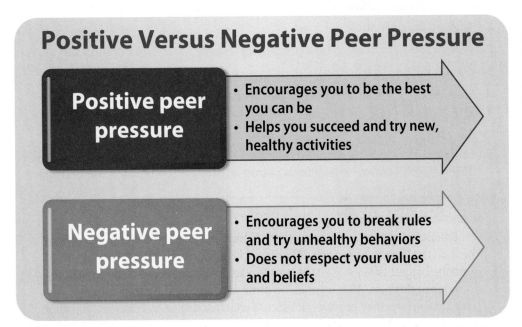

Figure 15.26
Peer pressure may include encouragement of risky behaviors, but it can also include support for healthy activities.

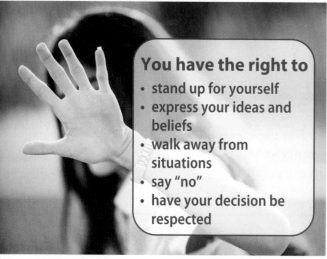

You have the right to
- stand up for yourself
- express your ideas and beliefs
- walk away from situations
- say "no"
- have your decision be respected

kckate16/Shutterstock.com

Figure 15.27 If a person is trying to pressure you into risky behaviors, this person is not truly your friend. This person does not have your health and well-being at heart.

In healthy friendships, this type of negative peer pressure does not occur. True friends respect each other's choices. If you are experiencing negative peer pressure, you have the right to stand up for what you believe, and to walk away from situations that make you uncomfortable (**Figure 15.27**). If a friend ends a relationship with you over this choice, the person does not respect you and your friendship. Standing up to peer pressure is especially important when friends are doing something that could hurt you or someone else.

What can you do to stand up to peer pressure? Strategies you can use to respond to negative peer pressure include the following:

- Focus on your own thoughts, feelings, and values. Use a good decision-making process to make sure your actions reflect your core beliefs.
- Have the strength and self-confidence to walk away from a situation or from people who make you uncomfortable.
- Refuse to join in teasing someone because this person acts or looks different.
- Choose friends who have values similar to yours. People who share your values, goals, and beliefs will probably support the decisions you make.
- Support other people when they resist peer pressure. Sometimes, having just one other person say, "I agree, this is a bad idea," is all it takes to change a group's behavior.
- If peer pressure continues over time, talk to someone you trust—a parent or guardian, teacher, or school counselor.

Lesson 15.3 Review

1. Who are online friends?
2. **True or false.** One way to be a good friend is to celebrate your friend's successes.
3. What is the best way to deal with jealousy in a friendship?
4. Pressure to _____ is an example of positive peer pressure.
   - **A.** tease your friend
   - **B.** vape
   - **C.** skip class
   - **D.** study for a big exam
5. **Critical thinking.** Why do you think face-to-face interactions are important for building and maintaining relationships instead of relying on online communication?

Hands-On Activity

Brainstorm acts of kindness that your friends and peers would enjoy receiving. These do not have to be big acts of kindness. In relationships, little things can make the biggest difference. List at least five acts of kindness you could realistically do and then do them. After completing these acts, write a few paragraphs summarizing how they positively impacted your friendships and peer relationships.

Dating Relationships

Learning Outcomes

After studying this lesson, you will be able to

- **describe** the characteristics of a healthy dating relationship.
- **identify** strategies to set boundaries for physical intimacy before and during a dating relationship.
- **follow** strategies for forming a healthy dating relationship.
- **describe** healthy ways to handle the end of a dating relationship.

Key Terms ☞

casual dating way of getting to know how you interact with and feel about another person

infatuation intense romantic feelings for another person that develop suddenly and are usually based on physical attraction

passion powerful feeling based on physical attraction

exclusive committed to being romantically involved with only one dating partner

intimacy closeness

group dating going out with a group that includes the person one is interested in rather than dating as a couple

breakup end of a romantic relationship

Graphic Organizer

Dating Need-to-Know

On a separate piece of paper, draw a heart like in the example shown. Skim this lesson and write the main headings in a circle around the heart. As you read the lesson, take notes under each heading. Then, identify the five most important facts you learned in this lesson and write them in the middle of the heart.

Kochneva Tetyana/Shutterstock.com

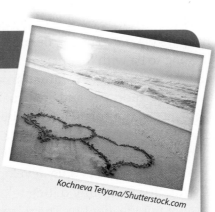

Characteristics of Healthy Dating Relationships
- Attraction—infatuation without closeness
- Closeness

1.
2.
3.
4.
5.

The End of a Dating Relationship

Strategies for Forming Healthy Dating Relationships

Physical Intimacy and Abstinence

Heart: popular business/Shutterstock.com

- learn about yourself and others
- get along with others
- form good peer relationships
- evaluate personalities
- learn about the give-and-take involved in relationships

Figure 15.28 Dating can help build interpersonal skills as well as communication skills.

Dating relationships are a new type of relationship for many young people. The decision to begin dating is personal, and different people feel ready to begin dating at different times. Some young people are interested in and ready for dating earlier than their peers. These people may feel attracted to a person in a romantic way and decide to act on those feelings. Other young people may not yet feel this type of attraction for someone else. Some families may have rules that limit or forbid dating until a certain age.

A couple can go out on a date without being in a dating relationship. **Casual dating** is a way of getting to know how you interact with and feel about another person. It can help you learn more about yourself (**Figure 15.28**). A *dating relationship* exists when two people date on a regular basis.

Characteristics of Healthy Dating Relationships

All types of healthy relationships share similar qualities, such as honesty and trust, mutual respect, safety, care, and commitment. Healthy dating relationships also have the following qualities:

- **Attraction.** Attraction refers to the physical and emotional connection that draws people together. Being attracted to someone means it is exciting to be with that person. Attraction without closeness is sometimes infatuation. **Infatuation** describes intense romantic feelings that develop suddenly and are usually based on physical attraction. A *crush* is an example of an intense, but short-lived, infatuation.
- **Closeness.** Closeness arises because two people share personal feelings and thoughts that they do not share with others. When they share with each other, these two people develop a bond.
- **Individuality.** In healthy dating relationships, each person maintains their own unique identity. The relationship does not redefine a person. Each person's core values, beliefs, and sense of self remain the same.
- **Balance.** People in a healthy dating relationship see each other regularly, but make time for friends and family members. In a healthy dating relationship, people also share time and activities equally and fairly (**Figure 15.29**).
- **Open communication, honesty, and respect.** Both people in a relationship should feel comfortable expressing their likes, dislikes, goals, values, and thoughts. In a healthy dating relationship, the couple can discuss these topics openly, honestly, and with respect.
- **Support.** In a healthy dating relationship, both people should support each other's successes, happiness, talents, interests, and goals.

Over time, love may develop in a dating relationship. *Love* describes an intense affection for and attachment to another person. Love develops gradually as people get to know each other on a more intimate level. This should not be confused with feelings of passion. **Passion** can be very powerful and exciting, but is typically short-lived because it is based in physical attraction.

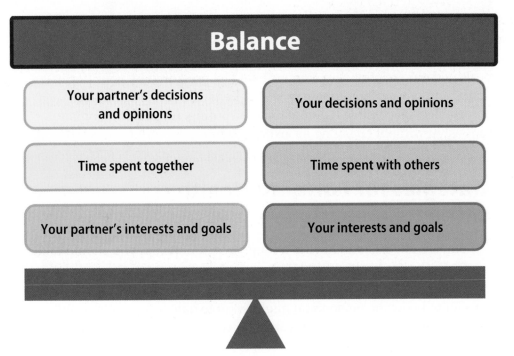

Balance

Your partner's decisions and opinions	Your decisions and opinions
Time spent together	Time spent with others
Your partner's interests and goals	Your interests and goals

Figure 15.29
In a healthy dating relationship, people should spend time with their dating partners as well as others, hear their opinions, and let them make some decisions.

As love develops, couples may decide to commit to be **exclusive**, or romantically involved with only one dating partner. Being exclusive means that the couple agrees to work together at maintaining the relationship. It also means the couple is willing to work through issues instead of ending the relationship when conflict occurs.

Physical Intimacy and Abstinence

Dating relationships often include some type of physical **intimacy**, or closeness, such as holding hands and kissing. Before you start dating, you should know how you feel about being physically intimate with another person (**Figure 15.30**). It is better to know your boundaries before you are in a situation that requires a quick decision. Be sure to enforce these personal boundaries and your affirmative consent during the relationship.

Many factors, including your values, religion, and judgment, will influence decisions you make about physical intimacy. *Abstinence*, or the commitment to refrain from sexual activity, is a healthy choice for young people. Abstinence is the only method that is 100 percent effective in preventing sexually transmitted infections (STIs), HIV/AIDS, and pregnancy. It also prevents emotional consequences such as guilt over keeping sexual activity a secret. Finally, it avoids social consequences related to being exclusive.

Questions to Ask About Physical Intimacy and Consent

- Am I comfortable hugging?
- Am I comfortable holding hands?
- Am I comfortable putting my arm around my partner? with my partner putting an arm around me?
- Am I comfortable sitting on my partner's lap? with my partner sitting on my lap?
- Am I comfortable being alone with my partner?
- Am I comfortable kissing?

Figure 15.30 These are examples of topics people can ask themselves about how comfortable or not comfortable they are with physical intimacy in a relationship. *Identify three factors that can influence decisions you make about physical intimacy.*

As with physical intimacy, you should consider your own boundaries related to abstinence before starting a dating relationship. When you start dating, communicate these boundaries and stick to them (**Figure 15.31**). In a healthy dating relationship, you will not feel pressured by your partner to engage in physically intimate or sexual behavior that does not feel comfortable. It is possible to maintain a rewarding, fun, healthy romantic relationship without engaging in sexual activity.

Strategies for Forming Healthy Dating Relationships

If you are interested in having a romantic relationship, you should take steps to ensure it is healthy. Strategies you can use for forming a healthy dating relationship include the following:

- Get to know the person you might want to date before dating. Talk to this person at school, during an activity, or on the phone before going out with this person. This will help you figure out if you share common interests.
- Go out with a group that includes the person in whom you are interested. **Group dating** is a good way to get to know a possible dating partner. Group dating reduces the pressure of having to keep a conversation going with someone you are just getting to know. It is also a good way to stay safe, especially if you do not know the person very well.
- Find ways to cope with your nerves. You may feel nervous about interacting with the person you may want to date. These feelings are normal. In fact, the other person will probably be nervous, too. If talking makes you nervous, plan activities that do not require much conversation, such as seeing a movie or attending a concert.

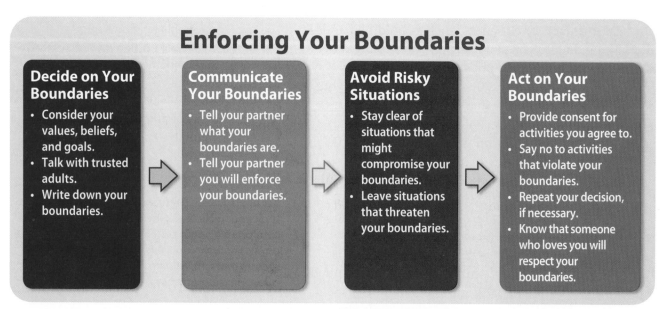

Enforcing Your Boundaries

Decide on Your Boundaries
- Consider your values, beliefs, and goals.
- Talk with trusted adults.
- Write down your boundaries.

Communicate Your Boundaries
- Tell your partner what your boundaries are.
- Tell your partner you will enforce your boundaries.

Avoid Risky Situations
- Stay clear of situations that might compromise your boundaries.
- Leave situations that threaten your boundaries.

Act on Your Boundaries
- Provide consent for activities you agree to.
- Say no to activities that violate your boundaries.
- Repeat your decision, if necessary.
- Know that someone who loves you will respect your boundaries.

Figure 15.31 It is important to formally decide what your boundaries are before you are confronted with a risky situation. This way you can be more prepared to enforce these boundaries.

Travis's First Date?

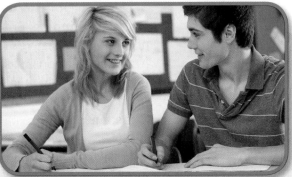

Today, Travis was asked by Casey to go on a date. Travis finds Casey attractive, both in her physical appearance and personality. Travis and Casey have been in some classes together and have some mutual friends, but they did not know each other before this year. Travis is definitely interested in getting to know Casey better.

Travis's older sister has a boyfriend and seems happy about it, but Travis is not sure if he is ready for a dating relationship. Travis participates in many extracurricular activities and is still trying to make friends at his middle school and in his community. He worries that having a dating relationship with Casey will keep him from making more friends. Travis is not 100 percent sure how his parents would feel about him dating at his age, but he thinks they would accept it. According to Travis's classmates, Casey is very interested in having a dating relationship with Travis.

Monkey Business Images/Shutterstock.com

Thinking Critically

1. What factors are influencing Travis's decision to go out with Casey? Which of these factors are internal and which are external?

2. What information do you think Travis should gather before trying to make this decision? How should he go about gathering this information?

3. Imagine that Travis ultimately decides not to go out with Casey. Write a script for a healthy, realistic conversation in which Travis tells Casey about his decision.

4. Why do you think it is sometimes difficult for young people to say "no" to activities their peers want them to do?

The End of a Dating Relationship

Many dating relationships between young people eventually end in a **breakup**, or the end of a romantic relationship. These relationships often do not last long. This is partly because young people's goals and beliefs are still forming and changing as they try to figure out their own identities. These changes can lead to one or both partners realizing that the relationship no longer works.

Breakups can be emotionally painful, especially for the person who does not want to end the relationship. It is important, however, to recognize when a relationship is not working. Someone ready to end a relationship should talk to the other person honestly—and with understanding. It is not fair to string the other person along.

No matter how a relationship ends, both people involved will probably find it difficult to cope. When a relationship ends, people commonly feel sad, angry, lonely, and even physically ill. These feelings are a normal reaction to the end of a relationship and will heal over time.

Some people try to cope with the loss of a dating relationship by quickly beginning a new relationship. By doing this, however, they do not allow themselves time to process their feelings about the end of their previous relationship. Some of these feelings can spill over into the new relationship, which is unfair to new dating partners. New partners deserve to be with someone who is focusing on the new relationship. **Figure 15.32** lists some healthy strategies for coping with the end of a dating relationship.

Figure 15.32
A person can use various techniques to help manage with the end of a dating relationship. *What is the end of a dating relationship called?*

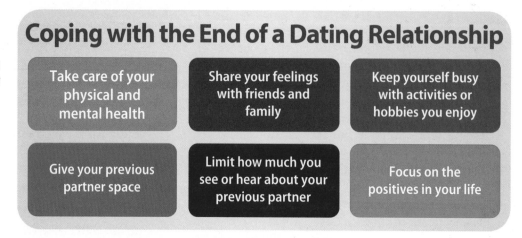

Coping with the End of a Dating Relationship

Take care of your physical and mental health

Share your feelings with friends and family

Keep yourself busy with activities or hobbies you enjoy

Give your previous partner space

Limit how much you see or hear about your previous partner

Focus on the positives in your life

Lesson 15.4 Review

1. What is the difference between casual dating and a dating relationship?
2. Which of the following is characteristic of a healthy dating relationship?
   A. Pressure.
   B. Individuality.
   C. Infatuation.
   D. Teasing.
3. **True or false.** Group dating can make it easier to get to know someone you do not know well.
4. Why do many dating relationships among young people eventually end?
5. **Critical thinking.** How does abstinence prevent the negative physical, emotional, and social consequences of early sexual activity?

Hands-On Activity

Even if dating is still years away for you, it is a good idea to think about what your rights and responsibilities in a dating relationship might be. Imagine you are in a dating relationship. Answer the following question based on what you learned in this lesson, your experiences, and your opinions. Reach out to trusted adults who have experience in healthy dating relationships to help you complete the activity. Do you believe dating partners should have a conversation about this information? If so, when and how should they discuss? If not, why not? Discuss your opinions about dating relationships with a trusted adult.

- What are my rights in the relationship? What are my responsibilities?
- What are my partner's rights in the relationship? What are my partner's responsibilities?

Summary

Lesson 15.1 **What Is a Healthy Relationship?**

- Relationships affect a person's health and well-being. Some relationships meet basic human needs. Relationships also meet the need to feel connected and loved.
- Healthy relationships are characterized by honesty, trust, mutual respect, care and commitment, emotional control, understanding, safety, and good interpersonal skills.
- You can communicate effectively by using active listening, clearly expressing yourself, being assertive, using I-statements, watching your nonverbal communication, and using online communication wisely.
- Conflict is normal, even in healthy relationships. Good conflict resolution involves the negotiation process. Some schools offer peer mediation to help with this.

Lesson 15.2 **Family Relationships**

- Family relationships serve the unique functions of providing for physical needs, meeting mental and emotional needs, and educating and socializing children.
- Communities offer many resources to help families fulfill their functions.
- Good communication and conflict resolution skills can help you maintain healthy relationships with parents or guardians as well as siblings.
- Families can experience both positive and difficult changes over time. Using effective strategies for maintaining family relationships will help family members handle changes.

Lesson 15.3 **Peer Relationships**

- Friendships include close friends, casual friends, acquaintances, and online friends. Celebrating diversity will help you strengthen your friendships.
- Strategies for building healthy friendships include making time for relationships, meeting friends face-to-face, and being a good friend.
- Common issues in friendships include cliques, jealousy, and changes over time.
- Peer pressure can be positive or negative. If you encounter negative peer pressure, you can stand up to it by sticking to your own beliefs and values.

Lesson 15.4 **Dating Relationships**

- Healthy dating relationships have the characteristics of attraction; closeness; individuality; balance; open communication, honesty, and respect; and support.
- Before a dating relationship, you need to consider your boundaries regarding physical intimacy. Sexual abstinence is a healthy choice for young people in dating relationships.
- Strategies for forming healthy dating relationships include getting to know the person you want to date, dating in groups, and coping with nerves.
- The end of a dating relationship is difficult for both partners. Usually, people need time to heal and examine the past relationship.

Check Your Knowledge

Record your answers to each of the following questions on a separate sheet of paper.

1. What are the characteristics of a healthy relationship?
2. **True or false.** Effective communication uses you-statements to express feelings.
3. Which of the following is a good skill for conflict resolution?
    A. Behave passively.
    B. Interrupt the other person.
    C. Keep calm.
    D. Insist on your way.
4. What does it mean to socialize children?
5. Explain why parents or guardians and young people often have conflicts during adolescence.
6. **True or false.** Identifying a personal space for each sibling is an example of a strategy that can help ease conflict and strengthen a relationship between siblings.
7. It is important to form and maintain friendships through _____ interactions.
8. What is a clique?
9. Which of the following is a good strategy for resisting negative peer pressure?
    A. Focus on your own thoughts, feelings, and values.
    B. Choose friends with different values.
    C. Join in teasing other people.
    D. Stay in uncomfortable situations.
10. **True or false.** In a dating relationship, a person's core values should change.
11. Why is sexual abstinence a healthy choice for young people?
12. **True or false.** Group dating can help you get to know a potential dating partner.

Use Your Vocabulary

acquaintances	feedback	passion
active listening	friendship	peer mediation
affirmative consent	group dating	relationship
breakup	immediate family	rituals
casual dating	infatuation	sibling rivalry
clique	interpersonal skills	socialize
communication process	intimacy	stereotypes
diversity	nonverbal	traditions
exclusive	communication	verbal communication
extended family	online friends	

13. Consider your prior exposure to each of the terms above. Read the text passages that contain each of the terms above. Then, write the definition of each term in your own words. Double-check your definitions by rereading the text and using the text glossary.

Think Critically

14. **Identify.** Identify a character in a book, movie, or television show who has healthy relationships with family members and friends. What makes the character's relationships healthy? Explain.

15. **Assess.** Assess your communication skills by analyzing your communication with family members and friends. In what areas of communication are you doing well? What areas do you need to improve?

16. **Compare and contrast.** Compare and contrast positive and negative peer pressure. Explain how each type of peer pressure can cause or solve issues in a friendship.

17. **Determine.** Compare and contrast healthy friendships and healthy dating relationships. Some people say that a healthy friendship is the foundation of a healthy dating relationship. Do you agree or disagree? Why?

DEVELOP Your Skills

18. **Communication skills.** Start a conversation with your parents or guardian or another trusted adult about expectations for relationships at this point in your life. Express your thoughts and discuss the types of people who make good friends, appropriate and inappropriate activities to do with friends, information that should be shared with trusted adults, the appropriate time to start dating, and the characteristics of an appropriate date.

19. **Advocacy, teamwork, and technology skills.** Work with a small team to identify the most important topic in this chapter that you would like to advocate for to promote the health of your peers. Write a conversational blog post for people your age about the importance of the topic. Enhance your blog post with information from valid and reliable print, digital, or in-person sources.

20. **Goal-setting skills.** Choose a relationship in your life that needs improvement. Identify what you can realistically do to improve it. Use the strategies discussed in this chapter and previous chapters and set a goal for yourself to improve, change, or end the relationship. Implement your plan and write a journal entry reflecting on what you learned about yourself and relationships.

21. **Accessing information.** Many resources are available to help young people navigate relationships. It is important that people who are struggling with relationships reach out to gain help. Spend time searching online for valid and reliable websites that help young people build healthy relationships and deal with relationship struggles. Then, identify adults in your life whom you could comfortably go to for help with improving your relationships. Finally, identify professionals in your community who help people improve and manage relationships. Make a list of all these resources and then highlight the top three you would use if you needed assistance with the relationships in your life.

Preventing and Responding to Violence

Essential Question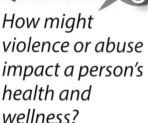

How might violence or abuse impact a person's health and wellness?

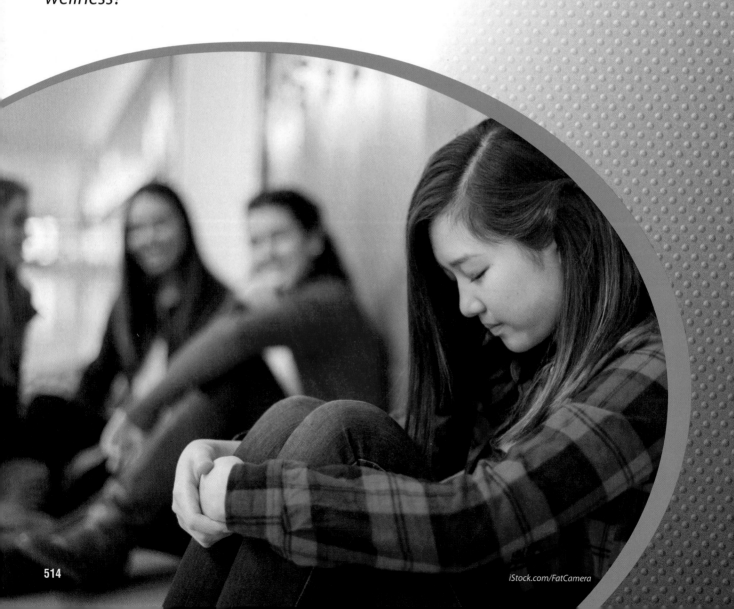

iStock.com/FatCamera

Reading Activity

As you listen to your teacher present the information in the chapter, write any comments or questions you may have about the content on a separate sheet of paper. Then review your comments and questions with a partner. Try to answer each other's questions. If you have any questions you cannot answer, discuss them with the rest of the class to pursue the answers to your questions.

How Healthy Are You?

In this chapter, you will be learning about violent behaviors. Before you begin reading, take the following quiz to assess your current understanding of how violent behaviors affect a person's health and well-being.

Health Concepts to Understand	Yes	No
Do you consider intimidating a friend or spreading rumors about a classmate examples of violent behavior?		
Do you think harassment and hazing are types of bullying?		
Do you believe that there is never a good reason to bully others?		
Are you aware of strategies you can use to respond to and stop bullying?		
Do you avoid using fake screen names online?		
Do you only say things to someone online that you would be willing to say in person?		
Are you aware of strategies you can use to respond to cyberbullying?		
Do you believe that all types of abuse are wrong, no matter who is committing the abuse and who is being abused?		
If your school has a violence-prevention program, do you follow the rules of the program?		
Are you aware of community resources to help reduce gang violence?		
Do you celebrate differences in others and encourage other people to do the same?		

Count your "Yes" and "No" responses. The more "Yes" responses you have, the more you understand the effects of violent behaviors. Now, take a closer look at the questions with which you responded "No." Develop your health literacy skills by accessing valid information about each of the concepts you do not understand. Evaluate any health websites you find using the information in Figure 1.16 of this text. If you do not understand the instructions, ask for clarification from your teacher.

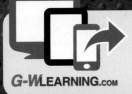

Click on the activity icon or visit www.g-wlearning.com/health to access online vocabulary activities using key terms from the chapter.

G-WLEARNING.com

Bullying and Cyberbullying

Key Terms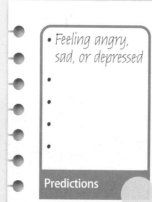

bullying repeated aggressive behavior toward someone that causes the person injury or discomfort

peer abuse violent mistreatment of one peer by another

harassment type of bullying that targets a particular part of a person's identity, such as race, religion, or sex

stalking following and repeatedly contacting someone in a way that causes the person to feel scared, nervous, or threatened

hazing use of pressure by a group to make someone do something embarrassing or even dangerous to be accepted by a group

bystanders people who are present at an event, but do not intervene

bystander effect situation in which a bystander is less likely to intervene because the person thinks someone else will

upstander person who recognizes when a behavior is wrong, takes steps to intervene and stop the behavior, and promotes positive change; also called an *ally*

cyberbullying form of bullying that uses electronic means

Learning Outcomes

After studying this lesson, you will be able to

- **discuss** what violent behavior is.
- **contrast** bullying, cyberbullying, harassment, and hazing.
- **describe** the consequences of bullying.
- **evaluate** strategies for responding to bullying.
- **identify** the consequences of cyberbullying.
- **explain** ways of responding to cyberbullying.
- **list** strategies for bullying prevention.

Graphic Organizer

Bullying Affects Your Health

Before reading this lesson, try to answer the following question: "How do you think bullying and cyberbullying affect your overall health?" In an organizer like the one shown, list at least five predictions of bullying-related consequences based on your current knowledge and experience. After reading the lesson, write at least five bullying-related health consequences and five strategies for responding to bullying. An example is provided for you.

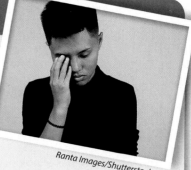

Ranta Images/Shutterstock.com

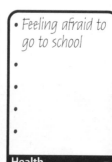

• Feeling angry, sad, or depressed	• Feeling afraid to go to school	• Tell a trusted adult
•	•	•
•	•	•
•	•	•
Predictions	**Health Consequences**	**Strategies for Responding**

When you think of the word *violence*, you may not think of intimidating a friend or spreading rumors about a classmate. Both of these actions, however, are examples of violent behavior. Isabela and Sofia are sisters who go to the same school. Sofia likes to play sports and is outgoing, but Isabela is quiet in class. Sofia's friends like to make fun of Isabela for being shy, and when Sofia sees them gossiping online about her sister, she feels uncomfortable. Isabela avoids many of her classmates and feels nervous going to school. Because of her anxiety, Isabela dropped out of the school play. She feels bad because she regrets her decision, but she does not want to spend more time with her classmates.

The actions of Sofia's friends are violent behavior. *Violent behavior* is the intentional use of words or actions that cause or threaten to cause injury to someone or something. An example of violent behavior might be hitting someone, forcing someone to do something, or destroying someone's belongings. Although violent behavior often involves the use of physical force, it is not always physical. Violent behavior can also refer to behavior that results in *psychological injury*, or injury to a person's social or emotional health. Many factors can lead to violence, but violent behavior is always a personal choice (**Figure 16.1**).

Violent behavior among peers often happens in schools and takes the form of bullying and cyberbullying. In this lesson, you will learn about these types of violent behavior and ways to respond to and prevent them.

Risk Factors for Violent Behavior

Individual risk factors

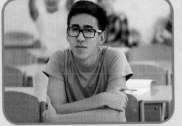

Africa Studio/Shutterstock.com

- Lack of control over behavior and anger
- History of early aggressive behavior
- Exposure to violence, abuse, and conflict in the family
- Use of tobacco, alcohol, or drugs
- Rejection of social values or institutions
- Immaturity
- *Prejudice*, or unfair negative beliefs about a group of people
- Discrimination and bias
- Stressful events
- Physical or mental health condition

Family risk factors

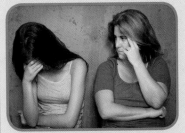

Kamira/Shutterstock.com

- Authoritarian parenting style (one that demands strict obedience)
- Discipline for breaking rules that is either too harsh, lenient, or inconsistent
- Poor supervision of children
- Low level of involvement and emotional attachment in family
- Low level of family education and income
- Use of tobacco, alcohol, or drugs in the family
- Criminal record
- Violent behavior in the family
- Access to weapons

(Continued)

Figure 16.1
Several factors can affect whether a person or group chooses violence. These risk factors can be related to the individual who chooses violence, the family, peers, and the community. The presence of risk factors does not necessarily mean that a person will act violently. Still, one of the best ways to understand and prevent violence is to pay attention to its risk factors.

Risk Factors for Violent Behavior *(Figure 16.1 Continued)*	
Peer and social risk factors 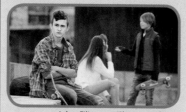 *Iakov Filimonov/Shutterstock.com*	• Rejection by peers • Peer pressure • Little interest or involvement in school • Involvement in gangs • Poor academic performance • Violent behavior among peers
Community risk factors 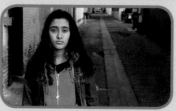 *AJR_photo/Shutterstock.com*	• Lack of economic opportunities • Poverty • Lack of community groups and social services • High crime and unemployment rates • Lack of healthy families in the community • High rate of families moving out of the community

Bullying

Bullying is a type of repeated aggressive behavior toward someone that causes the person injury or discomfort. Bullying involves a power imbalance, which means someone uses power to control or harm others. Bullying is also called **peer abuse** because it involves ongoing violent behavior toward a peer. You will learn more about abuse in the next lesson.

Bullying can be physical, emotional, or social. For example, a bully might hit, push, corner, or shove someone, which are forms of physical bullying.

Examples of emotional bullying include insulting or mocking a person, making fun of someone, or taking someone's belongings. Spreading *gossip*, or hurtful rumors, is a form of social bullying. Social bullying also includes excluding someone, sharing someone's secrets, or making someone feel isolated or rejected.

Other forms of bullying include harassment, stalking, and hazing. **Harassment** targets another person because of a particular part of the person's identity. It may target a person's race, religious beliefs, or sex, for example. Harassment is a form of discrimination, making it illegal. Examples include using racial slurs or displaying symbols or words that communicate hatred toward others. Excluding or making fun of someone because of the person's religious beliefs or sex is also harassment.

Stalking is a type of bullying that involves following and repeatedly contacting someone. Stalking tries to control or scare someone and makes the person being stalked feel nervous, afraid, or threatened. For example, if someone starts showing up places you visit after you say you do not want to talk, this is stalking. Stalking is a crime and can also occur online.

Hazing is a type of bullying that uses group pressure to make someone do embarrassing or dangerous activities to be accepted. For example, a group may force someone to do something risky, uncomfortable, or illegal to fit in.

Embarrassing someone or making someone endure physical violence to become part of a club are also examples of hazing. Because hazing is dangerous, many states have laws against it.

Bullying is always the fault of the person bullying others. Usually, the person bullying others has personal negative feelings or insecurities that lead to hurting others. There is never a good reason to bully, even if a person acts or looks different from you (**Figure 16.2**).

BUILDING Your Skills

Rumor Has It

Rumors are (unfortunately) a common part of young people's lives. People often spread unkind gossip to gain popularity or status. Sometimes, people spread gossip just because others are doing it, even though it is hurtful. If you have ever had a rumor spread about you, then you know the pain it can cause. If you have ever spread a rumor, then you probably know the uneasy feeling that spreading it causes. Spreading rumors is a form of bullying. So, what can you do if you hear a rumor?

Strategies for Responding to Rumors

- **Just STOP it.** When you hear a rumor about another person, do not tell anyone else. Remember that this rumor is about a real person, and spreading this rumor will only hurt that person more. A rumor will only last as long as people continue to talk about it.

- **Do not be part of the audience.** Simply listening to a rumor makes you part of the rumor. If the person spreading the rumor does not get attention or a reaction, that person will be less likely to spread rumors in the future. It can be hard to resist an interesting story, but make an effort to say, "I'm not interested in hearing mean gossip, thanks."

- **Reverse the pressure.** Ask the person who is spreading the rumor, "How do you know this is true?" or "Is this your information to spread?" This will make the person stop and hopefully quit spreading information about another person.

- **Talk with the subject of the rumor.** Find a private time and place to talk to the person about whom you heard a rumor. Tell the person what you heard. Perhaps the person can set the record straight or at least become aware of what is being said. You could offer to help the person go talk with a trusted adult to show support.

Stopping the spread of rumors is a difficult task, especially because it often feels like everyone talks about other people. You can, however, be an inspiration to others. Try practicing these strategies. Which do you think you are most likely to use? Why? How would you respond to hearing a rumor if you were alone? How would you respond to hearing a rumor if you heard it with a group of friends? You can be the first in your group of friends, and maybe even in your school, to stop the spread of rumors that harm other people. Imagine that a rumor was going around school about someone you know. Create a realistic role play that demonstrates the use of at least two of the strategies.

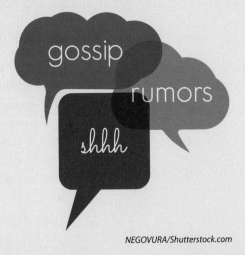

NEGOVURA/Shutterstock.com

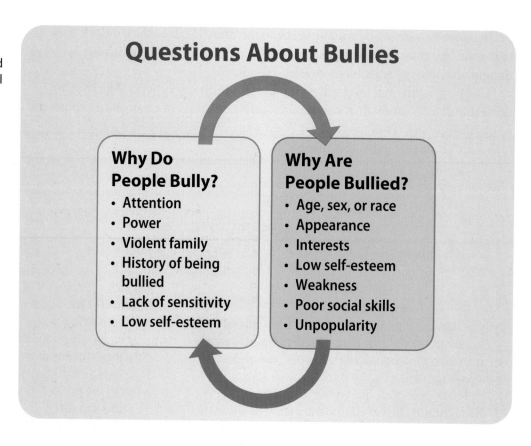

Questions About Bullies

Why Do People Bully?
- Attention
- Power
- Violent family
- History of being bullied
- Lack of sensitivity
- Low self-esteem

Why Are People Bullied?
- Age, sex, or race
- Appearance
- Interests
- Low self-esteem
- Weakness
- Poor social skills
- Unpopularity

Consequences of Bullying

Bullying can have severe and lasting consequences. Young people who are bullied may change their behavior, worry about going to school, or have trouble concentrating on homework. They might stop hanging out with friends after school or going to parties. They might even quit playing a sport or some other activity to avoid the bullying. People who are bullied can become seriously depressed. They can have difficulty sleeping and feel fearful of other people.

Some common signs that a person is being bullied include the following:

- feeling angry, sad, lonely, and depressed
- feeling bad about one's self
- wanting to hurt someone else or one's self
- feeling helpless to stop the bullying
- feeling afraid to go to school or use digital devices

Bullying does not just hurt the person being bullied. It also hurts the person bullying others and other people. By bullying, someone does not deal with personal deeper issues. Young people who are not bullied do not like seeing violent, bullying behavior. They may worry that the person will start picking on them next. Bullying creates an environment in which stress and violence seem normal, causing harm to everyone involved.

Strategies for Responding to Bullying

Bullying is never the fault of the person being bullied. You and others have a right to feel safe at school and in the community. If you are being bullied or if you see someone being bullied, you can use the following strategies to respond to and stop the bullying:

- If you see someone bullying another person, do not participate. Instead, tell the person to stop and ask how you can help the person being bullied.
- Do not respond to anyone who bullies you. People who bully others feel more powerful when people react to their meanness. Acting like you do not even notice or care can discourage bullying behavior.
- Be assertive. People who bully others often pick on people who seem scared or weak. Sometimes, simply standing up can get someone to change the behavior. Tell the person to leave you alone calmly and loudly. Then, just walk away.
- Avoid bullying back. Even if you are angry, do not respond by hitting, yelling, or gossiping. This can encourage the person to continue the bad behavior. It can also get you in trouble.
- Tell an adult. It is important to talk to a trusted adult if you or someone you know is being bullied. Teachers, principals, school nurses, school counselors, and other adults can help stop bullying. This helps keep you and other people safe.

When others are being bullied, you may want to ignore the behavior and not get involved. People who witness an event without intervening or getting help are called **bystanders**. Often, bystanders are waiting for someone else to act. Bystanders may think others are responsible for speaking up. This feeling of not having any responsibility to act is the **bystander effect**.

When bystanders stay quiet, bullying can continue. Instead of being a bystander, try to be an upstander. When you are an **upstander**, or *ally*, you recognize wrong behavior and do something to stop it, help the person being hurt, and promote positive change. An upstander might tell the person bullying others to stop or help the person being bullied get out and find help. An upstander might also alert an adult to the bullying (**Figure 16.3**).

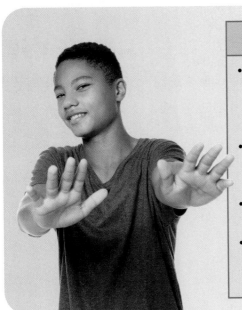

Ways to Be an Upstander

- Interrupt the situation by providing a distraction or helping the person being bullied escape the situation.
- Tell the person bullying others to stop. Use a direct, assertive, respectful voice.
- Recruit allies by getting support from people around you.
- Support the person being bullied and assist the person in getting help.

Africa Studio/Shutterstock.com

Figure 16.3
Most middle school students think bullying is a bad idea, but may not speak up to stop it. You can reduce bullying in your school by being an upstander and ally.

Cyberbullying

Cyberbullying is a form of bullying that uses electronic communication. In some ways, cyberbullying is similar to traditional bullying. Both cause emotional harm. In other ways, cyberbullying can be worse than traditional bullying. Electronic communication can spread far and quickly. Because people can hide behind fake screen names online, they can say things they would not say in person.

Sometimes, cyberbullying happens unintentionally. One person might post a joke about someone else and not realize that it was hurtful. Cyberbullying that happens repeatedly over time, however, is not accidental. Cyberbullying can involve embarrassing, harassing, or threatening peers in any of the ways shown in **Figure 16.4**.

Consequences of Cyberbullying

Cyberbullying can have serious and lasting consequences. Some of these consequences include the following:

- anxiety and depression
- loneliness and isolation
- low self-esteem
- lower grades
- aggressive actions
- withdrawal from friends and social activities
- changes in sleep, appetite, and behavior
- anxiety before, during, or after using digital devices
- avoidance of digital devices
- thoughts of hurting one's self or others

Figure 16.4
Cyberbullying can occur in many settings, including social media, texting or e-mail, chat rooms, gaming, and websites. *In what way is cyberbullying similar to traditional bullying?*

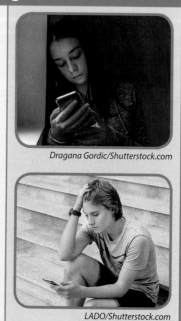

What Is Cyberbullying?

- Sending aggressive, mean, or threatening e-mails or messages
- Sharing hurtful or embarrassing messages, photos, or videos about someone on social media
- Blocking people's e-mail addresses or unfriending them on social media for no reason
- Spreading personal or embarrassing information or rumors about people
- Hacking into people's e-mail accounts or social media pages
- Impersonating others and *catfishing* (pretending to be someone to trick a person into a fake relationship)
- *Cyberstalking*, which can include sending inappropriate content or continuing to contact someone who does not want to talk
- Creating websites or documents to ridicule or embarrass other people

Dragana Gordic/Shutterstock.com

LADO/Shutterstock.com

How to Spot Cyberbullying

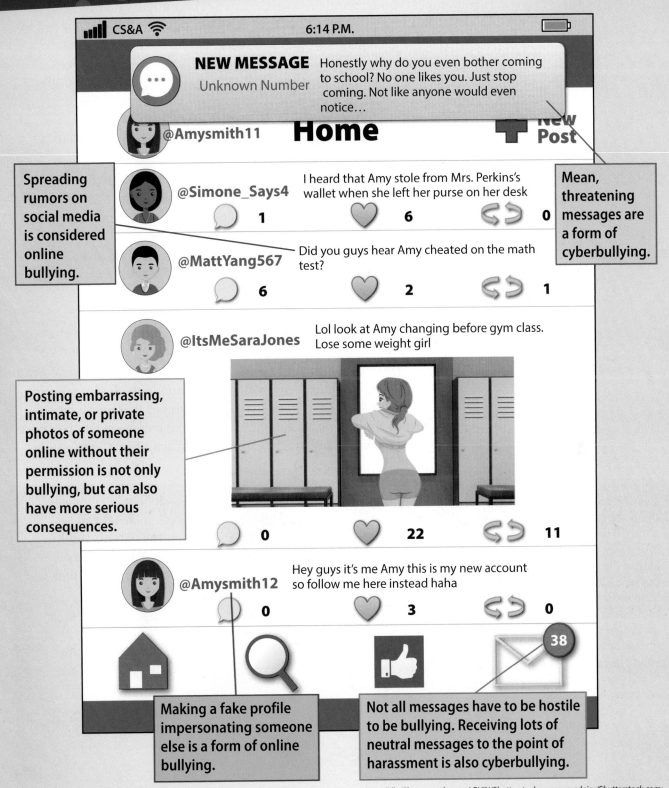

NEW MESSAGE Unknown Number — Honestly why do you even bother coming to school? No one likes you. Just stop coming. Not like anyone would even notice…

@Amysmith11   **Home**   New Post

Spreading rumors on social media is considered online bullying.

@Simone_Says4 — I heard that Amy stole from Mrs. Perkins's wallet when she left her purse on her desk
💬 1   ❤️ 6   🔁 0

Mean, threatening messages are a form of cyberbullying.

@MattYang567 — Did you guys hear Amy cheated on the math test?
💬 6   ❤️ 2   🔁 1

@ItsMeSaraJones — Lol look at Amy changing before gym class. Lose some weight girl
💬 0   ❤️ 22   🔁 11

Posting embarrassing, intimate, or private photos of someone online without their permission is not only bullying, but can also have more serious consequences.

@Amysmith12 — Hey guys it's me Amy this is my new account so follow me here instead haha
💬 0   ❤️ 3   🔁 0

Making a fake profile impersonating someone else is a form of online bullying.

Not all messages have to be hostile to be bullying. Receiving lots of neutral messages to the point of harassment is also cyberbullying.

Top to bottom: Hermin/Shutterstock.com; WEB-DESIGN/Shutterstock.com; VectorZilla/Shutterstock.com; LOVIN/Shutterstock.com; maradaisy/Shutterstock.com; ankudi/Shutterstock.com; Lorelyn Medina/Shutterstock.com

Cyberbullying is difficult to escape. Most young people spend a lot of time using their phones, computers, or tablets. Because of this, cyberbullying can happen any time of day or night.

Strategies for Responding to Cyberbullying

Sometimes, young people who experience cyberbullying do not want to tell anyone. They may feel embarrassed about the messages, videos, or photos shared about them (**Figure 16.5**). They may also worry that their parents or guardians will take away their phones, tablets, or computers. In these situations, it is important to remember that cyberbullying is the fault of the person bullying others and never the fault of the person being bullied.

The following strategies can help you respond to cyberbullying:

- If you see someone being cyberbullied, do not participate. Instead, ask how you can help the person being bullied.
- If someone is cyberbullying you, block that person's ability to contact you.
- Do not respond to the person's messages in any way. Responding will reinforce the behavior.
- Save or screenshot the person's messages, videos, or photos. Also, screenshot any hurtful messages posted online. This evidence can help prove you are being cyberbullied.
- Communicate with a trusted adult about the cyberbullying. The adult can intervene and help stop this behavior. You can also report cyberbullying by flagging content as inappropriate on social media or contacting your Internet service provider.

If you see someone being cyberbullied, do not participate. Instead, be an upstander and ally and ask how you can help. Remember that many school districts have rules about cyberbullying. Students who engage in this behavior can be suspended or kicked off sports teams or other activities. Certain types

Figure 16.5
Even if someone has shared embarrassing photos or videos online, cyberbullying is never the fault of the person being bullied. Cyberbullying can have serious effects on your health. It is important that you report it to a trusted adult. *Why might young people not want to tell anyone that they are being bullied?*

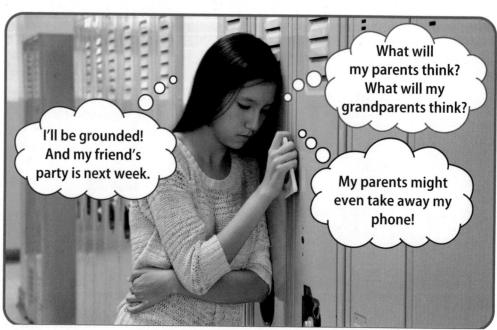

of cyberbullying are even against the law, especially if the cyberbullying results in self-harm.

Bullying Prevention

Bullying is a serious issue in many schools. In addition to hurting people who are bullied, it can cause stress and fear for all students. Schools often have programs for preventing bullying. Participating in these programs can help you learn about bullying and ways to respond. You can also take action on your own to prevent bullying in your school and among your peers. The following strategies can help stop bullying before it begins:

- Pay attention to yourself and your behaviors to recognize if you are bullying others. Often, bullying arises from people's insecurities. Address your insecurities by building self-esteem and healthy relationships. Practice empathy for others and get help if you find yourself acting aggressively toward others.
- Focus on your own beliefs and build your confidence. People who bully others sometimes target people who seem weak or insecure. Being comfortable with yourself can keep them away (**Figure 16.6**).
- Celebrate your peers' differences. Appreciating differences and diversity can create a positive environment and help people feel better about themselves.
- Avoid those who bully others whenever possible. If someone who bullies others is nearby, sit in a different part of the cafeteria or hang out in a different place after school.
- Use the buddy system. Try to be with a friend whenever you might run into someone who bullies others. This might prevent the person from acting.

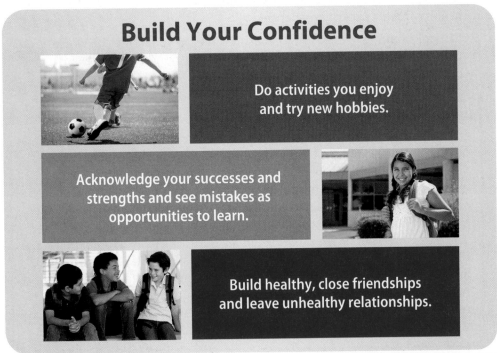

Build Your Confidence

Do activities you enjoy and try new hobbies.

Acknowledge your successes and strengths and see mistakes as opportunities to learn.

Build healthy, close friendships and leave unhealthy relationships.

Figure 16.6
Building your confidence can help prevent bullying.

Top to bottom: matimix/Shutterstock.com; Andy Dean Photography/Shutterstock.com; Monkey Business Images/Shutterstock.com

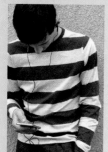

Think Before You Post

- Would I say this to someone's face?
- Am I trying to get attention or make people like me?
- How would this make the person involved feel?
- Is it private? Is it *actually* private? Will it stay private?
  - Do I have permission to share this?
  - Will this embarrass the person involved?
  - Will it hurt the reputation of the person involved?
  - Could this be interpreted in a way I do not intend?
  - Will I feel good about posting this later?
  - Does it contain anything inappropriate?

Jevanto Productions/Shutterstock.com

Figure 16.7
Asking these questions before you post can help you prevent cyberbullying behavior.

- Never share the passwords to your computer, phone, or social media accounts with anyone. This way, others cannot impersonate you online.
- Do not send or post anything online that you would not want shared with others (**Figure 16.7**).
- If you see signs of bullying behavior, tell a trusted adult. A trusted adult can help address the situation before it gets worse.

In addition to these strategies, communicating regularly with a trusted adult can help protect you from bullying. If you tell an adult about your relationships at school and online, that adult can help you with difficult situations. The adult can also advocate for you if bullying does occur.

Lesson 16.1 Review

1. **True or false.** Violent behavior always includes the use of physical force.
2. Because it involves ongoing violent behavior toward a peer, _____ is also called *peer abuse*.
3. Which type of bullying targets a particular part of a person's identity?
4. Loneliness, lower grades, aggressive actions, and anxiety using technology are all health consequences of experiencing _____.
5. **Critical thinking.** Explain why cyberbullying can sometimes be worse than traditional bullying. What can you do to respond to and prevent cyberbullying?

Hands-On Activity

On a piece of paper, draw a square and then draw something that you like inside of it. For example, you could draw your favorite animal or your favorite video game character. Then, sit in a circle with three other students. Going around the circle, describe hurtful things that you have heard said in your school or that have been said to you. Each time a hurtful statement is said, use a different-colored marker to color in the square over your drawing. Continue doing this until your time is up. What did the hurtful statements your group discussed do to your drawing? Can the layers of marker be taken back? Would apologizing to your drawing remove the layers of marker? Why do people say hurtful things to and about others? How can you promote kindness toward others? Discuss the power of words, both positive and negative, in your group. Within your group, take turns saying genuinely kind statements to each other.

Abuse and Neglect

Learning Outcomes

After studying this lesson, you will be able to

- **identify** the types of abuse.
- **explain** what intimate partner violence is.
- **summarize** the effects of child abuse and the results of reporting it.
- **list** forms of sibling abuse and elder abuse.
- **discuss** the cycle of abuse and ways of responding to abuse.
- **identify** strategies for preventing abuse.

Graphic Organizer

Abuse and Neglect Wheel

To record your notes for this lesson, draw a wheel like the one shown on a separate piece of paper. In the middle of the wheel, write the phrase *Abuse and Neglect*. As you read the lesson, assign a category to each section based on a different topic covered in the lesson. Write that topic at the top of each section. Fill the wheel with your notes on different types of abuse and neglect.

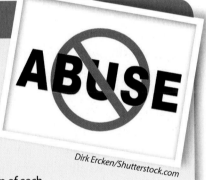

Dirk Ercken/Shutterstock.com

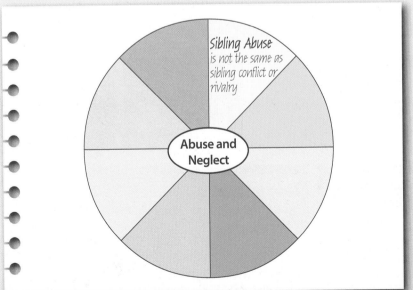

Sibling Abuse is not the same as sibling conflict or rivalry

Abuse and Neglect

Key Terms

abuse violent behaviors that cause physical, emotional, sexual, or financial harm to another person

physical abuse behaviors that cause physical harm to a person

emotional abuse attitudes or controlling behaviors that harm a person's mental health

sexual abuse sexual activity to which one person does not or cannot consent

financial abuse use of money to show power in a relationship and make others act in certain ways

intimate partner violence abuse that involves couples who are or were in a romantic relationship

child abuse any act an adult commits that causes harm or threatens to cause harm to a child

neglect type of child abuse in which a child's basic physical, emotional, medical, or educational needs are not met by parents or guardians

sibling abuse violent behaviors that one sibling inflicts on another sibling

elder abuse behaviors or neglect that cause harm to someone 60 years of age or older

There is no place for violent behavior or abuse in healthy relationships. Consider, for example, Sofia and Isabela from the previous lesson. Sofia and Isabela have healthy relationships with their family. Their friend Tad, however, is always fighting with his mother. Sometimes, his mother calls him names and shoves him out of the house. Sofia and Isabela are unsure how to help their friend. Tad thinks the way his mother behaves is normal. Sofia and Isabela know, however, that all types of abuse are wrong, no matter the circumstances.

Types of Abuse

Abuse refers to the consistent, violent mistreatment of a person. For example, hitting someone whenever you are angry is abuse. Shaking a sibling is also abuse. Like violent behavior, abuse is not always physical. People can use words, attitudes, and behaviors to abuse another person (**Figure 16.8**). The following are types of abuse:

- **Physical abuse** involves actions that cause physical harm to another person. Physical abuse may involve hitting, kicking, choking, slapping, biting, shaking, or burning someone.
- **Emotional abuse** (also called *mental*, *verbal*, or *psychological abuse*) involves attitudes or controlling behaviors that harm a person's mental and emotional health. It includes making threats, calling someone names, delivering insults, ridiculing someone's identity, withholding love, and isolating a person in person and online.
- **Sexual abuse** involves sexual activity to which one person does not or cannot consent. Sexual abuse can include physical behaviors such as unwanted sexual activity. It can also include sexual harassment, taking nude pictures, or exposing one's self.
- **Financial abuse** is the use of money to show power in a relationship. Examples include stealing, giving gifts or money and expecting something in return, and withholding money to meet basic needs.

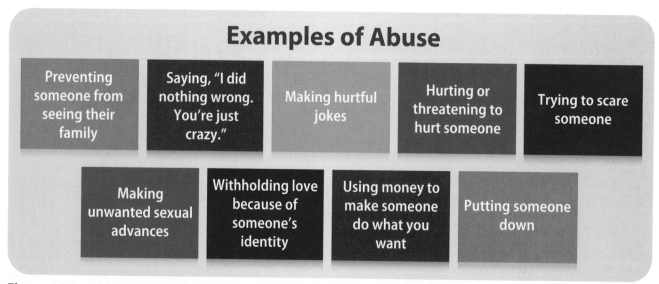

Examples of Abuse

| Preventing someone from seeing their family | Saying, "I did nothing wrong. You're just crazy." | Making hurtful jokes | Hurting or threatening to hurt someone | Trying to scare someone |

| Making unwanted sexual advances | Withholding love because of someone's identity | Using money to make someone do what you want | Putting someone down |

Figure 16.8 Many different actions can be considered abuse, but all are part of a violent, consistent mistreatment of another person. *What are the types of abuse?*

Abuse can occur in families, between friends, among classmates, or between dating partners. In all of these settings, abuse has serious physical and emotional consequences and can sometimes be a crime (**Figure 16.9**). Often, people try to make those they abuse feel responsible for the abuse. This is *never* the case. No matter the situation, the person committing the abuse is *always* responsible for the abuse. Some examples of abuse are intimate partner violence, child abuse, sibling abuse, and elder abuse. As you learned in the previous lesson, bullying is a type of peer abuse.

Intimate Partner Violence

Intimate partner violence is abuse between two people who are or were married, dating, or in a romantic relationship. It occurs when one or both partners try to dominate or control each other through physical, emotional, sexual, or financial abuse. Intimate partner violence is also called *domestic violence, spousal violence,* or *dating violence.* It can occur in person or electronically.

Intimate partner violence often starts with emotional abuse. Over time, this behavior leads to physical attacks (**Figure 16.10**). People who have experienced intimate partner violence may have physical injuries, such as bruises or broken bones. They may also experience depression, anxiety, fear, and shame. People who experience intimate partner violence may feel socially isolated and alone, partly because they do not want to tell anyone.

Violent Crimes Common in Abuse	
Crime	**Description**
Assault	The threat of physical injury to another person
	The threat of sexual activity without consent to another person
Battery	The physical injury of another person
Rape	Sexual activity to which another person does not or cannot consent (for example, due to age or condition)

Figure 16.9 Abuse is a criminal action and can have serious legal consequences, as with assault, battery, and rape.

Signs of Intimate Partner Violence

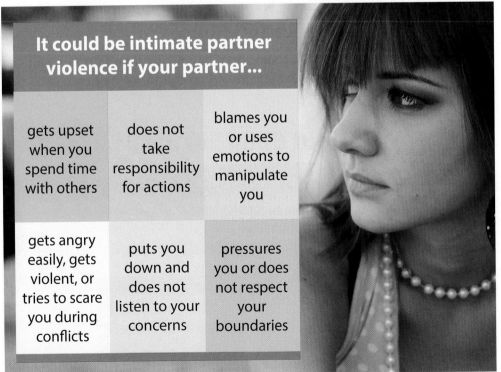

It could be intimate partner violence if your partner...

gets upset when you spend time with others

does not take responsibility for actions

blames you or uses emotions to manipulate you

gets angry easily, gets violent, or tries to scare you during conflicts

puts you down and does not listen to your concerns

pressures you or does not respect your boundaries

Figure 16.10 Intimate partner violence often starts with emotional abuse and then escalates to physical abuse. It can occur in any romantic relationship, whether partners are dating or married.

Ardelean Andreea/Shutterstock.com

Abuse and violence are not part of a healthy relationship. If a partner behaves violently even once, no matter the reason given, the other person should leave the relationship and seek help. There is no good excuse for violent behavior in a healthy relationship. It is essential to get out of a relationship the *very first time* violence occurs.

Child Abuse

Each year in the United States, nearly 700,000 children experience some form of abuse or neglect. Nearly 1,700 children die from abuse or neglect each year. **Child abuse** refers to any intentional act an adult commits that causes harm or threatens to cause harm to a child.

Types of Child Neglect and Abuse

Child abuse can take many forms. For example, withholding love, ignoring a child, and being emotionally distant are examples of emotional abuse. *Child sexual abuse* is a specific type of abuse in which an adult engages a child in any sexual activity. This may include kissing, touching, having the child view sexual images, or looking at the child sexually (**Figure 16.11**). Child sexual abuse may involve the use of pressure, force, or deception.

Another type of child abuse is neglect. **Neglect** occurs when an adult fails to meet a child's basic physical, emotional, medical, or educational needs. Neglect also includes the failure to protect a child from harm. For example, the child may be supervised inadequately or exposed to a dangerous living situation. A child who does not have enough food or clothes suited to the season also experiences neglect. Some specific risk factors related to child abuse and neglect are listed in **Figure 16.12**.

Effects of Child Neglect and Abuse

A child's sense of well-being comes from having the love, support, and respect of family members and caregivers. When children experience abuse or

Figure 16.11
Young people under a certain age cannot consent to sexual activities. This means that any adult who engages in sexual activity with a child can be charged with rape or sexual abuse.

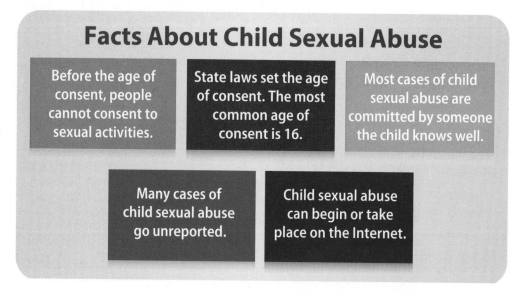

Facts About Child Sexual Abuse

Before the age of consent, people cannot consent to sexual activities.

State laws set the age of consent. The most common age of consent is 16.

Most cases of child sexual abuse are committed by someone the child knows well.

Many cases of child sexual abuse go unreported.

Child sexual abuse can begin or take place on the Internet.

Risk Factors for Child Abuse and Neglect

- Expensive or unavailable healthcare
- Unplanned pregnancy
- Teen pregnancy
- Emotional immaturity
- Difficult family relationships
- Lack of knowledge about parenting and child development
- Many children in the home or very young children
- Use of physical punishment for discipline
- Premature birth or low birthweight
- Dislike of child
- Disobedience and arguing
- Frequent crying

Figure 16.12 The risk factors for child abuse and neglect are similar to the risk factors for violent behavior, which you learned about in the previous lesson. Some additional, specific risk factors are listed here. *What is neglect?*

neglect, their sense of well-being is shattered. Not surprisingly, this can have serious consequences on children's health.

Physical consequences of child abuse or neglect can range from severe bruises to broken bones, burns, brain damage, and delayed development. Children who are abused also have an increased risk of developing health conditions and diseases as adults. Children who are abused or neglected are more likely to behave in unhealthy ways. They have an increased risk of using tobacco, abusing alcohol or drugs, doing poorly in school, and committing crimes.

Children who are abused or neglected also have a greater risk of mental health conditions. These include depression, anxiety, eating disorders, and post-traumatic stress disorder (PTSD). Ongoing abuse may cause children to develop learning, attention, and memory issues.

Child abuse or neglect can lessen a person's ability to establish and maintain healthy relationships in adulthood. People who do not experience love, trust, and support in their early years may have trouble building healthy relationships with others later.

Paying attention to the signs of child abuse and neglect can help people identify when this violent behavior is occurring (**Figure 16.13**).

Sibling Abuse

Sibling abuse is the violent mistreatment of one sibling by another. Sibling abuse can be

Signs of Child Abuse and Neglect

Type of Abuse	Signs
Physical abuse	<ul><li>Injuries, such as broken bones or severe bruises</li><li>Many injuries on different parts of the body</li><li>Several injuries that occurred at different times</li></ul>
Sexual abuse	<ul><li>Bruises in the pelvic area</li><li>Difficulty or pain when walking or sitting</li><li>Torn clothing</li></ul>
Emotional abuse	<ul><li>Withdrawn attitude and unwillingness to talk to others</li><li>Anxiety and worry</li><li>Difficulty sleeping</li><li>Aggressive or inappropriate behavior</li></ul>
Neglect	<ul><li>Underweight</li><li>Poor physical development</li><li>Lack of cleanliness</li></ul>

Figure 16.13 Sometimes, children and young people who are abused blame themselves. It is important to remember that the person being abused is *never* responsible for abuse.

physical, emotional, or sexual and has serious health consequences. According to some studies, sibling abuse is one of the most common types of family abuse. Sibling abuse most often occurs in families where other unhealthy relationships exist.

Some conflict or rivalry is normal between siblings, but abuse is not. Unlike rivalry, abuse is part of an ongoing, chronic pattern. Sibling abuse is typically one-sided and aims to dominate the person being abused.

Elder Abuse

Elder abuse is the abuse of an older adult and occurs in older adults' homes, nursing homes, or other living situations. Typically, family members or paid caregivers commit elder abuse. This abuse can take the following forms:

- physical abuse, including inappropriate use of medications or restraints
- emotional abuse, including ignoring calls for help or saying cruel words
- sexual abuse
- financial abuse, including the theft of money or property
- neglect, including failure to provide food, water, medications, and basic hygiene

Many cases of elder abuse go unreported. Older adults who are abused and neglected often feel helpless, lonely, and distressed. They also tend to die earlier than older adults who have not been abused (**Figure 16.14**).

CASE STUDY

Aarav and Rajesh: Boys Will Be Boys

Aarav is 12 years old, and he is scared of his older brother Rajesh. Rajesh always taunts Aarav about his weight, calling him "fatty" or "doughboy" and pinching the fat around his waist or on his arms. Aarav became very upset one day and told his dad about Rajesh's mean comments and actions. His father told Rajesh to stop teasing his brother, but it did not work, and Rajesh's teasing only got worse.

Often, Aarav's parents work late into the evening, which means that Rajesh is in charge at home after school. Rajesh yells at Aarav to do all of the chores, and if Aarav resists, Rajesh will hit, kick, and push him until he obeys. Aarav tries his hardest to stay out of his brother's way and not anger him. Rajesh tells Aarav that he will hurt him more if he tells anyone about their fights. A few times, Aarav has had to hide the scrapes and bruises from his parents and people at school.

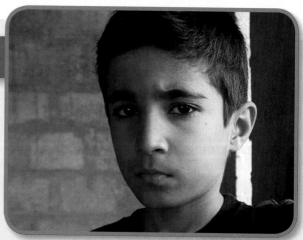

iStock.com/danishkhan

Thinking Critically

1. Are Rajesh's actions toward Aarav abuse? If yes, which type(s) of abuse?

2. What can Aarav do to stop his brother's actions? Whom should he talk to about his situation?

3. What are some possible health consequences for Aarav due to his brother's actions?

Preventing and Responding to Abuse

Many communities take steps to help prevent abuse. Programs educate people about abuse. Some schools hold campaigns to prevent peer abuse. Online resources and government agencies also share information. You can help prevent abuse using the following strategies.

Promote Health

One way to help prevent abuse is to promote health for yourself, your family, and your community. You can do this in the following ways:

- If you have experienced abuse, seek help from a mental health professional. People who have experienced abuse can sometimes abuse others.
- Develop skills in communicating effectively and resolving conflicts.
- Surround yourself with healthy relationships.
- Find ways to value diversity and show respect for others.
- Seek treatment for mental health conditions and illnesses.

Report Abuse

Recognizing abuse is the first step to stopping it. Some laws require children and teens to be educated about signs of abuse. For example, Erin's Law requires that children and teens be taught about body safety to recognize sexual abuse and to speak up if they are being abused.

Reporting abuse can get authorities involved. Anyone who thinks a person is being abused should report this to an authority (for example, a police officer or organization) or other trusted adult.

Several hotlines help people trying to report abuse and leave abusive situations (**Figure 16.15**). People can also report abuse through local or state departments of human services, law enforcement, and state hotlines.

Some professionals are required to report abuse. These workers, called *mandated reporters*, include teachers and other school personnel, social workers and child welfare workers, and healthcare professionals.

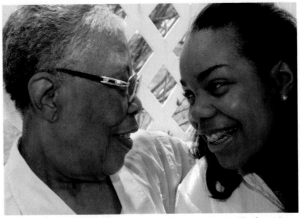

iStock.com/nano

Figure 16.14 Many older adults are dependent on their families or caregivers to help them meet their daily living needs. These older adults require the support of loved ones to help protect themselves against harm. If this care is not provided, older adults can be severely hurt by abuse or neglect. *What are the emotional consequences of elder abuse?*

Abuse Hotlines

Childhelp National Child Abuse Hotline
Call 1-800-422-4453

National Domestic Violence Hotline
Call 1-800-799-SAFE (7233)
Visit www.thehotline.org

National Teen Dating Abuse Hotline
Call 1-866-331-9474
Text *loveis* to 22522
Visit www.loveisrespect.org

vladwel/Shutterstock.com

Figure 16.15 Abuse hotlines can help people report abuse, leave abusive situations, and stay safe.

Once abuse is reported, a state organization, such as a child welfare agency or law enforcement, will talk with anyone who might have information. If the organization finds abuse has occurred, it may make arrests. In the case of child abuse, it may take the child away from the parents or guardians and place the child in foster care. *Foster care* is an arrangement in which adults agree to care for children who are not biologically theirs.

Those who commit abuse may be required to receive therapy and treatment. They may be charged and, if found guilty, sent to prison.

Break the Cycle

No matter the type, abuse is a pattern. This means that abuse continues over time. Abusive behavior usually follows a cycle of four stages (**Figure 16.16**). These four stages, called the *cycle of abuse*, include the following:

- tension building
- incident
- reconciliation
- calm

The cycle of abuse repeats as long as abuse continues. The abuse does not stop unless someone acts to break the cycle.

Steps for breaking the cycle of abuse include the following:

1. **Recognize** the abusive situation. Do not make excuses for the person who is being abusive. There is never a good reason for engaging in abusive behavior. Talking with a trusted adult could help you identify if a situation is abusive.

2. **Remember** that abuse may seem to stop during the calm stage in the cycle of abuse. This does not mean the abuse is over. Do not let this convince you that the abuse is not real. Even if the person acting abusively is being nice, the abuse still needs to be addressed.

3. **Do not try to change** the person committing the abuse. You cannot change another person. People who abuse others need professional help.

4. **Leave** or help someone leave the abusive relationship or situation. Sometimes it may seem unsafe to leave an abusive situation. Talk with a trusted adult or call a hotline about this and try to leave when it is safe. Crisis shelters are available to help some people who have experienced abuse. Sometimes, you may also need to block the person who is being abusive from communicating with you.

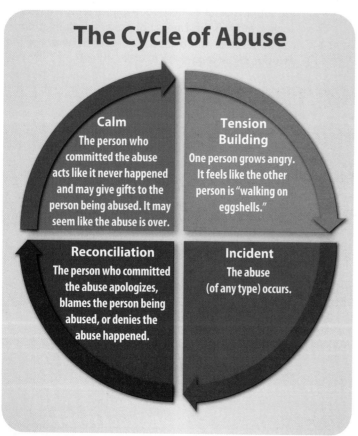

The Cycle of Abuse

Calm
The person who committed the abuse acts like it never happened and may give gifts to the person being abused. It may seem like the abuse is over.

Tension Building
One person grows angry. It feels like the other person is "walking on eggshells."

Reconciliation
The person who committed the abuse apologizes, blames the person being abused, or denies the abuse happened.

Incident
The abuse (of any type) occurs.

Figure 16.16 The cycle of abuse repeats even if it seems like the abuse has ended in the calm stage. The only way to stop abuse is to break the cycle.

Get Help and Treatment

If you experience abuse or are helping someone who has been abused, seek medical treatment for any injuries from the abuse. For example, you could go to a hospital or urgent care center. A crisis shelter can provide safety after you leave an abusive situation.

Seeking professional help after escaping abuse is an important part of moving forward. Mental health therapy sessions provide a safe space to share feelings, thoughts, and fears. Therapists can help people work through experiences, manage bad memories, and cope with anxiety, anger, and fear. This process can help people have healthier relationships. If you or someone you know has experienced abuse, talk to an adult you trust, such as a teacher, school counselor, or nurse. That person can help you find help from a trained professional.

People who commit abuse or neglect also need professional help. Specific types of treatment may benefit these people. For example, in the case of parents or guardians who abuse children, treatment could include education on appropriate parenting techniques. For people who commit sexual abuse, treatment may include training to increase empathy for others and self-control.

Lesson 16.2 Review

1. Making threats and calling someone names is a form of _____ abuse.
   A. physical
   B. emotional
   C. sexual
   D. sibling

2. _____ _____ violence occurs when one person in a romantic relationship abuses, controls, or dominates the other person.

3. **True or false.** Just as some sibling rivalry is normal between siblings, so is sibling abuse.

4. What are the four stages of the cycle of abuse?

5. **Critical thinking.** List two short-term and two long-term health consequences of child abuse for children.

Hands-On Activity

Learning about abuse is often very difficult. Perhaps you have seen abuse in your own family or that of a close friend. Perhaps you have never witnessed it. Either way, information about abuse can be shocking and hard to process. On a separate piece of paper, summarize what you believe are the five most important facts from this lesson. Talk about your summary with a classmate and discuss the similarities and differences between the facts you chose. Although it is never fun, talking about abuse can make people more likely to speak up and reach out for help. If you had concerns that someone was being abused, what would you do?

16.3

Other Types of Violence

Key Terms 👉

school violence any violent behavior that occurs on school property, at school-sponsored events, or on the way to or from school or school events

gangs groups of people who carry out violent and illegal acts

human trafficking form of modern slavery in which people are forced or pressured to perform some type of job or service against their will

hate crimes threats or violence against someone because of the individual's race, ethnic origin, disability, sex, or religion

homicide crime of killing another person

terrorism use of violence and threats to frighten and control groups of people to further an ideological aim

Learning Outcomes

After studying this lesson, you will be able to

- **explain** what school violence is and how schools prevent it.
- **describe** the reasons for and consequences of people joining gangs.
- **list** ways to protect yourself from human trafficking.
- **describe** how hate crimes can be prevented.
- **discuss** the consequences of homicide.
- **identify** ways to help prevent terrorism.
- **explain** what you can do to help prevent violence.

Graphic Organizer

Other Types of Violence

You learned about abuse, neglect, bullying, and cyberbullying in the previous lessons. In this lesson, you will learn about other types of violence. Create a KWL chart like the one shown. Before reading this lesson, write what you know and what you want to know about topics related to violence. After studying the lesson, write what you have learned.

iQoncept/Shutterstock.com

K What I **K**now	W What I **W**ant to Know	L What I Have **L**earned
Violent behavior and threats should be reported to a trusted adult	What are other ways to prevent or reduce violence?	Practicing conflict resolution skills, building healthy relationships, and practicing safety at home are all ways to help prevent violence

Lately, Sofia from the previous lessons has been watching the news with her parents. The more she learns about the world, the more she fears violence that could impact her community. Stories about gang violence and terrorism sometimes make Sofia afraid of going to public events. She wishes someone would tell her how to avoid and prevent these types of violence.

Violence can occur in many places, even in places where people should feel safe. You have already learned about bullying and abuse, two types of violence. In this lesson, you will learn about other types of violent behavior and ways to respond to and prevent them.

School Violence

School violence is any violent behavior that occurs on school property, at school-sponsored events, or on the way to or from school or school events (**Figure 16.17**). School violence can include bullying and cyberbullying. It also includes fighting and the use of weapons at school.

School should be a safe place for all students, but school violence puts students in danger. For example, a fight might seem like it only affects two students, but if a fight gets out of control, even uninvolved students can get hurt. Even if they are not physically injured, students who are exposed to violence can feel depressed, anxious, and fearful. If a student brings a weapon to school, many people can be hurt and even die. Violent behavior in schools can also have serious school and legal consequences. Fighting with another student can lead to detention, suspension, or expulsion. Attacking another student can lead to arrest by the police.

Many schools establish violence-prevention programs to help create a culture that does not tolerate violent behaviors. This means that the school

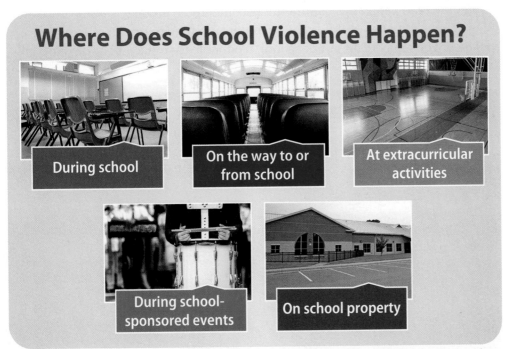

Where Does School Violence Happen?

During school

On the way to or from school

At extracurricular activities

During school-sponsored events

On school property

Left to right: cozyta/Shutterstock.com; Suzanne Tucker/Shutterstock.com; stockvideofactory/Shutterstock.com; Rattanapon Ninlapoom/Shutterstock.com; vincent noel/Shutterstock.com

Figure 16.17
School violence can happen at school, but can also occur in other locations for school-related events. *Is violence on the school bus considered school violence? Why or why not?*

takes violence seriously and tries to prevent it. Schools often use the following strategies to prevent and reduce violence:

- Select strong, positive, responsible student leaders who act appropriately and are not afraid to speak out against violence.
- Develop positive team-building activities, such as community service work, to strengthen bonds among students.
- Treat violent behavior as a serious offense. Any acts of violence result in consequences.
- Have a buddy system, with older students looking out for younger students.
- Encourage students to report any violent acts they observe immediately (Figure 16.18).
- Enforce rules regarding keeping school doors locked.
- Ensure a weapon-free school. Communicate rules about weapons and search students' belongings as necessary.
- Offer peer mediation programs to prevent conflicts from escalating.

To help reduce violence, students can cooperate with these programs and rules. For example, obeying rules about locking school doors can help keep dangerous people out of the building. Students have an important role in school strategies for violence prevention.

Gang Violence

Gang violence is violent behavior carried out in a gang. **Gangs** are groups of people who commit violent and illegal acts. These actions can include selling drugs, stealing, attacking others, and damaging others' property. Some young people join a gang to feel like part of a group and gain a sense of identity. Others do so because of peer pressure, the desire to make money, or the hope of protecting themselves and their families.

People who join gangs commonly become involved in acts of violence and other crimes. Because of this, gang members often go to prison or experience violence. They may drop out of school, be unable to find a job, or develop an

Figure 16.18
When young people quickly alert adults about violent behaviors, adults can prevent or stop dangerous situations. Some schools offer anonymous, online reporting systems.

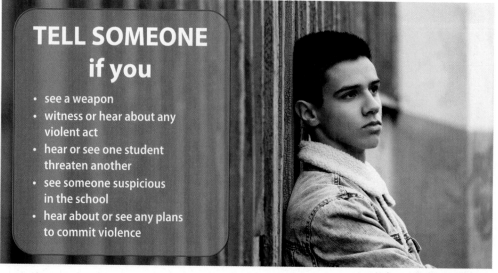

TELL SOMEONE if you
- see a weapon
- witness or hear about any violent act
- hear or see one student threaten another
- see someone suspicious in the school
- hear about or see any plans to commit violence

Malivan_Iuliia/Shutterstock.com

addiction to drugs. Committing a crime can severely impact a person's future. Many gang members also lose their lives to gang violence.

Communities often have resources that help reduce the amount of gang violence. For example, officials in cities take steps to limit the size and reach of gangs. To be successful, city workers and police officers have to be deeply engaged in the community and build trust. **Figure 16.19** lists some strategies you can use to protect yourself and avoid gang violence.

Human Trafficking

Human trafficking is a form of modern slavery in which people are forced or pressured to perform some job or service. In *labor trafficking*, employers use threats to force people to work. In *sex trafficking*, people are forced to engage in sexual activity. Traffickers use threats, violence, drugs, and coercion to make people do what they want.

Sometimes, trafficking begins with kidnapping. More often, people trick others with promises. For example, a person may reach out to someone on social media and ask to meet. Human trafficking can also begin in a relationship. One family member or partner may force another to work or engage in sexual activity.

Human trafficking has serious consequences. During and even after trafficking, people may experience fatigue, pain, and health conditions such as injuries, infections, and unwanted pregnancy. Mentally and emotionally, people who are trafficked may be depressed or anxious and have substance use disorders or PTSD. Often, people who are trafficked are isolated from supportive relationships.

Practicing safety precautions can help you avoid human trafficking. Lock the doors and windows at home. Do not go anywhere with someone you do not know well or meet someone you know online in person without supervision. Do not give out your personal information and avoid using substances such as drugs and alcohol.

If someone offers you a job that seems too good to be true, talk to an adult. If someone gives you gifts or money or makes promises, be aware that these behaviors may be *grooming* (building a relationship with the intent of taking advantage of a person). If you feel unsafe in a relationship, or are in a relationship where the other person has more power, leave the relationship. Reach out to a trusted adult or community resource for help.

Knowing the signs of human trafficking can help you identify if you or others are being trafficked. It is important to report any suspected cases of human trafficking (**Figure 16.20**).

Hate Crimes

Hate crimes are threats or volence against someone because of the person's race, ethnic origin, disability, sex, or religion. Hate crimes include damaging someone's property, making threats, and carrying out emotional and physical attacks.

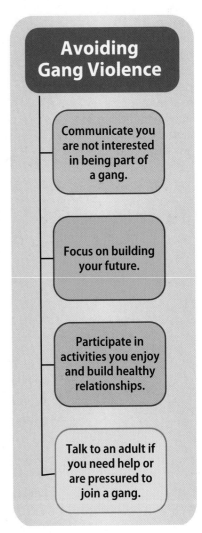

Avoiding Gang Violence

- Communicate you are not interested in being part of a gang.
- Focus on building your future.
- Participate in activities you enjoy and build healthy relationships.
- Talk to an adult if you need help or are pressured to join a gang.

Figure 16.19
Many communities have resources to help young people put these strategies for avoiding gang violence into action.

Signs of Human Trafficking

- Unexplained, regular school absences
- Running away from home
- Regular travel
- Bruises or other physical injuries
- Lack of control over schedule
- Hunger
- Sudden changes in behavior or hygiene
- Dodging questions or lying
- Older romantic partner
- Lack of concentration
- Anxiety, anger, and depression

STOP HUMAN TRAFFICKING

If you suspect **human trafficking**, **talk** to a trusted adult, **visit** humantraffickinghotline.org/chat, **call** the National Human Trafficking Hotline (1-888-373-7888), or **text** HELP to BeFree (233733)

ria_airborne/Shutterstock.com

People who experience hate crimes can suffer injury or loss of property. They may be emotionally scarred by the crime. Hate crimes also tend to hurt a community. This is because people who commit hate crimes see the person they attack as a symbol of a larger group.

Most states have laws against hate crimes. These laws increase the punishment for hate crimes, such as personal violence or property damage. Committing a hate crime can result in school consequences, such as suspension or expulsion. It can also result in legal consequences such as juvenile criminal charges.

Appreciating diversity and discouraging violent behavior can help reduce hate crimes. Hate crimes are usually motivated by prejudice and bias. Do not engage in these ideas. Instead, celebrate differences and encourage others to do the same.

Homicide

Killing someone is an extremely serious crime called a **homicide**. Homicides occur through physical injury. For example, attacking another student and causing death can lead to homicide. So can using a weapon at school. Whether intentional or unintentional, homicides lead to serious, lasting consequences.

Homicide robs another person of life. It devastates families, friends, and communities. No one deserves to be killed, and homicide only makes the issues in a person's life worse. Homicide leads to serious criminal charges. In some states, young people who commit homicide are treated as adults. These young people can be sentenced to life in prison.

The most important step in preventing homicide is reporting violent behavior to trusted adults. If a person threatens to kill someone, take this seriously and tell a school official, teacher, or other adult. You should also immediately report any weapons or violent situations you see at school or in your community. Reporting these situations can allow an adult to intervene before a homicide can occur.

Terrorism

Terrorism is the use of violence and threats to frighten and control groups of people. Terrorism is ideologically motivated. This means it aims to punish people for or convince people of certain ideas. Some examples of terrorism are killing or injuring people to promote a political or religious view. Terrorism often leads to the loss of many lives and creates fear in communities. It is a serious crime that does nothing to validate a person's viewpoint.

Most terrorism is a result of violent extremism. *Violent extremism* refers to beliefs that support the use of violence to promote an idea. For example, a violent extremist view might support hurting people who practice a particular religion.

The best way to prevent terrorism is to report any suspicious activity to the police (**Figure 16.21**). If you report suspicious activity, you should describe what you saw, when and where you saw it, and why it is suspicious. Another way to prevent terrorism is to celebrate the differences among people. Celebrating differences and encouraging others to do the same can reduce violent extremism.

What to Do If You Experience Violence

Unfortunately, violence sometimes occurs. In these situations, knowing how to respond is important. Violence can have serious physical and emotional effects, such as physical injuries and feelings of helplessness. Your actions immediately following violent behavior can affect your well-being and the well-being of others. The following strategies can help you respond to violent behavior:

- If someone in a relationship uses or threatens you with violence, tell a trusted adult and get out of that relationship as soon as possible. There is no excuse for violent behavior.
- If you witness or suspect violence of any kind, tell a trusted adult.
- If you are tempted to act violently, get out of the situation and talk to a trusted adult. You may need professional help to work through your feelings.
- If you experience violence, get medical help for any physical injuries. Report the violence to a trusted adult, such as a parent or guardian, school official, or the police. Seek professional help for dealing with the emotional impact of the violence.

What Is Suspicious Activity?

Unusual objects or situations
- An unfamiliar car parked in a strange location
- An unattended suitcase in a lobby
- A person lingering outside a school

Requesting information
- A person who wants to know how to get into your school
- A person who wants to know your club's exact schedule and location

Observation
- A person who sits in a car outside your school every day
- A person measuring and taking pictures of a community facility

Figure 16.21 There are certain activities that make people suspects for terrorism. If you witness a person doing anything suspicious, such as the examples listed here, immediately report this to the police.

Violence Prevention

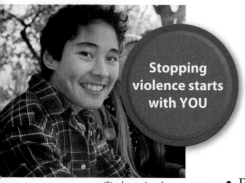

Stopping violence starts with YOU

iStock.com/gradyreese

Figure 16.22
By behaving in a nonviolent way and inspiring others to do so, by standing up against violence, and by practicing healthy conflict resolution, you can help reduce and prevent violent behaviors in your community. *What should you do if you witness any threats or violent behavior?*

Everyone in a community has a role in reducing and preventing violent behavior. This includes you. Behaving in a nonviolent manner is one way you can reduce violence (**Figure 16.22**). You can also recognize the signs of violence and reduce risk factors. The following strategies are ways you can help prevent and reduce violence:

- Resist the pressure to hurt others or join gangs. Focus on your values and beliefs and find healthy ways to feel good about yourself.
- Practice healthy conflict resolution. Use the negotiation process and keep calm.
- Give support to others who resist the pressure to act violently.
- Learn self-control to prevent yourself from becoming violent. Encourage others to use self-control, too.
- Choose your friends carefully. Build healthy relationships that are free from violence.
- Do not pick up a gun or other weapon. Report unsecure guns or weapons to a trusted adult.
- Practice safety when home alone and in public places. For example, lock the doors and windows at home. Do not give out your personal information.
- If you are tempted to act violently, seek help from a trusted adult.
- Talk to a trusted adult if you witness any threats or violent behavior.

Taking these personal steps to prevent violence can help build a community in which violence is less common. This type of community is better for you and others.

Lesson 16.3 Review

1. Which of the following is part of school violence?
   - **A.** Teasing from a sibling at home.
   - **B.** A parent neglecting a child.
   - **C.** Bullying on the bus.
   - **D.** All of the above.

2. What form of violence could include an employer forcing employees to work long hours for very little money?

3. **True or false.** Hate crimes are threats or attacks against someone for no reason.

4. Practicing healthy _____ resolution, such as negotiating, is one way to prevent or reduce violence.

5. **Critical thinking.** People often join gangs to feel like part of a group. What positive actions could young people take instead to get this feeling? What consequences of gang involvement should they consider when making a decision?

Hands-On Activity

Search online for a reliable article about an act of violence that influenced your community. Read the article and identify the risk factors that led to violence and the type of violence. With a partner, describe how the violence affected the person who experienced violence, the person who behaved violently, and the community. Share this summary with the class and lead a discussion about what could have prevented the violence.

Summary

Lesson 16.1 Bullying and Cyberbullying

- Violent behavior is the intentional use of words or actions that cause or threaten to cause injury to someone or something. Violent behavior results in physical or psychological injury.
- Bullying is repeated aggressive behavior that causes a person physical or emotional injury or discomfort. It includes harassment, stalking, and hazing.
- If you witness bullying, do not participate. Be an upstander, tell the person to stop, and avoid bullying back. Tell an adult if you or someone you know is being bullied.
- Cyberbullying is a form of bullying that uses electronic communication. Since young people spend so much time online, cyberbullying can be difficult to escape.
- Schools often have programs to teach you how to respond to bullying and prevent it.

Lesson 16.2 Abuse and Neglect

- The consistent, violent mistreatment of a person is abuse. Abuse can be physical, emotional, sexual, or financial. People who abuse others often try to make them feel responsible for the abuse, but this is never the case.
- Intimate partner violence involves couples who are or were married or in a romantic relationship. Child abuse refers to intentional acts that cause harm or threaten to cause harm to a child.
- Sibling abuse is the mistreatment of one sibling by another. This can be physical, emotional, or sexual, and is one of the most common types of family abuse. Older adults who are mistreated experience elder abuse.
- If you witness any type of abuse, tell a trusted adult. Abuse typically follows a pattern called the *cycle of abuse*, which includes four stages that repeat as abuse continues.

Lesson 16.3 Other Types of Violence

- Any emotionally or physically violent behavior that occurs in locations or events related to school is school violence. Schools do not tolerate violence due to its harmful effects on students.
- Gang violence is carried out by groups of people who commit violent and illegal acts. Human trafficking involves forcing people to perform a job or service against their will. Threats or violence against someone because of race, ethnic origin, disability, sex, or religion are hate crimes.
- Killing someone is called *homicide* and can be punished with life in prison, even for adolescents. The use of violence and threats to frighten or control groups of people is terrorism.
- If you experience violence or if you witness violence, tell a trusted adult. Get professional help for physical or emotional injuries from the impact of violence. To help reduce and prevent violent behavior, practice healthy conflict resolution and build healthy relationships free from violence.

Check Your Knowledge

Record your answers to each of the following questions on a separate sheet of paper.

1. A(n) _____ injury harms a person's social or emotional health.
2. What kind of violent behavior includes hazing, harassing, spreading rumors, and forming cliques?
3. Which of the following is *not* a sign that a person is being bullied?
   - **A.** Feeling angry, sad, or lonely.
   - **B.** Wanting to hurt someone else or one's self.
   - **C.** Having improved self-esteem.
   - **D.** Feeling helpless to stop the bullying.
4. _____ is a form of bullying that uses electronic communication.
5. _____ abuse may involve hitting, kicking, biting, or burning someone.
6. **True or false.** A child who does not have enough food or clothes suited to the season may be experiencing neglect.
7. Giving an older adult an inappropriate amount of medications is one form of _____ _____.
8. **True or false.** People who experience abuse can come to abuse others if they do not resolve their emotional issues.
9. What are groups of people who commit violent and illegal acts?
10. What are three signs of human trafficking?
11. Which form of violence aims to punish people for or convince people of certain ideas?
12. **True or false.** There are sometimes acceptable excuses for violent behavior in a relationship.

Use Your Vocabulary ↗

abuse	gangs	peer abuse
bullying	harassment	physical abuse
bystander effect	hate crimes	school violence
bystanders	hazing	sexual abuse
child abuse	homicide	sibling abuse
cyberbullying	human trafficking	stalking
elder abuse	intimate partner violence	terrorism
emotional abuse	neglect	upstander
financial abuse		

13. With a partner, choose two words to compare from the list above. Create a Venn diagram to compare your words and identify differences. Write one term under the left circle and the other term under the right. Where the circles overlap, write three characteristics the terms have in common. For each individual term, write characteristics in its respective outer circle.
14. For each of the terms above, identify a word or group of words describing a quality of the term—an *attribute*. Pair up with a classmate and discuss your list of attributes.

Think Critically

15. **Determine.** Is spreading rumors a form of violence? Why or why not?

16. **Compare and contrast.** Describe the similarities and differences between bullying and cyberbullying. What are the effects of each?

17. **Cause and effect.** Why do you think experiencing abuse makes a person more likely to abuse others? How can abuse be a cycle over generations?

18. **Draw conclusions.** Often, people remain silent about difficult situations that involve abuse. How can silence about abuse in relationships allow the abuse to keep happening?

19. **Identify.** Why is it important to report any suspicious activity you witness?

DEVELOP Your Skills

20. **Goal-setting skills.** Review the risk factors for violent behavior in Figure 16.1. What risk factors are present in your life? in your family and community? Identify two risk factors you want to reduce and set SMART goals for changing them.

21. **Accessing information skills.** Working with a partner, choose one key term in this chapter. Watch a video, listen to a podcast, or read an article about the type of violence and its legal consequences in your state. Make sure the source you access is reliable. Find information about whether the type of violence can lead to arrest, fines, or time in prison. In a digital presentation, summarize what you learned and share it with your classmates. Incorporate other key terms when relevant.

22. **Communication, conflict resolution, and teamwork skills.** Working in a team, plan and script a role play about standing up to violence or abuse. Your role play should end healthfully and should include the use of assertive communication skills. It should confront and address the violence in a way that ensures everyone's safety physically, socially, and mentally. As you develop the role play, pay attention to each team member's verbal and nonverbal communication. If someone is uncomfortable, show empathy and rework the role play. Enlist the help of your teacher, if needed, and perform the role play for the class.

23. **Advocacy and accessing information skills.** Identify 10 agencies in your community that assist people affected by violent behavior. These can be people who experience violence, people who commit abuse, or family members. Create a resource list with each agency's name, mission, and contact information.

24. **Advocacy and teamwork skills.** Working in a team, choose one type of violence discussed in this chapter. Then, review the information in this chapter about avoiding and preventing this type of violence. Take notes about this information and do additional research to learn about avoidance and prevention strategies. Design a campaign to reduce this type of violence in your community using the information from the chapter and additional resources as your supporting details. Put the campaign into action and summarize how successful it was.

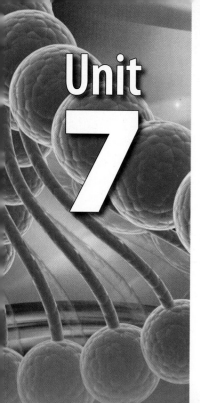

Unit 7

Human Development and Reproductive Health

Chapter 17 Human Development

Chapter 18 Sexually Transmitted Infections and HIV/AIDS

Warm-Up Activity

Ask Angelique: Going to the Doctor

Angelique is a popular social media presence in your community and age group. She focuses on helping teens through tough stuff. One of the ways she connects with her audience is through a Question and Answer blog. Angelique posts questions or situations that teens send her and asks other teens to provide advice based on their own experiences.

Read the post below and respond to Anonymous on a separate sheet of paper. Find a partner and review each other's responses.

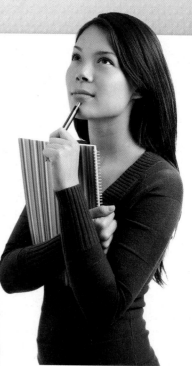

Maridav/Shutterstock.com

> Dear Angelique,
>
> How old does someone need to be to go into a doctor's appointment alone, without parents? I am 14 and I feel like I want to talk to my doctor about issues without my parents hearing. I trust my parents and they are great, but I worry that they might react strongly and embarrass me in front of my doctor. I know that I can talk with my parents, but sometimes I just want to be independent. If it is OK for me to go into my appointments alone, how do I tell my parents that is what I want?
>
> Thanks,
> Anonymous

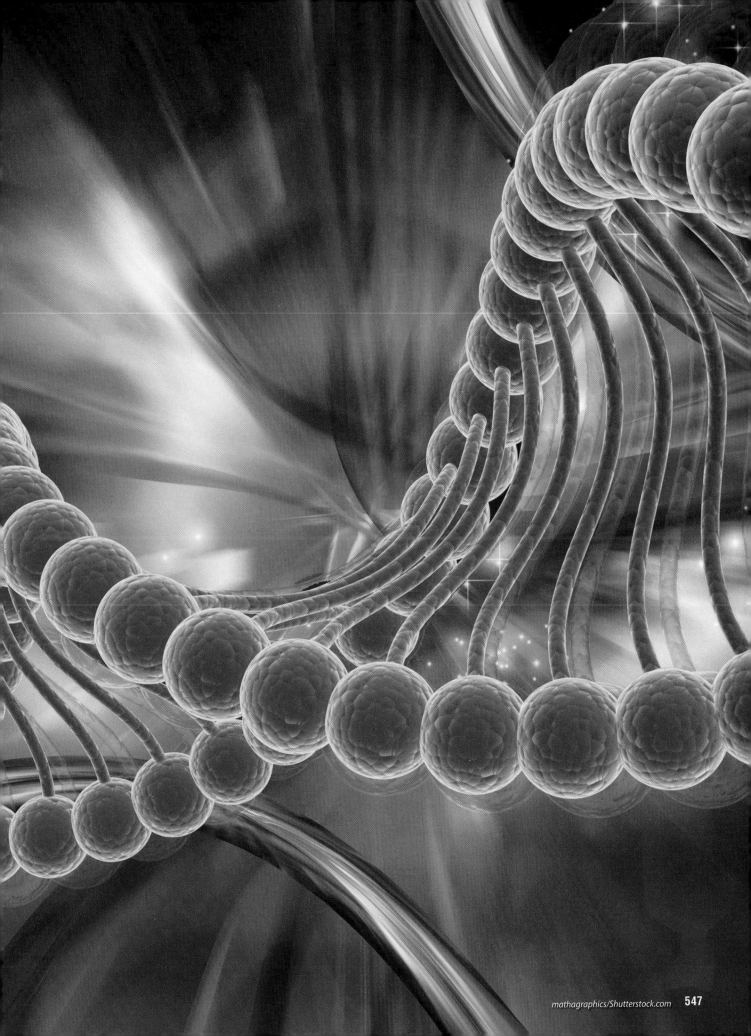

Chapter 17

Human Development

Essential Question ❓

What intellectual, emotional, and social developments occur during each stage of the life span?

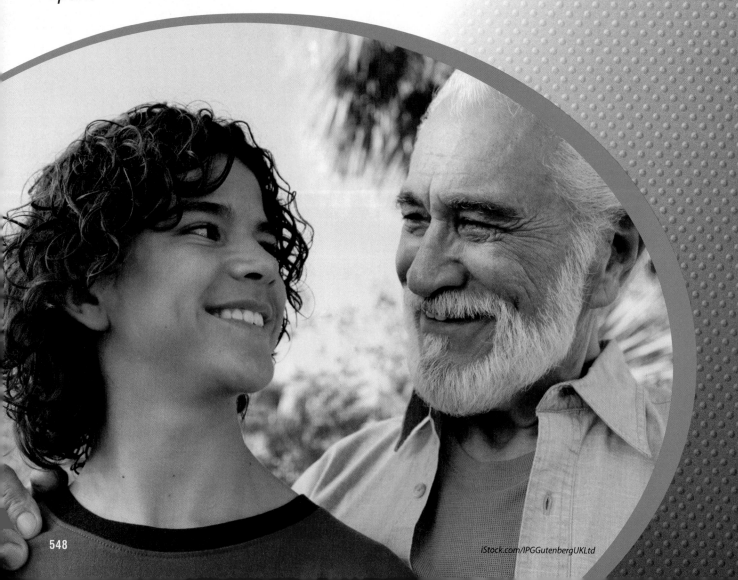

Reading Activity

Before reading this chapter, scan the chapter title. Write a paragraph describing what you know about this topic. As you are reading the chapter, compare and contrast the information in the chapter with your prior knowledge about the human life cycle. After reading, consider how prior knowledge of the subject matter helped you understand human development.

How Healthy Are You?

In this chapter, you will be learning about human development. Before you begin reading, take the following quiz to assess your understanding of human development, and how health needs change throughout the life span.

Health Concepts to Understand	Yes	No
Do you understand the functions of the male and female reproductive systems?		
Do you know the differences among the germinal, embryonic, and fetal stages of pregnancy?		
Can you name each of the developmental stages of a person?		
Can you name the milestones typical in the infancy, toddler, preschool, and middle childhood life stages?		
Do you know the physical changes that accompany puberty in males and females?		
Do you understand how the adolescent brain can be more susceptible to risky behaviors?		
Do you understand that as teens grow, so does their need to establish independence and rely on their own judgment?		
Do you understand how the body and a person's health needs change during adulthood?		
Do you understand what it means to grieve the loss of a loved one?		

Count your "Yes" and "No" responses. The more "Yes" responses you have, the more you understand human development. Now, take a closer look at the questions with which you responded "No." Develop your health literacy skills by accessing valid information about each of the concepts you do not understand. Evaluate any health websites you find using the information in Figure 1.16 of this text. If you do not understand the instructions, ask for clarification from your teacher.

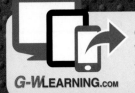

Click on the activity icon or visit www.g-wlearning.com/health to access online vocabulary activities using key terms from the chapter.

G-WLEARNING.com

The Beginning of Life

Key Terms 🖝

reproductive system body system that consists of a group of organs working together to make the creation of new life possible

ovulation release of an egg from one of the follicles into the uterus

menstruation discharge of some blood and tissues from the uterus

fertilization process by which the sperm and egg combine to create a zygote

zygote egg that has been fertilized by a sperm

obstetrician/gynecologist (OB/GYN) type of doctor who specializes in pregnancy, labor, and delivery

prenatal development period of growth that occurs from conception to birth

embryo term that describes a developing baby during the embryonic stage of prenatal development

fetus term that describes a developing baby during the fetal stage of prenatal development

Learning Outcomes

After studying this lesson, you will be able to

- **describe** the male and female reproductive systems.
- **explain** what the menstrual cycle is.
- **explain** what causes fertilization to take place.
- **summarize** the changes in a pregnant person's body.
- **describe** what happens to the developing child in the three stages of fetal development.

Graphic Organizer

Human Reproduction

Creating a baby is a complex process that involves the body systems, sexual activity, and healthy development. Create a graphic organizer like the one shown to increase your knowledge of human reproduction. As you read this lesson, fill in your organizer with notes about the process.

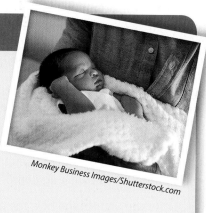
Monkey Business Images/Shutterstock.com

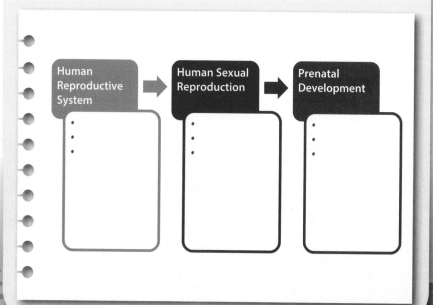

Human Reproductive System

Human Sexual Reproduction

Prenatal Development

The story of your life began as a single cell. This cell was created from the merging of two cells—one cell from each parent. The combination of these two cells produced you—a unique human being unlike any who ever has or ever will exist. One such unique human being is 10-year-old Xavier. He was created from the merging of one cell from each biological parent (**Figure 17.1**). In this lesson, you will learn how this amazing process works.

The Human Reproductive System

The human **reproductive system** is a body system in which organs work together to make the creation of new life possible. An *organ* is a body part with a specific function. For example, the heart is the organ that pumps blood throughout the body. Unlike other body systems, the reproductive system does not begin to work at birth. It does not become capable of working until *puberty*, which is when the body reaches sexual maturity. Also unlike other body systems, the reproductive system is different in males and females. (You will learn more about puberty and care of the reproductive systems later in this chapter.)

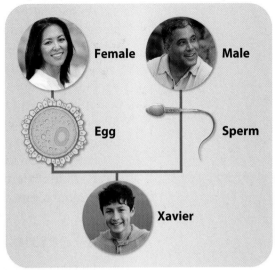

Rows: digitalskillet/Shutterstock.com; Fotoluminate LLC/Shutterstock.com; Double Brain/Shutterstock.com; Designua/Shutterstock.com; Digital Media Pro/Shutterstock.com

Figure 17.1 A human person is created from a combination of a female's egg and the sperm of a male. *Which body system works to create a human life?*

The Male Reproductive System

The male organs of reproduction produce and transport hormones and *sperm*, or male sex cells (**Figure 17.2**). Male sex organs include the testes and penis, seminal vesicles, bulbourethral gland, prostate, and vas deferens. These organs grow and mature as males enter puberty. The *testes* produce sperm and the hormone *testosterone*. The *scrotum*, a saclike structure, holds the testes.

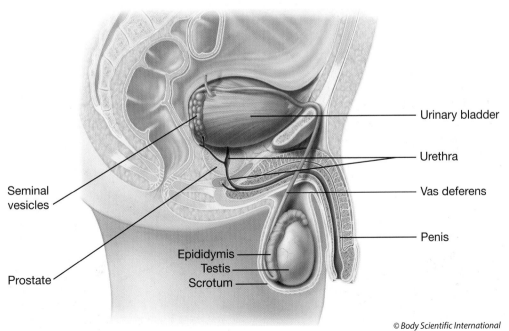

Seminal vesicles

Prostate

Epididymis

Testis

Scrotum

Urinary bladder

Urethra

Vas deferens

Penis

Figure 17.2
This illustration shows the side view of the male reproductive organs. Sperm form in the testes (one *testis* shown) and are carried to the penis by the vas deferens. The seminal vesicles, bulbourethral gland (not shown), and prostate secrete a fluid that mixes with sperm to form *semen*.

© Body Scientific International

As the sperm mature, they enter the *epididymis*. This structure is a coiled tube along the outer wall of the testes. It leads into another tube, the *vas deferens*. This tube carries sperm to the *penis*, the male organ used in sexual intercourse.

The penis contains tissues that can fill with blood. When that happens, the penis becomes stiff. This is called an *erection* and happens when a male is sexually excited. Intense stimulation causes the epididymis and vas deferens to contract and send sperm into the urethra. The *urethra* is a tube within the penis that has an opening at the outer end.

Before sperm leave the body, the *seminal vesicles*, *bulbourethral gland*, and *prostate* secrete fluids to form *semen*. Semen protects and nurtures sperm. *Ejaculation* occurs when more contractions force the semen out through the opening of the urethra.

The Female Reproductive System

The female reproductive organs have several functions (**Figure 17.3**). The *ovaries* produce female sex cells, or eggs (*ova*), and the hormones *progesterone* and *estrogen*. There are two ovaries, which are small, almond-shaped organs in the lower abdomen. Each ovary contains thousands of immature eggs. A *follicle*, which is a single layer of nurturing cells, surrounds each egg.

Once a female reaches sexual maturity, a single egg and its follicle grow toward maturity each month. They leave the ovary and enter the nearby opening of the *fallopian tube*. One fallopian tube leads from each ovary to one side of the *uterus*. That structure is a hollow organ lined with a tissue called *endometrium*. The walls of the uterus contain strong muscles and many blood vessels. During pregnancy, a baby develops within the uterus.

The *vagina* is a tube-like structure lined with a moist membrane. It connects to the uterus at the *cervix* and leads to an outer opening between the female's legs. A baby is delivered by leaving the uterus and passing through the vagina. The vaginal opening is protected by the *labia minora* and *majora* (singular

Figure 17.3
This illustration shows the side view of both the external and internal female reproductive organs. *What term describes the release of an egg from a follicle into the uterus?*

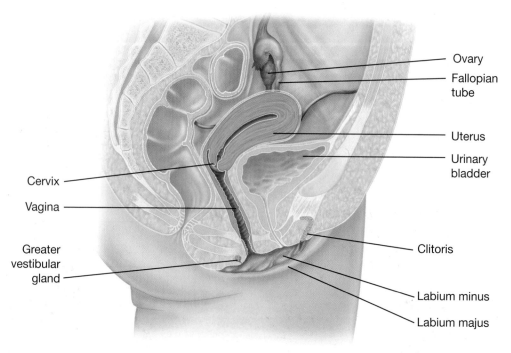

© *Body Scientific International*

labium minus and *majus*). Like the penis, the *clitoris* fills with blood during sexual excitement. The *greater vestibular gland* secretes fluid to lubricate the vagina.

When females reach puberty, they begin to have a menstrual cycle each month. At the start of the cycle, a follicle develops within an ovary. The follicle grows and develops with its egg. At the midpoint of the menstrual cycle, ovulation occurs. **Ovulation** is the release of an egg from a follicle into the uterus. When this happens, the lining of the uterus thickens. This change prepares the uterus to accept a fertilized egg. If that does not occur, menstruation begins. **Menstruation** is the discharge of some blood and tissues from the uterus (**Figure 17.4**). It marks the end of a menstrual cycle, and is followed by the beginning of a new menstrual cycle.

Females have menstrual cycles each month for many years. They do not have a cycle during pregnancy, however. Each menstrual cycle lasts around 28 days. That time span can vary from person to person and even from month to month for the same person. Just before or during menstruation, a female may feel some discomfort, called *cramps*. How much discomfort is felt also varies from female to female.

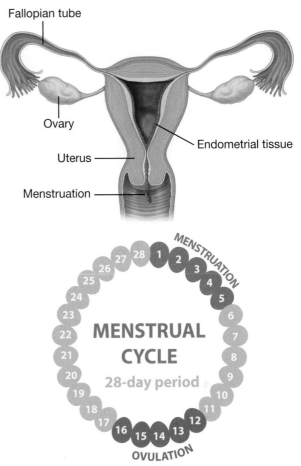

Top to bottom: © Body Scientific International; Photoroyalty/Shutterstock.com

Figure 17.4 Eggs are produced in the ovaries and are then released into the uterus. If a pregnancy does not occur during ovulation, menstruation begins. This is the discharge of some blood and tissues from the uterus. *How long does one menstrual cycle last?*

Human Sexual Reproduction

Humans reproduce through sexual intercourse. For pregnancy to take place, a male's sperm must enter the female's vagina. The sperm then swim from the vagina to the fallopian tube, where an egg may be located. There, one sperm and the mature egg combine in a process called **fertilization**.

When fertilization takes place, a single sperm breaks through the outer layers of the egg. The fertilized egg is called a **zygote** (**Figure 17.5**). At that point, pregnancy begins.

During pregnancy, the female's body releases hormones. They stop any more eggs from being released. They also prevent menstruation from occurring. Therefore, the first sign of pregnancy is often a missed menstrual period. A female can confirm pregnancy by having a pregnancy test.

During pregnancy, a female should make regular visits to an **obstetrician/gynecologist (OB/GYN)**. This type of doctor specializes in pregnancy, labor, and delivery. The doctor ensures that the pregnant person and the developing baby are both healthy during pregnancy. The doctor can also look for signs of possible difficulties. An OB/GYN can help the pregnant person have a healthy diet. It is very important for a pregnant person to receive this care.

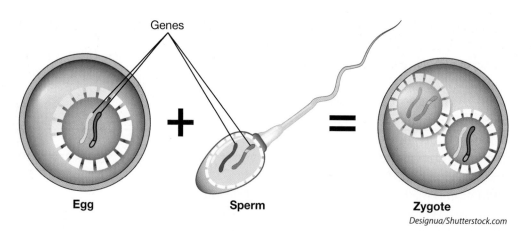

Genes

Egg + Sperm = Zygote

Designua/Shutterstock.com

Prenatal Development

Doctors measure pregnancies in weeks. Most babies are born 36 to 40 weeks after fertilization. During a pregnancy, the developing baby changes dramatically and rapidly. This period of change is known as **prenatal development**. It consists of three stages.

Germinal Stage

The *germinal stage* of prenatal development begins at fertilization and lasts about two weeks. In this phase, the single-celled zygote goes through a process of dividing itself into many cells. First, the single cell divides into two. These two cells then each divide, producing four cells. Those cells also divide, and so on. In five days, the zygote divides seven times, forming a ball of 128 cells. Meanwhile, this ball of cells has traveled to the uterus. After eight to ten days, it implants itself in the lining of the uterus. This implanted mass of cells is called an **embryo**.

Embryonic Stage

The *embryonic stage* of prenatal development lasts about six weeks. It is a critical period. During this time, the embryo begins to form the various tissues and organs that make a human. Systems that will help the embryo develop also take shape during this stage (**Figure 17.6**). They include the following:

- A membrane grows and surrounds the embryo implanted in the uterus.
- An organ called the *placenta* forms in the uterus. Rich in blood vessels, it helps support the embryo. The placenta removes waste products of the embryo and supplies needed hormones to the embryo. It also prevents bacteria from reaching the embryo. The placenta blocks some—but not all—harmful substances from reaching the embryo as well. Chemicals such as alcohol, nicotine, and many drugs can still pass from the pregnant person to the developing baby. The placenta cannot block them. These substances can be very harmful to the baby.
- The *umbilical cord* also forms. This tube is full of blood vessels. It connects the placenta to the developing baby at its abdomen. The cord carries food and oxygen from the pregnant person to the embryo.

During the embryonic stage, the body's major organs also begin to take form. Around three weeks, heartbeat begins.

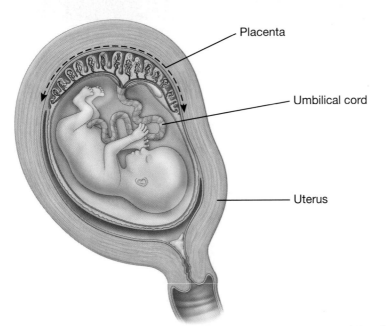

Placenta

Umbilical cord

Uterus

© Body Scientific International

Figure 17.6
After the ball of cells implants itself in the lining of the uterus, the embryo begins to form the various tissues and organs that make a human. *Which stage of prenatal development involves this formation of tissues and organs?*

Fetal Stage

The ninth week of pregnancy marks the beginning of the *fetal stage*. At this stage, the baby is now called a **fetus**. This stage lasts until the baby is born. During the fetal stage, the fetus grows considerably. By the fourth month, the fetus has grown enough that the pregnant person looks pregnant. After nine months, most of the organs, bones, and muscles of the fetus have completed their development. When that occurs, the baby is ready to be born.

Lesson 17.1 Review

1. When does the reproductive system become capable of working?
2. In the female reproductive system, _____ is the release of an egg into the uterus.
3. **True or false.** The placenta and umbilical cords are formed during the germinal stage of pregnancy.
4. Which stage of pregnancy starts at the ninth week and lasts until the baby is born?
5. **Critical thinking.** Explain the process of human sexual reproduction, from sexual intercourse to pregnancy.

Hands-On Activity

It can be uncomfortable to talk about reproduction, especially when using words that you do not use in "normal conversation." The best way to become more comfortable talking about human development and sexual health is through practice. Using appropriate vocabulary and maturity, explain how life begins to a classmate. Start with ovulation and end with the birth of the baby. As you describe this process, your classmate should listen carefully, take notes on your explanation, and ask questions when something does not make sense or whenever appropriate.

Lesson 17.2

Child Development

Key Terms ⤴

human life cycle sequence of developmental stages a person experiences from birth through adulthood

milestones important events that occur in each of the developmental stages of the human life cycle

life span actual number of years a person lives

life expectancy estimate of how long a person in a particular society is likely to live

early childhood period of time from infancy through the preschool years

temper tantrum toddler's episode of emotional upset that often includes yelling, crying, hitting, kicking, or even biting

middle childhood period of time when children are between five and 12 years of age; also called the *school-age years*

Learning Outcomes

After studying this lesson, you will be able to

- **identify** the different areas of development in the human life cycle.
- **describe** the factors that influence development.
- **summarize** the different ways a child develops during early childhood.
- **explain** the different ways a child develops during middle childhood.

Graphic Organizer

The Developing Child

Throughout the human life cycle, a person will experience physical, intellectual, emotional, and social changes. As you read this lesson, use an organizer like the one shown to take notes about the various developments that occur during a person's early childhood years and middle childhood years. Examples are provided for you.

Tanya Little/Shutterstock.com

Early Childhood Years
- Physical
- Intellectual — *Learning to speak*
- Emotional
- Social

Middle Childhood Years
- Physical
- Intellectual
- Emotional
- Social — *Development of friendships outside family*

A human life is made up of stages like a book is made up of chapters. The opening chapter of a book sets the stage for the following chapters. The story of a life unfolds in the same way that chapters build on each other. Each new chapter brings new elements to the plot. In this lesson, you will learn about the many changes that occur during the first chapters, or the early years, of life.

For example, Xavier from the first lesson remembers watching his little brother grow from an infant into a toddler and learn how to walk and talk. Xavier also recognizes the changes that he has gone through himself in middle childhood. He has grown several inches, learned how to be a good friend, and started to build his self-esteem.

The Human Life Cycle

When a baby is born, the **human life cycle** begins. This cycle carries a person through a series of developmental stages. With each new stage, the person begins a new phase of life. The human life cycle includes four developmental stages (**Figure 17.7**).

Each developmental stage of the human life cycle includes **milestones**, or important events. Some people reach a milestone earlier or later than others in the same stage. For example, a major developmental milestone of childhood is learning how to walk. The exact age at which a child begins to walk, however, differs from one child to the next. You will learn about adolescence and adulthood in the last two lessons of this chapter. This lesson will focus on early childhood and middle childhood.

Not all people experience every stage in the human life cycle. Some people have a much shorter life span than others. A person's **life span** is the actual number of years the individual lives. Each person's life span depends on family background, environment, and lifestyle. People age at different rates, which can affect their life spans. This is because aging carries with it risks for disease and disability that can shorten a life span.

As the health of a society improves, so does the life expectancy of its people. **Life expectancy** is an estimate of how long a person in a particular society is

Stages of the Human Life Cycle

Stage	Description
Early childhood 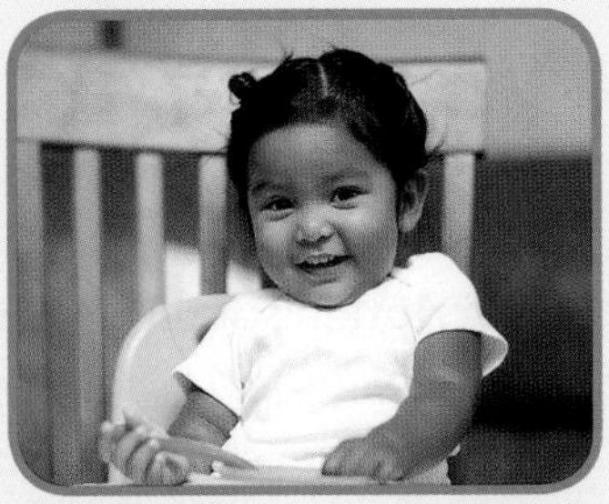 *Marlon Lopez MMG1 Design/Shutterstock.com*	Infancy (from birth to one year of age), the toddler years (from one to three years of age), and the preschool years (from three to five years of age)
Middle childhood 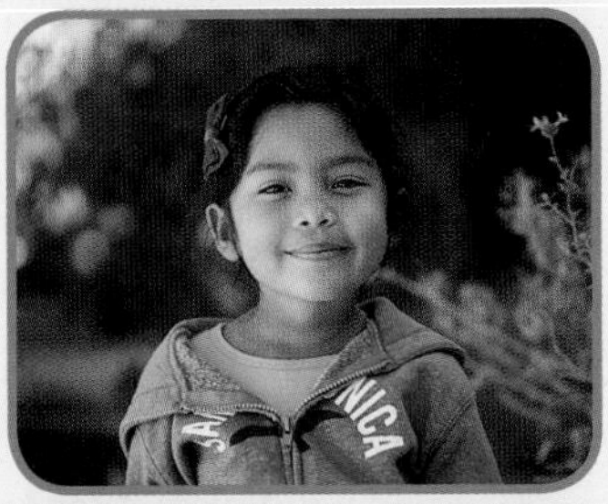 *Marlon Lopez MMG1 Design/Shutterstock.com*	Five to 12 years of age
Adolescence 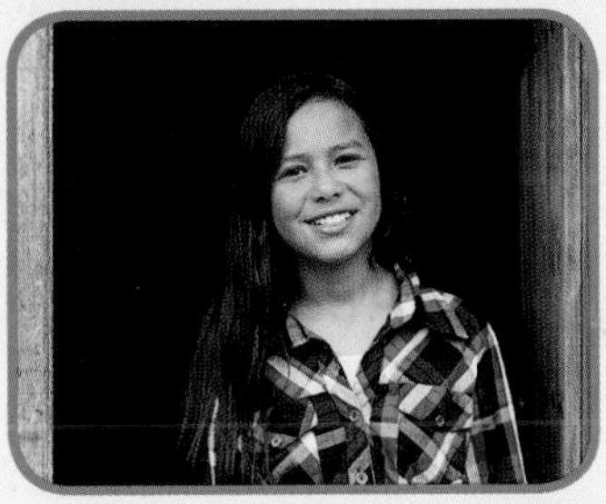 *santypan/Shutterstock.com*	Twelve to 19 years of age
Adulthood 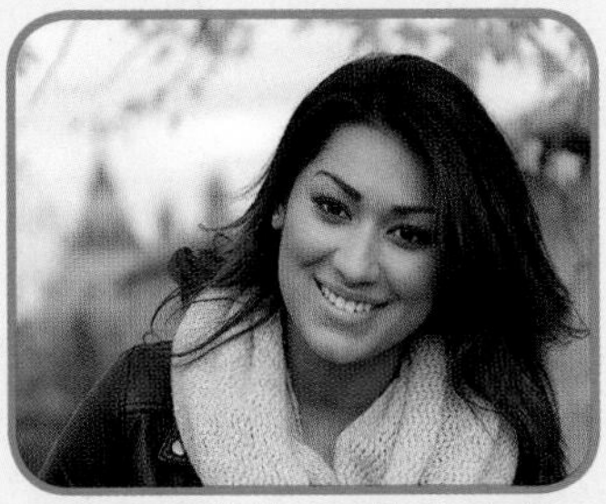 *Click Images/Shutterstock.com*	Twenty years of age and older

Figure 17.7 Looking at your baby pictures and school photos together will show how dramatically you changed throughout childhood.

likely to live. In the United States, the average life expectancy is 76.1 years for males and 81.1 years for females. Life expectancy differs from one country to another. It can also differ for groups in the same country (**Figure 17.8**).

Types of Human Development

People develop physically, intellectually, emotionally, and socially. These types of development are related and affect each other. Following are descriptions of the types of development:

- *Physical development* includes growth of the body and body parts. The other aspects of human development build on the basis of these physical changes. For instance, the brain develops and grows more complex in structure. These changes allow a child to process information, learn, and think in more complex ways.
- *Intellectual development* describes the growth of a person's ability to think. This includes how a person processes information and responds to the world. This type of development also includes learning to speak.
- *Emotional development* refers to a person's ability to form an identity and personality. It includes the ability to act and react independently and to have self-esteem.
- *Social development* refers to the ability to interact with others in acceptable ways. Social and interpersonal skills develop throughout a person's life. Much of the foundation for these skills is laid in childhood.

Influences on Development

Many factors influence how a person develops. Some are internal, meaning they come from inside a person. Others are external, or outside the person (**Figure 17.9**).

One key factor that influences development is the person's genetic makeup. A person's genetic makeup is the special combination of characteristics that come from the individual's biological parents.

Figure 17.8
Certain factors can change a person's life expectancy. *What is the average life expectancy for males and females in the United States?*

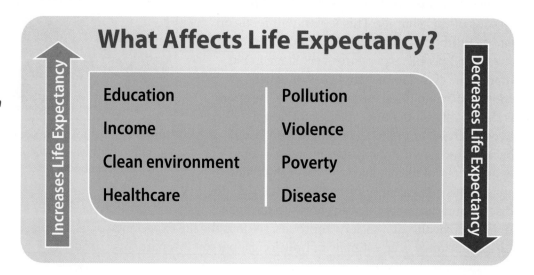

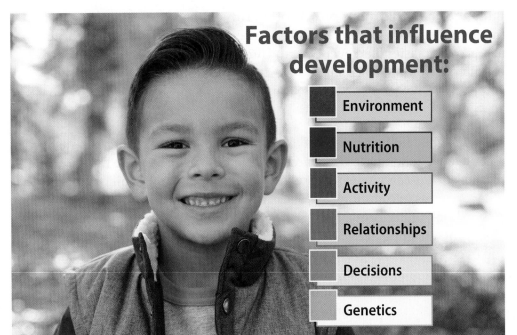

Factors that influence development:

- Environment
- Nutrition
- Activity
- Relationships
- Decisions
- Genetics

Figure 17.9
A person's level of physical activity, behavior, and family environment are all examples of influences that can affect how a person develops.

iStock.com/monkeybusinessimages

Each person's genetic makeup is unique, except in the case of identical twins, who have the same genetic makeup. A person's genetic makeup sets many physical traits, such as hair and eye color. It also gives a person certain tendencies, such as being tall or short.

Genetic makeup is not the only influence on physical appearance, however. The food a child eats when developing can affect height, for instance. A childhood illness can affect physical development as well.

Family is one of the most important influences on development and health. This influence is seen in a person's genetic makeup. People in some families are at greater risk to develop certain diseases, for instance. The childhoods that parents had can influence how they raise their children. That can affect the development of those children.

The environment a person lives in also affects development and health. Growing up in a small town is different from growing up in a large city. Each type of place provides a different set of experiences. Those experiences can influence how a child develops. The healthcare that a person receives is an important part of the environment, too.

The decisions that a person makes have a major impact on development. How a person talks and acts with other people shapes the types of friendships formed. The friends a person chooses to spend time with can have an impact, too. Friends who are responsible, caring people will influence a person to be that way also. People who make risky choices can influence someone to make similar unwise choices.

The Early Childhood Years

The term **early childhood** describes the period of time from infancy through the preschool years. During this time, infants learn many new skills. They then become toddlers, who are always on the move. Toddlers next turn into engaging and curious preschoolers. During the preschool years, children immerse themselves in life, soaking up everything they encounter, learning and growing faster than ever before. Throughout the magical years of early childhood, children reach many milestones.

Infancy

During the first year of life, *infants* learn how to adapt to life. Infants rely completely on their parents, guardians, and other caregivers to meet all of their needs. As caregivers respond promptly to an infant's smiling, crying, or other attempts to communicate, they reassure that the baby is safe and loved. As a result, infants form a strong attachment to their caregivers.

As infants grow, they achieve many milestones. They learn how to roll over, explore and grasp objects, and respond to voices. By the end of infancy, some children will say their first recognizable words. Others may not speak until they are toddlers. Even children who do not speak can show signs that they understand many words and phrases. When children do say their first words, they have reached a major developmental milestone.

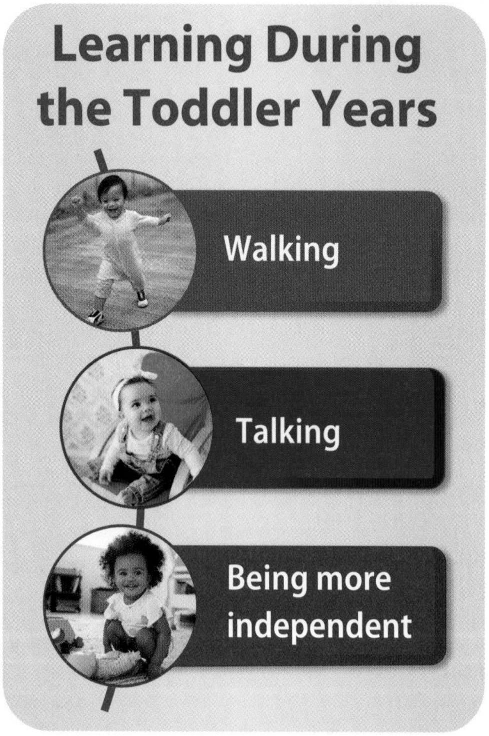

The Toddler Years

Toddlers are one to three years of age. Much growth and development occurs in these years (**Figure 17.10**).

Physically, toddlers begin to lose some of the baby fat they had as infants. They also develop more teeth, which helps them feed themselves. A major physical milestone of toddlers is taking their first steps. Once toddlers learn how to walk, they are constantly on the go and exploring everything.

A toddler's language skills are a sign of intellectual growth and development. A child's first words are typically simple ones such as *dada* or *mama*. Once children begin to speak, their language skills grow quickly. By the end of the toddler years, children can often say several hundred words.

Toddlers become more independent, and they often focus on doing what they want to do. If parents, guardians, or other caregivers prevent them from doing what they want, toddlers often react with frustration and anger. This is called a **temper tantrum**, and it includes yelling, crying, hitting, kicking, or even biting. These reactions are normal and are simply the way toddlers test limits. Temper tantrums usually occur less frequently as children learn those limits.

Learning During the Toddler Years

- Walking
- Talking
- Being more independent

Top to bottom: Bplanet/Shutterstock.com; Dusan Petkovic/Shutterstock.com; Monkey Business Images/Shutterstock.com

Figure 17.10 Learning to walk, talk, and become more independent are milestones that humans typically experience during development in the toddler years. *What is the term for negative behavior that tests the limits of a toddler's independence?*

The Preschool Years

Preschoolers are children between three and five years of age. During this stage of development, children are usually very active. They show rapid development of two kinds of motor skills (**Figure 17.11**).

Because of preschoolers' improved motor skills, they can interact with more objects and engage in more activities than toddlers. Brain development enables preschoolers to observe more and develop more ideas about their world. Language skills also continue to improve at a rapid rate among preschoolers.

In the preschool years, children engage in more social activities than ever before. This enables preschoolers to form relationships with new adults and friends. Preschoolers seek to please others, especially parents, caregivers, family members, familiar adults, and friends. Children this age are forming their first friendships. Preschoolers also begin to develop empathy. *Empathy* is a sense of how another person may be feeling. This is an emotional milestone because it prepares children to form healthy, close relationships.

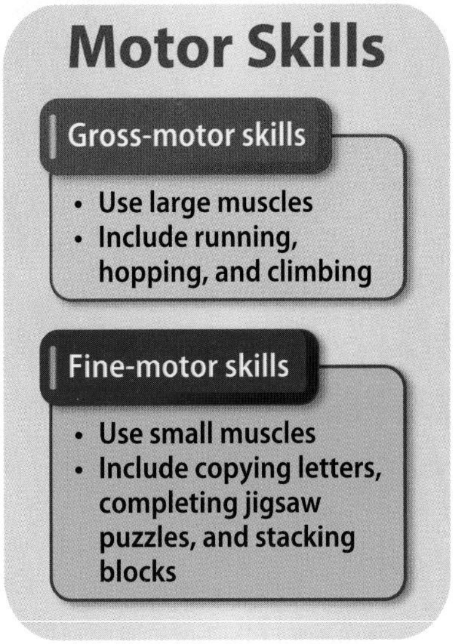

Motor Skills

Gross-motor skills
- Use large muscles
- Include running, hopping, and climbing

Fine-motor skills
- Use small muscles
- Include copying letters, completing jigsaw puzzles, and stacking blocks

Figure 17.11
Children develop many gross- and fine-motor skills during the preschool years. *What are these large muscle movement skills called?*

The Middle Childhood Years

Middle childhood, or the school-age years, refers to the period of time when children are between five and 12 years of age. This stage includes another major milestone—children begin going to school. During these years, important physical, intellectual, emotional, and social growth and development take place.

Physical Development

Children tend to grow at a slow and steady pace during the school-age years. By the end of this period, though, growth may alternate between periods of quick development and slow change. This is why the height and weight of children who are the same age can be very different.

Children who eat too many calories and are not active enough physically can experience overweight. Children who experience overweight or obesity often have a difficult time losing weight as they mature. Establishing healthful habits of eating and physical activity can help children be healthy throughout their lives.

Being physically active also helps children improve their motor skills. It increases their ease of movement as well. Many school-age children enjoy playing organized sports, such as baseball or soccer. Children who are active develop muscle strength and coordination faster than children who are less active.

Intellectual Development

Children encounter many new learning opportunities in the school years. Schoolwork increases their language and problem-solving skills. Advances in brain development enable school-age children to become logical thinkers who learn from their previous experiences. Children apply knowledge they have gained in the past to solve current problems.

During the school-age years, children think about their world in a concrete way. This means that they think about the present and generally do not think about the future. School-age children often do not link today's actions to

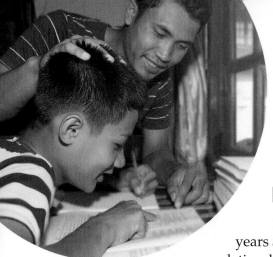

i am way/Shutterstock.com

Figure 17.12
Since school-age children have difficulty planning in a concrete way, parents and guardians often help their children plan for future needs and consequences.

future effects. They have not yet developed the skill of planning because they cannot yet think abstractly (**Figure 17.12**).

In addition, school-age children generally think about issues as black or white, right or wrong, and good or bad. They seek answers that are simple and straightforward, and do not yet see the complexity of problems very easily.

Emotional and Social Development

School-age children have an expanding social network. These years are characterized by the development of friendships and other relationships outside the family. Children make friends and learn how to be a good friend.

During the school-age years, children also develop their *self-esteem*. This is a person's sense of worth, purpose, security, and confidence. Healthy self-esteem develops when children have supportive family and friends. It also develops from having accomplishments. When children successfully deal with mistakes and accomplish projects at school, they learn to feel confident about their abilities. Handling arguments with friends and adapting to changes at home can also build self-esteem.

Lesson 17.2 Review

1. Important events in the development of a human life, such as learning how to walk, are called _____.

2. What are the four types of human development?

3. What is the difference between gross-motor skills and fine-motor skills?

4. During what stage do children begin going to school?
   A. Middle childhood.
   B. Toddler years.
   C. Infancy.
   D. Early childhood.

5. **Critical thinking.** What developments occur for children during middle childhood? Explain physical, intellectual, social, and emotional developments.

Hands-On Activity

Talk with your parents, guardians, or other trusted adults about your childhood, from infancy through your middle childhood years. Ask about your milestones as well as all aspects of your development (physical, intellectual, emotional, and social). Combine the information from this conversation with your memories to create a timeline of your childhood so far. Use images and pictures if you can. Are there times that are harder for you to remember? What about for the adults in your life? How do your memories compare to theirs?

Adolescence and Puberty

Learning Outcomes

After studying this lesson, you will be able to

- **describe** the physical changes that occur in males during puberty.
- **explain** the physical changes that occur in females during puberty.
- **summarize** the intellectual, emotional, and social growth and development that occurs during adolescence.
- **identify** common health and wellness issues that affect adolescents.

Key Terms 📲

adolescence period of development between 12 and 19 years of age

puberty stage of life when the body reaches sexual maturity

primary sexual characteristics changes to the sex organs during puberty

secondary sexual characteristics features that appear during puberty, but do not directly affect the sex organs

testosterone hormone that triggers growth and development of the male sex organs

estrogen hormone that triggers growth and development of the female sex organs

Graphic Organizer

Adolescent Development

On a separate sheet of paper, create a graphic organizer like the one shown. As you read this lesson, take notes on each type of development that humans experience during adolescence. List as many details as you need to fill out the organizer. An example is provided for you.

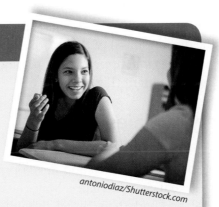

antoniodiaz/Shutterstock.com

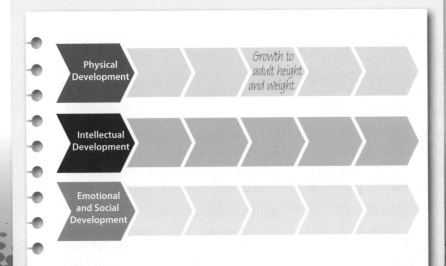

Physical Development — Growth to adult height and weight

Intellectual Development

Emotional and Social Development

A child's body and mind transform during adolescence. No longer children, but not yet adults, adolescents undergo physical changes that prepare their minds and bodies for adulthood. On their way to adulthood, adolescents also experience many intellectual, emotional, and social changes. These changes begin with puberty, when the reproductive system starts to mature.

Xavier looks forward to becoming a teen. He hopes that he will get taller and grow a beard. He is excited to go to high school, get a job, and learn how to drive. You will learn about these changes and other aspects of adolescence in this lesson.

Physical Development and Puberty

Physical changes are the trademark of **adolescence**, or the period of development between 12 and 19 years of age. During this time, males and females complete most of their physical growth. They achieve their adult height and weight. Their sexual organs also mature, which means they become capable of sexual reproduction. **Puberty** is the period of time during which all of these physical changes are taking place. Everyone goes through puberty, so it helps to know what changes to expect during this time.

Sex hormones drive the physical and emotional changes of puberty. Puberty is triggered when brain hormones affect the testes in males and the ovaries in females. The testes and ovaries then release hormones that affect the development of primary and secondary sexual characteristics. **Primary sexual characteristics** refer to the development of the sex organs. **Secondary sexual characteristics** are other features that appear during puberty, such as body hair, a deep voice, or breast development (**Figure 17.13**).

Puberty in Males

Puberty begins in males around 10 to 14 years of age. The hormone **testosterone** triggers growth and development of the male sex organs and male secondary sexual characteristics. Male secondary sexual characteristics include pubic, facial, and body hair; broad shoulders; and increased muscle mass. A male's voice deepens as the larynx grows and may crack as the body adjusts.

Figure 17.13
Both males and females will experience physical growth and sexual maturation during puberty. *During which stage of the life span does puberty begin?*

Primary and Secondary Sexual Characteristics

Primary sexual characteristics

Males: Growth of the testes and penis; erections start to occur

Females: Growth of the ovaries, vagina, and labia; menstruation begins

Secondary sexual characteristics

Males: Pubic, facial, and body hair; deeper voice; broad shoulders; increased muscle mass; and more oil production on skin

Females: Breast development, pubic and underarm hair, widening of the hips, more body fat in hips and buttocks, and more oil production on skin

Puberty: What to Expect

Males:
Starts between ages 10–14

Females:
Starts between ages 8–14

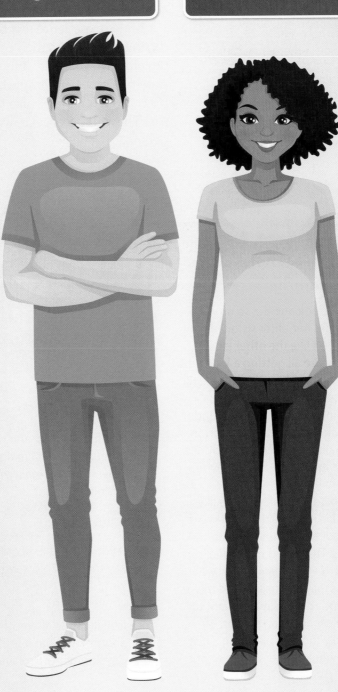

Males:

- Voice deepens, but may crack occasionally
- Shoulders broaden
- Facial, body, pubic hair growth begins
- Muscle mass increases
- Increase in height up to 4 inches per year
- Weight gain
- Acne breakouts may appear on face, shoulders, and back

Females:

- Increased oil production in skin and scalp may lead to acne
- Breasts develop
- Underarm, leg, and pubic hair growth begins
- Menstruation begins
- Increase in height up to 3 inches per year
- Weight gain, and additional fat concentrated in hips, thighs, and buttocks
- Hips widen

Volhah/Shutterstock.com

Caring for the Male Reproductive System

Problems	Care
Hernia	Get medical care.
Sexually transmitted infections (STIs)	Practice abstinence and get medical care.
Testicular cancer	Check the testes for any swelling or lumps.
Testicular injury	Wear protective equipment.
Testicular torsion	Seek emergency care.

Figure 17.14 Listed are possible conditions of the male reproductive system and care procedures. In addition to these care procedures, males should practice good reproductive hygiene. They should keep the organs of the reproductive system clean and protected.

During puberty, males also grow taller and gain weight quickly. Their growth rate may even double, and males can grow 4 inches in one year. By the time puberty ends, a male may have grown 14 inches and gained 40 pounds.

Another change that happens during puberty is increased oil production on the skin and scalp. This extra oil can lead to acne on the face, shoulders, back, and chest. Sometimes, males experience swelling in their breasts. This development is normal and usually goes away as adolescence continues.

Males experience erections and sexual desires during puberty. As their reproductive systems develop, they should start paying attention to possible issues and important care procedures (**Figure 17.14**). Males also become curious about sex. They may feel sexually attracted to another person.

CASE STUDY

Akiko Feels Left Behind

"Why does everyone look and act so much older than me?" Akiko asks her older sister. Akiko is in eighth grade and feels like the other kids, especially the other girls, are all getting a lot taller and more mature than she is. Akiko thinks she still looks like a little kid. There are girls in her class who have started wearing bras and shaving under their arms. Some of her friends have even gotten their periods already. Akiko feels like her body looks the same as it has for years, except maybe she is a little taller.

Akiko is not ready to be an adult yet. She likes the freedom of being a kid, but she does not want to be left behind. Some of her friends have started to ask boys out on dates. There is someone Akiko thinks she likes, but she does not really know what that means. Akiko thinks maybe she just likes this person because her friends do. She might want to have a boyfriend, but she is also kind of grossed out by the idea, especially the idea of kissing a boy. Akiko is pretty sure she would rather just hang out with her friends watching videos, creating new and

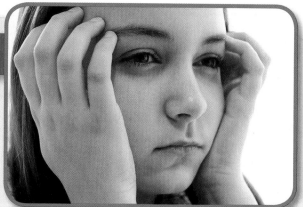

Monkey Business Images/Shutterstock.com

amazing food dishes, and playing outside. Akiko is so confused about life right now that she does not know what she really wants. She thinks being 13 years old is tough!

Thinking Critically

1. If you were Akiko's older sister, what would you say to Akiko? How would you say it? When would be the best time and place to have this conversation?

2. Is Akiko's social-emotional development abnormal? What about her physical development? Explain.

Puberty in Females

Females begin puberty earlier than males. The first sign of puberty in females is breast development, which occurs around 8 to 14 years of age. In females, the hormone **estrogen** triggers growth and development of the female sex organs. Estrogen also causes development of female secondary sexual characteristics. These include breast development and growth of pubic, underarm, and leg hair. During puberty, a girl's hips also widen, and fat is added to the hips and buttocks.

During puberty, a female's body grows quickly as well. Girls can grow up to 3 inches per year. By the end of puberty, a female may have grown 10 inches and gained 25 pounds.

Females also begin menstruating during puberty. The *menarche*, or first menstrual period, may be upsetting to a young female. Family members or a doctor can help an adolescent female understand what menstruation means and how to prepare for this monthly cycle. As their reproductive systems develop, females should start paying attention to possible issues and important care procedures (**Figure 17.15**).

Like males, females experience increased oil secretion on the skin and scalp. They may also develop acne. With these physical changes, females also grow curious about sex and may experience sexual attraction.

Intellectual Development

During adolescence, the brain is still developing. Young adolescents think in concrete terms, as they did in childhood. They often view the world in black-and-white terms and may fail to see the complexity of many situations. Adolescents may be unable to imagine future consequences that could arise from their actions. As a result, young adolescents may act without thinking and take risks that can harm their health, such as experimenting with alcohol or drugs.

As adolescents mature, they develop the ability to think more abstractly and to see more than two sides of issues. This ability helps them handle more

Caring for the Female Reproductive System	
Problems	**Care**
Breast cancer	Check the breasts for any lumps or swelling.
Ovarian cysts	Get medical care.
Premenstrual syndrome (PMS)	Treat cramps with medication, if necessary.
Sexually transmitted infections (STIs)	Practice abstinence and get medical care.
Toxic shock syndrome	Change tampons every four hours.
Yeast infection	Keep the reproductive area clean, change sanitary napkins every four hours, and get medical care.

Figure 17.15
Listed are possible conditions of the female reproductive system and care procedures. *How can a female better understand and prepare for a monthly period?*

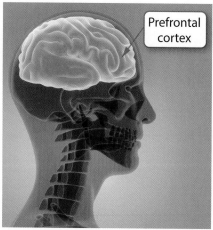

Magic mine/Shutterstock.com

Figure 17.16 Because the prefrontal cortex is still developing during adolescence, young people may have trouble practicing good judgment.

challenging situations. They can think through issues that are more complex. They can understand different points of view.

Over time, adolescents gain the ability to think about more abstract concepts. Even older adolescents, however, may occasionally fail to predict the consequences of their actions. They may still take risks. They can participate in risky behaviors when they ignore what they have learned intellectually and focus on what they see as emotional and social needs. For example, adolescents sometimes engage in risky behavior in the hopes of winning the acceptance or respect of peers. This is because their brains are still developing. One of the last portions of the brain to fully develop is the prefrontal cortex, which is responsible for rational thinking and decision-making (**Figure 17.16**). The prefrontal cortex usually has not fully developed until age 25.

Emotional and Social Development

Adolescents feel the need to establish their independence, be on their own, and rely on their own judgment. School activities and friends offer plenty of opportunities to gain independence. The chance to make independent decisions and explore life is important for adolescents' emotional growth.

Some adolescents emphasize their independence by distancing themselves from their parents or guardians. They might not be as affectionate as they were in childhood. This change can be upsetting to parents or guardians. Some adolescents say less to their parents or guardians about their day at school than they did when younger. They often do this out of a desire to maintain privacy and to show their independence.

While adolescents seek independence, they also have a strong need to feel that they belong. During adolescence, a person's social world expands beyond the family and even close friends. The social world becomes increasingly important to them. Adolescents' relationships will include new friends, friends of the opposite sex, dating partners, teachers, and coaches. As their social life grows, adolescents get a taste of what adult life is like and learn skills for maintaining social connections.

Adolescents are typically concerned about being accepted by their peers. They may seek their peers' approval and try to fit into a group of peers at school or in the neighborhood. Peers can be a source of support and fun. Unfortunately, adolescents can also be negatively influenced by peers. That influence may cause them to engage in behaviors they might not otherwise choose.

Another important change in adolescence is development of a sense of personal identity. Adolescents ask questions like "Who am I?" and "What am I really like?" They may act, talk, and relate to others in different ways over time. These changes are often an attempt to try out different personalities. Adolescents are looking for the one that feels right, when they feel true to themselves. Over time, adolescents come to have a surer sense of who they are. They can base that sense of identity on the values they hold, the goals they have, and the ways of acting that feel most right to them.

Health and Wellness Issues

Adolescents face health and wellness issues that are not common in childhood. They also face issues not usually seen in adulthood. Some of these issues arise because of newly acquired independence. For instance, having the ability to go to the mall with friends means they now face decisions about how to do so safely.

Handling Peer Pressure

Some health and wellness issues result from new pressures from peers. Adolescents might see someone being bullied. Then, they face the choice between standing up for the person being bullied or being a bystander. To make this choice, they need to call on their sense of what is right. They may

BUILDING Your Skills

Peer Pressure Throughout the Life Span

During childhood and adolescence, peers become a major source of stress. (Remember, the stress from peers can be good!) Peers are people around the same age and they have a big influence on a person's decisions, behaviors, and life, especially through childhood and adolescence, but even throughout adulthood.

Sometimes, peers will explicitly ask or tell another person to do something (external peer pressure). Other times, the pressure is internal, meaning the individual wants to do something that others are doing because they want to fit in. The desire to fit in and belong with others is a natural and powerful feeling. Both types of peer pressure (internal and external) can be positive and persuade people to do great things. Both can also be negative, however, and push people to behave in ways that do not promote physical, social, or mental and emotional health.

Role-Play: Positive and Negative

In small groups, choose a stage of life to focus on: early childhood, middle childhood, adolescence, or adulthood. Then, plan and perform two role play situations for the class, both based on the stage of life you chose. The first role play should involve the person dealing healthfully with positive peer pressure. The second role-play situation should involve the person dealing healthfully with negative peer pressure. Once you have performed your role plays, answer the following questions:

1. What similarities in peer pressure across life stages are present? What differences?

2. What strategies are effective at dealing with peer pressure? Are these the same for both positive and negative peer pressure? Explain.

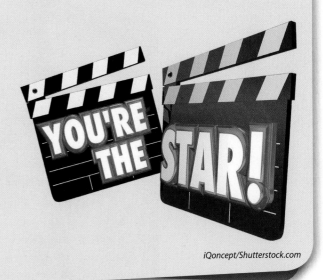

iQoncept/Shutterstock.com

also have to take safety into account. Adolescents not sure of how to handle situations like this can talk to a trusted adult.

Adolescents can also be pressured to join with others in risky behaviors. Adolescents who think about their own identity and values can resist this kind of negative peer pressure. Thinking about the consequences of these risky behaviors can help as well.

Using a decision-making process can help adolescents prepare for resisting peer pressure (**Figure 17.17**). Good decision making starts with identifying the decision. Then you need to brainstorm options. Once you identify possible outcomes, you weigh the costs and benefits of each option. Use your values and goals to help you analyze these costs and benefits. Then choose the option that has the best balance of costs and benefits. Taking this approach can help you resist negative peer pressure.

Teen Pregnancy

One possible consequence of giving in to negative peer pressure is teen pregnancy. Since adolescents have reached sexual maturity, they run the risk of pregnancy if they engage in sexual activity.

Pregnancy can cause serious health conditions for adolescents since their bodies are still developing (**Figure 17.18**). The demands of a growing fetus can interfere with growth during puberty. It is very important that a pregnant adolescent get good prenatal care.

Being a parent poses challenges to adolescents, too. Adolescent parents are at risk of dropping out of school. This can limit their chances to build the

Figure 17.17
Using the decision-making process can help young people, who are learning what they think is right and wrong, stand up for their beliefs and values.

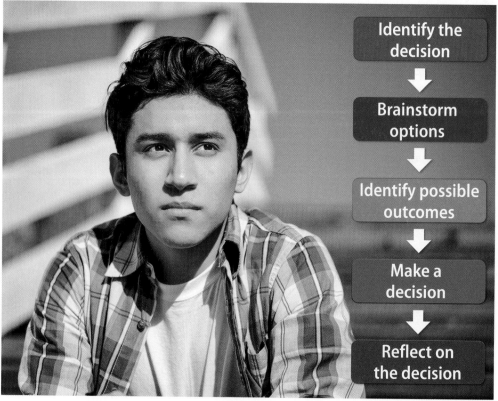

Identify the decision

⬇

Brainstorm options

⬇

Identify possible outcomes

⬇

Make a decision

⬇

Reflect on the decision

mdurson/Shutterstock.com

future they want for themselves. Adolescent parents are at risk of living in poverty as well.

Adolescent parents also face emotional difficulties. Parenting is hard work, full of responsibilities. Adolescents who are still trying to sort out their own lives can feel overwhelmed by meeting the demands of a baby. They can feel depressed and alone. Adolescent parents also face changes to relationships that can cause difficulties. Some experience strained relations with family members. Others find that they no longer see their friends because they have to spend so much time caring for a child or because they are no longer in school.

Some adolescents who become pregnant choose to give their babies up for adoption. They feel unable to meet the demands of parenting. State agencies can help a teen with that choice. States also have *safe haven laws* (also called *safe surrender laws*) that allow people to leave their babies at certain facilities with no questions asked. These laws protect innocent and vulnerable babies from the dangers of abandonment.

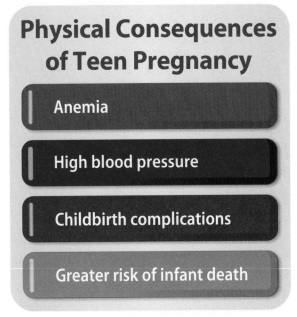

Physical Consequences of Teen Pregnancy

- Anemia
- High blood pressure
- Childbirth complications
- Greater risk of infant death

Figure 17.18 Adolescents, in particular, are at an increased risk of physical complications and illnesses during pregnancy. *What kind of medical care is important for adolescents who become pregnant?*

Lesson 17.3 Review

1. What is the time period in adolescence during which physical growth and sexual development occur?

2. The hormone _____ causes the development of male sex organs and secondary sexual characteristics, such as facial hair and a deep voice.

3. **True or false.** Relationships with friends, coaches, dating partners, and teachers help adolescents feel that they belong.

4. Thinking about their values and identity can help adolescents resist negative

   _____ _____.

5. **Critical thinking.** How can emotional and social development during adolescence cause conflict between the adolescent and the adolescent's parents or guardians? What changes are occurring?

Hands-On Activity

Create a Venn diagram to compare and contrast puberty and adolescence in females and males. Be sure to include all aspects of health and development as you complete the diagram. After it is complete, share your Venn diagram with a classmate and work together to draw conclusions about puberty and adolescence for teens in general.

Adulthood and Aging

Key Terms

young adulthood stage of human development that occurs from 20 to 40 years of age

middle adulthood stage of human development that occurs from 40 to 65 years of age

older adulthood stage of human development that begins at 65 years of age

sandwich generation adults who care for their parents as well as their own children

hospice care type of care given to people who are dying that provides comfort and support to them and their families

Learning Outcomes

After studying this lesson, you will be able to

- **identify** and **describe** the stages of adulthood.
- **describe** how people can adapt to the changes that occur during aging.
- **summarize** types of care people may need as they approach the end of life.
- **explain** the stages of grief and how people can cope with grief and loss.

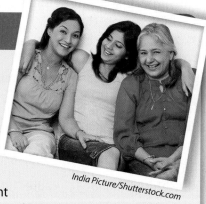

India Picture/Shutterstock.com

Graphic Organizer

The Effects of Aging

As you learned earlier in the chapter, growth and development begins before a baby is even born. Once a baby is born, growth and development occur rapidly throughout childhood and into adolescence when puberty begins. In this lesson, you will learn that development continues into adulthood. As you are reading this lesson, use an organizer like the one shown to take notes about the development and changes that occur during adulthood.

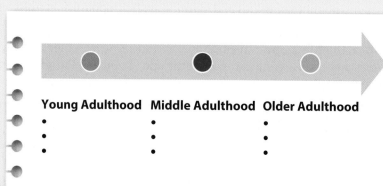

Young Adulthood   **Middle Adulthood**   **Older Adulthood**

How do you know when you have become an adult? Do you become an adult when you reach a certain age—18 or 21, for example? Does a particular event such as getting a driver's license, graduating from high school or college, or getting married make you an adult?

Xavier, from the previous lessons, wonders about adulthood. His older cousins are in their 20s, his parents are in their 40s, and his grandparents are in their 60s. Xavier is curious about what to expect as he grows older.

In this lesson, you will learn about the different stages of adulthood. You will also learn about changes that occur during each of these stages and how these changes affect health. Some health changes that occur in adulthood are unavoidable. You can influence other changes by making decisions that enhance health today and throughout life.

The Mature Adult

Adulthood is defined in many different ways. In the United States, state and federal governments see most people as adults when they become 18 years old. In most states, people are able to vote and marry without a parent's or guardian's permission once they reach that age. When a person turns 18, that individual can also be treated as an adult in a court of law.

Another definition of adulthood is based on physical maturity. Young adults have reached their mature height and weight, possess their greatest strength and endurance, and enjoy their sharpest thinking ability. Adolescents must mature in many other ways, however, to be considered adults. Perhaps most importantly, they must gain intellectual, emotional, and social maturity (Figure 17.19).

Stages of Adulthood

Adults continue to change and develop through various stages of adulthood. **Young adulthood** occurs from 20 to 40 years of age, **middle adulthood** occurs

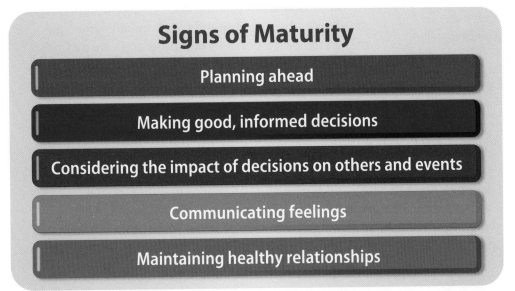

Signs of Maturity

- Planning ahead
- Making good, informed decisions
- Considering the impact of decisions on others and events
- Communicating feelings
- Maintaining healthy relationships

Figure 17.19
Certain character traits, like good communication and decision-making, are signs that a person has reached full maturity and would be considered an adult.

from 40 to 65 years of age, and **older adulthood** is considered 65 years of age and older. Adults in each stage share many experiences, rewards, and challenges.

Young Adulthood

Young adulthood is a period of transition and preparation for adulthood. It can be an exciting stage full of personal growth. Young adults achieve some goals or take steps toward some of their life goals.

People achieve full physical maturity in young adulthood. Adults who are 20 to 40 years of age possess their greatest strength, endurance, and cognitive abilities. Their sensory organs and reflexes have reached peak performance. In addition, the brain completes development in the early years of young adulthood.

In the United States, many young adults become fully responsible for their lives. This can mean having an income and living independently or with others. There is no "typical" young adult in the United States. Young adults may be single, married, or divorced. They may or may not have children. Some live alone or with their parents or guardians, and some live with other young adults.

During young adulthood, many people make decisions about entering a committed relationship or marriage. *Marriage* is a formal, committed relationship with a defined, legal status. Married couples share resources and legal responsibility for any children they have. In the United States, the age of marriage has risen steadily. Today, many adults are not married. Those who do marry often wait until they are older and more mature (**Figure 17.20**).

Divorce can occur during any stage of adulthood. Some 40 to 50 percent of marriages end in divorce. A divorce profoundly changes a person's life. It affects income, living arrangements, and home ownership. Divorce also causes relationships with children, other family members, and friends to change. Divorce has a major effect on a person's emotions and sense of self. Unmarried young adults with long-term relationships may experience breakups that can cause as many changes as a divorce.

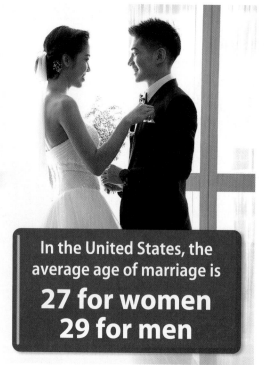

In the United States, the average age of marriage is

27 for women
29 for men

sippakorn/Shutterstock.com

Figure 17.20 Fewer Americans today are getting married, and more people are waiting to do so until they are older, more financially stable, and more mature. *What percent of marriages end in divorce?*

Middle Adulthood

In the United States, adults who are 40 to 65 years of age tend to be fairly healthy and active. Today's adults are not only living longer, but also have more healthy and productive days over their lifetime. After years of experience, middle-aged adults may make some of their greatest achievements. Compared with younger adults, middle-aged adults tend to be more flexible and adapt well to change.

Physical and health changes during middle adulthood are slow, and most middle-aged adults adapt well to their changing bodies. Though strength, coordination, and endurance begin to decline, thinking skills and memory usually remain strong. Adults can adjust to changes in vision and hearing by adapting behavior or using reading glasses or hearing aids.

Middle-aged adults may have adolescent or adult children. As these children grow up, adults adjust to new relationships with their children. Middle-aged adults also often have more work responsibilities.

Some middle-aged adults care for aging parents or family members who need help. This can be difficult, especially for adults who also have children. Adults who care for their parents and their own children are called the **sandwich generation** (Figure 17.21). Many communities have resources to help middle-aged adults in the sandwich generation. These include healthcare professionals; after-school activities and care for children; and counseling to help middle-aged adults balance responsibilities.

Older Adulthood

Advancing age brings rewards and new challenges. Many older adults show confidence, knowledge, and good judgment and maintain cognitive skills into old age. They have experience with life's hardships and are better able to manage emotions, make compromises, and understand viewpoints. These qualities lead many to consider older adults wise.

When older adults retire from work, they find time to pursue new jobs, hobbies, and other interests. These activities often lead to new friendships. Older adults may enjoy the company of grandchildren and adjust to new relationships with their adult children.

Naturally, older adults may also experience declining health and independence, reduced income, and loss of some aging friends and family. After retirement, older adults find ways to maintain a social life, feel productive, and remain active. Some ways retired adults can fulfill these needs include working part-time jobs; volunteering at schools, hospitals, or museums; or exploring new subjects.

Adaptations to Aging

A number of changes can be expected during aging. These changes are not necessarily the result of diseases or disorders. It is normal for many body functions to change as the body grows older (**Figure 17.22**).

By adapting to the changes caused by aging, adults can maintain an active, healthy life. Some older adults use technologies that make up for changing abilities. For example, hearing aids help older adults with hearing loss.

The Sandwich Generation

Top to bottom:
Monkey Business Images/Shutterstock.com;
pixelheadphoto digitalskillet/Shutterstock.com;
Lightfield Studios/Shutterstock.com

Figure 17.21 People in middle adulthood may care for their own children as well as their aging parents. This is known as being in the sandwich generation.

Health Changes During Adulthood

Body System	Possible Health Changes	Body System	Possible Health Changes
Sensory organs 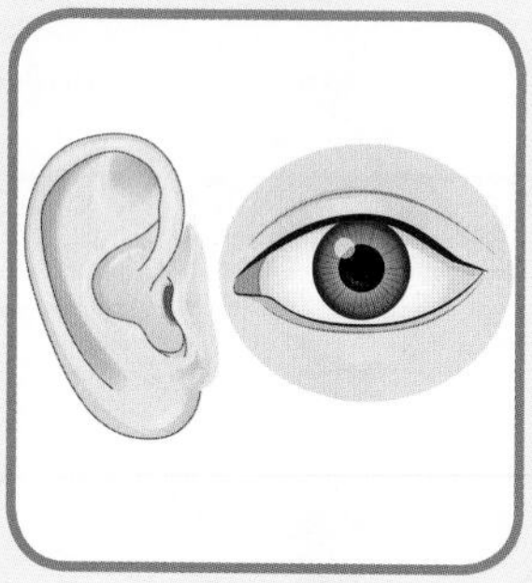 *solar22/Shutterstock.com*	• Wrinkles, age spots, and skin tags develop. • Older adults find it difficult to focus on close objects or read small print. • Hearing loss occurs.	**Respiratory system** 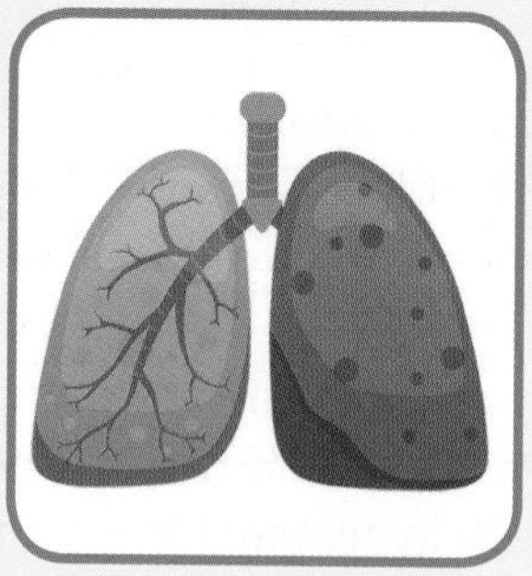 *Gaidamashchuk/Shutterstock.com*	• Chest and rib muscles weaken, leading to shortness of breath. • Risk of lung infection increases.
Digestive system 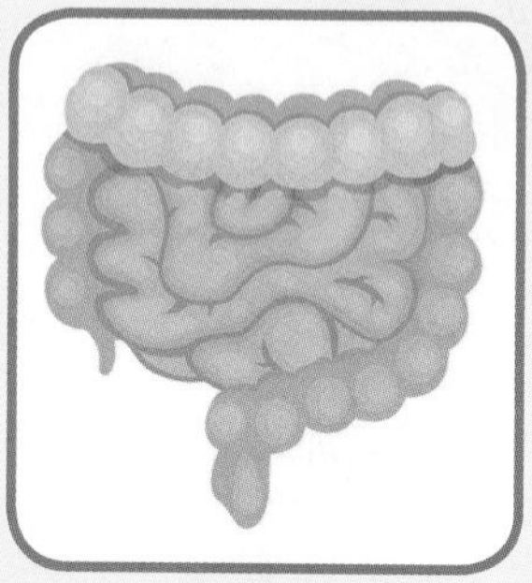 *Gaidamashchuk/Shutterstock.com*	• The mouth becomes dry, and cavities are more common. • Intestinal linings thin, slowing digestion. • Liver function decreases, increasing medication side effects.	**Reproductive system** 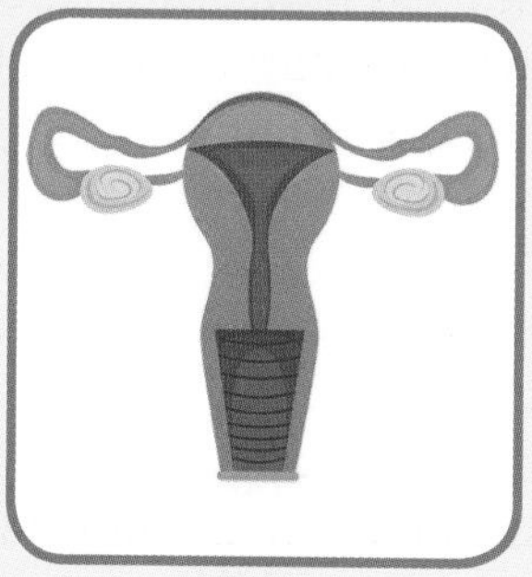 *Gaidamashchuk/Shutterstock.com*	• Women enter *menopause*, the end of the reproductive years. • The prostate can grow larger, causing infection.
Urinary system 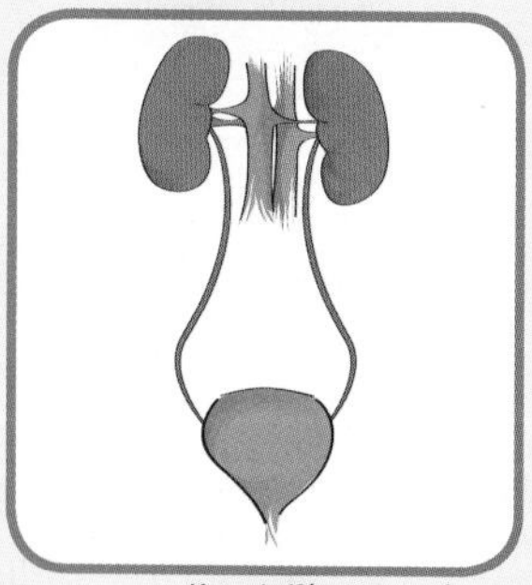 *Kateriz/Shutterstock.com*	• Kidney function decreases, leading to dehydration. • *Incontinence*, or the inability to control urination, sometimes develops. • The risk of urinary tract infections increases.	**Muscles and bones** 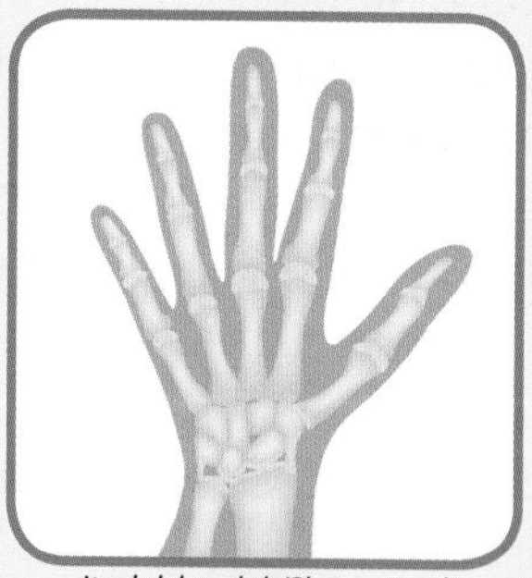 *gritsalak karalak/Shutterstock.com*	• Muscle mass and strength decrease. • Bones lose density, strength, and mass. • Joints become stiff and sometimes painful.
Circulatory system 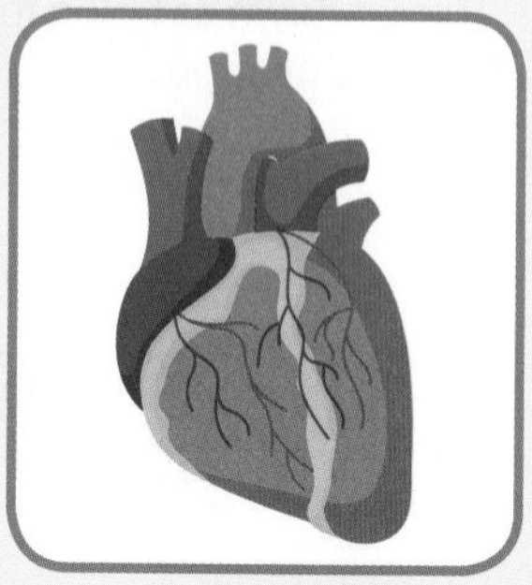 *EgudinKa/Shutterstock.com*	• Blood vessels stiffen and narrow, increasing risk for hypertension. • Risk of heart disease increases.	**Nervous system** 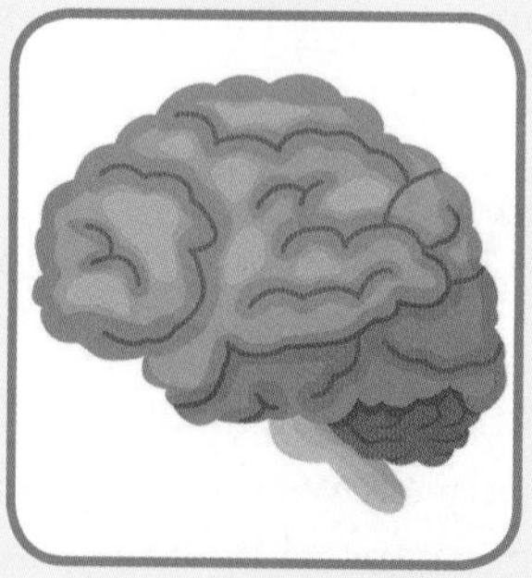 *Gaidamashchuk/Shutterstock.com*	• Memory may lapse. • Reflexes and reaction time decline.

Figure 17.22 Changes occur in each body system during aging. *What is an example of a device that an older adult can use to adapt to reduced mobility, strength, and balance?*

Bifocals, a type of eyeglasses with extra lenses, and large fonts improve reading. Engaging in meaningful activities can help keep the mind sharp.

Some older adults have more difficulty than others with mobility, strength, and balance. These adults may use canes, wheelchairs, and other devices to remain active and mobile. At home, ramps can be built to replace steps to make going up or down a level easier. The home can be modified to reduce the risk of falls.

Adults can continue to be physically active by adapting as they age. Instead of running, older adults can walk, bike, or swim. These activities keep them active while lowering the impact on their joints and bones. If endurance becomes difficult, older adults can do activities more often, but for shorter periods of time.

Many older adults can live independently. Some older adults need small amounts of help. They may be unable to drive and need someone to take them places. Adults with serious health conditions, however, may require care. This can include daily care such as dressing, eating, bathing, and using the bathroom. It can also mean the need for healthcare. Older adults who need a great deal of care often cannot live alone. Luckily, there are housing options to help take care of these older adults (**Figure 17.23**).

The End of Life

The human life cycle ends in death. Death can occur at any time and can be sudden or expected. When it is expected, a person may receive hospice care in the months leading up to death. The goal of **hospice care** is to provide comfort for people who are dying and their families. During hospice care, dying people do not receive treatment for their disease. Instead, patients receive pain relief and emotional support and comfort.

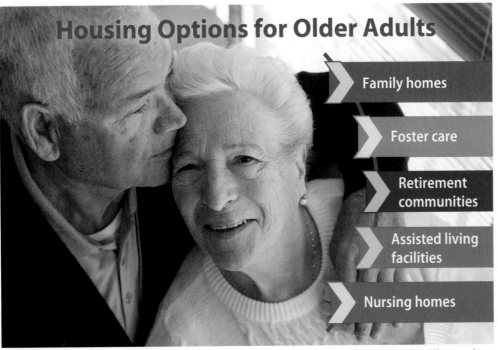

Housing Options for Older Adults

Family homes

Foster care

Retirement communities

Assisted living facilities

Nursing homes

La Vieja Sirena/Shutterstock.com

Figure 17.23
Different settings for older adult housing can provide different types of care. A nursing home, for example, can provide medical care, while assisted living facilities can provide relative independence for older adults.

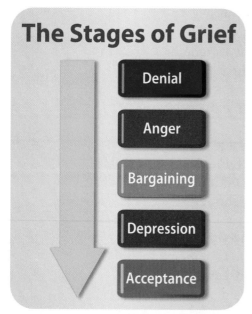

The Stages of Grief

Denial

Anger

Bargaining

Depression

Acceptance

Figure 17.24 When a loved one dies, it is normal to experience grief. Not everyone experiences all the stages of grief, and not in a precise order, but these are the general emotions associated with the grieving process.

The end of the human life cycle is often accompanied by grief. *Grief* is a complex emotional experience that includes a profound sense of loss and sadness. As you learned in Chapter 6, a grieving person has many feelings following the death of a family member, spouse, or friend (**Figure 17.24**).

Grieving is a normal and healthy process. People should be allowed to grieve through whatever means they feel is right. They might need to feel very sad and cry for a long time. They might also need to mark the loss with a ritual, such as a funeral. During the grieving process, people can practice the following healthy behaviors:

- Avoid isolation. Instead, share feelings with trusted people.
- Do not make difficult decisions or major life changes. If major decisions must be made, discuss with close family members.
- Seek help with personal care tasks. Get professional help for coping, if necessary. Not getting necessary help can lead to depression.
- Get good nutrition, physical activity, and adequate sleep.

Lesson 17.4 Review

1. Which of the following is a developmental stage of adulthood?
   A. Older adulthood.
   B. Young adulthood.
   C. Middle adulthood.
   D. All of the above.
2. **True or false.** A typical young adult is married, has children, and owns a home.
3. Adults who care for their parents as well as their own children are called the _____ generation.
4. What is the type of care given to people who are dying that provides comfort and support to them and their families?
5. **Critical thinking.** What are some examples of changes that occur throughout older adulthood? What are some ways that older adults can adapt to these changes to maintain an active, healthy life?

Hands-On Activity

Think about how you want your adulthood to look—consider all stages of adulthood. Draw, write, or create something that displays the picture in your mind. Include what health and behavioral choices you can and will make to promote health and wellness throughout adulthood. What decisions can you make now to help you achieve this vision? What kind of people will you need around you? What activities will you do? What situations do you and will you avoid? What decisions do you anticipate making that will impact your future? Share your drawing, writing, or creation with a classmate and with your family.

Review and Assessment

Summary

Lesson 17.1 The Beginning of Life

- The human reproductive system consists of a group of organs that begins working at puberty, when the body reaches sexual maturity. Male reproductive organs include the testes and penis, seminal vesicles, bulbourethral gland, prostate, and vas deferens. Female reproductive organs include ovaries (which produce ova), fallopian tubes, uterus, and vagina.
- The male reproductive organs produce and transport sperm. The female reproductive organs produce eggs. For pregnancy to occur, the sperm enters the vagina. There, one sperm and one egg form a zygote in a process called *fertilization*.
- Prenatal development refers to the developments of a baby during pregnancy. This consists of the germinal stage, embryonic stage, and fetal stage.

Lesson 17.2 Child Development

- The human life cycle carries a person through the developmental stages. Important events that occur throughout the life cycle are called *milestones*. A person's life span is the actual number of years lived. The estimate of life span is known as *life expectancy*.
- Human development includes physical, intellectual, emotional, and social development. Many factors influence human development. The early childhood years include the infant, toddler, and preschooler stages. Children between five and 12 years of age are in middle childhood.

Lesson 17.3 Adolescence and Puberty

- Young people between 12 and 19 years of age are in *adolescence*. During adolescence, people undergo significant physical changes as they enter puberty. Some of the changes during puberty include growth in height and weight, acne, sexual attraction, and sexual curiosity for both males and females.
- During adolescence, people develop the ability to handle challenging situations and more complex issues. Adolescents want to establish independence, rely on their own judgment, and maintain privacy. Social relationships become increasingly important. This means that peer pressure can become more of an issue.

Lesson 17.4 Adulthood and Aging

- People reach physical maturity in young adulthood (20 to 40 years old). People in this stage have many new privileges and responsibilities.
- In middle adulthood (40 to 65 years old), people remain healthy and active and make some of their greatest achievements.
- Older adulthood (65 years and older) brings joys as well as loss and grief. Older adults adapt to the decline in their bodies' functions, such as mobility and strength.
- The human life cycle ends in death. If a death is not unexpected, a person may receive hospice care to provide comfort. Grief involves a profound sense of loss and sadness.

Check Your Knowledge

Record your answers to each of the following questions on a separate sheet of paper.

1. What are the names of male and female sex cells?
2. A(n) _____ is a doctor who specializes in pregnancy, labor, and delivery.
3. What are the three stages of prenatal development?
4. What is the difference between life span and life expectancy?
5. **True or false.** The early childhood stage begins after infancy and ends after preschool.
6. Which stage of development involves children beginning to go to school?
7. Which of the following does *not* occur in puberty for both males and females?
   A. Growth of pubic hair.   C. Acne.
   B. Broadened shoulders.   D. Sexual attraction and curiosity.
8. **True or false.** During adolescence, people gain the ability to think about abstract concepts, which means they will no longer participate in risky behaviors.
9. Why can pregnancy cause serious health conditions for adolescents?
10. Which stage of adulthood involves reaching full physical maturity?
    A. Young.   C. Older.
    B. Middle.   D. None of the above.
11. Identify three things older adults can do to maintain their health.
12. List the stages of grief.

Use Your Vocabulary ↗

adolescence	middle adulthood	puberty
early childhood	middle childhood	reproductive system
embryo	milestones	sandwich generation
estrogen	obstetrician/gynecologist	secondary sexual
fertilization	(OB/GYN)	characteristics
fetus	older adulthood	temper tantrum
hospice care	ovulation	testosterone
human life cycle	prenatal	young adulthood
life expectancy	development	zygote
life span	primary sexual	
menstruation	characteristics	

13. In teams, create categories for the terms above and classify as many of the terms as possible. Then, share your ideas with the remainder of the class.
14. Classify the list of terms above into the following two categories: sexual reproduction and human development. Find a classmate to partner with and then together compare how you classified the terms. How were your lists similar? How were they different? Discuss your lists with the class.

Think Critically

15. **Identify.** Compare the structures in male and female reproductive systems and describe how each performs similar functions.

16. **Draw conclusions.** Can anyone with a uterus get pregnant the first time having sexual intercourse? Can anyone with a penis get someone pregnant the first time having sexual intercourse? Explain.

17. **Make inferences.** What stage of life do you believe is the most difficult? Which is the easiest? Explain your reasoning based on the information in this chapter.

18. **Predict.** "With freedom comes responsibility." How does this quote by Eleanor Roosevelt relate to your life right now? How will it relate to your life as you move through adolescence and all stages of adulthood?

DEVELOP Your Skills

19. **Access information.** What are the main questions that most people your age have about puberty, adolescence, reproduction, or the life span? What rumors have you heard that you are not sure are correct? Write your questions and then find correct answers from valid and reliable sources. List the sources you used.

20. **Literacy and communication skills.** Interview a trusted older adult about human development and the human life span. Develop at least five questions about adulthood that interest you and ask them, using proper vocabulary and maturity. During the interview, ask for clarification on any words or explanations you do not understand. Write an essay reflecting on the conversation and the information you heard. Before turning your essay in to your teacher, be sure to have the person you interviewed review it and check your essay for accuracy, proper grammar, and spelling.

21. **Decision-making and goal-setting skills.** What is most important to you? What do you value? What do you believe? Who are you, to your core? Are you able to answer these questions easily? It is all right if you cannot, but these are important questions to think about as a young person. Take some time to think about the answers to these questions and create a mission statement for your life. Post this mission statement somewhere you will see it every day. Let this serve as a reminder of who you are and what you want out of life. How can knowing your values and your self-identity improve your ability to resist negative peer pressure?

22. **Teamwork skills.** Using effective communication skills with a partner, draw a timeline that portrays the life span of a human. Start with prenatal development and continue all the way to the end of life. At various ages on the timeline, mark as many milestones and aspects of development as you can. Write a short explanation of human development portrayed in your timeline.

Chapter 18

Sexually Transmitted Infections and HIV/AIDS

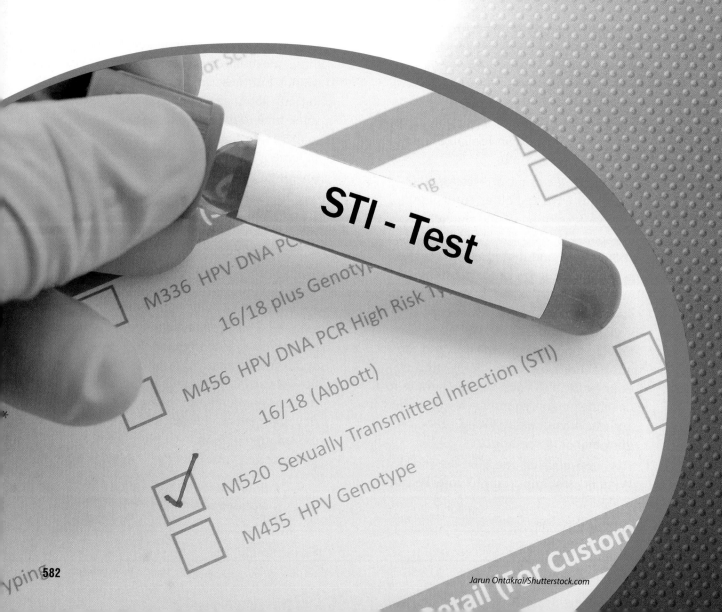

Jarun Ontakrai/Shutterstock.com

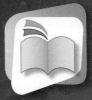

Reading Activity

Before reading, scan the chapter to find italicized words or phrases. Create a list of the italicized terms. On a piece of paper, write definitions for each word or phrase by looking at how it is used within its sentence and paragraph. Then, use the Internet to look up the terms and their meaning. Make any adjustments to your list.

How **Healthy** Are You?

In this chapter, you will be learning about sexually transmitted infections (STIs) and HIV/AIDS. Before you begin reading, take the following quiz to assess your current understanding of STIs and HIV/AIDS as well as prevention and treatment methods.

Health Concepts to Understand	Yes	No
Do you know how sexually transmitted infections (STIs) spread among people?		
Are you aware that many people with STIs do not show any symptoms?		
Do you know how to get testing for STIs?		
Do you understand how different STIs are treated?		
Are you aware that sexual abstinence is the only 100 percent effective method of preventing STIs?		
Do you know the difference between HIV and AIDS?		
Do you know what resources offer testing for HIV?		
Do you understand precautions you can take to help prevent HIV transmission?		
Are you aware of how PrEP and PEP reduce risk for HIV transmission?		

Count your "Yes" and "No" responses. The more "Yes" responses you have, the more you understand about STIS and HIV/AIDS. Now, take a closer look at the questions with which you responded "No." Think about how you can increase your understanding of issues in these areas. Develop your health literacy skills by accessing valid information about each of the concepts you do not understand. Evaluate any health websites you find using the information in Figure 1.16 of this text. If you do not understand the instructions, ask for clarification from your teacher.

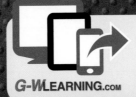

Click on the activity icon or visit www.g-wlearning.com/health to access online vocabulary activities using key terms from the chapter.

Sexually Transmitted Infections (STIs)

Learning Outcomes

After studying this lesson, you will be able to

- **understand** how people contract sexually transmitted infections (STIs).
- **describe** the most commonly reported STIs.
- **identify** potential STI resources.
- **explain** treatment methods for STIs.

Graphic Organizer

STI Cause and Effect

As you listen to your teacher present this lesson, use a graphic organizer similar to the one shown to visually organize your notes about the most common STIs. Identify whether the cause of the STI is a bacterium, virus, or protozoa. Then, identify the effects and possible treatments for each STI. An example is provided for you.

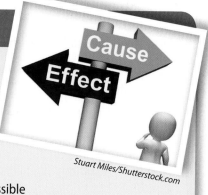

Stuart Miles/Shutterstock.com

STI	Cause	Health Effects	Treatment
Chlamydia	Bacteria	Silent disease with few or no symptoms; progresses quietly to severe bacterial infection; can cause infertility	Antibiotics prescribed by doctor

Communicable diseases are diseases that spread among living things and objects. These diseases are caused by pathogens. You learned about several types of communicable diseases in Chapter 12. In this chapter, you will learn about a type of communicable disease called a *sexually transmitted infection (STI)*. **Sexually transmitted infections (STIs)** spread from one person to another during sexual activity. According to the World Health Organization (WHO), more than one million STIs are contracted each day around the world (**Figure 18.1**).

How People Contract STIs

Just as with other communicable diseases, bacteria, viruses, and protozoa cause STIs. These pathogens live in and on the surfaces of the reproductive organs. Depending on the type of STI, they may also reside in the mouth, rectum, blood, and other bodily fluids.

STIs spread when people engage in *sexual activity*, or actions that involve contact with a person's reproductive organs. This can include sexual touching and *sexual intercourse*, which is any sexual activity that involves the insertion of a body part or object into another body part. STIs can affect people of all sexes, ages, races, nationalities, and ethnic origins. Sometimes, STIs are called *sexually transmitted diseases (STDs)*.

Engaging in sexual activity one time with just one sexual partner who has an STI is all it takes to contract an STI. People with more sexual partners have greater chances of getting an STI. Although it is possible for a person with certain *oral* (appearing on the mouth) STIs to transmit the infection by kissing, other STIs are not transmitted this way. Casual contact, such as using the same toilet seat, does not transmit STIs.

Common STIs

The most commonly reported STIs include chlamydia, gonorrhea, syphilis, trichomoniasis, genital herpes, and human papillomavirus (HPV). As you read the following sections, you will learn about the signs, symptoms, and treatments for each of these STIs.

Chlamydia

Chlamydia, a common STI caused by bacteria, is a "silent" disease because it has few or no symptoms (**Figure 18.2**). If symptoms do occur,

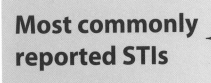

Most commonly reported STIs

- Chlamydia
- Gonorrhea
- Syphilis
- Trichomoniasis
- Genital herpes
- Human papillomavirus (HPV)

Figure 18.1
The most commonly reported STIs are chlamydia, gonorrhea, syphilis, trichomoniasis, genital herpes, and human papillomavirus (HPV). Of these, the most common is HPV.

Due to its lack of symptoms, the Centers for Disease Control and Prevention (CDC) reports that more than

ONE MILLION

cases of chlamydia go undiagnosed each year.

tulpahn/Shutterstock.com

they are often mild, such as nausea or a burning sensation during urination. Chlamydia poses a serious threat to female reproductive health. The "silent" nature of the disease allows it to quietly progress to a severe bacterial infection of the female reproductive organs. This condition, called *pelvic inflammatory disease (PID)*, can cause *infertility*, or the inability to have children. Chlamydia can be treated and cured with prescription antibiotics.

Gonorrhea

Gonorrhea is a bacterial infection that primarily affects the genitals, rectum, and throat. According to the CDC, gonorrhea is a very common STI, especially among people between 15 and 24 years of age. Like chlamydia, gonorrhea causes few or no symptoms in many people. Symptoms, however, do develop in some cases of gonorrhea (**Figure 18.3**). Doctors often prescribe two kinds of antibiotics to treat gonorrhea.

Figure 18.3
While most cases of gonorrhea present few or no symptoms, the symptoms that do develop vary between males and females.

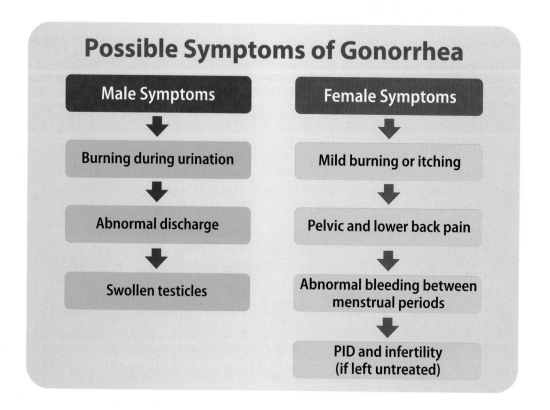

Possible Symptoms of Gonorrhea

Male Symptoms	Female Symptoms
Burning during urination	Mild burning or itching
Abnormal discharge	Pelvic and lower back pain
Swollen testicles	Abnormal bleeding between menstrual periods
	PID and infertility (if left untreated)

Syphilis

Syphilis is a bacterial infection that can cause extremely serious health conditions and disability. This STI progresses through several stages, which include the following:

- **Primary syphilis.** During this first stage, sores develop at the site of the infection. Direct contact with a syphilis sore during sexual activity is what spreads syphilis. The sores are not painful, do not itch, and heal after a few weeks.
- **Secondary syphilis.** The secondary stage of syphilis develops days, weeks, or even months after the primary stage. In the secondary stage, a red or copper-color rash appears, mainly on the palms of the hands and soles of the feet, but sometimes elsewhere. The rash heals, but the person still has syphilis and enters the next stage (**Figure 18.4**).
- **Latent syphilis.** During the latent syphilis stage, a person still has syphilis, but there are no signs or symptoms of the disease.
- **Late-stage syphilis.** In this final stage of syphilis, an internal infection that does not have obvious external signs is present. It is characterized by damage to the brain in the form of *dementia* (deteriorating mental function), paralysis, and fatal damage to the heart, liver, and blood vessels.

Syphilis is most treatable during the early stages. Antibiotics can most effectively cure syphilis in its primary and secondary stages. Even if late-stage syphilis is cured, the organ damage remains permanent.

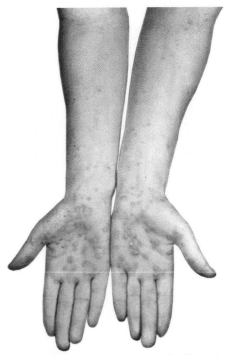

Courtesy of the Centers for Disease Control and Prevention

Figure 18.4 The secondary stage of syphilis includes a red or copper-color rash. This rash will go away on its own, but that does not rid a person of the syphilis infection. *During the secondary stage of syphilis, where does the rash typically develop?*

Trichomoniasis

Trichomoniasis is an infection caused by protozoa. Trichomoniasis often has no symptoms, and it is considered to be the most curable common STI (**Figure 18.5**). Some females with trichomoniasis will experience itching, burning, and pain during urination. Trichomoniasis is easily cured with prescription medications.

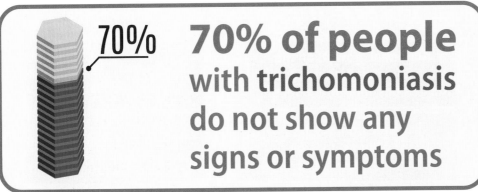

70%

70% of people with trichomoniasis do not show any signs or symptoms

Figure 18.5
When an STI shows no symptoms, infection can go undiagnosed and untreated. This means that people are more likely to infect their sexual partners.

bbgreg/Shutterstock.com

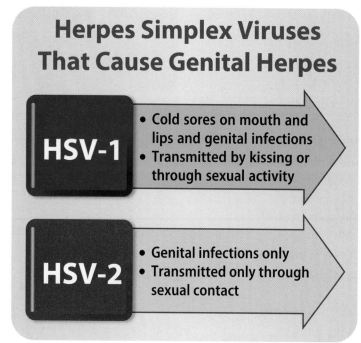

Herpes Simplex Viruses That Cause Genital Herpes

HSV-1
- Cold sores on mouth and lips and genital infections
- Transmitted by kissing or through sexual activity

HSV-2
- Genital infections only
- Transmitted only through sexual contact

Figure 18.6 The two kinds of herpes simplex virus (HSV) are caused by different types of direct contact and cause different infections. *Which type of HSV causes genital infections only?*

Because males often have no symptoms, their infection may go undiagnosed and untreated, making it easy to reinfect their partners. Therefore, both partners must be treated to control reinfection.

Genital Herpes

Two kinds of herpes simplex virus (HSV) cause infections: *HSV type 1* and *HSV type 2* (**Figure 18.6**). **Genital herpes** is very common in the United States among people between 14 and 49 years of age.

A person with genital herpes usually has mild or no symptoms. Blisters arise at the site of infection, burst, and heal after a few weeks. Typically, these blisters return, but in a milder form, sometimes with swollen lymph nodes and fever. This recurrence of genital herpes is called an *outbreak*. No cure exists for herpes, but medication can control the frequency and severity of outbreaks.

Human Papillomavirus

Human papillomavirus (HPV) is the most commonly contracted STI. HPV infects cells in skin and membranes, causing them to grow abnormally. At least 40 kinds of HPV can cause genital infections. Some types can cause cancer.

Almost all sexually active people carry HPV at one time or another. Luckily, most HPV infections do not cause health conditions because the body fights and eliminates the viruses. Some types of HPV, however, cause genital warts, and other types can cause cervical cancer (**Figure 18.7**).

If a person develops visible genital warts from an HPV infection, a doctor may prescribe skin treatments, prescription medication, or surgical removal.

Figure 18.7
The body easily fights and eliminates most types of HPV. Some types of HPV, however, can cause genital warts or cervical cancer.

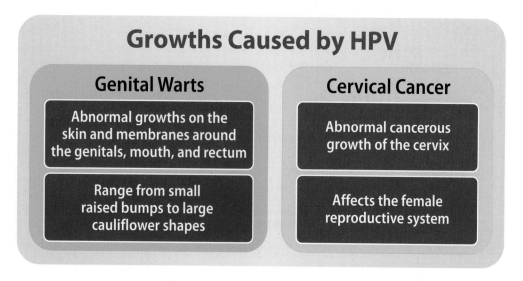

Growths Caused by HPV

Genital Warts
- Abnormal growths on the skin and membranes around the genitals, mouth, and rectum
- Range from small raised bumps to large cauliflower shapes

Cervical Cancer
- Abnormal cancerous growth of the cervix
- Affects the female reproductive system

Treatments for cancer caused by HPV vary depending on the severity and location of the cancer.

A vaccine exists to reduce the risk for HPV infection. The vaccine is recommended for females and males from 11 to 12 years of age. The vaccine is given in three shots over a six-month period of time. If people do not get all of the vaccine at this age, they can still receive the vaccination between 13 and 26 years of age.

Preventing STIs

STIs have many unpleasant symptoms (**Figure 18.8**). Although treatments exist for these conditions, it is easier to prevent STIs than it is to treat them. Two of the most effective methods for preventing STIs include sexual abstinence and the use of condoms.

Practicing Abstinence

Because people contract STIs through sexual activity, the most effective way to prevent STIs is to practice sexual abstinence. Sexual **abstinence** is the

CASE STUDY

Aiden's "Perfect" Relationship

Bryan has always looked up to his older brother Aiden. Aiden taught him to throw a baseball, lift weights, and play video games. He seemed invincible—until recently. This image shattered when Aiden was diagnosed with an STI, and his relationship began to crumble.

Bryan adored Aiden's girlfriend, Ellie. They seemed perfect for each other. Together, they all played soccer and enjoyed working out. Ellie and Aiden often helped Bryan with his homework. Then, one day, Ellie stopped coming over, and Aiden seemed distant and angry. After one week, Aiden confessed to Bryan what was happening. Aiden was experiencing swollen testicles and burning when he urinated. Hoping for answers, Aiden had turned to Ellie, but she was argumentative and defensive.

Finally, Aiden told his mother. Aiden began to question why he started having sex as a teen and whether it was really worth it. After seeing the doctor, Aiden was diagnosed and treated for gonorrhea. After going through this experience, Aiden and Bryan have decided it is better to just wait to have sex.

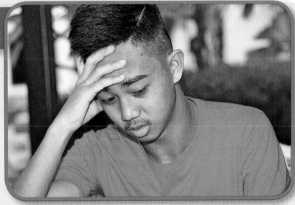

cheapbooks/Shutterstock.com

Thinking Critically

1. Do you think Aiden considered the consequences of sex prior to making the decision to have sex? Why or why not?

2. What were the physical, social, and emotional consequences of Aiden deciding to have sex?

3. Do you think Aiden will succeed at staying sexually abstinent in future relationships? Defend your answer.

4. What advice would you give Aiden about future sexual relationships?

While it is possible that an STI will not show any noticeable symptoms, most STIs show some symptoms. *Which STI is characterized by hair and weight loss in later stages?*

Sexually Transmitted Infections

Name	Symptoms
Chlamydia	• Vaginal or penile discharge, painful urination, fever • If left untreated, may damage reproductive organs and cause infertility
Gonorrhea	• Vaginal or penile discharge, painful or frequent urination, fever, abdominal pain • If left untreated, may damage reproductive organs and cause infertility
Syphilis	• Early stage: small, painless sore on affected area • Later stages: body rash, fever, hair and weight loss, headache, sore muscles • If left untreated, may cause permanent internal damage and death
Trichomoniasis	• For males: itching and burning in the urethra, discharge from the penis • For females: yellow-green vaginal discharge with a foul odor, burning, itching, and pain during urination and sexual intercourse
Genital herpes	• Blisters or sores around the affected area with pain and itching
HPV	• Warts on genitals, painful urination • Cervical and other types of cancer

commitment to refrain from sexual activity. Abstinence is the only 100 percent effective method for preventing STIs and has many other benefits.

There are certain obstacles, such as peer pressure, that may discourage people from practicing abstinence. Friends or partners may try to persuade a person to engage in sexual activity. The use of alcohol and drugs can impair judgment and lower *inhibition* (feelings of restraint), increasing risk for early or unwanted sexual activity. By avoiding risky situations that may include drugs and alcohol, a person can make responsible decisions involving the choice to maintain abstinence.

Committing to abstinence may require a person to use refusal skills. As you learned in Chapter 9, refusal skills can help someone stand up to peer pressure. Planning and even practicing refusal skills for refusing sex, drugs, and alcohol can help people become familiar with words and actions they can use if risky situations occur (**Figure 18.9**).

Using Condoms

A correctly used condom can also reduce the chances of contracting STIs. A **condom** is a device that provides a barrier to pathogens that cause STIs. Condoms may be external or internal. An *external condom* fits over an erect penis. An *internal condom* fits inside the vagina or rectum. External and internal condoms should *not* be used together.

Planning and Practicing Refusal Skills

Practice

- Before you are presented with a risky situation, consider the words you might use.
- What if you are invited to an unsupervised party where alcohol or drugs may be present?
- What if your dating partner is pressuring you to have sex?

Refuse

- Verbally refuse the risky behavior. Be assertive and honest. Keep your response short, clear, and simple.
- If verbally refusing is not enough, walk away from the situation.

Seek Advice

- Remember that you do not need to face this stress alone.
- Find guidance for handling specific situations from a parent, teacher, counselor, or other trusted adult.

Figure 18.9
You can decrease your chances of being pressured or convinced to participate in risky behaviors by preparing your refusal skills in advance.

Most condoms are made of latex, which reduces the risk of STI transmission. Some nonlatex condoms, such as those made of polyurethane or polyisoprene, also help prevent STI transmission. Condoms made of natural materials (for example, *lambskin condoms*) do not help prevent STIs. This is because they contain tiny holes through which pathogens can pass.

To be effective, a condom must be applied correctly, must fit well, must be used for each sex act from beginning to end, and must be removed correctly. A condom can be used only once, and a new one must be used each time a person has sex. Any condom that has expired, has holes or tears, or has dried out must be thrown away because it will not work. In fact, a person should only use unexpired condoms from a reliable source, such as a clinic nurse. Condoms may become damaged if stored in places that become very cold or hot, such as in a car, or where they could be crushed, such as in a wallet.

Treatment of STIs

Many STIs are easily treated, especially in their early stages. For example, bacterial STIs are treatable, even curable, with antibiotics prescribed by a doctor. Being cured, however, does not mean that people cannot contract those STIs again. Even after receiving treatment, exposure to an STI will result in another infection.

Viral infections cannot be treated with antibiotics, but they can be controlled with a number of antiviral medications. Viral infections are not curable, however. Antiviral medications simply control the virus, sometimes

Testing and Treatment

Young people often do not know where to go to ask questions about their sexual health, not to mention seeking testing or treatment for an STI. Some young people feel comfortable asking their parents or guardians questions. Others would rather talk to another trusted adult.

Fortunately, many community resources are available to help young people trying to take care of their sexual health. Public health departments, private and nonprofit organizations, doctors' offices, and even some schools offer resources to help educate young people about sexual health and STIs. Some of these organizations may also offer testing and treatment. Minors (people under the age of 18) can even access many of these resources on their own.

Learning about these community resources can help you remember them if you ever do have questions about your sexual health or need to get testing or treatment for an STI.

Access Community Resources

Do you know what resources are available to educate young people and provide STI testing and treatment in your community? In this activity, you will identify these resources and keep a list for your future reference.

To identify community resources, do research using valid and reliable sources. You can also talk with a parent, guardian, trusted adult, or school nurse. The community resources you identify should support sexual health, answer sexual health questions, educate people about ways to prevent STIs, and provide treatment options.

Create a flyer, brochure, public service announcement, or advertisement to highlight resources in your community. Provide the following information on your product: name of the resource, contact information, and services provided. Include information on three or more options within your community.

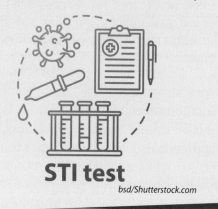

STI test

bsd/Shutterstock.com

greatly reducing the severity and frequency of symptoms. **Figure 18.10** shows treatments for STIs.

STI Resources

Community resources are available to help people who suspect they might have an STI. Doctors can provide tests to determine whether someone has an STI, and treatment if necessary. Public health departments often provide diagnosis, treatment, and prevention programs. Private and nonprofit organizations may also offer assistance or online testing. Some schools may even provide sexual health and wellness programs.

Those who need additional emotional support may find counseling services and support groups in their communities. People may also find support through their friends and family. People can learn more about resources available to them by searching the Internet or by asking a doctor or nurse. Getting help when necessary is a good way to promote overall health and well-being.

Treatment for STIs

Chlamydia	Prescribed antibiotics
Gonorrhea	Prescribed antibiotics
Syphilis	Prescribed antibiotics or penicillin injection
Trichomoniasis	Prescribed antibiotics
Genital herpes	No cure, but prescribed medication can control breakouts and symptoms
HPV	No cure, but prescribed medication can ease symptoms

Figure 18.10
While bacterial infections are treatable and usually curable with antibiotics, viral infections such as genital herpes and HPV cannot be cured. Treatment options for viral infections include easing symptoms and controlling breakouts.

Lesson 18.1 Review

1. _____ are communicable diseases spread from one person to another during sexual activity.
2. **True or false.** Genital herpes is a bacterial infection that can cause pelvic inflammatory disease (PID) and lead to infertility.
3. What causes the spread of syphilis?
4. Name two ways to help prevent STIs.
5. **Critical thinking.** Are all STIs curable? Explain your response.

Hands-On Activity

Interview an important, trusted adult in your life about that person's knowledge of sexually transmitted infections. Be sure to prepare quality, in-depth questions in advance. Compare the person's answers to the information provided in the text. Did your trusted adult provide accurate information? Would you consider this person a good resource for sexual health information? How did you feel talking with this person about STIs? Why did you feel that way? What other questions do you have now about STIs?

HIV/AIDS

Learning Outcomes

After studying this lesson, you will be able to

- **distinguish between** HIV and AIDS.
- **understand** the transmission of HIV.
- **describe** the signs and symptoms of HIV/AIDS.
- **explain** testing procedures for diagnosing HIV.
- **identify** treatment methods for HIV/AIDS.

Graphic Organizer

KWL Chart: Learning About HIV/AIDS

Create a chart like the one shown. Before you read the lesson, outline what you know and what you want to know about understanding HIV/AIDS. After reading the lesson, outline what you have learned. An example is provided for you.

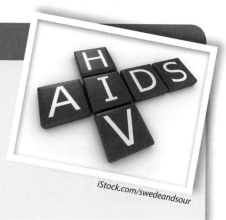

iStock.com/swedeandsour

K	W	L
What I <u>K</u>now	**What I <u>W</u>ant to Know**	**What I Have <u>L</u>earned**
HIV infects and kills cells, weakening the body's immune system	Does everyone infected with HIV develop AIDS?	AIDS is a condition in which the body cannot fight infections/disease; can develop later after HIV onset

A round the world, more than 37 million people are living with HIV/AIDS. Since this epidemic began, the World Health Organization (WHO) estimates 35 million people have died from AIDS-related causes. HIV/AIDS knows no national boundaries. It affects people of all sexes, ages, races, nationalities, and ethnic origins. HIV transmission is most common among people ages 13–34.

In this lesson, you will learn about what HIV/AIDS is. You will also learn about the transmission of, signs and symptoms of, testing for, and prevention and treatment of HIV/AIDS.

Understanding HIV and AIDS

To understand HIV and AIDS, you must first know what each term means (**Figure 18.11**). **Human immunodeficiency virus (HIV)** infects and kills white blood cells, weakening the body's immune system. At a certain point, HIV can completely wear down the immune system. This leads to **acquired immunodeficiency syndrome (AIDS)**, a health condition in which the body cannot fight infections and diseases.

AIDS can develop later, perhaps many years after the onset of HIV. Treatment can slow the progression of HIV into AIDS and help people with AIDS live longer. Many people who have HIV/AIDS can live long, healthy lives if they receive regular treatment. Treatment also greatly reduces the risk for HIV transmission.

A person tests positive for HIV if a laboratory test detects the presence of HIV *antibodies* in the person's blood. *Antibodies* are proteins the body's immune system produces to detect and destroy certain harmful substances, such as HIV. If HIV antibodies are in a person's blood, the person's blood must contain HIV. Testing positive for HIV means that a person has HIV, but it does not necessarily mean that a person has AIDS.

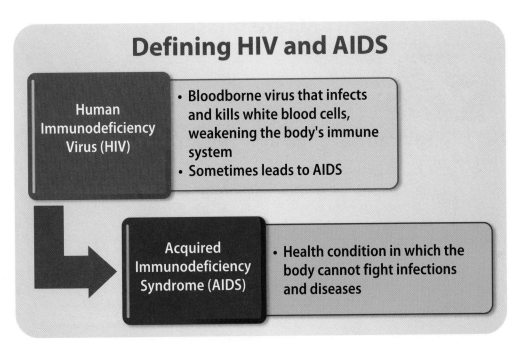

Defining HIV and AIDS

Human Immunodeficiency Virus (HIV)
- Bloodborne virus that infects and kills white blood cells, weakening the body's immune system
- Sometimes leads to AIDS

Acquired Immunodeficiency Syndrome (AIDS)
- Health condition in which the body cannot fight infections and diseases

Figure 18.11
HIV is a virus that infects cells and weakens the body's immune system. Sometimes, perhaps many years after the onset of HIV, a person can develop AIDS, in which the body cannot fight infections and diseases. *Can HIV be cured with antibiotics? Why or why not?*

HIV Transmission

There are certain ways HIV *can* and *cannot* be transmitted (**Figure 18.12**). HIV is found in certain bodily fluids, including blood, semen, vaginal fluids, and breast milk. HIV is *not* found in tears, saliva, or sweat. HIV can be transmitted through sexual activity. It can also be transmitted if someone who has HIV gives birth to or breastfeeds a baby.

HIV can also be transmitted through contaminated needles used for drugs or medications, tattoos, or body piercings. At one time, HIV was often transmitted in *blood transfusions*, or procedures in which people receive donated blood. In the United States, however, the blood supply is now screened for HIV, so transfusions are usually very safe.

HIV is *not* transmitted by mosquitoes or by kissing, spitting, shaking hands, sharing food, or using the same toilet seat. Healthy, intact skin provides an effective barrier against HIV. HIV transmission is possible through open sores on skin, in the mouth, or on genitals.

Certain factors increase the risk for HIV transmission. People who abuse drugs are more likely to share hypodermic needles, increasing their risk of exposure to blood with HIV. Having other STIs also increases the risk for contracting HIV. Sores and inflammation associated with other STIs damage the intact skin that protects against HIV. This means a person with STIs is more at risk for HIV transmission.

Signs and Symptoms of HIV/AIDS

The signs and symptoms of HIV and AIDS depend on how far HIV has progressed. Without treatment, HIV progresses through three stages, the last of which is AIDS.

Figure 18.12
HIV can be transmitted in certain bodily fluids such as blood and semen, but not through other fluids such as saliva or sweat.

HIV Transmission

HIV can be found in

- blood (including needles for drugs or medications, tattoos, or piercings)
- semen
- vaginal fluids
- breast milk
- open sores on skin, in the mouth, or on genitals

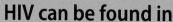

HIV is *not* found in

- tears
- saliva (kissing, spitting, sharing food)
- sweat
- mosquitoes
- healthy, intact skin (for shaking hands, using the same toilet seat, etc.)

- **Stage 1: Acute HIV infection.** The first signs and symptoms of HIV usually develop two to four weeks after HIV transmission. Even though there is a large amount of the virus in the blood during this stage, symptoms are usually minor and may not be recognized. Some people may not experience them at all. Early symptoms resemble a flu-like illness with fatigue and swollen, painful lymph nodes. Because of this, many people in this stage do not know they have HIV at all (**Figure 18.13**).
- **Stage 2: Latency.** A person may experience no symptoms at all, and levels of HIV in the blood are low. This stage can last 10 or more years, though some people may progress through the stage more quickly. Some people, called **long-term non-progressors**, pass through this stage very slowly. Treatment can extend this stage, sometimes by several decades or indefinitely. At the end of this stage, immunity begins to decrease, leading to AIDS.
- **Stage 3: Acquired immunodeficiency syndrome (AIDS).** In AIDS, HIV has severely damaged the immune system. The immune system cannot fight off infections that would not normally harm the body. In AIDS, unusual or normally harmless pathogens attack the body, causing **opportunistic infections**. These infections take advantage of the body's weakened immune system and can result in death (**Figure 18.14**). Other signs and symptoms of AIDS include severe weight loss, diarrhea, fever and chills, and nausea.

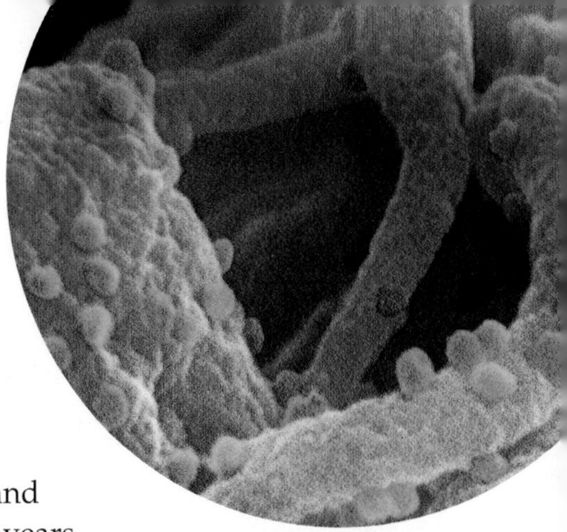

Courtesy of the Centers for Disease Control and Prevention

Figure 18.13
HIV (shown here in green) weakens the body's immune system by infecting and killing cells (shown in red).

Testing for HIV

HIV testing is critical for personal and community health. Testing examines a blood sample for the presence of HIV antibodies. Recall that the presence of HIV

Figure 18.14
With the body's immune system weakened, opportunistic infections attack the body and can cause death.

HIV damages the immune system, making it vulnerable to opportunistic infections such as these:

- *Pneumocystis pneumonia*, an infection of the lungs that the immune system can usually stop.
- Yeast infections in the mouth (called *thrush*), throat, lungs, and vagina.
- *Tuberculosis*, a bacterial lung infection.
- Infections of the intestines, skin, eyes, and nervous system.
- Brain infections and *meningitis* (infection of the membranes around the brain and spinal cord).
- Blood vessel tumors (*Kaposi's sarcoma*).

antibodies means the presence of HIV. A person may not develop HIV antibodies until weeks or months after exposure to HIV. Therefore, if a person gets a negative blood test, but still suspects exposure to HIV within the past three months, HIV testing should be repeated after three more months have passed.

Test results are available in a few days, or the rapid version of the test gives results in 20 minutes. Though tests are typically performed in doctors' offices and hospital labs, they may be done in other locations as well. HIV test sites can be found by searching the Internet or by contacting the Centers for Disease Control and Prevention (CDC).

A home version of the HIV test is available without a prescription. The test is inexpensive, fast, painless, and private. If the home test indicates the presence of HIV, the person should see a doctor for a test to confirm the results.

HIV testing is the key to controlling HIV transmission within society. Sexually active people should be tested every year and every time they switch sexual partners. Sadly, some people with HIV do not know they have it (**Figure 18.15**). If each affected individual knew, steps could be taken to prevent further transmission of the virus. Increased testing could significantly reduce HIV transmission.

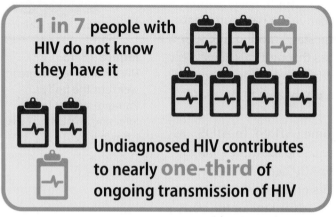

Telman Bagirov/Shutterstock.com

Figure 18.15 Sexually active people who have undiagnosed HIV can unknowingly transmit the virus to others.

HIV Test Results Are Confidential and Private

The *Health Insurance Portability and Accountability Act (HIPAA)* is a federal law that requires confidentiality for HIV test results, just as it does for other medical records. This means the results of a person's HIV test must be kept secret under the law. If an HIV test is positive, healthcare providers must report the results to the state. This is because states track and study the number of HIV cases. The results, however, are reported with no identifying personal information to protect the identity of the individual.

Although healthcare providers and states must keep HIV test results private, people living with HIV are encouraged to share their results with certain people. HIV is easily transmitted between sexual partners, so individuals should share their test results to protect their partners. Some cities and states have partner-notification laws requiring individuals with HIV or their doctors to notify sexual or needle-sharing partners.

Protecting Individuals with HIV from Discrimination

Individuals living with HIV often face discrimination in society and in their workplaces. *Discrimination* is the unfair treatment of a certain group of people. Some employers might refuse to hire people with HIV, worrying that they will take many sick days. Others might make assumptions about the person's lifestyle and disapprove of the individual's situation. This can also lead to discrimination. The federal government seeks to prevent this type of discrimination.

Two important laws protect the rights of people with HIV. The *Americans with Disabilities Act (ADA) of 1990* and the *Rehabilitation Act of 1973* prohibit discrimination against people with HIV. This means that people with HIV cannot be denied jobs, benefits, education, services, or other rights because of their HIV status. These laws also protect the families of people living with HIV.

Treatment for HIV/AIDS

In the 1980s, there was no effective treatment for people living with HIV/AIDS. People began to think HIV/AIDS was an untreatable, fatal disease. Today, this view of HIV/AIDS is untrue. Treatments have improved the health and quality of life for people living with HIV.

The treatment for people living with HIV is **antiretroviral therapy (ART)**, a combination of medications, sometimes called a *cocktail*, that interfere with HIV reproduction. People with HIV should start ART as soon as possible.

The aim of ART is to reduce the amount of HIV in a person's blood. Today, ART can reduce the amount of HIV to the point of being undetectable. People using ART regularly also do not transmit HIV. Some people taking ART never develop AIDS.

HIV Prevention

Understanding the activities that can cause transmission is the best way to avoid contracting HIV. These activities involve contact with a person's blood, semen or pre-seminal fluids, vaginal fluids, or breast milk. In the United States, HIV is most commonly spread through sexual activity and needle sharing.

Since HIV can spread through sexual activity, methods of preventing other STIs also help prevent HIV (**Figure 18.16**). The only 100-percent effective method of preventing HIV transmission through sexual activity is sexual abstinence. Using a condom also reduces the risk of HIV transmission.

HIV transmission can also occur if people share needles. If you take a medication you need to inject, never share needles with another person. Be sure to use a new, sterile needle for each injection. If you get a piercing or tattoo, make sure the piercer or tattoo artist is licensed and uses a new, sterile needle and new ink for each customer.

Certain medications can also reduce a person's risk of contracting HIV. These include the following:

- **Pre-exposure prophylaxis (PrEP)** is a course of ART that can protect a person from contracting HIV. It comes as a pill that must be taken every day. PrEP is intended for people who have a high risk of contracting HIV. When taken properly, PrEP reduces a person's risk of contracting HIV from sexual

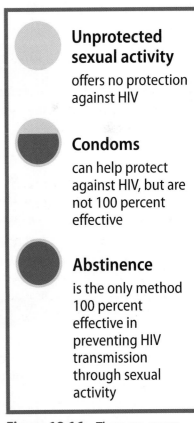

Unprotected sexual activity offers no protection against HIV

Condoms can help protect against HIV, but are not 100 percent effective

Abstinence is the only method 100 percent effective in preventing HIV transmission through sexual activity

Figure 18.16 There are many methods to prevent STIs, but abstinence is the only method that is 100 percent effective.

activity by more than 90 percent. When combined with other prevention methods, PrEP reduces the risk to near-zero. PrEP also reduces the risk of contracting HIV from shared needles by more than 70 percent. PrEP does not prevent other STIs.

- **Post-exposure prophylaxis (PEP)** is a course of ART a person can take within 72 hours of exposure to HIV to help prevent transmission. PEP is only intended for emergency situations. There are two kinds of PEP: oPEP and nPEP. *Occupational post-exposure prophylaxis (oPEP)* is used by healthcare professionals after HIV exposure from a needle injury or contact with bodily fluids. People can use *nonoccupational post-exposure prophylaxis (nPEP)* after HIV exposure outside the workplace, such as through sexual activity or shared needles (**Figure 18.17**).

Figure 18.17
PrEP and PEP can help prevent HIV transmission.

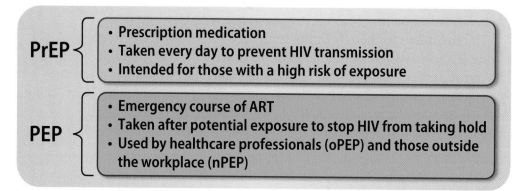

PrEP
- Prescription medication
- Taken every day to prevent HIV transmission
- Intended for those with a high risk of exposure

PEP
- Emergency course of ART
- Taken after potential exposure to stop HIV from taking hold
- Used by healthcare professionals (oPEP) and those outside the workplace (nPEP)

Lesson 18.2 Review

1. **True or false.** The presence of HIV antibodies in the blood indicates a person has HIV.
2. Each of the following is a bodily fluid source of HIV *except* _____.
   - **A.** blood
   - **B.** semen
   - **C.** saliva
   - **D.** breast milk
3. List two types of opportunistic infections.
4. Why is HIV testing critical to community health?
5. **Critical thinking.** What is discrimination? What laws protect the rights of people with HIV against discrimination? How can people promote respect for those living with HIV?

Hands-On Activity

Create a Venn diagram. Label one of the circles "People living *with* HIV/AIDS" and the other "People living *without* HIV/AIDS." Complete the Venn diagram. List examples of everyday activities that these groups of people can and cannot do. The center, where the circles overlap, indicates what activities both groups of people can or cannot do. When complete, review your information. Draw conclusions about what people living with HIV/AIDS can and cannot do. What do your conclusions show about misconceptions people may have about those who are living with HIV/AIDS?

Review and Assessment

Summary

Lesson 18.1   Sexually Transmitted Infections (STIs)

- Sexually transmitted infections (STIs) are communicable diseases that spread from one person to another during sexual activity, including sexual touching and sexual intercourse. They are caused by pathogens.
- STIs are sometimes called *sexually transmitted diseases (STDs)*.
- Common STIs include chlamydia, gonorrhea, syphilis, trichomoniasis, genital herpes, and human papillomavirus (HPV).
- Sexual abstinence, or refraining from sexual activity, is the only 100 percent effective method for preventing STIs. Using a condom during sexual activity can also reduce a person's risk of contracting an STI.
- Some STIs are easily treated and curable, and others are not. People can receive STI testing from doctors, public health departments, and organizations offering in-person or online services.

Lesson 18.2   HIV/AIDS

- Human immunodeficiency virus (HIV) is a bloodborne virus that infects and kills white blood cells, weakening the immune system.
- HIV can progress into acquired immunodeficiency syndrome (AIDS), a health condition in which the body's immune system cannot fight infections and diseases.
- HIV is found in bodily fluids such as blood, semen, vaginal fluids, and breast milk. Activities that involve contact with these fluids, such as sexual activity and needle sharing, can transmit HIV.
- Signs and symptoms of HIV/AIDS depend on how far HIV has progressed.
- Testing for the presence of HIV antibodies involves examining a sample of blood. HIV testing is an important part of community and public health.
- Antiretroviral therapy (ART) is the main treatment for HIV/AIDS. With early treatment, a person living with HIV may never develop AIDS.
- HIV prevention involves using precautions during activities that can transmit HIV. For example, sexual abstinence prevents HIV transmission through sexual activity. Using a condom also lowers this risk.
- Certain medications can also lower risk for transmission of HIV. These include pre-exposure prophylaxis (PrEP) and post-exposure prophylaxis (PEP).

Check Your Knowledge

Record your answers to each of the following questions on a separate sheet of paper.

1. **True or false.** STIs are noncommunicable diseases.
2. What activities can transmit an STI?
3. Chlamydia can lead to a severe bacterial infection of the female reproductive organs, called ____.
4. What is the most commonly contracted STI?
   A. Syphilis.
   B. Genital herpes.
   C. Chlamydia.
   D. Human papillomavirus (HPV).
5. What is the most effective way to prevent STIs?
   A. Condoms.
   B. Respiratory etiquette.
   C. Sexual abstinence.
   D. Hand washing.
6. Name two STIs that are incurable.
7. **True or false.** AIDS is the virus that leads to HIV.
8. Why does having other STIs increase risk for HIV transmission?
9. Which stage of HIV is characterized by flu-like symptoms?
10. **True or false.** Even with treatment, HIV will always progress to AIDS.
11. What is the main treatment method for HIV/AIDS?
    A. Abstinence.
    B. Antiretroviral therapy (ART).
    C. Pre-exposure prophylaxis (PrEP).
    D. Post-exposure prophylaxis (PEP).
12. ____ can be taken within 72 hours of exposure to HIV to help prevent transmission.

Use Your Vocabulary ↗

abstinence	genital herpes	post-exposure prophylaxis (PEP)
acquired immunodeficiency syndrome (AIDS)	gonorrhea	pre-exposure prophylaxis (PrEP)
antiretroviral therapy (ART)	human immunodeficiency virus (HIV)	sexually transmitted infections (STIs)
chlamydia	human papillomavirus (HPV)	syphilis
condom	long-term non-progressors	trichomoniasis
	opportunistic infections	

13. Find a video, podcast, or article from a reliable source that discusses one of the key terms from the list above. Create a digital presentation to summarize your findings, incorporating other key terms when relevant. Present it to the class and answer any questions your classmates may have. Be sure to cite your media source.
14. With a partner, make flash cards of the chapter terms. On the front of the card, write the term. On the back, write the phonetic spelling as written in a dictionary. Practice reading aloud the terms, clarifying each other's pronunciations where needed.

Think Critically

15. **Cause and effect.** What are the potential consequences, for personal health and the health of others, if someone engages in unsafe sexual behaviors and does not regularly get tested for STIs or HIV?

16. **Identify.** What agencies and resources are available in your community for accessing sexual healthcare services (such as STI testing)? Identify at least two.

17. **Analyze.** Based on the information you read in this chapter, why is STI testing, including testing for HIV, critical for personal and community health?

18. **Draw conclusions.** What might be the social consequences of contracting an incurable STI or HIV? How could this diagnosis impact future relationships?

DEVELOP Your Skills

19. **Teamwork and advocacy skills.** With a partner, role-play the following situation: A teen must explain to a friend the benefits of practicing sexual abstinence. One student plays the role of the teen; the other acts as the friend. Use your own words to explain how abstinence can prevent STIs, HIV, pregnancy, and other consequences. Incorporate key terms as they are relevant. As the teen explains the benefits of abstinence, the friend should ask questions if the explanation is unclear. Switch roles and repeat the activity. After reviewing your role play with your teacher, present it to the class to advocate for abstinence.

20. **Communication skills.** Imagine you are hanging out with a group of friends at night in your neighborhood park. Several are flirting. Your best friend talks about leaving the group for a while, implying the intention to have sex. You are immediately worried, knowing this is not only a bad decision, but also unplanned. How could you respond to convince your friend not to make this decision? Write your response in essay form. Then, share and discuss your response with the rest of the class.

21. **Advocacy, access information, and technology skills.** In groups of three, review this chapter and do additional research to learn about community resources available to support sexual health. Then, create a public service announcement (PSA) video to encourage teens to abstain from risky sexual behaviors. In your PSA, encourage abstinence, educate others on ways to prevent STIs and HIV, and include community resources to help support sexual health. Share your video with the teacher. With teacher permission, post it to the class website for peer review.

22. **Analyze influences.** Social media, TV shows, and music often portray risky sexual behaviors with little to no consequences. Analyze these messages and determine whether the risk of STIs or HIV was stated or implied in the message. Discuss your findings in essay form. Include how these messages impact the way adolescents view the risk of contracting an STI or HIV.

23. **Communication and accessing information skills.** Imagine you are a writer for a middle school newspaper or website. Write an editorial, article, or advice column targeted at middle school students. Choose a topic related to STIs or HIV. Be sure the information is relevant and interesting to your audience. Likewise, be sure the information you provide is accurate. In addition to this chapter, use other valid and reliable sources to add more detail to your writing. Cite your sources.

Human Sexuality

Chapter 19   Understanding Sexuality

Chapter 20   Making Responsible Sexual Decisions

Warm-Up Activity

What Do You Know About Sexuality?

Throughout this unit, you will learn about sexuality and birth control methods. You may already know some information about these topics. Maybe you have heard about sexuality from friends, healthcare providers, parents or guardians, or other trusted adults. Perhaps you learned more about these topics from television, social media, or websites. No matter the source, you need accurate information to promote your own health.

Before reading this unit, complete a table like the one shown. Identify what you already know, what you want to learn, and what questions you may have about sexuality and birth control methods.

After reading the chapters in this unit, reread your lists from this activity. Decide if the information you already knew was accurate. Correct the information, if needed. Write down any information you wanted to and did learn. Finally, answer the questions you had about sexuality and birth control methods. If any of your questions were not answered, talk about them with a trusted adult.

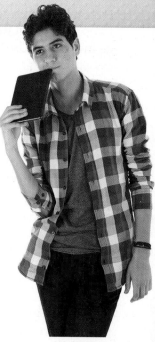

Ebtikar/Shutterstock.com

What I Know	What I Want to Learn	What Questions I Have
• •	• •	• •

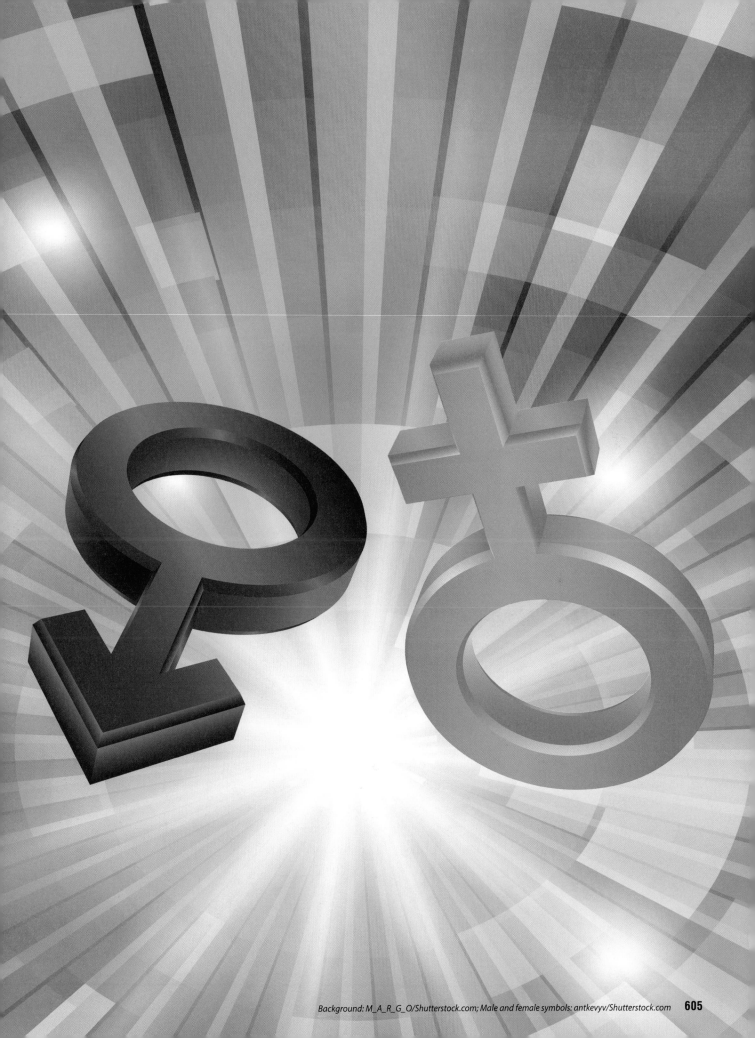

Chapter 19

Understanding Sexuality

Essential Question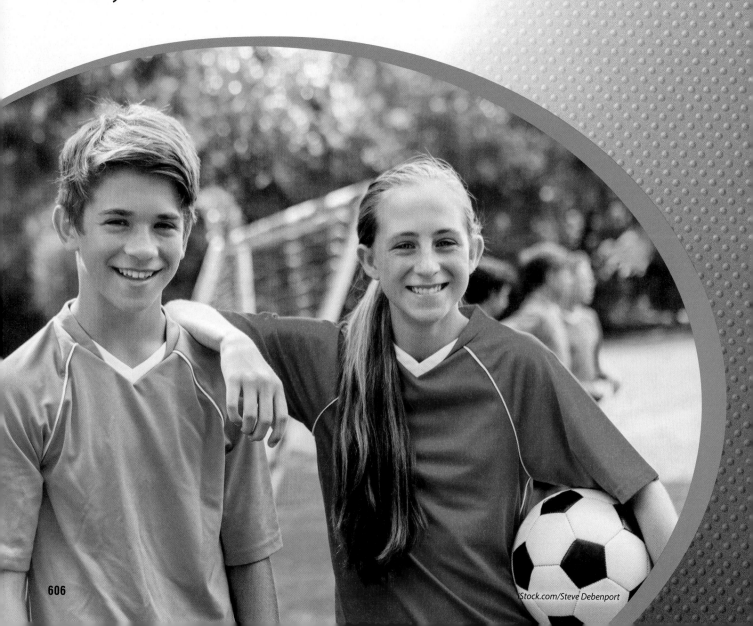

Why is it important for adolescents to understand sexuality?

iStock.com/Steve Debenport

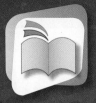

Reading Activity

Before reading this chapter, write down the key terms. Using these terms, write two paragraphs summarizing what you already know about human sexuality. If you do not know how a key term relates to the concept of sexuality, write the term below your paragraphs. After you finish reading the chapter, explain how that term relates.

How Healthy Are You?

In this chapter, you will be learning about human sexuality. Before you begin reading, take the following quiz to assess your current level of understanding about human sexuality.

Health Concepts to Understand	Yes	No
Do you know what is included in sexuality?		
Can you explain how chromosomes determine biological sex?		
Do you understand the difference between gender and gender identity?		
Can you explain the different types of sexual orientations?		
Do you understand the changes that occur during puberty and how puberty leads to sexual feelings?		
Do you know the consequences of sexual activity?		
Can you explain how sexual abstinence is a healthy choice for young people?		
Do you know what sexual harassment is?		
Can you explain how lack of consent is central to the definition of sexual assault?		
Do you understand the impact of sexual assault on physical, emotional, and social health?		
Can you list ways to prevent and respond to sexual assault?		

Count your "Yes" and "No" responses. The more "Yes" responses you have, the more knowledge you possess of human sexuality. Now, take a closer look at the questions with which you responded "No." As you read this chapter, look for these topics to increase your understanding. Develop your health literacy skills by accessing valid information about each of the concepts you do not understand. Evaluate any health websites you find using the information in Figure 1.16 of this text. If you do not understand the instructions, ask for clarification from your teacher.

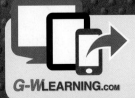

Click on the activity icon or visit www.g-wlearning.com/health to access online vocabulary activities using key terms from the chapter.

What Is Sexuality?

Learning Outcomes

After studying this lesson, you will be able to

- **recognize** the different aspects of sexuality.
- **explain** the concept of biological sex.
- **describe** how gender is identified and expressed.
- **identify** various sexual orientations.
- **understand** the challenges associated with homophobia.

Idea.s/Shutterstock.com

Graphic Organizer

Aspects of Sexuality

On a separate sheet of paper, draw a circle and write *Sexuality* in the middle. Then, draw four circles around the middle circle and label them *Biological Sex*, *Gender*, *Sexual Orientation*, and *Sexual Experiences and Thoughts*. As you read this lesson, organize your notes around the appropriate circles. An example is shown.

Biological Sex — Determined by sex chromosomes

Do not have to be sexually active to undertand sexuality

Sexual Experiences and Thoughts

Sexuality

Gender

Sexual Orientation

You have probably heard the word *sexuality,* but do you know what it means? This year is not the first time Carter has heard the word *sexuality.* Still, he does not understand how the word applies to him. Last month, Carter's older sister told their parents that she identified as homosexual. Now, Carter's friend Alia is saying that she is not sure about her sexual orientation. Carter does not feel attracted to anyone at school yet, and he wonders what it will feel like when he is attracted to someone. He questions whether he has a sexuality, since he does not want to have sex.

Sexuality is about more than your thoughts, attractions, or experiences. You do not have to be sexually active or even interested in sex to understand your sexuality. Sexuality is also more than your sexual anatomy, chromosomes, or body parts. The word *sexuality* means more than all these things. **Sexuality** includes factors such as a person's biological sex, sexual expression and feelings, orientation, and gender identity (**Figure 19.1**). In some people, these are separate aspects of sexuality. In other people, some of these aspects of sexuality interact.

Sexuality is an important part of a person's identity. It includes how a person looks, feels, thinks, and acts. It also affects how other people perceive and treat a person and what roles the person plays in family and society. Understanding sexuality is an important part of knowing and learning about yourself.

Biological Sex

The first aspect of sexuality is biological sex. **Biological sex** refers to whether an individual is genetically and physically a male or female. It is determined by a person's sex chromosomes. These chromosomes are inherited from a person's biological parents. The two sex chromosomes are X and Y.

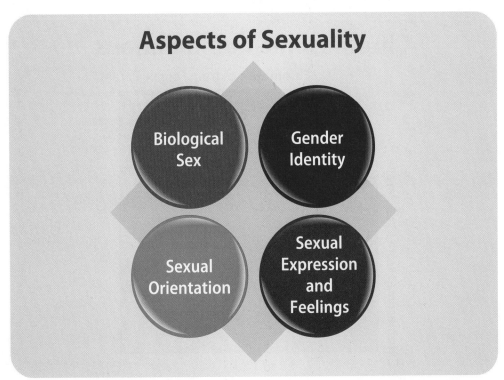

Aspects of Sexuality

Biological Sex

Gender Identity

Sexual Orientation

Sexual Expression and Feelings

Figure 19.1
Sexuality is an important part of a person's identity, which includes the way people think of themselves as well as how others perceive them. There are four main aspects to a person's sexuality.

Males inherit a Y chromosome from the male parent and an X chromosome from the female parent. Females inherit an X chromosome from each parent (**Figure 19.2**). These chromosomes direct the development and growth of sex organs and other sexual characteristics.

By about the seventh week of prenatal development, a fetus' biological sex can be determined by a doctor through a blood test. After the eighteenth week, the sex organs of a fetus can be seen using ultrasound. At birth, biological sex is usually obvious by the appearance of the external sex organs. Based on this anatomy, babies are assigned a biological sex of male or female at birth.

Some babies are born with an unclear biological sex, however. This condition is called a **disorder of sex development (DSD)**. It is also known as *difference of sex development (DSD)* or *intersex*. DSDs are relatively common, occurring in as many as 1–2 percent of live births. Babies with DSDs have external sex organs that are not obviously male or female. This does not mean that babies with DSDs possess both male and female organs. Rather, organs have not developed fully and cannot be identified. For example, male organs may appear smaller or resemble female organs. Due to this, babies with DSDs cannot be assigned a biological sex at birth based on anatomy alone.

In other cases, external sex organs may not match a baby's chromosomes. For example, a baby with XY chromosomes may be born with female characteristics. A baby with XX chromosomes may develop male characteristics. Some babies have one X chromosome from one parent and no sex chromosome from the other parent. Some males may have two X chromosomes and one Y chromosome. Babies born with these conditions may not have an unclear biological sex at birth. Instead, unclear sexual traits may appear during puberty. These conditions make clear that being male or female is more complicated than having certain sexual anatomy or sex chromosomes.

Figure 19.2
Females have the chromosome combination XX, and males have the chromosome combination XY. Each baby inherits one sex chromosome from each parent. The female parent always donates an X chromosome. The male parent can donate either an X or a Y chromosome. *Which aspect of sexuality is determined by a person's sex chromosomes?*

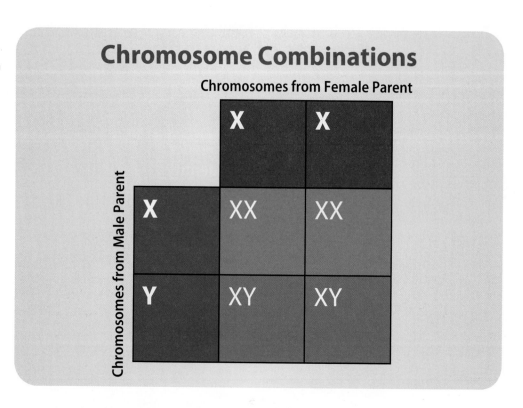

Gender

The second aspect of sexuality is gender. **Gender** refers to the characteristics a society associates with a particular biological sex. As a result, ideas about gender are constantly changing. Behavior and appearance, such as clothing and accessories, often influence the perception of gender.

Gender Expectations

Definitions of gender vary among societies and cultures and change over time. So do **gender roles**, which are behaviors society considers "appropriate" for a certain gender. In the United States, gender is often described as *masculine* or *feminine*. Characteristics commonly described as masculine or feminine are generally extreme opposites. For example, people may associate aggressiveness with men and passiveness with women. This distinction is an example of the *gender binary*, or the idea that the genders of man and woman are entirely opposite.

It is impossible to be completely aggressive or passive. Most people's behavior lies somewhere in between the two extremes (**Figure 19.3**). In addition, no person possesses only masculine or feminine traits. For example, a boy can be a highly competitive athlete and still take care of a younger sibling. A girl can be a great friend and still be dedicated to pursuing a career as a computer programmer.

For these reasons, gender can be a source of insecurity for adolescents. Because they are still developing, adolescents often feel insecure about how others see them. They may also feel pressured to act a certain way based on gender stereotypes. *Gender stereotypes* are preconceived ideas, roles, and characteristics people associate with a certain gender. They may think they have to be entirely masculine or feminine, not realizing these are just imagined norms. In truth, many people do not conform to typical gender expectations or roles. Part of understanding sexuality is knowing yourself and your own gender identity.

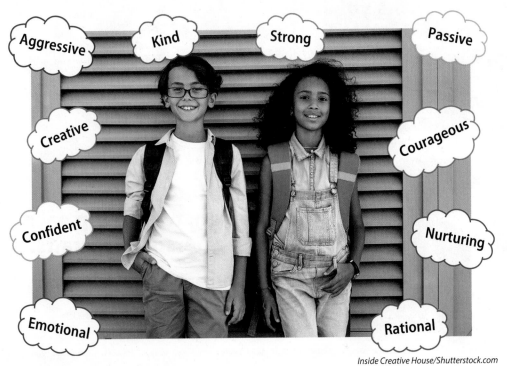

Figure 19.3
No one is completely masculine or completely feminine. Most people possess both masculine and feminine characteristics. *From the characteristics listed, which ones do you think describe you?*

Aggressive Kind Strong Passive
Creative Courageous
Confident Nurturing
Emotional Rational

Inside Creative House/Shutterstock.com

Breaking the Myth of Gendered Personality Traits

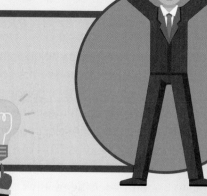

Personality traits are often described as either "masculine" or "feminine."

Example: aggressive or assertive

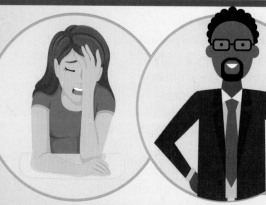

These gendered traits tend to be polar opposites.

Example: emotional versus rational

No one is fully one extreme or the other, and the traits you have are not determined by your biological sex.

Example: courageous or powerful

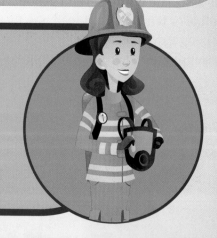

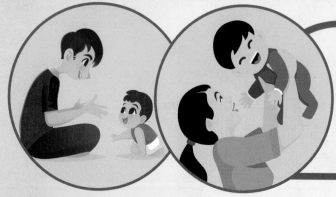

Everyone has the potential, as a person, to develop each of these personality traits.

Example: parental and nurturing

Gender Identity

Gender identity is your internal, deeply held thoughts and feelings about gender. It includes how you feel and think about your gender. Gender identity influences *gender expression*, or the way you outwardly display your gender. This includes the clothes you wear and your physical appearance and behaviors. Gender identity often develops very early in life. In fact, most three-year-olds easily identify themselves as boys or girls. A child's sense of individual gender usually becomes well-established around five years of age (**Figure 19.4**).

Gender identity is taught when parents identify a baby's biological sex at birth and raise the baby as a boy or girl. As a result, a child learns to identify as a boy or girl. As they grow older, people may realize they do not entirely identify with an assigned gender. These people may revise how they see and express their gender identity.

Some people may not be comfortable with the gender assigned to them. This happens for many reasons. For example, a person with female external organs may be raised as a girl, but identify as a boy. He may assume the roles and behaviors associated with boys. A person who has a gender opposite of the individual's biological sex is considered **transgender**.

Because of social and cultural expectations, some people who are transgender are confused about their gender identity for many years. They choose to change their appearance, clothing, and name to match the gender they feel they really are (**Figure 19.5**). Another example of gender identity is being *nonbinary*. This means having a gender identity that falls outside the categories of man or woman. People who are nonbinary may identify with neither gender (*agender*) or both genders (*bigender*).

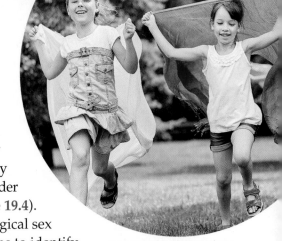

Robert Kneschke/Shutterstock.com

Figure 19.4
During childhood, most boys play with other boys, and girls play with other girls. This may be a way that children solidify and support their own sense of gender. It is normal, however, for some children to role play as the opposite sex or prefer playing with children of the opposite sex. *Around what age does a child's sense of individual gender become well-established?*

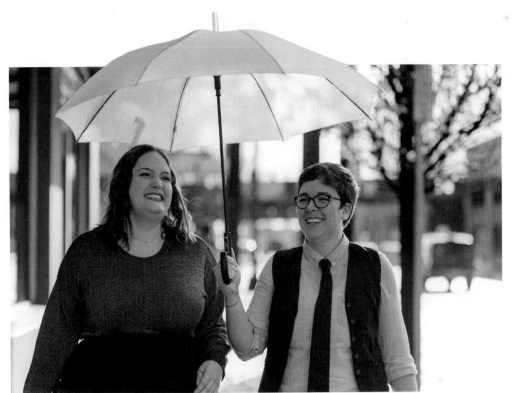

iStock.com/FatCamera

Figure 19.5
People who are transgender choose to change their appearance to match the gender they feel they really are.

Unfortunately, people who are transgender or nonbinary may face discrimination and rejection. If people are confused about their gender identity or identify with another gender, friends should be supportive and recognize the difficulties the person may experience. Talking to a counselor or a trusted adult is also a good source for additional support.

Sexual Orientation

Another aspect of sexuality is sexual orientation. **Sexual orientation** describes the continuing pattern of a person's romantic and/or sexual attraction to other people. Feelings of attraction develop during puberty, so not all adolescents know what this feels like. Different people develop feelings of attraction at different times. Examples of different types of sexual orientation include the following:

- **Heterosexual.** People who are heterosexual are romantically and physically attracted to people of the opposite gender.
- **Homosexual.** People who are homosexual are romantically and physically attracted to people of their own gender. The term *gay* can refer to both homosexual men and women. Women who are gay may also refer to themselves as *lesbian*.
- **Bisexual.** People who are bisexual are romantically and physically attracted to people of both genders. A person who is bisexual is attracted to both the same gender and the opposite gender.
- **Asexual.** People who are asexual may feel romantic or physical attraction, but are not sexually attracted to either gender.

People of all sexual orientations can be found in all races, ethnicities, cultures, countries, and social and economic backgrounds. Many factors, some unknown, influence the development of a person's sexual orientation (**Figure 19.6**). Sexual orientation develops in adolescents at various times as well. Some adolescents

Figure 19.6
Known factors that influence sexual orientation include a person's genes, environment, and experiences.
Which sexual orientation involves a person who is physically attracted, but not sexually attracted, to either gender?

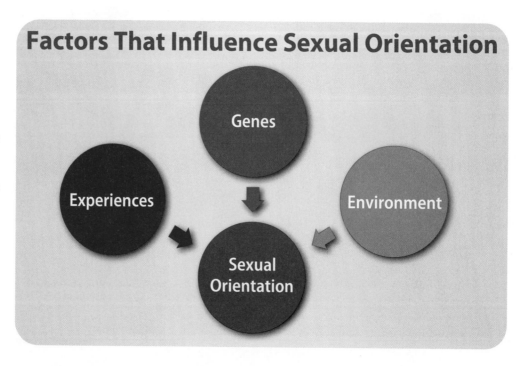

Factors That Influence Sexual Orientation

recognize that they are homosexual or bisexual early in puberty. Some people may know as early as childhood.

LGBT+ stands for *lesbian*, *gay*, *bisexual*, and *transgender*. LGBT+ is a common abbreviation used to identify people of nonheterosexual orientations or gender identities that do not match biological sex. The plus sign indicates the inclusion of other sexual orientations and gender identities as well. For example, the acronym *LGBT* is sometimes expanded to include *Q* (queer or questioning), *I* (intersex), and *A* (asexual). Some people of this community are active in trying to make sure LGBT+ people are treated fairly and have the same basic rights as all people.

Questions About Sexual Orientation

Adolescents often have questions about their emerging sexuality. It is normal for some adolescents who are heterosexual to feel confused about their sexual orientation. At times, some adolescents who are heterosexual may feel attracted to the same gender. This does not necessarily mean they are homosexual or bisexual. For example, a girl might develop a crush on another girl or on a female celebrity. This feeling is fairly common due to increased hormone levels in puberty. In time, most adolescents sort out their feelings as they discover and understand their sexual orientation.

Adolescents who are LGBT+ are also exploring their sexuality and sexual orientation. People who are LGBT+ often think about and want to discuss their romantic feelings, dating experiences, and sexuality. They may feel they need to hide this part of themselves, however.

From a young age, people who are LGBT+ notice that most people are heterosexual. This may make some adolescents who are LGBT+ feel out of place and unaccepted by others (**Figure 19.7**).

If you want to learn more about sexual orientation, turn to valid and reliable sources. Ask the school nurse, a doctor, a counselor, or a therapist. Visit websites provided by government agencies or experts in the field.

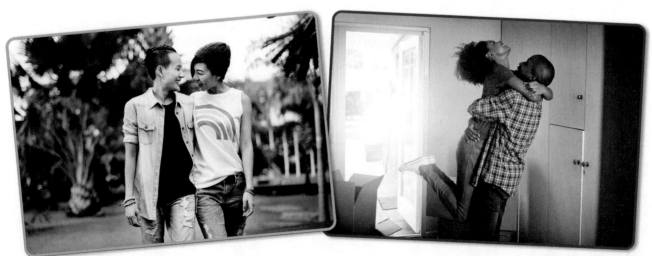

Left to right: iStock.com/Rawpixel; iStock.com/Peopleimages

Figure 19.7   Movie and television portrayals of characters with certain sexual orientations can influence how people perceive this aspect of sexuality. It is important to remember that these fictional people are created for entertainment purposes, however. The truth is that people—no matter their sexual orientation—are people. Each one is an individual, and each one may dress and behave in very different ways from others of the same orientation. ***What is the abbreviation used to identify people who are transgender, homosexual, or bisexual?***

Homophobia

People who are LGBT+ sometimes experience unfair treatment. The term **homophobia** was first used in 1969 to describe an irrational fear of homosexuality. Today, it refers to hostility, anger, exclusion, and violence directed at individuals who are LGBT+. People who are LGBT+ often have to deal with other people's negative attitudes and actions, sometimes on a daily basis. The negative attitudes may even come from the family members of the individual who is LGBT+.

Because of these attitudes, adolescents who are LGBT+ are at a greater risk for developing depression and anxiety. They are also at a higher risk of dropping out of school and running away from home. To avoid harassment, some people who are LGBT+ hide their sexual orientation or gender identity. Doing so, however, can be difficult and painful to deny this basic part of who they are.

BUILDING Your Skills

Promoting Acceptance, Tolerance, and Unity

Has anyone ever teased or treated you badly because of your biological sex, gender identity, or sexual orientation? Have you ever witnessed this type of harassment or discrimination? If so, you probably know how negative words and actions can hurt a person's self-esteem and confidence.

Discrimination and harassment of any kind are wrong. It is important to stand up and use your voice to speak out against them in any form. Schools around the world have been proactive in battling discrimination and harassment. Many have created student clubs or safe zones to promote acceptance, tolerance, and unity among people of all sexualities. Even if you are not part of a student club, you play a part in encouraging unity and tolerance. Owning this part and speaking up can help people of all sexualities feel accepted.

Improve Your School Climate

To play your part in promoting acceptance, tolerance, and unity, you can start by assessing your school climate. Your school climate refers to how well your school promotes acceptance, tolerance, and unity among people of all sexualities. It includes how students are treated by school staff and other students. Use the following steps to improve your school climate:

1. In small groups, discuss ways to improve the school climate for all students, regardless of sexual orientation or gender identity to feel accepted. One student in the group should take notes about these suggestions.

2. As a class, share these suggestions. Choose three to five suggestions that are realistic for your school.

3. Relay your class suggestions to a student club that promotes acceptance, tolerance, and unity. If a club like this or a safe zone does not exist at your school, consider creating one. Work with the club to implement your suggestions.

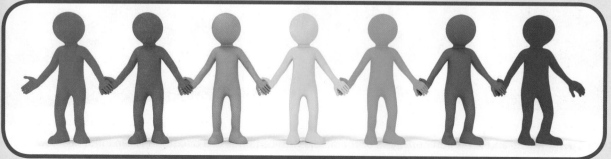

Markus Gann/Shutterstock.com

Despite discrimination, many people who are LGBT+, especially those who have good support systems, do feel comfortable with themselves. Many feel relieved when they tell trusted family members and friends about their sexual orientation or gender identity.

Support for Youth Who Are LGBT+

It is important for youths who are LGBT+ to have a supportive and accepting group of people around them. To create such a group, many schools have created student organizations, as well as safe zones, for students who are LGBT+ and those who support them (**Figure 19.8**).

Laws help protect people who are LGBT+ from discrimination and persecution. Federal laws, including the *Civil Service Reform Act of 1978* and the *Civil Rights Act of 1991*, prohibit employers from discriminating against workers because of their sexual orientation.

As you learned in Chapter 16, *hate crimes* are criminal acts motivated by differences in race, religion, disability, ethnicity, or sexual orientation. People who are LGBT+ may experience these crimes. The *Matthew Shepard and James Byrd, Jr. Hate Crimes Prevention Act* protects people from crimes motivated by sexual orientation and race.

Safe Zones...

- help people in the LGBT+ community feel welcomed.
- are spaces where students know they will be accepted.
- increase inclusiveness and support.
- lead to greater feelings of safety, tolerance, and respect for students who are LGBT+ as well as the community.

Figure 19.8 Safe zones are designated parts of a school as spaces where people in the LGBT+ community feel welcomed and accepted.

Lesson 19.1 Review

1. What is sexuality?
2. **True or false.** Females inherit two X chromosomes from their female parents.
3. Explain how gender identity develops.
4. Which of the following orientations involves attraction to both genders?
   - **A.** Asexual.
   - **B.** Homosexual.
   - **C.** Heterosexual.
   - **D.** Bisexual.
5. **Critical thinking.** Why are the characteristics associated with each gender constantly changing?

Hands-On Activity

Working with a partner, choose one topic related to sexuality that was discussed in this lesson. Your goal will be to educate others about your chosen topic and promote acceptance. Using the information in this lesson, create a flyer about your chosen topic. On your flyer, include a slogan about acceptance and an explanation of your chosen topic. Also, include a community resource that can provide support and answer questions about sexuality. With teacher permission, hang your flyers in the halls of your school for students to view.

Lesson 19.2

Sexual Feelings and Behavior

Learning Outcomes

After studying this lesson, you will be able to

- **identify** the physical changes that occur in puberty.
- **explain** what sexual intercourse is.
- **describe** the results of sexual activity.
- **explain** the benefits of abstinence.
- **develop** refusal skills that can help avoid sexual activity.

Graphic Organizer

Understanding Sexual Feelings

Before reading this lesson, divide a piece of paper into three columns. Use three different colors to label the columns *Puberty*, *Sexual Activity*, and *Abstinence*. An example is shown. As you read this lesson, take notes in each column. Use the color you chose for each column. At the bottom of each column, write the two most important facts you learned.

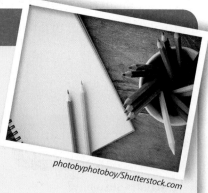

photobyphotoboy/Shutterstock.com

Puberty	Sexual Activity	Abstinence
Period of time for reaching sexual maturity *Triggered by hormones*		
Most important facts: 1. 2.	**Most important facts:** 1. 2.	**Most important facts:** 1. 2.

Y ou will learn more about the changes that occur during puberty in this lesson. Carter from the previous lesson has experienced these changes firsthand. His voice is deeper than it was last year, and hair has started growing under his arms. He is catching up to his friend Alia in height. This year, Alia confided in him that she feels sexually attracted to some of Carter's friends. Carter knows that Alia's feelings are normal and wonders if anyone is attracted to him. He also knows that sexual relationships carry risks that young people can find difficult to handle.

Puberty

Puberty, or the period of time in which the body reaches sexual maturity, plays a major role in people's sexual development. In Chapter 17, you read about the physical changes that occur as children go through puberty and adolescence. During puberty, hormones transform a child's body into that of an adult (**Figure 19.9**). These hormones also trigger powerful sexual feelings and drive the emotional changes of puberty.

The Importance of Sex Hormones

Hormones are specialized chemical messengers that glands produce and release into the blood. Because hormones travel through blood, they can carry messages to nearly every cell in the body. Each type of hormone affects only the activity of the body parts it targets. For example, *growth hormone* affects only bone, muscle, and connective tissue.

Some hormones target body parts related to sexual maturity and reproduction. These *sex hormones* are present in the body before puberty, but at low levels. Puberty begins when the brain releases *gonadotropin-releasing hormone*, which affects the pituitary gland in the brain. This hormone signals the pituitary gland to begin producing other hormones that affect the development of sex organs.

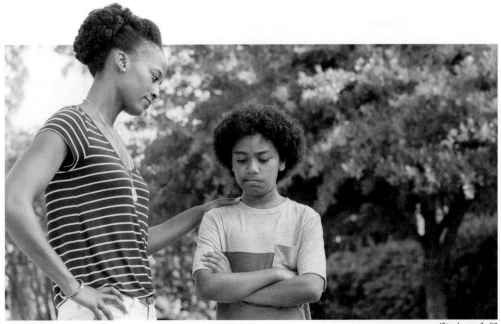

iStock.com/kali9

Figure 19.9
During puberty, adolescents grow quickly. Some adolescents may feel embarrassed about growing faster or slower than most of their friends and peers. It is normal for each person to grow at different rates. ***Which hormone affects bone, muscle, and connective tissue development?***

Hormones released by the pituitary gland affect the testes in males and the ovaries in females. The testes respond by increasing secretion of the hormone testosterone. *Testosterone* triggers growth and development of the testes, penis, and other male sexual characteristics. The ovaries respond by producing higher amounts of the hormone estrogen. *Estrogen* triggers growth and development of the ovaries, breasts, and other female sexual characteristics (**Figure 19.10**).

Physical Changes

As you learned in Chapter 17, both males and females go through dramatic physical changes during puberty (**Figure 19.11**). Some changes occur abruptly, and others happen gradually. Some adolescents experience a **growth spurt**, in which they quickly grow taller. Adolescents may repeatedly outgrow their clothes and shoes. The growth spurt is one of the most obvious external changes that occurs during puberty. Another physical change during puberty is weight gain. Males gain weight due to muscle development. Females gain weight due to the development of necessary body fat and muscle.

During puberty, males and females also develop primary and secondary sexual characteristics. *Primary sexual characteristics* relate to the sex organs. In males, the testes and penis grow. In females, the ovaries, vagina, and labia mature and grow.

Secondary sexual characteristics concern other parts of the body and are signs that the body is maturing. For example, in males, the shoulders broaden, muscles develop, and the voice deepens. Males also grow hair on their faces and other parts of their bodies, especially under the arms and around the genitals. Males may have *erections*, in which the penis lengthens and hardens. Erections can occur in response to sexual excitement or for no reason at all.

The bodies of females change shape, too. In females, the hips widen and body fat develops, especially at the hips and breasts. Breasts and nipples grow, sometimes unevenly and with feelings of soreness. *Menstruation*, or the

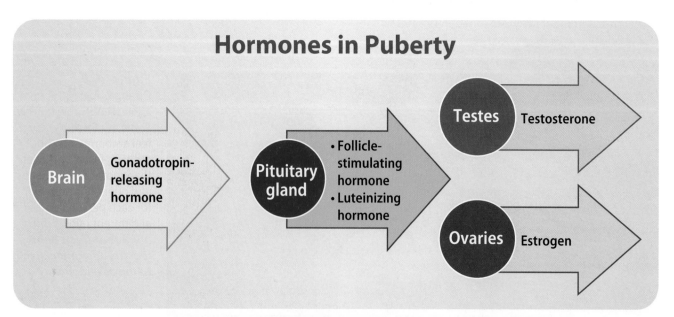

Figure 19.10 Puberty begins when the brain releases gonadotropin-releasing hormone. This hormone signals the pituitary gland to release follicle-stimulating hormone and luteinizing hormone. These hormones affect the testes in males and the ovaries in females. They cause the testes to release testosterone and the ovaries to release estrogen.

monthly shedding of blood and tissue from the uterus, begins about two years after the breasts develop. This change signals that a female's body is releasing *eggs*, or female sex cells. Vaginal secretions increase, and females also develop hair under the arms, on the legs, and around the genitals.

Different Rates of Development

The physical changes of puberty take place at different times and rates for different people (**Figure 19.12**). Some adolescents notice the signs of puberty earlier than others. Adolescents who look more physically mature than others can stand out. These adolescents may feel uncomfortable about their differences. Adolescents who understand the changes of puberty are less likely to feel uncomfortable as their own body changes or tease classmates going through these changes.

To learn more about the changes of puberty, seek valid information. For example, you can talk to the school nurse or a trusted doctor for accurate medical information. You can also get helpful, factual information from some websites. Choose websites carefully, though. Only visit the websites of government health agencies or valid health organizations.

Early Sexual Feelings

Elevated hormone levels affect adolescents emotionally. They can cause males or females to become sensitive, emotional, easily angered, and sexually attracted to others. Because these feelings are new, many adolescents ask themselves questions such as, "Am I normal?" and "Should I feel this way?" Like the physical changes of puberty, these emerging sexual feelings are perfectly normal.

The physical and emotional changes of puberty lead to curiosity about sex in males and females. Sexual excitement, or **arousal**, is normal and can be caused by sexual thoughts, daydreams, or images. Many adolescents find themselves thinking about sex often or having sexual dreams and fantasies about celebrities or people they know. Males may also experience erections and **wet dreams**, or ejaculations that occur during sleep.

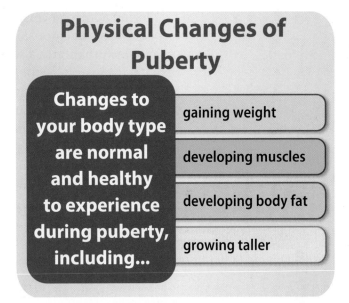

Physical Changes of Puberty

Changes to your body type are normal and healthy to experience during puberty, including...

- gaining weight
- developing muscles
- developing body fat
- growing taller

Figure 19.11 Physical changes like gaining weight or growing taller are normal to experience during puberty. *What develops during puberty that causes weight gain?*

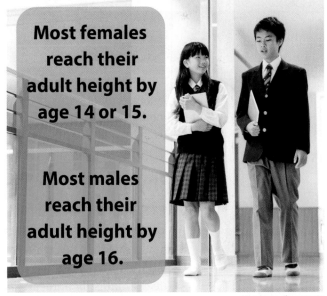

Most females reach their adult height by age 14 or 15.

Most males reach their adult height by age 16.

iStock.com/ferrantraite

Figure 19.12 An adolescent's rate of growth depends on individual genes and environment. It also depends on when puberty begins. *What is the term for a period in which a person quickly grows taller?*

During adolescence, males and females might begin masturbating in response to sexual arousal. **Masturbation** is the self-stimulation of the sex organ. Masturbation is a sexual activity that allows people to safely release sexual tension.

Some adolescents may feel embarrassed or guilty about masturbating because they have heard it is wrong or shameful. They may have heard that masturbation can cause acne, blindness, or other conditions. These beliefs are myths. Masturbation does not cause these issues. Masturbation is a normal and common response to sexual excitement. Adolescents who have questions about masturbation can talk with a doctor, nurse, parent or guardian, or other trusted adult.

Sexual Activity

As adolescents grow, they may start to develop a curiosity about sexual activity. They may want to talk about sex and make sexual comments. Some young people may be tempted to *sext*, or send sexual content in the form of actual text, pictures, or videos. Not sexting is the best way to avoid legal, professional, and social consequences (**Figure 19.13**).

Some adolescents may develop feelings of physical attraction to others that may arise during puberty. You may already be experiencing these feelings or you may eventually. The combination of romantic and physical attraction can feel new, complicated, and intense. It is a normal part of human development. Some adolescents may engage in sexual activities and intercourse. **Sexual intercourse** is any sexual activity that involves *penetration*, or the insertion of a body part or object into another body part. Engaging in sexual activities has serious consequences which should be thoughtfully considered.

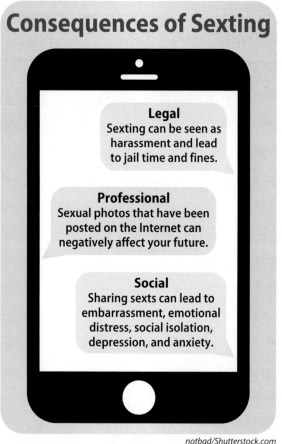

Consequences of Sexting

Legal
Sexting can be seen as harassment and lead to jail time and fines.

Professional
Sexual photos that have been posted on the Internet can negatively affect your future.

Social
Sharing sexts can lead to embarrassment, emotional distress, social isolation, depression, and anxiety.

notbad/Shutterstock.com

Figure 19.13 Sexting has various consequences. If someone sends you a sext, immediately delete the sext and tell a trusted adult.

Physical Consequences

Sexual activity can have many long-lasting physical consequences. These consequences can alter a person's goals and future decisions and opportunities. Having vaginal sex even once, and even for the first time, can lead to pregnancy and the birth of a baby (**Figure 19.14**). Becoming a teen parent changes a person's life dramatically and can lead to health conditions for the pregnant person and baby. You will learn more about teen pregnancy and parenthood in Chapter 20.

Sexual activity of any kind puts people at risk for STIs. Because some STIs do not show symptoms, some people do not know they have an STI. Even so, STIs can lead to infertility and other health conditions such as abnormal discharge or genital warts. While some are easily treated, others stay for the rest of a person's life.

Emotional and Social Consequences

For people in committed relationships, sexual feelings may lead to sexual activities that increase physical and emotional intimacy. Sexual feelings can solidify these relationships and bring people closer. Sexual activity can also bring intense emotion and stress to romantic relationships and can complicate lives in ways for which adolescents are unprepared.

Sexually active adolescents face emotional and social challenges that may have painful and unhappy consequences. Experts agree that adolescents are not emotionally mature enough to handle the consequences of sexual activity. **Figure 19.15** shows some examples of potential consequences that can occur from sexual activity.

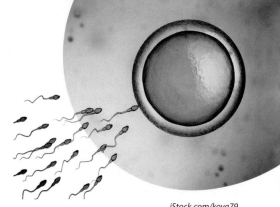

iStock.com/koya79

Figure 19.14
Fertilization occurs when a sperm enters an egg. Fertilization can result in pregnancy if the fertilized egg implants in the female's uterus.

Abstinence

Many adolescents recognize the potential consequences of early sexual activity and choose abstinence. *Abstinence* is the decision not to engage in sexual activity. Abstinence is recommended for adolescents for many reasons. For example, continuous abstinence is the only strategy that is 100 percent effective for preventing pregnancy. Abstinence also protects people from STIs, including HIV/AIDS. Because sexual activity may cause emotional issues, abstinence also promotes adolescents' emotional and social growth.

There are many ways to express romantic feelings for another person without sexual activity. Holding hands, hugging, and kissing are ways to show physical affection without sexual activity. Providing emotional support, pursuing common interests, trying each other's favorite activities or hobbies, and ensuring each partner feels important and respected can help strengthen relationships on an emotional level. Simply telling a partner that you care for them or exchanging compliments can show affection.

Figure 19.15
Adolescents should consider some of the risks that may result from engaging in sexual activity.

Emotional and Social Consequences of Sexual Activity

Jealousy
Becoming possessive of a partner can weaken the relationship.

Loss of Trust
Breaches in trust can end a relationship.

Feelings of Guilt or Shame
These feelings are difficult to experience and may hurt a person's relationship.

Less Personal Growth
Partners may exclude other relationships or responsibilities.

Reasons People Choose Abstinence

- Follow personal, moral, religious, or other beliefs and values
- Wait until they feel ready for sexual activity
- Wait until they find the right partner
- Enjoy a partner's company without having to deal with sexual activity
- To get over a breakup
- Focus on school, hobbies, or other extracurricular activities
- To recover from an illness, infection, or medical procedure
- Avoid pregnancy and STIs

Figure 19.16 Choosing abstinence allows people to focus on their personal growth.

Choosing Abstinence

According to experts, abstinence is a healthy decision adolescents can make regarding sexual activity. It promotes adolescent health and helps a person grow socially and emotionally. There are many reasons why people choose abstinence (**Figure 19.16**). Knowing the reasons you want to abstain from sexual activity will help you stick to your decision. Be confident in your decision and clear in your own mind about the reasons you choose to abstain so you can explain your decision to others.

To support your decision, avoid situations that will make abstinence difficult. For example, dating in groups or avoiding unsupervised parties can reduce the risk of sexual activity occurring. Avoiding alcohol and drugs, which can reduce good judgment, is another approach. Talk to your partner before a potential sexual encounter rather than in the moment.

If you are not sure how to make a decision about a sexual relationship, talk to a parent or guardian, adult sibling, doctor, counselor, teacher, or other trusted adults. Trusted adults can help you understand your concerns so you can make a well-reasoned decision. Your decision to abstain from sexual activity is entirely your own. It is a sign of your confidence and maturity to stand by your decision (**Figure 19.17**).

Talking to an adult about these matters might make some adolescents feel uncomfortable. The issue is too important to ignore, however. To talk effectively about these issues, choose an adult you trust. Set aside a quiet time and place to talk. Think about what you want to ask. Speak clearly and honestly about your feelings and worries. Listen fully to what your advisor has to say. Bear in mind that you might need to have more than one talk about the subject.

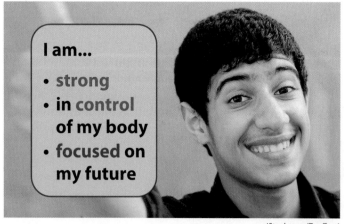

I am...
- **strong**
- **in control of my body**
- **focused on my future**

iStock.com/ZouZou1

Figure 19.17 Abstinence from sexual activity is a sign of confidence and maturity.

Dealing with Sexual Pressure

Adolescents may encounter many outside pressures and conflicting messages about sexual activity. Romantic partners may pressure adolescents to have sex. Friends and peers may say that "everyone is doing it." This is not true, however. In reality, most adolescents do not have sex.

Many conflicting messages about sexual activity come from the media. Advertisements, films, and other media often portray young people in sexual relationships. The implied message is that sex is a common part of adolescent relationships. In reality, millions of young people choose abstinence. In addition, media portrayals of sexual relationships often make them seem casual, with little or no risk or emotional fallout. While these scenes in the media create interesting storylines, the messages they convey are not realistic.

CASE STUDY

Marla and Nathan: A Not-So-Magical Relationship

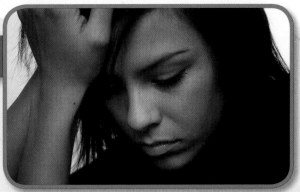

iStock.com/BCFC

Marla always imagined that her first real relationship would be magical. Her boyfriend would treat her like a princess and love spending time with her family. Marla recently started dating Nathan, and their relationship is good but not great. After three months, the relationship does not feel magical. Marla wonders if she had an unrealistic expectation of a relationship.

Marla and Nathan enjoy going to the movies and playing soccer together. Nathan will hang out with Marla's family, but only if she begs him. Generally, Marla enjoys Nathan's company, but she does not feel like a princess. She feels uncomfortable when he talks to her about doing sexual things or pressures her to send inappropriate text messages. Lately, the pressure has intensified. Marla wants to talk with her family about her feelings, but does not know how to start the conversation and fears disappointing them.

Thinking Critically

1. If you were Marla's friend, what advice would you give her about dating Nathan?

2. Why do you think Marla continues to stay in the relationship? If she stays in the relationship and gives into Nathan's demands, how could this affect her future relationships and decision-making?

3. If Marla chooses to send Nathan inappropriate text messages, what are the possible consequences of sexting?

4. If you were Marla, whom would you talk to about this situation? How would you start the conversation?

To resist sexual pressure, remember that the actions of others are not what determine your health. Only *you* can make choices to promote your health and well-being. Also, practice the words and actions you would use if pressured to engage in sexual activity. Knowing what you will say or do will make dealing with sexual pressure easier (**Figure 19.18**). Sometimes, you may have to physically leave a situation or walk away from people who are pressuring you. Finding a group of supportive people who understand your decision to remain abstinent can also help you resist sexual pressure.

Using Refusal Skills

As you learned in Chapter 1, *refusal skills* can help you respond to peer influences without going against your own goals, values, and health. Refusal skills can help when you are being pressured to do something you think is wrong, unhealthy, or against your values. With these skills, you can make independent, informed decisions.

Everyone has the right to refuse sexual activity at any time. The best way to refuse sexual activity is to clearly state you are not interested. Speak assertively and leave the situation, if needed. This can reduce the other person's ability

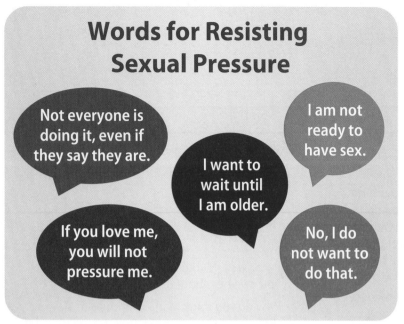

Words for Resisting Sexual Pressure

Not everyone is doing it, even if they say they are.

I want to wait until I am older.

I am not ready to have sex.

If you love me, you will not pressure me.

No, I do not want to do that.

Figure 19.18 A great way to resist sexual pressure is by practicing what you might say in certain situations. *When do you have the right to refuse sexual activity?*

to pressure you. Clearly giving consent can help state your views of sexual activity. You will learn more about consent in the next lesson.

Partners have the responsibility to respect each other's decisions about sexual activity. If one partner does not want to engage in sexual activity, the other partner should not do or say anything that applies pressure. Partners should accept each other's decisions and avoid pressuring each other. This shows true caring and respect.

If you are being pressured to engage in sexual activity, talk to a trusted adult for help. Negative pressure is a sign of an unhealthy relationship. You might need to end the relationship to end the pressure.

Lesson 19.2 Review

1. Which of the following triggers the development of male sexual characteristics?
   A. Insulin.
   B. Testosterone.
   C. Growth hormone.
   D. Estrogen.
2. **True or false.** Masturbation can cause acne, blindness, and other conditions.
3. Explain how early sexual activity can lead to less personal growth.
4. **True or false.** Abstinence promotes adolescents' social and emotional growth.
5. **Critical thinking.** Why are portrayals of sexual activity in the media not realistic?

Hands-On Activity

Consider the messages about sexual activity in your life. Create a three-column table on a separate sheet of paper. Include the following information in your table:

- Label the left column *Influences* and add rows for each of the following: television, social media, music, friends, family, and religious organizations.
- Label the middle column *Messages*. In this column, state the message you receive related to your sexual health or sexual activity.
- Label the right column *Positive or Negative*. Identify whether the messages you receive are positive or negative. Positive messages promote abstinence, and negative messages encourage risky sexual behaviors.

Choose one positive message and turn it into a text, tweet, or social media post that encourages abstinence. With teacher permission, hang your positive messages around the room or in the halls of your school.

Unwanted Sexual Activity

Learning Outcomes

After studying this lesson, you will be able to

- **explain** the meaning of affirmative consent.
- **define** sexual harassment.
- **describe** types of sexual assault.
- **identify** consequences of sexual assault.
- **develop** refusal skills that can help avoid unwanted sexual activity.
- **describe** steps for helping someone who experienced sexual assault.

Key Terms 📇

age of consent age at which a person can legally agree to engage in sexual activity

sexual harassment verbal or nonverbal sexual attention that occurs without consent

sexual assault act of threatening, pressuring, or forcing someone into sexual activity

rape sexual intercourse that occurs without consent

statutory rape crime that takes place when someone over the age of consent engages in sexual intercourse with someone under the age of consent

Graphic Organizer

Violence and Harassment

Before you read this lesson, fold a piece of paper into four sections. Cut along the folds to create four smaller pieces of paper. Label the smaller pieces *Sexual Harassment*, *Sexual Assault*, *Results of Sexual Assault*, and *Preventing and Responding to Sexual Assault*. As you read the lesson, take notes on the front and back of the appropriate piece of paper. Flip through the four pieces after reading to review the lesson.

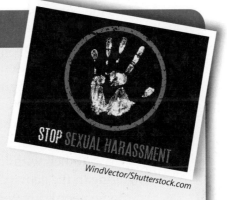

STOP SEXUAL HARASSMENT

WindVector/Shutterstock.com

Sexual Harassment	Sexual Assault
Unwanted attention of sexual nature Verbal or nonverbal	
Results of Sexual Assault	**Preventing and Responding to Sexual Assault**

Sexual harassment and assault are serious issues. Although they can happen to anyone at any age, adolescents are especially vulnerable. This is partly because adolescents' physical, emotional, and sexual development are all at different levels. People who are more sexually experienced may take advantage of adolescents. Some adolescents may have poor judgment or decision-making skills, increasing their risk for violence. No matter the situation, sexual harassment and sexual assault are always harmful and are serious crimes.

What Is Consent?

A key part of a healthy relationship and sexual activity is affirmative consent. As you learned in Chapter 15, *affirmative consent* is a direct, verbal, freely given agreement that occurs when someone clearly says *yes*. Consent is direct. This means it clearly communicates agreement and does not show hesitation. An example of consent is saying "Yes, I want to do that" while making eye contact and smiling.

Consent is also verbal. This means it uses words, not just body language or how a person is dressed. Consent does *not* occur if someone says *no* or nothing at all. People cannot and should not assume a person agrees to a behavior unless the person specifically, verbally says *yes*. In addition, if a person gave consent to a past sexual activity, this does not mean the consent applies to future activities. A person must freely give consent every time.

Consent is freely given. Consent does *not* occur if a person feels pressured into saying *yes* or hesitantly says *yes* (**Figure 19.19**). It also means consent can be changed at any time. For example, a person can agree to a sexual activity but then withdraw the consent by saying *no* before engaging in the activity.

Some people are not legally capable of giving consent to sexual activity. Only someone who fully understands what the agreement is can give consent. People cannot give consent to sexual activity if they are one of the following:

- being pressured or coerced by someone else
- under the influence of drugs or alcohol
- affected by certain disabilities or disorders, such as a cognitive disability
- asleep or unconscious
- younger than the **age of consent**, which is the age at which a person can legally agree to engage in sexual activity; it is 16 years of age in most states

Some people believe that if two people are in a romantic relationship, any kind of sexual activity must be consensual. This is false. No one, not even a long-term romantic partner, has the right to pressure someone to engage in sexual activity (**Figure 19.20**). If sexual activity occurs without consent, the person who committed the sexual assault is entirely to blame. The person who experienced the assault is *never* to blame. Without *mutual consent*, or

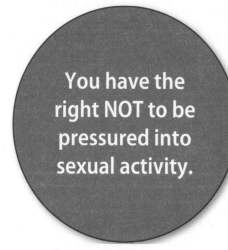

You have the right NOT to be pressured into sexual activity.

Figure 19.19 Affirmative consent is the difference between sexual activity and sexual harassment or assault. Sexual activity without consent is sexual violence and is wrong and illegal.

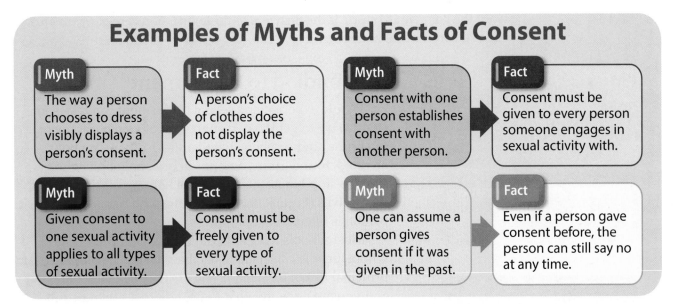

Examples of Myths and Facts of Consent

Myth
The way a person chooses to dress visibly displays a person's consent.

Fact
A person's choice of clothes does not display the person's consent.

Myth
Consent with one person establishes consent with another person.

Fact
Consent must be given to every person someone engages in sexual activity with.

Myth
Given consent to one sexual activity applies to all types of sexual activity.

Fact
Consent must be freely given to every type of sexual activity.

Myth
One can assume a person gives consent if it was given in the past.

Fact
Even if a person gave consent before, the person can still say no at any time.

Figure 19.20 Consent must be freely given each time and can never be assumed or coerced.

consent by both people, sexual attention is sexual harassment, and sexual activity is sexual assault.

Sexual Harassment

As adolescents grow curious about sexual activity, they may want to talk about sex and make sexual comments. If these comments are not wanted, however, they can be sexual harassment. **Sexual harassment** is unwanted sexual attention, or sexual attention that occurs without consent. Both males and females can commit and experience sexual harassment (**Figure 19.21**).

Recognizing Harassment

Sexual harassment can be verbal or nonverbal. *Verbal sexual harassment* includes the use of words, gossip, and threats. People who tell sexual jokes, make inappropriate or intimidating sexual comments, or spread sexual rumors in person or on social media are guilty of sexual harassment. Sexual harassment can also include sexual comments just spoken in the presence of a person who feels uncomfortable with the comments. Even pressing someone to say *yes* after the person said *no* to a date is considered sexual harassment.

Nonverbal sexual harassment occurs when people make sexual gestures at or about someone. This type of sexual harassment includes pinching, rubbing, or brushing up against someone in an unwanted way. It also includes whistling in a sexual way at someone or staring at someone's body.

If you are not sure whether a behavior counts as sexual harassment, ask yourself these questions: Does it make me feel uncomfortable? Do I

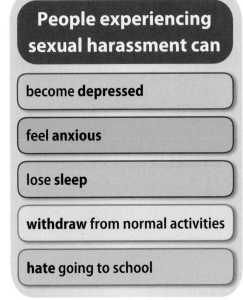

People experiencing sexual harassment can

become **depressed**

feel **anxious**

lose **sleep**

withdraw from normal activities

hate going to school

Figure 19.21 Unwanted sexual attention can cause negative health consequences for people experiencing it, including depression, anxiety, and insomnia. *What are the two types of sexual harassment?*

want the behavior to stop? If the answers to these questions are *yes*, you are experiencing sexual harassment.

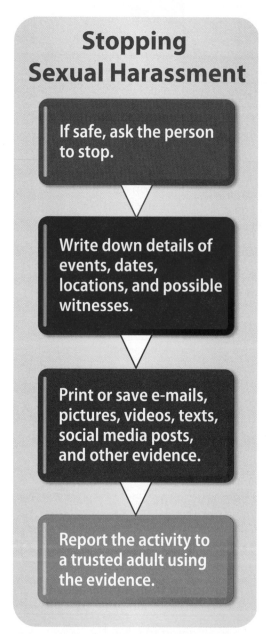

Stopping Sexual Harassment

If safe, ask the person to stop.

Write down details of events, dates, locations, and possible witnesses.

Print or save e-mails, pictures, videos, texts, social media posts, and other evidence.

Report the activity to a trusted adult using the evidence.

Figure 19.22 It can be intimidating to ask a person to stop harassing behavior. In these cases, try telling a trusted adult or asking a friend to accompany you. Only confront the person if you believe doing so is safe. Otherwise, talk to a trusted adult.

Responding to Harassment

People experiencing sexual harassment can take some steps to try to get the person to stop. Sexual harassment is a crime, and someone who harasses others can be arrested, found guilty, and put in prison. People who take steps to stop harassment could be helping more than just themselves (**Figure 19.22**). Someone who harasses one person is likely to harass others.

Most schools have a sexual harassment policy. At school, people can speak with their teachers, counselors, or principal to ask for help. If you are ever sexually harassed and you are not sure what to do, talk to a trusted adult.

If you see someone being sexually harassed, you can take steps to be an upstander or ally and help. Speak up and tell the person who is harassing someone to stop. Try to get the person experiencing the harassment away. If you feel unsafe or uncomfortable getting involved, tell a teacher or principal. Upstanders and allies play an important role in stopping sexual harassment. In addition, creating awareness of what sexual harassment is and promoting a safe and respectful environment can help reduce harassment.

Sexual Assault

Threatening or forcing someone into sexual activity is **sexual assault**. Sexual assault is a type of *sexual violence*, or sexual behaviors that occur without consent. Other examples of sexual violence are intimate partner violence, sexual abuse, and stalking. Sexual assault is illegal and occurs whenever there is sexual activity without consent. One example of a sexual assault crime is **rape**, or sexual intercourse that happens without consent. **Figure 19.23** states additional examples of behaviors that are sexual assault.

Laws prohibit sexual activity between older people and adolescents considered incapable of giving consent. The crime of **statutory rape** occurs when someone over the age of consent has sex with someone under the age of consent. The older person can be charged with statutory rape even if the younger person agrees to have sex. For example, if the age of consent in a state is 16, a 17-year-old who has sex with someone under the age of consent could be charged with statutory rape.

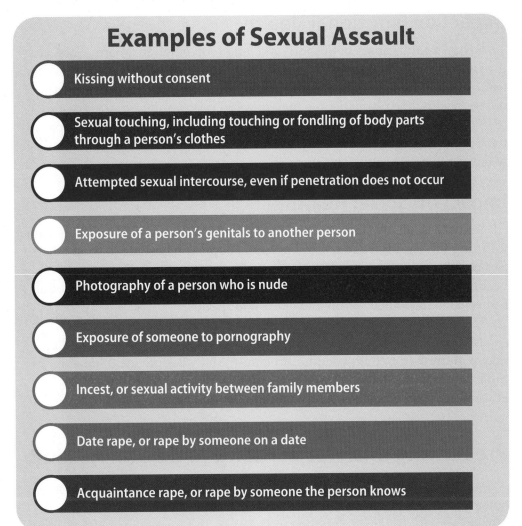

Examples of Sexual Assault

- Kissing without consent
- Sexual touching, including touching or fondling of body parts through a person's clothes
- Attempted sexual intercourse, even if penetration does not occur
- Exposure of a person's genitals to another person
- Photography of a person who is nude
- Exposure of someone to pornography
- Incest, or sexual activity between family members
- Date rape, or rape by someone on a date
- Acquaintance rape, or rape by someone the person knows

Figure 19.23
All of these examples are sexual assault if they occur without consent that is clearly and freely given.

Although sexual assault involves violence of a sexual nature, experts say that it is not an act of sex, but an act of power and aggression. People who commit sexual assault use force, violence, weapons, or alcohol and drugs to make people submit to sexual acts. More males than females carry out sexual assault, and more females than males experience sexual assault. Both males and females, however, can commit sexual assault or experience sexual assault.

Effects of Sexual Assault

Sexual assault can harm the health and well-being of people who experienced the assault, not just immediately but for years. Sexual assault can also have lasting and harmful effects on a person's family, friends, and community.

Impact on Physical Health

Sexual assault can lead to physical health conditions. Physical injuries can include bruises, broken bones, and pain in affected parts of the body. People who experienced the assault might develop frequent headaches and have difficulty sleeping. Finally, sexual assault can lead to an unwanted pregnancy or an STI.

Impact on Emotional Health

Sexual assault causes both short- and long-term emotional harm. Soon after the attack, many people who experienced sexual assault feel shock, denial, fear, anxiety, shame, guilt, and confusion. These symptoms may disappear or lessen with time. Some people may develop post-traumatic stress disorder (PTSD) or become depressed (**Figure 19.24**). Some people attempt to cope with the trauma by engaging in risky behaviors. By doing so, they increase the risk of having further health conditions.

Impact on Social Health

Sexual assault also harms a person's social health, especially if the person inflicting the assault was a trusted person. People can hesitate to trust others as a result of sexual assault. This hesitance can prevent them from forming healthy, intimate relationships. Some people who experienced sexual assault feel isolated from their family members and friends.

Though they are not to blame for sexual assault, some people who experienced it feel shame and guilt. Their self-esteem goes down, and they may withdraw from their friends and family. Many people fear blame or punishment if they tell others. As a result, they do not report the assault to law-enforcement officials, friends, and family members.

Preventing and Responding to Sexual Assault

You are in charge of your health and the decisions that promote it. Others, however, can exert a powerful influence on your decisions. The best way to prevent sexual assault is to understand consent and treat others with respect (**Figure 19.25**). Additional methods include avoiding risky situations and knowing how to respond to sexual assault.

Avoiding Risky Situations

Avoid situations that increase the risk of sexual assault. An example is being alone with someone in an unfamiliar place or without adult supervision,

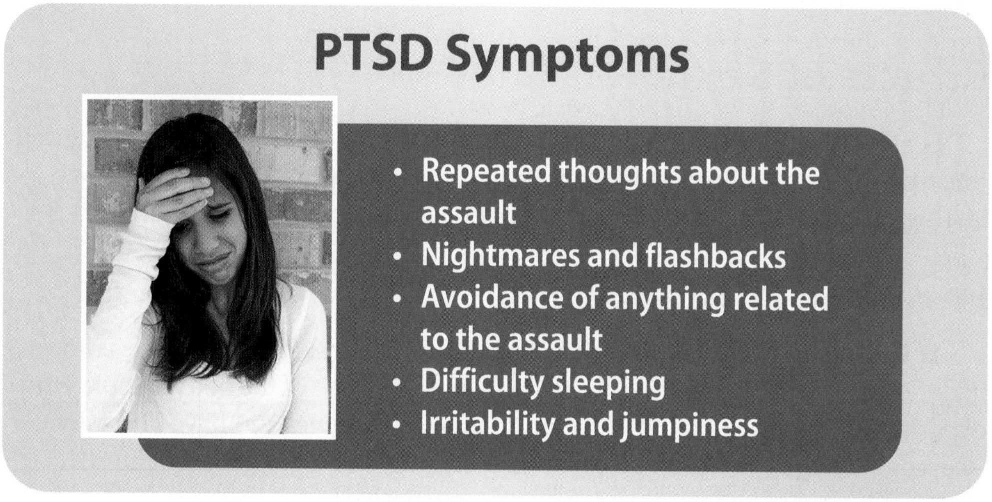

Figure 19.24
Anxiety, depression, shame, confusion, and shock are all possible symptoms for a person who experienced sexual assault. In some cases, a person may even develop PTSD. *What response to trauma can increase the risk of further health conditions?*

PTSD Symptoms

- Repeated thoughts about the assault
- Nightmares and flashbacks
- Avoidance of anything related to the assault
- Difficulty sleeping
- Irritability and jumpiness

Tracy Whiteside/Shutterstock.com

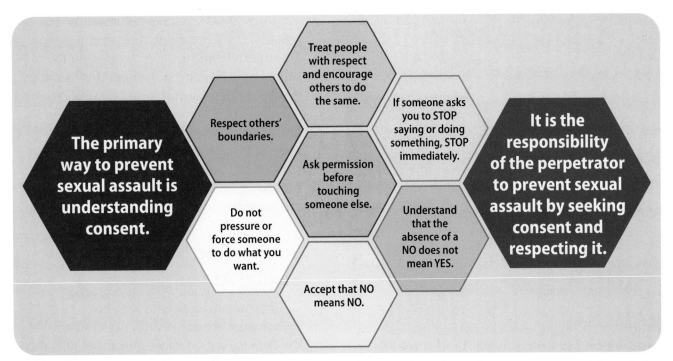

Figure 19.25 Seek consent by asking permission before touching someone else, and respect that person's boundaries by not pressuring them to do what you want.

whether you know the person or not. Never go alone to unfamiliar, isolated places with people you do not know well. If a situation makes you uncomfortable or you are pressured to do something you do not want to do, leave the situation and call a friend, parent or guardian, or other trusted adult immediately.

Another risky situation involves the use of alcohol or drugs. These substances weaken a person's ability to think clearly, sense danger, and to resist or understand consent. They also weaken *inhibitions*, or the limits placed on behavior by one's values or conscience. Staying away from situations that involve alcohol and drugs is a good way to avoid this risk.

Responding to Sexual Assault

If people experience or are threatened with sexual assault, they can try to fight back. If possible, they should run away from their attackers and try to get help. Otherwise, they may be able to scare off their attacker by struggling against them or attacking back. Physical and verbal resistance greatly reduce the risk of injury during sexual assault.

In the event of a sexual assault, a person should immediately get to a safe place and call 911 or the National Sexual Assault Hotline (800-656-4673) for help. It is important to get medical attention right away at a hospital or clinic. The person will receive an examination, treatment for physical injuries, and tests for STIs. Medication can be given to decrease the risk of an STI or pregnancy.

Sexual assault is a crime and should be reported to law enforcement. Police can only arrest the person who committed the assault if they know what occurred and can collect evidence. As a result, a person who experiences sexual assault should not change clothes or shower before going to the police station or hospital. Professionals can gather evidence from clothes and hair.

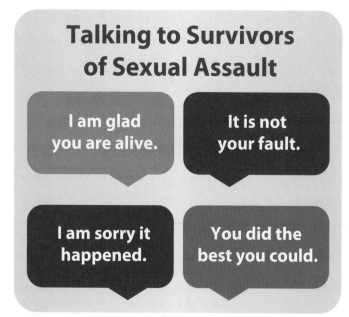

Talking to Survivors of Sexual Assault

I am glad you are alive.

It is not your fault.

I am sorry it happened.

You did the best you could.

Figure 19.26 Sometimes, it can be hard to know what to say to a survivor of sexual assault. The messages in this illustration can be helpful and can convey that you care. *Who is never to blame for an attack of sexual assault?*

Many people who experienced sexual assault find it helpful to receive counseling. Some people find support by talking to others who have been through this trauma. A school nurse, doctor, or local crisis center can provide information about counselors and local support groups. People might also find it useful to talk to other adults they trust. Parents or guardians, a family physician, community leaders, and teachers are examples.

Supporting Survivors of Sexual Assault

If you know a person who has experienced sexual assault, understand that the person may or may not want to talk about the attack. Follow the person's lead and do not ask too many questions. Try to be a good listener and do not judge or blame the person for what happened (**Figure 19.26**). Encourage the person to seek professional help or talk to a trusted adult. Remember, the person who experienced sexual assault is never to blame.

Lesson 19.3 Review

1. _____ is a direct, verbal, freely given agreement that occurs when someone clearly says yes.
2. **True or false.** Spreading sexual rumors about a person is sexual harassment.
3. How does sexual assault impact physical health?
4. Why are situations that include drugs or alcohol risky?
5. **Critical thinking.** If someone asks to kiss your friend, and your friend looks away, is this consent? Why or why not?

Hands-On Activity

For this activity, imagine that you are in the scenarios below. On a separate sheet of paper, describe how you would respond to each scenario. Then, share your answers with a partner and discuss other ways to respond.

Scenario 1: At a party, your partner wants to escape together to a quiet room. Lately, your partner has been pressuring you to have sex. You care about your partner, but are not interested in having sex.

Scenario 2: In class, a student beside you starts to make sexual comments and compliments about you. The comments make you feel uncomfortable.

Review and Assessment

Summary

Lesson 19.1 **What Is Sexuality?**

- Sexuality is the expression of a person's gender through behavior and physical characteristics. It includes biological sex, gender and gender identity, sexual orientation, and sexual experiences and thoughts.
- Biological sex is determined by sex chromosomes (XX or XY). Some babies are born with a DSD. Sometimes, rare conditions can cause people to develop sex organs that do not match the sex chromosomes.
- Gender refers to the characteristics a society associates with a particular biological sex. A person's internal, deeply held thoughts and feelings about gender is gender identity. Gender identity develops early in life, and some people may be transgender or nonbinary.
- Sexual orientation refers to the continuing pattern of romantic and sexual attraction. Examples of some sexual orientations include heterosexual, homosexual, bisexual, and asexual.

Lesson 19.2 **Sexual Feelings and Behavior**

- During puberty, hormones change a child's body into that of an adult. Sex hormones target parts of the body related to sexual maturity. Early sexual feelings also emerge during puberty and can cause arousal.
- Physical consequences of sexual activity include pregnancy and STIs. Emotional and social consequences include loss of trust, less personal growth, jealousy, and feelings of guilt and shame.
- Abstinence is a healthy decision young people can make about sexual activity. It reduces negative consequences of sexual activity and helps a romantic relationship thrive. Refusal skills can help young people remain abstinent.

Lesson 19.3 **Unwanted Sexual Activity**

- Affirmative consent is a direct, verbal, and freely given agreement that occurs when someone clearly says *yes*. Consent is important in healthy relationships.
- Sexual harassment is unwanted sexual attention, or sexual attention that occurs without consent. It can be verbal or nonverbal. People can respond to sexual harassment by intervening or by documenting the person's actions.
- Sexual assault is threatening or forcing someone into sexual activity. It is illegal and a crime.
- Sexual assault has serious consequences for physical, emotional, and social health. It can cause physical injuries and can lead to intense anxiety and depression.
- Sexual assault is never the fault of the person who experienced it. One way to help prevent sexual assault is to avoid risky situations. If a sexual assault has occurred, the person should call 911 immediately and seek medical help. People can support survivors of sexual assault by listening and being supportive.

Check Your Knowledge

Record your answers to each of the following questions on a separate sheet of paper.

1. What are the four aspects of sexuality?
2. **True or false.** Babies with DSD have sex organs that are obviously male.
3. What does it mean to be transgender?
4. Which of the following is an irrational fear of homosexuality?
   A. Homophobia.
   B. Heterosexuality.
   C. Bisexuality.
   D. Masculinity.
5. Explain how hormones trigger the process of puberty.
6. Which of the following is a primary sexual characteristic?
   A. Breast development.
   B. Pubic hair.
   C. Muscle development.
   D. Ovary maturation.
7. **True or false.** Sexual intercourse can lead to pregnancy if a sperm fertilizes an egg.
8. Why is sexual abstinence a healthy choice for young people?
9. Under what circumstances can people *not* give consent?
10. ___ sexual harassment includes the use of words, gossip, and threats.
11. **True or false.** Some people who experience sexual assault develop PTSD.
12. Which of the following should a person who experienced sexaul assault do first?
    A. Change clothes.
    B. Take a shower.
    C. Call 911.
    D. Receive counseling.
13. **True or false.** A good way to support a person who has experienced sexual assault is to follow the person's lead in talking about the attack.

Use Your Vocabulary ↗

age of consent	gender roles	sexual intercourse
arousal	growth spurt	sexuality
biological sex	homophobia	sexual orientation
consent	masturbation	statutory rape
disorder of sex	rape	transgender
development (DSD)	sexual assault	wet dreams
gender	sexual	
gender identity	harassment	

14. Quickly write a word you think relates to each term shown in the list above. In small groups, exchange papers. Have each person in the group explain a term on the list. Take turns until all terms have complete explanations.
15. With a partner, choose two terms from the list above to compare. Create a Venn diagram. Write one term under the left circle and the other term under the right. List differences in each of the circles. Where the circles overlap, write three characteristics the terms have in common. Share your Venn diagram with another pair that chose different terms from yours. As a small group, discuss the differences and common characteristics for each set of terms.

Think Critically

16. **Cause and effect.** How do television, media, music, and pop culture shape expectations for gender in society? How do these expectations influence how people act and express their gender?

17. **Draw conclusions.** Why might it be challenging to accept others with sexualities different from yours? How can people overcome these prejudices and influences?

18. **Identify.** List the reasons that young people may find it awkward or difficult to talk about their sexuality or ask questions about their sexual health. How could young people and adults make these situations less awkward?

19. **Make inferences.** Why might it be difficult for a young person to refuse unwanted sexual activity in a relationship? Explain your answer.

DEVELOP Your Skills

20. **Communication skills.** It is normal to have questions about your sexual health. Asking questions can help you get accurate information. Create a list of at least five questions you have about your sexual health. Then, choose a trusted adult with whom you feel comfortable and ask these questions. If you do not feel comfortable initiating this conversation, write a letter to the trusted adult. In your letter, ask your questions and request a time to talk. Write a summary reflecting on the conversation and the information you learned.

21. **Accessing information skills.** Research local resources and reliable websites that provide accurate information about sexual health. Choose one local resource and one website to present to the class. Create a digital presentation describing your chosen resources and the benefits of using them. Then, present this information to the class.

22. **Advocacy skills.** Create a poster or flyer advocating for abstinence and healthy relationships. On your poster or flyer, list five benefits of abstinence, five ways of showing affection that do not involve sexual activity, and five qualities of a healthy relationship. With teacher permission, hang your poster or flyer in your classroom or in a school hall.

23. **Refusal skills.** Imagine that you are in a relationship. Your partner is trying to persuade you to have sex, but you are not ready. Your partner uses the statements below to convince you. With a classmate, write your response to each statement. Then, practice assertively responding to the statement with your classmate.

> Come on, everyone else is having sex.

> It's not that big of a deal. I love you, and we are going to be together forever.

> What are you waiting for? Sex is not that big of a deal.

> I'm with you. You should trust me. I'm not going to hurt you.

Chapter
20

Making Responsible Sexual Decisions

Essential Question

How can young people make responsible decisions about sexual activity?

Lesson 20.1 Pregnancy Prevention

Lesson 20.2 Teen Pregnancy and Parenthood

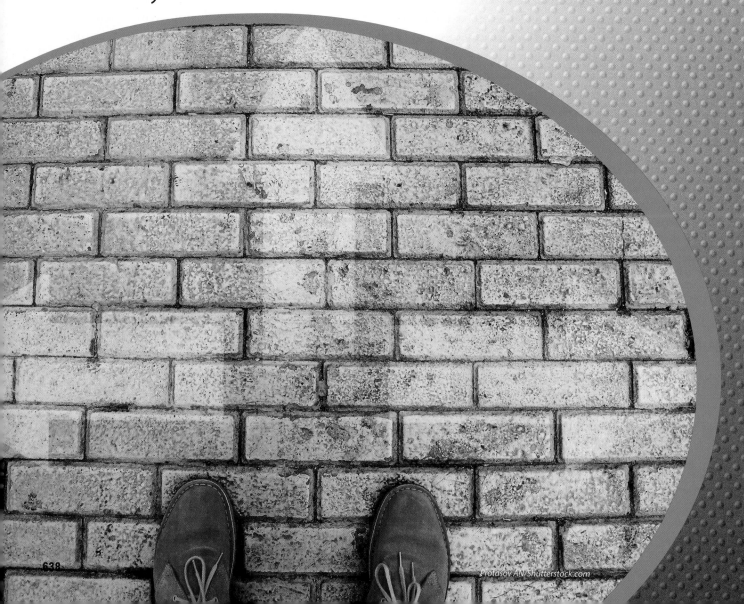

Protasov AN/Shutterstock.com

Reading Activity

Based on your own knowledge, list what you think are the best methods to prevent pregnancy. As you read this chapter, list the methods as noted in the text. After you finish reading the chapter, compare the two lists. In what ways are they similar and different? What do you think is the most effective method of preventing pregnancy? Write a paragraph to summarize your findings.

How Healthy Are You?

In this chapter, you will be learning about responsible sexual decisions, pregnancy prevention, and teen pregnancy and parenthood. Before you begin reading, take the following quiz to assess your current understanding of responsible sexual behavior.

Health Concepts to Understand	Yes	No
Do you understand how sexual intercourse leads to pregnancy?		
Can you differentiate between myths and facts about pregnancy prevention?		
Can you explain how abstinence is the most effective form of birth control?		
Do you know the difference between the external and internal condom?		
Can you explain how the birth control pill uses hormones to prevent pregnancy?		
Do you know why withdrawal is an ineffective form of birth control?		
Can you explain what options people have for unplanned pregnancy?		
Do you know the challenges of teen pregnancy for the parents and the child?		
Can you explain how teen parenthood affects parents, children, families, and society?		
Do you understand the benefits of abstinence?		

Count your "Yes" and "No" responses. The more "Yes" responses you have, the more you understand about making responsible sexual decisions. Now, take a closer look at the questions with which you responded "No." Think about how you can increase your understanding of issues in this area. Develop your health literacy skills by accessing valid information about each of the concepts you do not understand. Evaluate any health websites you find using the information in Figure 1.16 of this text. If you do not understand the instructions, ask for clarification from your teacher.

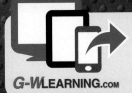

Click on the activity icon or visit www.g-wlearning.com/health to access online vocabulary activities using key terms from the chapter.

G-WLEARNING.com

Pregnancy Prevention

Key Terms 📤

contraception any method that reduces the risk of pregnancy resulting from sexual intercourse; also called *birth control*

external condom object worn over erect penis during sexual activity

internal condom device similar to a pouch, which is placed inside the vagina or rectum

oral contraceptives pills that contain hormones to reduce the likelihood of pregnancy

birth control patch thin, 2- to 3-inch, plastic patch applied to the skin that works like a birth control pill

vaginal ring small, flexible ring that releases hormones to stop ovulation

withdrawal natural birth control method based on the male pulling out of the female's vagina before ejaculation

emergency contraception contraceptive method used to prevent pregnancy when other contraception has failed

sterilization permanent birth control method in which a medical doctor performs a procedure on either a male or female to prevent sperm and egg from uniting

abortion procedure to end a pregnancy

Learning Outcomes

After studying this lesson, you will be able to

- **recognize** pregnancy prevention facts and myths.
- **identify** the benefits of continuous abstinence.
- **explain** how effective barrier methods are in preventing pregnancy.
- **identify** hormonal birth control methods.
- **describe** natural birth control methods.
- **determine** what options are available when contraception fails.
- **summarize** sterilization procedures.
- **identify** different options available for people who experience unplanned pregnancies.

Graphic Organizer

Birth Control

Before reading this lesson, draw a rectangle on a separate piece of paper. Write the words *Birth Control* in the rectangle. As you read, list general facts about birth control above the rectangle. Take notes about different methods of birth control below the rectangle. An example is shown.

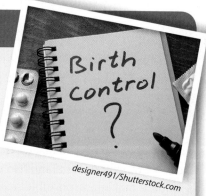

designer491/Shutterstock.com

Birth control is called <u>contraception</u>
Reliable information can come from healthcare professionals

Birth Control

Abstinence—refraining from sexual activity

Pregnancy and raising children can be among the most rewarding and meaningful experiences in a person's life. In fact, 13-year-old Esmeralda dreams of someday having her own family. She loves her baby brother and likes to babysit him and some other children in the neighborhood. Esmeralda looks forward to someday being a parent taking care of her own children. From talking with her parents, however, she knows that pregnancy and parenting are permanent decisions that require much thought and careful planning.

In her health class, Esmeralda learned that vaginal sexual intercourse always carries with it the risk of pregnancy. During vaginal sexual intercourse, a male's sperm can enter the female's vagina and reach an egg. The sperm may fertilize the egg, causing pregnancy (**Figure 20.1**). Sexually transmitted infections (STIs) are also a risk of any sexual intercourse. These physical consequences and other social and emotional consequences can significantly alter a person's life. To guard against these consequences, Esmeralda knows it is important to make responsible sexual decisions.

In this lesson, you will learn about pregnancy and contraception. **Contraception**, also called *birth control*, is any method that reduces the risk of pregnancy resulting from sexual activity. Many birth control methods exist. They differ, however, in how effective they are and in whether they also protect against STIs. Choosing a birth control method is a matter of understanding pregnancy prevention and making a careful decision.

Myths and Facts About Pregnancy Prevention

Many myths exist about pregnancy and sexual intercourse. A good way to avoid falling for myths is to learn the facts about reproduction and pregnancy prevention. **Figure 20.2** on the next page lists some common myths and facts about pregnancy.

The best way to learn the facts about birth control is to talk to a healthcare professional. These trained specialists will be able to discuss different methods honestly and objectively. A family doctor or school nurse can also answer some of these questions. When using other sources of information, such as a

Development of the Fetus

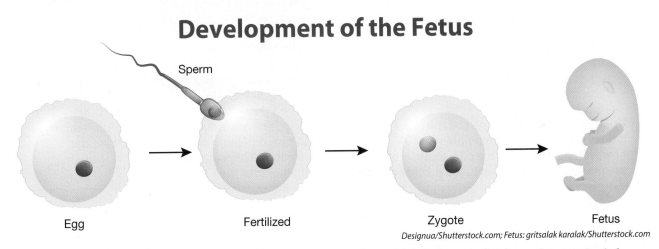

Sperm

Egg   Fertilized   Zygote   Fetus

Designua/Shutterstock.com; Fetus: gritsalak karalak/Shutterstock.com

Figure 20.1 During pregnancy, a fertilized egg develops into a fetus. *What is the term for the various methods for reducing the risk of pregnancy?*

Myths and Facts of Pregnancy Prevention

Myth

Females younger than 18 years of age cannot become pregnant.

Fact

Females younger than 18 years of age *can* and *do* become pregnant. A female who has begun menstruating can become pregnant regardless of the age.

Myth

A female cannot become pregnant the first time a couple has sex.

Fact

A female *can* become pregnant the first time the couple has sex.

Myth

A female who urinates after sex will not get pregnant.

Fact

Urinating after sex does *not* prevent pregnancy.

Myth

Pregnancy will not occur if a couple uses contraception during sex.

Fact

Using contraception reduces the risk of pregnancy. It does not completely eliminate that risk, however. Abstinence is the only method of pregnancy prevention that is 100 percent effective.

Myth

A female cannot become pregnant if the male withdraws the penis before ejaculating.

Fact

A female *can* become pregnant even if a male withdraws before ejaculation. The penis often releases some sperm before ejaculation.

Myth

Pregnancy will not occur if a female stands up during sexual intercourse.

Fact

A female *can* become pregnant no matter the position during sexual intercourse.

Myth

A female cannot become pregnant while menstruating.

Fact

A female *can* become pregnant while menstruating. It is unlikely, but possible.

Myth

A female who *douches*, or cleans the inside of the vagina, after sex will not get pregnant.

Fact

Douching after sex does *not* prevent pregnancy. In fact, douching can actually increase the likelihood of pregnancy by pushing semen deeper into the vagina.

Figure 20.2 Widespread myths about pregnancy can cause young people to be misinformed about their sexual health and can lead to unhealthy behaviors. *Who is the best person to speak to about the myths and facts of pregnancy?*

healthcare website, always assess each source's credibility (**Figure 20.3**). It is important to have accurate information about birth control.

Birth Control Methods

Birth control methods help prevent pregnancy, and some also protect against STIs. Each birth control method has its advantages and disadvantages. A person should consider personal goals when selecting a method. Cost and availability should also be considered. Some methods are inexpensive and can be obtained without a doctor's prescription. Other methods require a doctor's visit. Some people want to use a reversible method of birth control so they can choose to have children in the future. Others would prefer a permanent method.

Each method is effective only when used correctly every time. Because of this, ease of use is also an important factor. Some types of birth control include abstinence, barrier methods, hormonal methods and intrauterine devices (IUDs), natural methods, and sterilization. Only one of these methods is 100 perfect effective in preventing pregnancy and STIs.

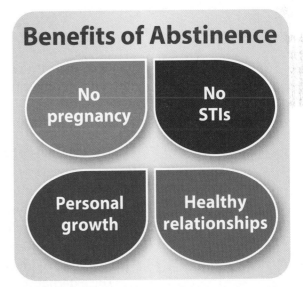

Finding Reliable Sources

Does the source have medical expertise?

What is the mission or objective of the source?

Does the source describe alternatives?

Is the source a profit-making organization?

Figure 20.3
Illustrated here are some questions you can ask to assess the reliability of a source.

Abstinence

The only contraceptive method that is 100 percent effective in preventing pregnancy is *abstinence*, which is the decision to not engage in sexual activity. Abstinence also prevents STI transmission and encourages young people's social and emotional growth. Abstinence helps young people pursue their goals and grow personally. Unlike other methods of birth control, it is free and always available. There are no risks involved in using abstinence, and abstinence is reversible, meaning that people can choose to have children later in life.

Abstinence has many benefits, which you learned about in the previous chapter (**Figure 20.4**). It helps romantic relationships thrive and helps young people focus on themselves and their future goals. Continuous abstinence is guaranteed to prevent pregnancy and STIs. Abstinence is a healthy, responsible sexual decision that young people can choose.

Benefits of Abstinence

No pregnancy

No STIs

Personal growth

Healthy relationships

Figure 20.4 Abstinence is a responsible sexual decision adolescents can make. Some of the benefits are listed here. *How effective is abstinence in preventing pregnancy?*

Barrier Methods

Barrier methods of birth control physically reduce the risk of fertilization by preventing sperm from reaching the egg. Each barrier method has its advantages and disadvantages, and some methods are more effective than others. Also, not all methods protect users from contracting STIs. Barrier

Aparna Chooses Abstinence

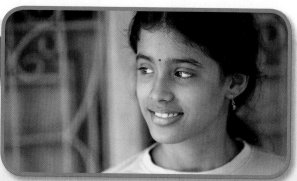

v.s.anandhakrishna/Shutterstock.com

Today, Aparna is choosing abstinence. She knows that her body is her own and is choosing not to have sex. Three months ago, Aparna started dating Juan, a classmate from school. After an open conversation, Aparna and Juan made the decision to start having sex. Everything was going well until Aparna missed her period. Due to the missed period, Aparna began to think she was pregnant. She immediately told Juan, and the two began to discuss the possibility of a child. They were both nervous of how this will affect their schooling and personal lives. They also discussed whether they would raise the child or place the child for adoption. A few days later, Aparna got her period.

Today, Aparna and Juan decided together to remain abstinent. They decided to wait to engage in sexual activity until they are both older and are more ready in the future. They are instead choosing to focus on themselves, school, friends, and family relationships. In addition, they are finding new ways to strengthen their relationship without sexual activity.

Thinking Critically

1. Why are Aparna and Juan choosing abstinence? Do you think they will succeed at staying abstinent? Why or why not?

2. If you were Aparna's friend, what advice would you give her about remaining abstinent in relationships?

3. If Aparna had been pregnant, how could her life have changed? How could Juan's life have changed?

4. What other ways can Aparna and Juan show affection in their relationship without engaging in sexual activity?

methods of birth control include external condoms, internal condoms, the contraceptive sponge, the diaphragm, and the cervical cap.

External Condom

The **external condom**, sometimes called the *male condom*, is worn over the penis during sexual intercourse. It is 85 percent effective in preventing pregnancy by catching the semen released during ejaculation and preventing sperm from reaching the egg. Condoms also protect against STIs. They are made from latex, *polyurethane* (forms of plastic), or *polyisoprene* (latex-free rubber). They can also be made of sheepskin or lambskin, but these condoms are not effective in reducing the risk of STIs.

The external condom fits over the erect penis and must be applied after an erection and before the penis touches the sexual partner's genitals (**Figure 20.5**). This is important because the penis can release fluids prior to ejaculation. Those fluids can contain sperm and microorganisms that cause STIs. Some condoms are coated with *spermicide*, a substance that stops sperm from swimming and reaching the egg.

Condoms cannot be reused. A new one must be used each time intercourse occurs. External condoms become dry, brittle, and ineffective over time. Because of this, each package comes with an expiration date. Damaged or expired condoms are not effective in reducing the risk of pregnancy or STIs.

Benefits of Abstinence from Sexual Activity

Allows time to wait until a person is ready

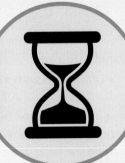

Prevents pregnancy

24/7

Always available

Prevents STI transmission; has no medical side effects

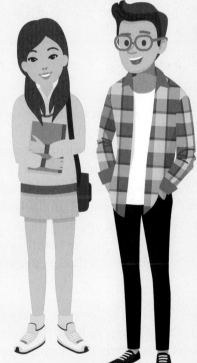

Promotes personal growth and healthy relationships

Does not cost any money

Girl: Irina Strelnikova/Shutterstock.com; Boy: Olga1818/Shutterstock.com; Icons, clockwise from top: Francois Poirier/Shutterstock.com; Suphalak Rueksanthitiwong/Shutterstock.com; Puckung/Shutterstock.com; 3D Vector/Shutterstock.com; CB studio/Shutterstock.com; A Aleksii/Shutterstock.com

Figure 20.5
People can practice applying the external condom by putting it over an object shaped like a penis.
What material makes a condom less effective in preventing the transmission of STIs?

Using the External Condom

The following steps are used to apply and remove an external condom:

1. Gently tear open the package at its edge. Do not use teeth or scissors to do this. If the package is wet or sticky, throw it out.
2. Determine which way the condom unrolls.
3. Pinch the condom tip to remove air. This prevents breakage when the condom fills with semen.
4. Place the condom at the tip of the erect penis and roll it to the base of the penis.
5. Apply some water-based lubricant if the condom is not lubricated. Never use petroleum-based lubricants with a latex condom. These substances will break down the latex barrier.
6. After intercourse, the penis must be removed from the partner's genitals before it softens. Otherwise, the condom can fall off and spill semen. When removing from the penis, hold the base of the condom securely while withdrawing. This will keep the condom from coming off the penis.
7. Pull off the condom and dispose of it in the trash. Wash your hands. Never reuse a condom.

The Internal Condom

The **internal condom**, sometimes called the *female condom*, is a device similar to a pouch, which is placed inside the vagina or rectum (**Figure 20.6**). They are made of plastic and must be inserted before the penis touches a partner's genitals. The internal condom reduces the risk of pregnancy by 79 percent by catching semen and preventing sperm from entering the vagina. It also forms a barrier against STIs. The effectiveness of internal condoms can be improved by using spermicide or by withdrawing the penis before ejaculation. It should not be worn with an external condom since friction between the two condoms reduces effectiveness.

Contraceptive Sponge

The *contraceptive sponge* reduces the risk of pregnancy by 88 percent for people who have never given birth. It helps block sperm from entering the uterus. The

Figure 20.6
The internal condom is the only female birth control method that prevents pregnancy and STIs.

Using the Internal Condom

The following steps are used to insert and remove an internal condom:

1. Apply spermicide to the end of the condom that will face the uterus.
2. Squeeze the inner ring at the closed end of the condom and push it into the vagina as deep as it will go. The outer ring should rest about 1 inch outside the vagina.
3. Hold the outer ring against the vaginal opening while the penis is inserted. Make sure the penis does not slide outside the internal condom.
4. After intercourse, hold the outer ring against the vaginal opening as the penis is withdrawn.
5. Twist the end of the condom to trap semen inside and prevent spillage.
6. Pull the condom out of the vagina and discard it in the trash. Never reuse a condom.

sponge contains spermicide, which stops sperm from swimming. It does not protect against STIs. Therefore, the female's partner should still wear a condom.

The sponge is made of plastic foam and is about 2 inches in diameter. The sponge is inserted into the vagina and covers the cervix. It can be inserted several hours before sexual intercourse and should be left in place at least six hours after intercourse. It can remain in the body for 30 hours.

Diaphragm

The *diaphragm* is a flexible, cup-shaped disk that covers the cervix and helps block sperm from entering the uterus. Unlike condoms and sponges, a diaphragm requires an exam and prescription. The diaphragm comes with directions for insertion, removal, and care. A person must use it each time intercourse occurs and cover it with spermicide before insertion. The diaphragm is 88 percent effective in preventing pregnancy. It does not protect against STIs, however.

Cervical Cap

The *cervical cap* is a flexible cup that covers the cervix (**Figure 20.7**). Like the diaphragm, the cervical cap helps block sperm from entering the uterus and requires a prescription from a doctor or other healthcare professional. It comes with directions for insertion, removal, and care. It must be covered with spermicide and inserted before intercourse. The cervical cap should stay in place at least six hours after intercourse, but should not remain in the body more than 48 hours. For people who have never given birth, it is 86 percent effective in preventing pregnancy.

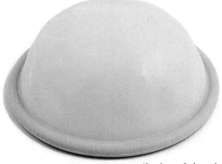

iStock.com/Lalocracio

Figure 20.7
The cervical cap is made of silicone and works best for people who have never given birth. *What is the maximum amount of time a cervical cap should remain in the body?*

Hormonal Methods and IUDs

Hormones are chemicals in the body that control many body functions, including reproduction. When used medically, the female hormones estrogen and progestin can inhibit ovulation and help prevent pregnancy. These hormones can also treat some medical conditions, such as severe menstrual pain. These methods use hormones to influence only the female reproductive system. Research is ongoing to identify hormonal methods for males, however.

Oral Contraceptives

Oral contraceptives, also called *birth control pills* or *the pill*, contain hormones that reduce the risk of pregnancy by preventing ovulation. If ovulation does not occur, there is no egg for a sperm to fertilize.

The pill is taken by mouth, or *orally*, at about the same time every day. It is 91 percent effective at preventing pregnancy if taken *exactly as prescribed by the doctor*. Skipping even one pill increases the chance of becoming pregnant. Oral contraceptives do not protect against STIs.

People must have a medical exam before using the pill. This is because females with certain medical conditions should not take the pill. A prescription written by a healthcare professional is needed to purchase the pill. The pill comes in two basic forms: the combination pill and the progestin-only pill (**Figure 20.8**).

Types of Birth Control Pills	
Type	**Description**
Combination pill (pack of 28)	A female using the 28-pill pack takes active pills for three weeks, then inactive pills for one week. The last seven pills have no effect. During the week a female takes inactive pills, menstruation should occur.
Combination pill (pack of 21)	A female using the 21-pill pack takes active pills for three weeks and then no pills for one week. Her period should begin during that week. After that week, she starts a new 21-pill pack.
Combination pill (pack of 91)	A female using the 91-pill pack only menstruates once every three months. She takes active pills for 12 weeks and then takes inactive pills for one week.
Continuous pill (pack of 365)	A type of combination pill that contains 365 active pills that are taken each day. Also known as *extended-cycle birth control*.
Progestin-only pill	The progestin-only pill comes in a 28-pill pack. All the pills contain active hormones.

Birth Control Patch

The **birth control patch** (often called the *patch*) is a thin, 2- to 3-inch, plastic patch applied to the skin like a bandage. The patch uses the hormones estrogen and progestin to prevent ovulation. It works like the birth control pill, except hormones are absorbed from the patch through the skin and into the blood. The patch comes with directions. A female typically wears one patch a week for three weeks. No patch is worn during the fourth week as menstruation should occur. The patch is 91 percent effective in pregnancy prevention.

Vaginal Ring

The **vaginal ring** is a small, flexible ring that releases estrogen and progestin to stop ovulation (**Figure 20.9**). It is inserted into the vagina and left in place for three weeks. Three weeks after insertion, the ring should be removed, ideally at the same time as it was inserted. The ring is discarded, and no ring is used during the fourth week. During this fourth week, menstruation should occur. The vaginal ring comes with directions for storage, insertion, and removal and is 91 percent effective in preventing pregnancy.

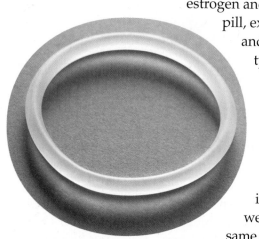

Image Point Fr/Shutterstock.com

Figure 20.9
The vaginal ring releases hormones that stop ovulation and thicken cervical mucus. *What happens during the week that the vaginal ring is not used?*

Birth Control Shot

The *birth control shot* is an injection of the hormone progestin. This injection stops ovulation and reduces the risk of pregnancy by 94 percent. A female must see a healthcare professional to receive the shot every three months. Depending on the type of shot, it can be given in the arm, in the buttocks, or under the skin.

Birth Control Implant

The *birth control implant* is a flexible, toothpick-sized rod that holds progestin. A doctor inserts the implant under the skin of the upper arm.

The implant releases progestin, which stops ovulation. It can be left in place for three years. The implant is 99 percent effective in preventing pregnancy.

Intrauterine Device (IUD)

An *intrauterine device (IUD)* is a small, T-shaped device that is inserted into the uterus by a doctor (**Figure 20.10**). Two types of IUDs exist: copper IUDs and hormonal IUDs. The copper IUD is thought to interfere with sperm movement, fertilization, and implantation. Hormonal IUDs thicken cervical mucus and inhibit ovulation. IUDs last for years, and hormonal IUDs can reduce menstrual cramps and significantly lighten or even stop menstruation. IUDs are 99 percent effective at preventing pregnancy. Both types of IUDs can be removed if a female wants to become pregnant.

Natural Methods

Natural methods of birth control do not use barriers or hormones. Some people prefer these natural methods. Natural methods include the fertility awareness method (FAM) and withdrawal.

Fertility Awareness Method (FAM)

The *fertility awareness method (FAM)* relies on the natural rhythm of a female's fertility. Couples use FAM to track when ovulation occurs and which days the egg can be fertilized. By not having intercourse on those days, they try to practice birth control.

The best way to determine when pregnancy is more likely to occur is to identify which day female ovulation occurs. A female can use several methods to know when ovulation will happen, such as tracking changes in body temperature or the mucus in the vagina. The female can also track menstruation dates on a calendar or app (**Figure 20.11**).

FAM is only somewhat helpful for preventing pregnancy. It requires females to pay careful attention to changes in their bodies. Many couples who use FAM do not use the methods regularly and correctly. As a result, about 25 out of 100 couples using FAM become pregnant. Furthermore, FAM does not prevent STIs. FAM is best for couples who are married or in a committed, exclusive relationship. For these reasons, FAM is not recommended for adolescents.

Withdrawal

Withdrawal, or *pulling out*, is one of the least effective birth control methods when used alone. A male using this method pulls the penis out of the female's vagina before ejaculating. This may keep sperm out of the vagina and reduce the risk of pregnancy.

Withdrawal is not an effective method of birth control. It is difficult to time and is not always easy for a male to withdraw during sexual excitement.

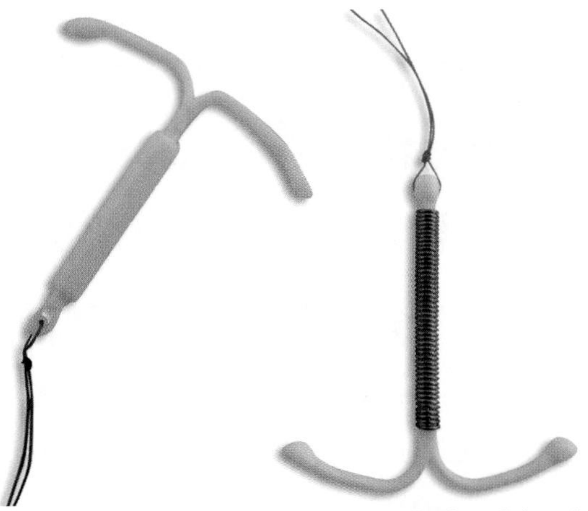

iStock.com/Lalocracio

Figure 20.10
IUDs fit inside the uterus. The two types of IUDs are hormonal (on the left) and copper (on the right). *Who inserts an IUD into the uterus?*

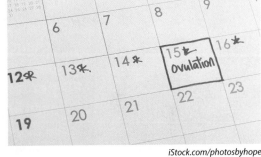

iStock.com/photosbyhope

Figure 20.11
Typically, a female can become pregnant three to five days before ovulation and on the first and possibly second day after ovulation. To avoid pregnancy, intercourse should not happen on these days. *Which form of pregnancy prevention requires this knowledge of fertility?*

Withdrawal is **not** an effective pregnancy prevention method.

According to the CDC, **22 out of 100** people experience an unplanned pregnancy using withdrawal.

Figure 20.12 Rates of pregnancy using withdrawal are high compared to rates using other birth control methods.

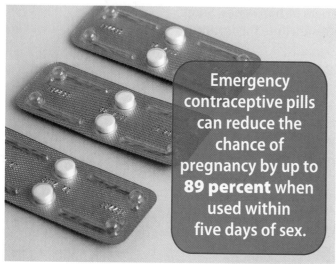

Emergency contraceptive pills can reduce the chance of pregnancy by up to **89 percent** when used within five days of sex.

Addyvanich/Shutterstock.com

Figure 20.13 Emergency contraception can help prevent pregnancy if other forms of pregnancy prevention fail. *Can emergency contraception stop or interrupt a pregnancy that has already occurred?*

Fluid containing sperm often leaks from the penis before ejaculation and can cause pregnancy (**Figure 20.12**). Withdrawal also does not protect people from STIs.

Emergency Contraception

Even when partners agree to use birth control and try to use it correctly, mistakes can happen. In these cases, a person might use **emergency contraception** to help prevent pregnancy (**Figure 20.13**). This method of birth control can only be used for a few days after sex, however.

One type of emergency contraception is the copper IUD. If inserted within five days of sexual intercourse, this IUD is the most effective method of emergency contraception.

Several types of emergency contraception pills are also available, including *ella®* and *Plan B One-Step®*. These pills contain hormones that prevent ovulation and thicken cervical mucus.

Emergency contraception is similar to other hormone-based birth control methods, but has a greater amount of the hormones. Emergency contraception pills prevent fertilization. They cannot stop or interrupt a pregnancy that has already occurred. Emergency contraception does not reduce the risk of STIs and should not be used regularly.

Sterilization

Sterilization is the only permanent birth control method. It is a procedure performed by a doctor that prevents the sperm and egg from uniting. Sterilization prevents pregnancy, but not STIs. Reversing sterilization is difficult and often unsuccessful. As a result, people considering sterilization must be sure they do not ever want children (**Figure 20.14**). Both males and females can receive sterilization.

Male Sterilization

Male sterilization involves a surgery called a *vasectomy*. During a vasectomy, the *vas deferens* are closed. This prevents any sperm from leaving the testes. Usually, a doctor performs a vasectomy in a hospital. The surgery involves a small incision or puncture in each side of the scrotum. A vasectomy is nearly 100 percent effective, making it the most effective in preventing pregnancies.

Choosing Sterilization

Reasons to Choose Sterilization	Reasons NOT to Choose Sterilization
• Adults know they do not want to have more children. • Other birth control methods or pregnancy may carry serious health risks to adults. • Adults have genetic diseases or disorders they do not want to pass onto children. • Adults know they are and will never be emotionally or financially able to raise a family.	• Adults might want children in the future. If there is any future possibility for children, sterilization is not an option. • Adults feel pressured to be sterilized. They should be free to make their own decisions. • Adults have other personal issues that need attention in the present. These issues may go away over time, sterilization will not.

Figure 20.14
There are various reasons why couples may or may not choose sterilization as a birth control method.

Most males recover quickly from a vasectomy with no side effects. Some males experience bruising, swelling, and discomfort after the procedure. After a vasectomy, the prostate and seminal vesicles continue to function. Males can ejaculate normally, and the testes continue to make testosterone. Males can have an erection and have sex as they did prior to the operation.

Female Sterilization

Female sterilization works by cutting the fallopian tubes and sealing or removing part of them. This surgery is called *tubal ligation* and makes it impossible for sperm to reach an egg. This means that tubal ligation is nearly 100 percent effective in preventing pregnancy. Doctors may perform tubal ligation in a hospital or outpatient surgery clinic. Three months after surgery, doctors view an X-ray to confirm the tubes were successfully blocked.

Sterilization does not affect the function of the ovaries. A female continues to make female hormones and ovulate after this procedure. Sterilization also does not affect a female's sexual characteristics, sexual arousal, or ability to have sex.

Unplanned Pregnancy

As you have learned, abstinence is the only contraceptive method that is 100 percent effective. With any other method, some pregnancies may still happen. When pregnancy occurs, people have several options. Some people choose to give birth to and raise the baby. Others choose to place the child for adoption, or in some cases, end the pregnancy.

Some people choose to become parents and raise the child. If people decide to parent their child, they must prepare and learn everything they can about parenthood. Parents have many responsibilities. They must provide for all of the child's physical needs, such as food and shelter. They must also provide for the child's emotional needs, such as interacting with the child.

Parents are a child's first teachers. From parents, a child learns language, communication, and social skills. Later, parents should be involved in the

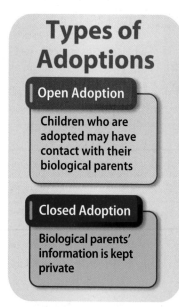

Types of Adoptions

Open Adoption

Children who are adopted may have contact with their biological parents

Closed Adoption

Biological parents' information is kept private

Figure 20.15
Adoption laws vary by state. People who choose to place a child for adoption have two options.

child's school education. Perhaps the most important responsibility of parenting is to be dependable and actively present in a child's life. This builds the child's trust, confidence, and self-esteem.

Some people may decide to give birth to the child and then place the child for *adoption* (**Figure 20.15**). People may make this choice for a variety of emotional, medical, and financial reasons. Parents who choose this route may feel some grief and loss following adoption, but this decision may be best for the child's future and help other couples have children.

Every state has *safe haven laws* (also called *safe surrender laws*) that allow people to leave their babies at certain facilities with no questions asked and with no legal consequences. These laws protect babies from the dangers of abandonment. Each state has age restrictions for a baby who is left at a safe haven. Safe havens include fire stations, police stations, and hospitals. Babies will be well cared for until they can be adopted.

In some cases, people who are not ready to give birth and raise a child choose to end the pregnancy with a procedure called **abortion**. Abortion is *not* a type of birth control. Birth control methods are designed to *prevent* pregnancy. Abortion *ends* a pregnancy that has already begun. A person who decides to have an abortion should do so at the earliest possible date to avoid potential health risks.

Many people are strongly opposed to abortion. Others believe it is a personal choice. If considering abortion, young people can benefit from a strong family support system. Counseling from doctors and advisors can also be helpful.

Lesson 20.1 Review

1. What is the only contraceptive method that is 100 percent effective in preventing pregnancy?

2. Which of the following blocks sperm from entering the female's vagina?

   A. Withdrawal.
   B. External condom.
   C. Birth control patch.
   D. Vaginal ring.

3. **True or false.** The birth control pill contains hormones that prevent ovulation.

4. Why is withdrawal not an effective method of birth control?

5. **Critical thinking.** Choose one source of information about contraception and explain why it is or is not reliable.

Hands-On Activity

Many school and community programs exist to promote sexual health. These programs encourage abstinence and help people make responsible sexual decisions. Working with a partner, research programs that advocate for the sexual health of young people. These programs may exist at the high school level or be run by the community. Identify one program and research it further. Create a blog post summarizing its mission, methods, and contact information. Share your blog post with the class.

Teen Pregnancy and Parenthood

Learning Outcomes

After studying this lesson, you will be able to

- **summarize** how sexual intercourse during adolescence could lead to teen pregnancy.
- **identify** risk and protective factors of teen pregnancy and parenthood.
- **describe** the challenges of teen pregnancy and parenthood and how they can be managed.
- **identify** resources for teen parents.
- **implement** the decision-making process to help make responsible sexual decisions.

Key Terms 📖

miscarriage spontaneous loss of the fetus

teen pregnancy pregnancy that occurs during the adolescent years when an adolescent's body is still developing and maturing

teen parenthood act or process of adolescent parents raising a child

prenatal care medical care during pregnancy

Graphic Organizer

Pregnancy During Adolescence

On a separate piece of paper, create four boxes as shown. Label each box with the main headings of the lesson in different colors. As you read the lesson, record the main points of each section. After reading, discuss the main points with a partner. Add any additional notes to your graphic organizer as needed.

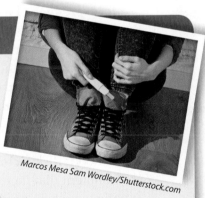

Marcos Mesa Sam Wordley/Shutterstock.com

Risk and Protective Factors	Challenges of Teen Pregnancy and Parenthood
Resources for Teen Parents	**Responsible Sexual Decision-Making**

A bstinence is the only 100 percent effective method of preventing pregnancy and avoiding sexually transmitted infections (STIs). As a result, Esmeralda from the previous lesson knows that abstinence is a healthy sexual choice she can make. She knows other birth control methods can reduce the risk of pregnancy, although sometimes pregnancies do occur. Esmeralda saw this firsthand when her older brother became a father in college. Esmeralda loves her niece, but she does not want to have children until she has finished school.

As you know, pregnancy occurs when a sperm from the male's semen fertilizes the female's egg. The fertilized egg becomes a zygote and divides rapidly. It implants in the female's uterus and slowly grows into a fetus. During pregnancy, the female's menstrual cycle stops. Sometimes, the female's body does not carry the fetus until birth. A **miscarriage**, or spontaneous loss of the fetus, may occur.

If the female does have a complete pregnancy, the birth of the baby will occur. Pregnancy and parenthood will change the lives of both parents. Knowing the facts about teen pregnancy and parenthood is important for helping young people make responsible sexual decisions.

Risk and Protective Factors

Teen pregnancy refers to a pregnancy that occurs during the adolescent years, when an adolescent's body is still developing and maturing. As you learned in the previous lesson, when pregnancy occurs, parents can choose to place the child for adoption or raise the child once the child is born. Adolescents who choose to raise their child start the journey of **teen parenthood**.

Several risk factors can lead to teen pregnancy and parenthood. Risk factors include the behaviors and environment that increase an adolescent's chance of experiencing teen pregnancy and parenthood. The factors can be either internal or external. **Figure 20.16** lists examples of potential risk factors that could increase these chances.

As with other aspects of health, various behaviors and environments can decrease an adolescent's chances of teen pregnancy and parenthood. These are protective factors. Adolescents can install protective factors into their personal life to decrease the chance of becoming parents at an early age. Examples of protective factors include the following:

- Discussion with parents or guardians about types of contraceptive methods and proper use. This discussion can also involve a healthcare professional.
- Parental or guardian support and a healthy family dynamic.
- Accurate knowledge of sexual health through healthcare professionals or valid resources.
- Continuous abstinence, or the commitment to refrain from sexual activity.

Risk Factors for Teen Pregnancy and Parenthood

- Limited knowledge of sexual health and contraceptive methods
- A parent who had a child before the age of 20
- Unprotected sexual activity
- Living in a home with frequent family conflict
- Use of alcohol and drugs
- Low self-esteem

Figure 20.16
Risk factors include the behaviors and environment that increase an adolescent's chances of teen pregnancy and parenthood.

Challenges of Teen Pregnancy and Parenthood

Adolescents who are pregnant or are adolescent parents may face various challenges. These challenges can affect the physical, emotional, and social health of adolescent parents, as well as their child. Adolescent parents may also face economic challenges (**Figure 20.17**). The challenges of teen pregnancy and parenthood can be managed in several ways.

Many of the physical challenges associated with teen pregnancy result from poor **prenatal care**, or medical care during pregnancy. Adolescent parents may neglect prenatal care due to the desire to keep a pregnancy secret, lack of knowledge about proper prenatal care, or other potential reasons. Poor prenatal care, however, can lead to serious health conditions for both the pregnant parent and the unborn child.

To ensure the safest possible pregnancy and the health of a developing baby, people should never keep a pregnancy secret. Instead, they should visit a doctor to begin prenatal care as soon as possible. This involves making regular visits to an obstetrician/gynecologist (OB/GYN) who specializes in pregnancy, labor, and delivery. During pregnancy, people need to prioritize their own health. Doctors can advise people how to care for themselves and their unborn child during pregnancy (**Figure 20.18**).

Challenges of Teen Pregnancy and Parenthood

Physical	
Parent	**Child**
• STIs contracted from sexual intercourse • Anemia • High blood pressure • Complications during childbirth	• Low birthweight • Death within the first year of life • Dependence on addictive substances • Slow growth • Infections
Social and Emotional	
• Balancing responsibilities as parents with relationships with family members and friends • Handling emotions and feelings of stress from new responsibilities of raising a child • Decrease time for social and extracurricular activities	
Economic	
• Completing school • Finding a job with a supportable income • Financial responsibilities of paying for food, clothing, housing, child care, health care, and education for the child	

Figure 20.17 Pregnant adolescents, adolescent parents, and their children may face various challenges.

Healthy Behaviors of Pregnancy

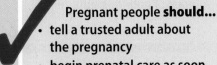

Pregnant people should...
- tell a trusted adult about the pregnancy
- begin prenatal care as soon as possible
- take prenatal vitamins
- get enough sleep each night
- eat whole grains, fresh fruit, vegetables, and lean meats
- drink plenty of water
- take precautions to prevent STIs
- get moderate physical activity

Pregnant people should not...
- keep pregnancy a secret
- vape or smoke
- drink alcohol
- use drugs
- eat junk food
- get excessive physical activity
- diet to lose weight

Figure 20.18 Consulting with a doctor can help pregnant people have a healthy pregnancy. *What is medical care during pregnancy called?*

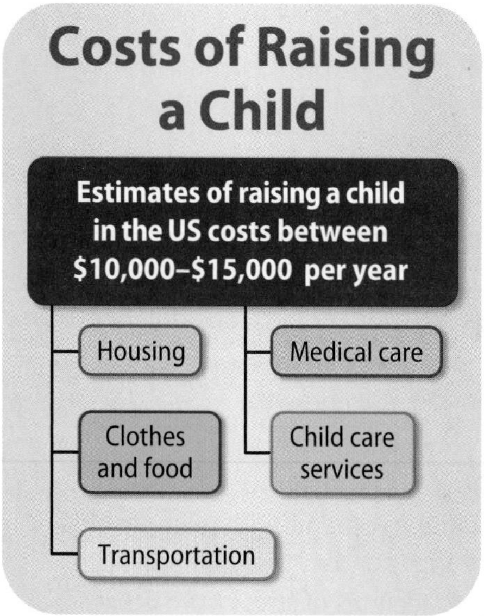

Costs of Raising a Child

Estimates of raising a child in the US costs between $10,000–$15,000 per year

- Housing
- Medical care
- Clothes and food
- Child care services
- Transportation

Figure 20.19 The expenses for raising a child involves various items, and both parents are required to contribute.

Throughout pregnancy and parenthood, maintaining healthy relationships is important. These relationships can include the relationship between the adolescent parents, family members, and friends and peers. Healthy relationships can provide adolescent parents with support and encouragement and satisfy different needs. For example, family members can assist with raising the child with the adolescent parents and provide emotional support.

Sometimes emotions and feelings can become overwhelming for an adolescent parent. Parents may feel angry or depressed as they realize how pregnancy has affected their goals and futures. They may also feel stressed due to new responsibilities. Adolescent parents can manage these feelings by taking care of their mental and emotional health and getting professional help, if needed.

It is also valuable for adolescent parents to complete their education. Not completing high school can lead to limited job opportunities, which can result in financial difficulties (**Figure 20.19**).

BUILDING Your Skills

Sexual Health Pledge

A *pledge* is a promise or agreement to do or refrain from doing something. As you think about and enter relationships, a pledge can help you protect your sexual health. It can help you create expectations and boundaries now, even if you are not in a relationship. By creating these boundaries, you show that you are in control of your body and decisions.

Today, design a sexual health pledge that puts *you* in control of your body and decisions. The example pledge shown can help you better understand the wording you can use. To design your pledge, use the following steps:

1. Consider the goals you have for your life and list them. Do you want to go to college? What kind of family and career do you want?

2. Brainstorm your own values related to sexual health and list them. Consider how your goals relate to your values and what influences have shaped your values.

3. Share your list of goals and values with a trusted adult. Then, talk with the trusted adult about expectations regarding sexual health. Seek input about what your pledge should say.

4. Use the decision-making process to help you decide what is most important to you about protecting your sexual health. Then, write your sexual health pledge based on your acquired knowledge, goals, and decisions.

5. Underneath your pledge, write specific steps you will take to protect your sexual health. Add an inspirational quote and illustrate your pledge with at least one image.

6. Sign your pledge.

7. Take your pledge home and put it in a special place in your room. Review the pledge often to remind yourself of your decision.

Sexual Health Pledge

I am choosing to be in control of my body!

I, _____, pledge
(person's name)

to make decisions that protect my sexual health.

Although it may be challenging to balance academics with the responsibility of raising a child, adolescents can turn to family for support. Family members can help care for the child while the adolescent parents are in school. If family members are not available, adolescent parents can seek out child care services. They can even look for night classes or online education courses. Receiving at least a high school diploma opens more employment opportunities for adolescent parents to help financially support their child. You will learn more about different resources for adolescents who are expecting or are currently parents in the next section.

Resources for Teen Parents

Adolescents who are expecting or currently raising a child may find themselves balancing their personal needs and the needs of their child. They may feel overwhelmed, depressed, or frustrated with the new responsibilities of raising a child. Adolescent parents are not alone when it comes to taking care of their child, however.

There are numerous resources available within a community to help adolescent parents (**Figure 20.20**). These resources can help adolescent parents and their families adjust to the life changes of raising a child. For example, adolescent parents can attend local pregnancy and parenting support groups to help them understand and meet the needs of raising a child. Support groups can provide pregnant adolescents and parents an opportunity to meet other adolescent parents and learn about child development and resources in the community.

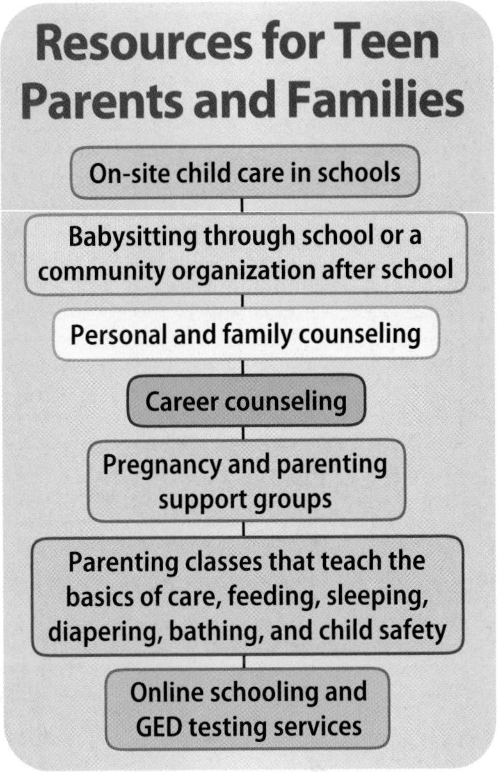

The government also provides resources for adolescents who are pregnant or are parents. For example, Medicaid can assist adolescents who are pregnant with getting the medical care they need to have a healthy pregnancy. Another organization is the *Special Supplemental Nutrition Program for Women, Infants, and Children (WIC)*. This program provides federal grants to states for supplemental foods, healthcare referrals, and nutrition education for pregnant people, parents who require assistance, and infants and children up to age five.

Resources for Teen Parents and Families

- On-site child care in schools
- Babysitting through school or a community organization after school
- Personal and family counseling
- Career counseling
- Pregnancy and parenting support groups
- Parenting classes that teach the basics of care, feeding, sleeping, diapering, bathing, and child safety
- Online schooling and GED testing services

Figure 20.20 Various resources exist for adolescent parents and their families within a community to help with raising a child.

Responsible Sexual Decision-Making

Knowing how to make responsible decisions concerning sexual activity can be difficult for adolescents, especially if they are feeling pressured by their peers or the media. You can use the decision-making process that you learned in Chapter 1 to help you make responsible sexual decisions. These skills are especially important when making difficult decisions that can affect your physical, social, and mental and emotional health. **Figure 20.21** shows an example of how you could use the decision-making process to determine how to practice abstinence.

It is important to remember that adolescents are still growing, both physically and emotionally. Practicing continuous abstinence, especially refusal skills, can be a way for adolescents to mature before worrying about a sexual relationship. Conducting proper research and asking trusted adults questions can also help you make safe sexual decisions. It is important to remember that making choices that allow you to pursue personal interests and goals are a part of promoting your personal health and wellness.

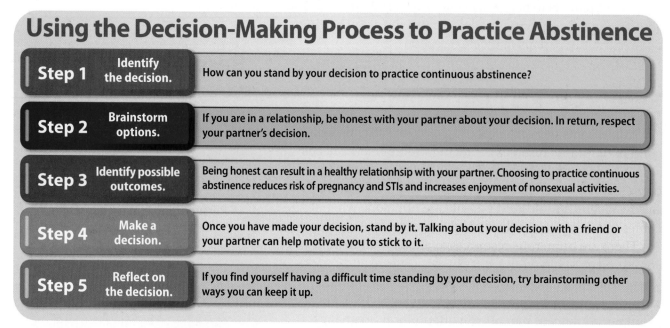

Using the Decision-Making Process to Practice Abstinence

Step 1	Identify the decision.	How can you stand by your decision to practice continuous abstinence?
Step 2	Brainstorm options.	If you are in a relationship, be honest with your partner about your decision. In return, respect your partner's decision.
Step 3	Identify possible outcomes.	Being honest can result in a healthy relationhsip with your partner. Choosing to practice continuous abstinence reduces risk of pregnancy and STIs and increases enjoyment of nonsexual activities.
Step 4	Make a decision.	Once you have made your decision, stand by it. Talking about your decision with a friend or your partner can help motivate you to stick to it.
Step 5	Reflect on the decision.	If you find yourself having a difficult time standing by your decision, try brainstorming other ways you can keep it up.

Figure 20.21 The decision-making process can be used to help adolescents make safe, responsible sexual decisions.

Lesson 20.2 Review

1. Which of the following is *not* an example of a protective factor?
   A. Continuous abstinence.
   B. Knowledge of contraceptive methods and proper use.
   C. Unprotected sexual activity.
   D. Parental or guardian support.

2. A(n) _____ is a healthcare professional who specializes in pregnancy, labor, and delivery.

3. Name two government organizations that provide resources for adolescents who are pregnant or are parents.

4. **Critical thinking.** How do you think teen pregnancy and parenthood affects a young person's relationships with peers?

Hands-On Activity

Imagine that you have a friend who is considering whether to become sexually active. Your friend knows that sexual activity can lead to pregnancy, but thinks it would not be difficult to have a child this early in life. Using the information you learned in this lesson, write a letter to your friend outlining how teen pregnancy and parenthood change a person's life. Recommend abstinence in the letter. Then, divide into small groups to discuss your letters and ways to make them more effective.

Summary

Lesson 20.1 Pregnancy Prevention

- Contraception, or birth control, is a method for reducing the risk of pregnancy. It is important to have accurate information about birth control. You can get accurate information from healthcare professionals, a doctor, or a school nurse.
- Abstinence is the most effective method of preventing pregnancy and STIs. Abstinence is affordable and reversible. It is a healthy sexual decision for young people.
- Barrier methods of birth control prevent sperm in semen from entering the female's vagina. These methods include the external condom, internal condom, contraceptive sponge, diaphragm, and cervical cap.
- Hormonal methods of birth control use the female hormones estrogen and progestin to inhibit ovulation. These methods include oral contraceptives, the birth control patch, the vaginal ring, the birth control shot, the birth control implant, and intrauterine devices (IUDs).
- Natural methods of birth control do not use barriers or hormones. The fertility awareness method (FAM) prevents pregnancy by scheduling intercourse around a female's ovulation. The withdrawal method involves withdrawing the penis before ejaculation. This method is not effective.
- When contraception fails, emergency contraception can help prevent pregnancy. Examples include the *ParaGard* copper IUD and emergency contraceptive pills.
- Sterilization is a permanent method of birth control. It involves a procedure called *vasectomy* for males and a procedure called *tubal ligation* for females.
- If a person becomes pregnant, the parents can give birth to and raise the child, place the child for adoption, or seek an abortion.

Lesson 20.2 Teen Pregnancy and Parenthood

- Pregnancy occurs when a sperm fertilizes an egg. Sometimes, a miscarriage can lead to the loss of a pregnancy. If the female has a complete pregnancy, the baby will be born and both parents lives will change.
- Risk factors include behaviors and environment that increase chances of teen pregnancy and parenthood. Protective factors decrease the chance of teen pregnancy and parenthood, such as accurate knowledge of sexual health and continuous abstinence.
- Challenges of teen pregnancy and parenthood can affect the physical, emotional, and social health of adolescent parents, as well as their child.
- Prenatal care and regular doctor visits can protect the health of the pregnant adolescent and baby. Having healthy relationships and completing an education can help manage social and economic challenges.
- Community and government sponsored resources are available to help adolescent parents in the raising of their child.
- Knowing how to make responsible sexual decisions that reflect your goals can help with your overall physical, mental and emotional, and social health.

Check Your Knowledge

Record your answers to each of the following questions on a separate sheet of paper.

1. What is the purpose of contraception?

2. **True or false.** Healthcare professionals are a good source of information about contraception.

3. Why should the external condom be applied before the penis touches a sexual partner's genitals?

4. Which of the following is a small, T-shaped device inserted into the uterus?
   - **A.** Birth control implant.
   - **B.** Vaginal ring.
   - **C.** Internal condom.
   - **D.** Intrauterine device (IUD).

5. **True or false.** The fertility awareness method (FAM) involves tracking a female's ovulation.

6. **True or false.** Emergency contraception contains hormones that can stop a pregnancy that has already begun.

7. **True or false.** Sterilization can be easily reversed.

8. If a pregnancy occurs, what are three options for the parents?

9. **True or false.** Pregnancy and parenthood can change the lives of both adolescent parents.

10. Teen pregnancy refers to a pregnancy that occurs during the _____ years, when a person's body is still developing and maturing.

11. Which of the following is *not* an example of a healthy behavior for pregnancy?
    - **A.** Take prenatal vitamins.
    - **B.** Eat whole grains, fresh fruit, vegetables, and lean meats.
    - **C.** Keep pregnancy a secret.
    - **D.** Take precautions to prevent STIs.

12. **True or false.** Making choices that allow you to pursue personal interests and goals is a part of promoting your personal health and wellness.

Use Your Vocabulary

abortion	internal condom	teen parenthood
birth control patch	miscarriage	teen pregnancy
contraception	oral contraceptives	vaginal ring
emergency contraception	prenatal care	withdrawal
external condom	sterilization	

13. Work with a partner to write the definitions of the terms above based on your current understanding before reading the chapter. Then, pair up with another team to discuss your definitions and any discrepancies. Finally, discuss the definitions with the class and ask your teacher for necessary correction or clarification.

14. For each of the terms above, identify a word or group of words describing a quality of the term—an *attribute*. Pair up with a classmate and discuss your list of attributes. Then, discuss your list of attributes with the whole class to increase understanding.

Think Critically

15. **Draw conclusions.** Is it easier for a young person to have sex or to have a conversation with a partner about sex, expectations, and contraceptive options? Defend your answer. Which option is better?

16. **Cause and effect.** What factors do you think impact a young person's decision to have sex or to abstain from sex?

17. **Identify.** Identify the pros and cons of sexual behavior at a young age.

18. **Compare and contrast.** Compare and contrast two forms of contraception. Why would a couple choose one form over another?

DEVELOP Your Skills

19. **Communication skills.** Open communication about sexual health can help you get accurate information and make responsible decisions. For this activity, talk with a parent, guardian, or other trusted adult about relationships, dating, and expectations for sexual activity. Discuss the following questions: What are the possible pros and cons of being in a romantic relationship? What are your family's expectations regarding dating, relationships, and sexual activity? Write a short reflection summarizing the conversation and the information you learned.

20. **Analyze influences.** Social media, television, and music surround young people with images and words that encourage risky sexual behaviors. For this activity, choose one image, television show, movie, or song that has a sexual message. Describe the sexual message and its portrayal. How could this message affect the decisions young people make about sexual health? Why do you think social media, television, and music send these messages? What messages should the media be sending to young people? Explain your answer.

21. **Access information.** Talk to a parent, guardian, trusted adult, or school nurse about ways and places to obtain contraception in your community. You can also do individual research to find this information. Create a brochure, public service announcement, billboard advertisement, flyer, or presentation summarizing ways to obtain contraception. Provide specific information, such as the name of a business or organization, contact information, and the services provided. Present this information to the class.

22. **Goal-setting skills.** Identify and write down at least four important goals you have for your future. Now, imagine that you are about to become an adolescent parent. You have made the decision to raise the child. What effect will your decision to be an adolescent parent have on your future goals? List each goal and describe how your decision will affect it. How would you adjust your goals to raise the child? Write a short reflection summarizing how you would feel if your goals were impacted in this way.

Body Mass Index-for-Age Percentiles

Body Mass Index for Boys

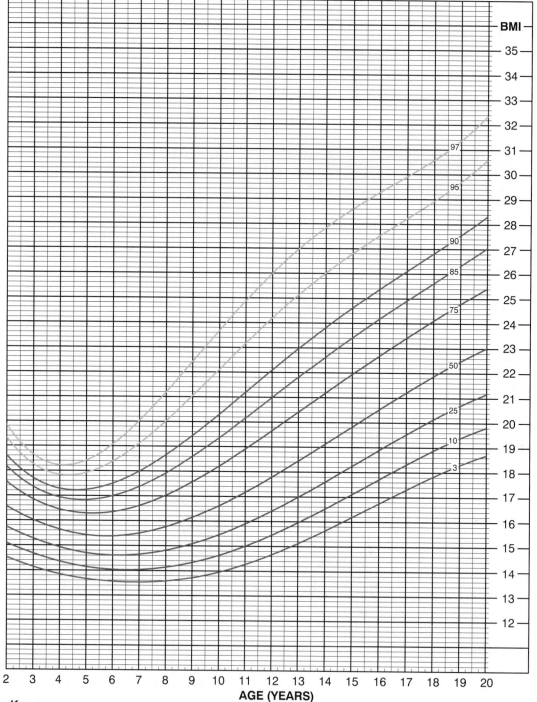

Key

Weight Status Category	Percentile Range
Underweight	Less than the 5th percentile
Healthy weight	5th percentile to less than the 85th percentile
Overweight	85th to less than the 95th percentile
Obese	Equal to or greater than the 95th percentile

SOURCE: Developed by the National Center for Health Statistics in collaboration with the National Center for Chronic Disease Prevention and Health Promotion

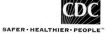

SAFER · HEALTHIER · PEOPLE™

Body Mass Index for Girls

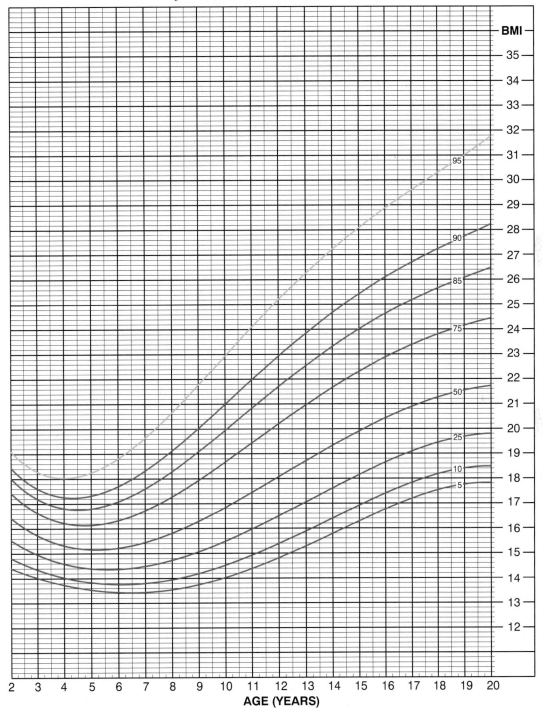

Key

Weight Status Category		Percentile Range
▬▬▬	Underweight	Less than the 5th percentile
▬▬▬	Healthy weight	5th percentile to less than the 85th percentile
▬▬▬	Overweight	85th to less than the 95th percentile
▬▬▬	Obese	Equal to or greater than the 95th percentile

SOURCE: Developed by the National Center for
Health Statistics in collaboration with the
National Center for Chronic Disease Prevention
and Health Promotion

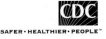

SAFER·HEALTHIER·PEOPLE™

Glossary/Glosario

English

A

abortion. Surgical procedure to end a pregnancy. (20.1)

abstinence. Commitment to refrain from sexual activity; only method that is 100 percent effective in preventing STIs. (18.1)

abuse. Violent behaviors that cause physical, emotional, sexual, or financial harm to another person. (16.2)

acid rain. Any form of precipitation that includes particles containing acid. (14.1)

acne. Skin condition in which inflamed, clogged hair follicles cause pimples. (3.1)

acquaintances. People you know and interact with, but may not consider friends. (15.3)

acquired immunodeficiency syndrome (AIDS). Health condition in which the body can no longer fight infections and disease; caused by the progression of human immunodeficiency virus (HIV). (18.2)

action plan. Detailed step-by-step method to reach a desired outcome; outlines what you are going to do, how you are going to do it, and when it will be done. (1.3)

active listening. Act of concentrating on person talking with the goal of understanding the message and the speaker's feelings about it. (15.1)

addiction. Physical and psychological need for a substance or behavior. (9.2)

adolescence. Period of development between 12 and 19 years of age. (17.3)

advocate. To take actions that show support. (1.3)

aerobic. Using oxygen to break down energy for use in the muscles. (8.2)

aerosol. Suspension of fine particles or droplets in the air. (9.1)

Español

A

aborto. Procedimiento quirúrgico para terminar un embarazo. (20.1)

abstinencia. Compromiso de abstenerse de la actividad sexual; único método que es 100 por ciento eficaz en prevenir los ITS. (18.1)

abuso. Patrón de maltrato físico, emocional, sexual o financiero con violencia hacia otra persona. (16.2)

lluvia ácida. Cualquier forma de precipitación que incluye partículas que contienen ácido. (14.1)

acné. Condición de la piel en que los folículos pilosos inflamados y obstruidos causan espinillas. (3.1)

conocidos. Personas con las que conoce e interactúa, pero no puede considerar amigos. (15.3)

síndrome de inmunodeficiencia adquirida (SIDA). Afección de salud en la que el cuerpo ya no puede combatir infecciones y enfermedades; causado por la progresión del virus de inmunodeficiencia humana (VIH). (18.2)

plan de acción. Método detallado paso por paso para lograr un resultado deseado; enumera lo que vas a hacer, cómo lo vas a hacer y cuándo lo realizarás. (1.3)

escucha active. Acto de concentrarse en la persona que habla con el objetivo de entender el mensaje y los sentimientos de esa persona respecto del mensaje. (15.1)

adicción. Necesidad física y psicológica para una sustancia o comportamiento. (9.2)

adolescencia. Período de desarrollo entre 12 y 19 años de edad. (17.3)

abogar. Realizar acciones que muestren apoyo. (1.3)

aeróbico. Uso del oxígeno para descomponer la energía para su uso en los músculos. (8.2)

aerosol. Suspensión de partículas finas o microgotas en el aire. (9.1)

Note: The numbers in parentheses following definitions represent the lesson in which the terms appear.

English

affirmative consent. Direct, verbal, freely given agreement that occurs when someone clearly says *yes*. (15.1)

age of consent. Age at which a person can legally agree to engage in sexual activity. (19.3)

agility. Ability to rapidly change the body's momentum and direction. (8.2)

Air Quality Index (AQI). Number that communicates to the public the level of pollutants in the air. (14.2)

Al-Anon Family Groups. Support group where family members and friends who have loved ones with an alcohol use disorder come together to share their experiences, receive encouragement, and learn ways to cope with challenges. (10.2)

Alateen. Support group where young people who have loved ones with an alcohol use disorder come together to share their experiences and learn ways to cope with challenges. (10.2)

alcohol. Addictive drug that alters brain function and affects a person's body, thinking, and behavior; known as a *depressant*. (10.1)

Alcoholics Anonymous (AA). Self-help program for people with an alcohol use disorder to help them change how they think about drinking. (10.2)

alcohol poisoning. Medical emergency that occurs when a large amount of alcohol enters the bloodstream in a short period of time. (10.1)

alcohol use disorder. Type of substance use disorder in which a person has an addiction to alcohol and continues to consume it despite negative health effects. (10.1)

anaerobic. Powering the body without the use of oxygen. (8.2)

anaphylaxis. Allergic response in which fluid fills the lungs and air passages narrow, restricting breathing. (13.3)

antibiotics. Substances that target and kill pathogenic bacteria. (12.1)

Español

consentimiento expreso. Acuerdo verbal, directo y voluntario que ocurre cuando alguien dice que *sí* con claridad. (15.1)

edad para dar consentimiento. Edad a la que una persona puede aceptar legalmente participar en actividades sexuales. (19.3)

agilidad. Capacidad para cambiar rápidamente la dirección y el impulso del cuerpo. (8.2)

Índice de Calidad del Aire (Air Quality Index, AQI). Número que comunica al público el nivel de contaminantes en el aire. (14.2)

Grupos de Familia Al-Anon. Grupo de apoyo donde familiares y amigos que tienen seres queridos con un trastorno por consumo de alcohol se unen para compartir sus experiencias, recibir ánimo y aprender maneras de enfrentarse a los desafíos. (10.2)

Alateen. Grupo de apoyo donde los jóvenes que tienen seres queridos con un trastorno por consumo de alcohol se unen para compartir sus experiencias y aprender maneras de enfrentarse a los desafíos. (10.2)

alcohol. Droga adictiva que altera la función cerebral y afecta el organismo, pensamiento y comportamiento de una persona; se conoce como un *depresor*. (10.1)

Alcohólicos Anónimos (AA). Programa de autoayuda para personas con trastornos por consumo de alcohol que las ayuda a cambiar cómo piensan respecto de la bebida. (10.2)

intoxicación por alcohol. Emergencia médica que se produce cuando una gran cantidad de alcohol ingresa al torrente sanguíneo en un período breve de tiempo. (10.1)

trastorno por consumo de alcohol. Tipo de trastorno por consumo de sustancias en el que una persona tiene una adicción al alcohol y continúa consumiéndolo a pesar de los efectos negativos sobre la salud. (10.1)

anaeróbico. Energizar el cuerpo sin el uso de oxígeno. (8.2)

anafilaxia. Reacción alérgica en la que fluidos llenan los pulmones y las vías aéreas estrechas, restringiendo la respiración. (13.3)

antibióticos. Sustancias que ataca y destruye las bacterias patógenas. (12.1)

English

antiperspirant. Product designed to stop or dry up sweat. (3.1)

antiretroviral therapy (ART). Treatment for HIV/AIDS in which a combination of drugs is given to interfere with HIV reproduction. (18.2)

anxiety disorder. Condition in which someone responds with extreme or unrealistic fear and dread to certain situations, experiences, or objects. (6.1)

appendix. Finger-shaped organ attached to the large intestine; made of lymphatic tissue. (2.3)

arousal. Sexual excitement. (19.2)

arteries. Blood vessels that carry oxygen-rich blood. (2.2)

arthritis. Condition that results in inflammation of the joints, causing pain and stiffness. (12.2)

astigmatism. Condition in which the eye does not focus light evenly onto the retina; objects appear blurry and stretched out. (3.2)

attention-deficit hyperactivity disorder (ADHD). Condition in which a person has difficulty paying attention and controlling behavior. (6.1)

attitudes. Set ways a person thinks or feels about someone or something. (5.1)

autoimmune disease. Condition that causes the body's immune system to attack and damage healthy body tissues. (12.2)

automated external defibrillator (AED). Rescue device that delivers a controlled, precise shock to the heart. (13.3)

B

beliefs. Ideas or thoughts a person knows to be true, based on real experiences, scientific facts, or what a person has learned from others. (5.1)

binge drinking. Consuming four drinks for females and five drinks for males on the same occasion. (10.1)

biodegradable. Able to break down without causing harm when thrown out. (14.2)

Español

antitranspirante. Producto diseñado para detener o secar el sudor. (3.1)

terapia antirretroviral (TARV). Tratamiento para el VIH/SIDA en el que se administra un combinación de drogas para interferir en la reproducción del VIH. (18.2)

trastorno de ansiedad. Condición en que alguien responde con temor y miedo extremo o poco realista a algunas situaciones, experiencias, u objetos. (6.1)

apéndice. Órgano con forma de dedo adjunto al intestino grueso; hecho de tejido linfático. (2.3)

excitación. Excitación sexual. (19.2)

arterias. Vasos sanguíneos que llevan la sangre rica en oxígeno. (2.2)

artritis. Condición que resulta en la inflamación de las articulaciones, causando dolor y rigidez. (12.2)

astigmatismo. Condición en que el ojo no enfoca la luz uniformemente a la retina; los objetos aparecen nublados y estirados. (3.2)

síndrome de déficit atencional (ADHD). Condición en que una persona tiene dificultad prestando atención y controlando comportamiento. (6.1)

actitudes. Maneras fijas en que una persona piensa o siente sobre alguien o algo. (5.1)

enfermedad autoinmune. Afección que hace que el sistema inmunológico del cuerpo ataque y dañe los tejido corporales saludables. (12.2)

desfibrilador externo automático (DEA). Dispositivo de rescate que ofrece una descarga controlada, precisa al corazón. (13.3)

creencias. Cosas una persona sabe que es cierto, basado en experiencias auténticos, hechos científicos, o que una persona he aprendido de otros. (5.1)

atracón de bebidas. Consumir cuatro bebidas, en el caso de hembras, y cinco bebidas, en el caso de varones, en la misma ocasión. (10.1)

biodegradable. Capaz de descomponer sin causar daño cuando tirado. (14.2)

English

biological sex. Individual's sex, male or female, as determined by the person's chromosomes. (19.1)

bipolar disorder. Condition characterized by periods of intense depression that alternate with periods of manic moods. (6.1)

birth control patch. Thin, 2- to 3-inch, plastic patch applied to the skin that works like a birth control pill. (20.1)

bladder. Organ that stores urine until it can be pushed out of the body. (2.3)

blood alcohol concentration (BAC). Percentage of alcohol in a person's blood. (10.1)

blue light. Type of light from many digital devices, such as phones, tablets, televisions, and computers, that produces large amounts of energy. (4.1)

body art. Permanent decorations that are applied to the body; examples include tattoos and piercings. (3.1)

body compassion. Feelings of acceptance, care, and kindness toward one's body. (7.4)

body composition. Ratio of the various components—fat, bone, and muscle—that make up a person's body. (7.3)

body image. Thoughts and feelings about how one's body looks. (7.4)

body mass index (BMI). Tool used to determine whether a person's weight is healthy for that person's height; BMI = weight (lbs.)/height (in.)^2 × 703. (7.3)

body neutrality. Focus on what the body can do, rather than how it looks. (7.4)

body positivity. Appreciation of diverse body types. (7.4)

body system. Collection of organs that work together. (2.1)

brain stem. Part of the brain that controls the heartbeat and breathing rate. (2.4)

breakup. End of a romantic relationship. (15.4)

Español

sexo biológico. Sexo de una persona, varón o hembra, según lo que determinan los cromosomas de esa persona. (19.1)

trastorno bipolar. Afección caracterizada por periodos de depresión intensa que se alternan con periodos de estados de ánimo maniáticos. (6.1)

parche anticonceptivo. Parche plástico fino, 2- a 3-pulgadas, aplicado a la piel que funciona como una pastilla del control de la natalidad. (20.1)

vejiga. Órgano que almacena la orina hasta puede ser empujado fuera del cuerpo. (2.3)

concentración de alcohol en la sangre (BAC). Porcentaje de alcohol en la sangre de una persona. (10.1)

luz azul. Tipo de luz de varios dispositivos digitales, como teléfonos, tabletas, televisores y computadoras, que produce grandes cantidades de energía. (4.1)

arte corporal. Decoraciones permanentes que se aplican al cuerpo; ejemplos incluyen tatuajes y piercings. (3.1)

compasión corporal. Sentimientos de aceptación, cuidado y bondad hacia el cuerpo. (7.4)

composición corporal. Proporción de los componentes varios—grasa, hueso, y músculo—que forman el cuerpo de una persona. (7.3)

imagen corporal. Pensamientos y sentimientos acerca de cómo luce el cuerpo de uno mismo. (7.4)

índice de masa corporal (IMC). Herramienta utilizada para determinar si el peso de una persona es saludable para su altura; IMC = peso (lb)/altura (pulg.)^2 × 703. (7.3)

neutralidad corporal. Foco en lo que el cuerpo puede hacer, en lugar de en cómo se ve. (7.4)

positividad corporal. Valoración de diversos tipos de cuerpos. (7.4)

sistema corporal. Colecciones de órganos que funcionan juntos. (2.1)

tallo cerebral. Parte del cerebro que controla el latido y la frecuencia respiratoria. (2.4)

rupture. Término de una relación romántica. (15.4)

English

bronchi. Two air passages, each of which connects the trachea to a lung. (2.2)

brownfield site. Land, such as an old factory or gas station, that contains hazardous waste. (14.2)

bullying. Repeated aggressive behavior toward someone that causes the person injury or discomfort. (16.1)

bystander effect. Situation in which a bystander is less likely to intervene and stop violent, harmful, or unsafe behavior because the person thinks someone else will. (16.1)

bystanders. People who are present at a situation, but do not participate or intervene. (16.1)

C

caffeine. Substance that increases energy, alertness, and attention, making it difficult to sleep. (4.3)

cancer. Complex disease that typically involves an uncontrolled growth of abnormal cells. (12.2)

capillaries. Small arteries that deliver oxygen and nutrients to cells and pick up cells' waste. (2.2)

carbohydrates. Major source of energy for the body; found in fruits, vegetables, grains, and milk products. (7.1)

carcinogens. Cancer-causing substances. (9.1)

cardiopulmonary resuscitation (CPR). Emergency procedure that uses chest compressions to restore heartbeat; may also involve mouth-to-mouth breathing. (13.3)

casual dating. Way of getting to know how you interact with and feel about another person. (15.4)

cavities. Holes in the teeth that occur when plaque eats into a tooth's enamel. (3.2)

cerebellum. Part of the brain that controls coordinated, smooth muscle activity. (2.4)

Español

bronquios. Dos vías aéreas, cada uno de los cuales conecta la tráquea a un pulmón. (2.2)

sitio previamente urbanizado. Tierra, tal como una fábrica o gasolinera, que contiene residuos peligrosos. (14.2)

intimidación. Comportamiento repetido y agresivo hacia alguien que causa herida o incomodidad de la persona. (16.1)

efecto espectador. Situación en la que un espectador tiene menos probabilidades de intervenir y detener un comportamiento violento, dañino o inseguro porque cree que alguien más lo hará. (16.1)

espectadores. Personas que están presentes en una situación, pero que no participan ni intervienen. (16.1)

cafeína. Sustancia que aumenta la energía, el estado de alerta y la atención, lo que dificulta dormirse. (4.3)

cáncer. Enfermedad compleja que típicamente consiste en crecimiento incontrolado de células anormales. (12.2)

capilares. Arterias pequeñas que entrega el oxígeno y los nutrientes a las células y recoge los residuos de las células. (2.2)

carbohidratos. Fuente importante de energía para el cuerpo; se encuentra en frutas, verduras, granos, y productos lácteos. (7.1)

carcinógenos. Sustancias que provocan cáncer. (9.1)

reanimación cardiopulmonar (RCP). Procedimiento emergencia que utiliza compresiones del pecho para devolver el latido; puede también consiste en respiración boca a boca. (13.3)

citas casuales. Manera de conocer cómo se interactúa con y se siente sobre otra persona. (15.4)

caries. Orificios en los dientes que ocurren cuando la placa carcome el esmalte de un diente. (3.2)

cerebelo. Parte del cerebro que controla la actividad de los músculos coordinados, lisos. (2.4)

English

cerebrum. Largest part of the brain, which interprets information from the sensory organs; controls muscle actions and is responsible for intelligence, memory, and personality. (2.4)

child abuse. Any act an adult commits that causes harm or threatens to cause harm to a child. (16.2)

chlamydia. Bacterial infection known as a "silent" disease because it has few or no symptoms. (18.1)

circadian rhythms. Naturally occurring physical, behavioral, and mental changes in the body that typically follow the 24-hour cycle of the sun. (4.1)

circulatory system. Body system formed by all the structures that move blood through the body; also called the *cardiovascular system*. (2.2)

clique. Small group of friends who deliberately exclude other people from joining or being a part of their group. (15.3)

club drugs. Several different types of drugs that young people may abuse at parties, bars, and concerts. (11.2)

cocaine. Drug that usually comes in the form of white powder made from the leaves of the coca plant. (11.2)

communicable disease. Condition someone can develop after coming into contact with living things or objects infected with the disease; also called *infectious disease*. (12.1)

communication process. Exchange of messages and responses between two or more people. (15.1)

composting. Process of gathering food scraps and organic waste into a bin and letting it decompose and then adding it to soil to help plants grow. (14.2)

concussion. Type of brain injury that results from a blow or jolt to the head or upper body. (8.3)

Español

cerebro. Parte más grande del cerebro, que interpreta información de los órganos sensoriales; controla acciones musculares y es responsable por la inteligencia, memoria, y personalidad. (2.4)

abuso infantil. Cualquier acción que un adulto comete que causa daño o amenaza causar daño a un niño. (16.2)

clamidia. Infección bacteriana conocido como una enfermedad "silencioso" porque tiene pocos o no síntomas. (18.1)

ritmos circadianos. Cambios físicos, conductuales, y mentales que ocurren naturalmente en el cuerpo que típicamente sigue el ciclo de 24 horas del sol. (4.1)

sistema circulatorio. Sistema corporal conformado por todas las estructuras que hacen circular la sangre a través del organismo; también llamado *sistema cardiovascular*. (2.2)

camarilla. Grupo pequeño de amigos que excluya deliberadamente otras personas de unirse o ser un parte de su grupo. (15.3)

drogas de club. Varios tipos diferentes de drogas que jóvenes pueden abusar en fiestas, bares, y conciertos. (11.2)

cocaína. Droga que usualmente proviene en la forma de polvo blanco hecho de las hojas de las plantas de coca. (11.2)

enfermedad transmissible. Afección que alguien puede contraer después de entrar en contacto con seres vivientes u objetos infectados con la enfermedad; también se llama *enfermedad infecciosa*. (12.1)

proceso de comunicación. Intercambio de mensajes y respuestas mientras dos o más personas. (15.1)

compostaje. Proceso en el que se recolectan restos de comida y residuos orgánicos en un recipiente y se dejan descomponer; luego son añadidos a la tierra para ayudar a las plantas a crecer. (14.2)

contusión cerebral. Tipo de lesión cerebral resultado de un golpe o impresión a la cabeza o cuerpo superior. (8.3)

English

condom. Device that provides a barrier to microorganisms that cause STIs. (18.1)

conflict resolution skills. Strategies for resolving disagreements in a positive, respectful way to promote healthy relationships. (1.3)

conjunctivitis. Viral or bacterial infection that causes inflammation of part of the eye; also known as *pinkeye*. (12.1)

contraception. Any method that reduces the risk of pregnancy resulting from sexual intercourse; also called *birth control*. (20.1)

co-occurring disorder. Two or more mental illnesses that occur together. (9.2)

culture. Beliefs, values, customs, and arts of a group of people. (1.2)

cyberbullying. Form of bullying that uses electronic means. (16.1)

D

dandruff. Dead skin that flakes off the scalp due to dryness, infrequent shampooing, or irritation. (3.1)

decision-making process. Process of making choices by identifying the decision, brainstorming options, identifying possible outcomes, making a decision, and reflecting on the decision. (1.3)

delayed sleep phase syndrome (DSPS). Condition that results from a delay in the sleep-wake cycle that affects a person's daily activities. (4.2)

deodorant. Product designed to cover up body odor. (3.1)

dependence. Effect that occurs when the body needs an addictive substance in its system to function normally or avoid cravings and anxiety. (9.2)

dermatologist. Skin specialist who diagnoses and treats skin conditions. (3.1)

dermis. Middle layer of the skin, which contains hair follicles. (2.1)

Español

condón. Dispositivo que proporciona una barrera para microorganismos que causan los ITS. (18.1)

habilidades de resolución de conflictos. Estrategias para resolver desacuerdos de una manera positiva y respetuosa con el fin de promover relaciones saludables. (1.3)

conjuntivitis. Infección vírica o bacteriana que causa inflamación en parte del ojo; también conocido como *pinkeye*. (12.1)

anticoncepción. Cualquier método que reduce el riesgo de embarazo como resultado de mantener relaciones sexuales; también se conoce como *control de natalidad*. (20.1)

trastorno concurrente. Dos o más enfermedades mentales que ocurren al mismo tiempo. (9.2)

cultura. Creencias, valores, costumbres, y artes de un grupo de personas. (1.2)

ciberacoso. Forma de intimidación que utiliza medios electrónicos. (16.1)

caspa. Piel muerta que desprende del cuero cabelludo por la resequedad, el champú poco frecuente, o la irritación. (3.1)

droceso de toma de decisions. Proceso mediante el cual se eligen opciones al identificar la decisión, aportar varias ideas, identificar los resultados posibles, tomar una decisión y reflexionar sobre la decisión. (1.3)

síndrome de fase de sueño retardado (DSPS). Condición que resulta de un retraso en el ciclo sueño-vigilia que afecta las actividades diarias de una persona. (4.2)

desodorante. Producto diseñado para cubrir el olor corporal. (3.1)

dependencia. Efecto que ocurre cuando el cuerpo necesita una sustancia adictiva en su sistema para funcionar normalmente o para evitar antojos y ansiedad. (9.2)

dermatólogo. Especialista en piel que diagnostica y trata afecciones cutáneas. (3.1)

dermis. Capa intermedia de la piel, que contiene folículos pilosos. (2.1)

English

detoxification. Process of completely stopping all alcohol use to remove the substance from the body. (10.2)

diabetes mellitus. Disease resulting from the body's inability to regulate glucose; commonly known as *diabetes*. (12.2)

diaphragm. Sheet of muscle beneath the lungs and above the abdomen that contracts and relaxes to help the chest expand so a person can inhale or shrink so a person can exhale. (2.2)

dietary fiber. Tough complex carbohydrate that the body is unable to digest. (7.1)

Dietary Guidelines. United States government recommendations for forming patterns of eating that will promote health. (7.2)

digestive system. Body system that breaks down food to provide nutrients and energy; also removes solid waste from the body. (2.3)

digital citizenship. Practice of taking responsible, healthy actions as part of the digital community. (13.2)

digital footprint. All of the content people share, access, or have shared about them online. (13.2)

dislocation. Serious injury in which bones move out of their normal position. (8.3)

disordered eating. Range of irregular eating behaviors with negative health consequences. (7.4)

disorder of sex development (DSD). Condition of having an unclear biological sex. (19.1)

distress. Stress that causes negative feelings and harmful health effects. (5.3)

diversity. Inclusion of people with different backgrounds. (15.3)

dopamine. Chemical released by the brain that produces feelings of pleasure. (9.1)

drug abuse. Use of addictive, illegal drugs. (11.2)

drugs. Medications and other substances that change the way the body or brain functions. (11.1)

Español

desintoxicación. Proceso de parar completamente todo uso de alcohol para quitar la sustancia del cuerpo. (10.2)

diabetes mellitus. Enfermedad resultante de la incapacidad del cuerpo a regular la glucosa; comúnmente conocido como *diabetes*. (12.2)

diafragma. Chapa de músculo bajo los pulmones y arriba del abdomen que contrae y relaja para ayudar el pecho expande para que una persona puede inhalar o encoge para que una persona puede exhalar. (2.2)

fibra dietética. Un carbohidrato complejo y duro que el cuerpo es incapaz de digerir. (7.1)

Pautas Alimentarias. Recomendaciones del gobierno de los Estados Unidos para formar patrones de comer que promoverá la salud. (7.2)

sistema digestivo. Sistema corporal que descompone la comida para proveer las nutrientes y la energía; quita los residuos sólidos del cuerpo. (2.3)

ciudadanía digital. Práctica de realizar acciones responsables y saludables como parte de la comunidad digital. (13.2)

huella digital. Todo el contenido que las personas comparten, acceden o han compartido sobre ellas en línea. (13.2)

dislocación. Lesión grave en que huesos mueven afuera de sus posiciones normales. (8.3)

alimentación desordenada. Serie de conductas alimentarias irregulares con consecuencias negativas para la salud. (7.4)

trastorno del desarrollo sexual (DSD). Afección en la que el sexo biológico no es claro. (19.1)

angustia. Estrés que provoca sentimientos negativos y efectos nocivos para la salud. (5.3)

diversidad. Inclusión de personas con orígenes diferentes. (15.3)

dopamine. Químico liberado por el cerebro que produce sentimientos de placer. (9.1)

abuso de drogas. Consumo de drogas adictivas e ilegales. (11.2)

drogas. Medicinas y otras sustancias que cambian la manera en que el cuerpo o cerebro funciona. (11.1)

English

E

early childhood. Period of time from infancy through the preschool years. (17.2)

eating disorder. Mental illness that causes major disturbances in a person's daily diet. (7.4)

eczema. Chronic condition that causes swollen, red, dry, and itchy patches of skin on one or more parts of the body. (3.1)

elder abuse. Behaviors or neglect that cause harm to someone 60 years of age or older. (16.2)

e-liquid. Substance made of nicotine or another drug and other chemicals; is heated during vaping. (9.1)

embryo. Term that describes a developing baby during the embryonic stage of prenatal development. (17.1)

emergency contraception. Contraceptive method used to prevent pregnancy when other contraception has failed. (20.1)

emergency preparedness. Knowing how to respond to a specific type of emergency. (13.1)

emotional abuse. Attitudes or controlling behaviors that harm a person's mental health; also called *verbal, mental,* or *psychological abuse.* (16.2)

emotional awareness. Skill of knowing which emotions you feel, and why. (5.2)

emotional intelligence (EI). Skill of understanding, controlling, and expressing your emotions and sensing the emotions of others. (5.2)

emotions. Moods or feelings you experience. (5.2)

empathy. Ability to put yourself in someone else's shoes, and to understand someone else's wants, needs, and viewpoints. (5.2)

enabling. Encouraging a person's unhealthy behaviors, either intentionally or unintentionally. (10.2)

endocrine system. Body system that produces chemical messengers called *hormones,* which regulate body processes. (2.4)

Español

E

primera infancia. Período de desarrollo desde la infancia hasta los años preescolares. (17.2)

trastorno alimentario. Enfermedad mental que causa grandes alteraciones en la alimentación diaria de una persona. (7.4)

eczema. Condición crónica que causa parches de piel hinchados, rojas, secas, y pruritos en uno o más partes del cuerpo. (3.1)

maltrato de ancianos. Maltrato físico, emocional, sexual o financiero o abandono de alguien mayor de 60 años de edad. (16.2)

e-líquido. Sustancia hecha de nicotina u otra droga y otras sustancias químicas; se calienta durante el vapeo. (9.1)

embrión. Término que describe un bebé en desarrollo durante la etapa embrionaria del desarrollo prenatal. (17.1)

anticoncepción de emergencia. Método anticonceptivo utilizado para prevenir el embarazo cuando otro método anticonceptivo ha fallado. (20.1)

preparación para emergencias. Saber cómo responder a un tipo específico de emergencia. (13.1)

abuso emocional. Actitudes o comportamientos dominantes que dañan la salud mental de una persona; también llamada *abuso verbal, mental,* o *psicológico.* (16.2)

conciencia emocional. Habilidad de comprender cuales emociones se siente y por qué. (5.2)

inteligencia emocional (emotional intelligence, EI). Habilidad de comprender, controlar, y expresar sus emociones y sentir las emociones de otras personas. (5.2)

emociones. Estados de ánimo y sentimientos experimenta. (5.2)

empatía. Capacidad de ponerse en los zapatos de otra persona, y comprender los deseos, necesidades, y puntos de vista de otra persona. (5.2)

posibilitar. Incentivando los comportamientos de mal salud, ya sea intencional o no accidental. (10.2)

sistema endocrino. Sistema corporal que produce los mensajeros químicos, llamadas *hormonas,* que controlan los procesos corporales. (2.4)

English

endorphins. Brain chemicals that improve mood; released during physical activity. (8.1)

endurance. Ability to continue performing a physical activity over time. (8.2)

environment. Circumstances, objects, or conditions that surround a person in everyday life. (1.2)

epidermis. Outermost layer of the skin. (2.1)

escape plan. Strategy that outlines safe routes and procedures for leaving the home in the event a fire occurs. (13.1)

estrogen. Hormone that triggers growth and development of the female sex organs. (17.3)

eustress. Positive stress that encourages growth and motivation. (5.3)

exclusive. Committed to being romantically involved with only one dating partner. (15.4)

exercise. Physical activity that is structured, planned, and has the purpose of increasing physical fitness. (8.1)

extended family. Distant relatives, including aunts, uncles, cousins, and grandparents. (15.2)

external condom. Object worn over erect penis during sexual activity. (20.1)

extinguish. Put out. (13.1)

F

fad diets. Stylish weight-loss plans that promise significant weight loss in short periods of time, often through cutting out food groups or buying premade meals. (7.3)

family therapy. Type of therapy in which all family members meet together with a therapist to build positive, healthy relationships. (6.2)

farsightedness. Condition in which distant objects are seen more clearly than nearby objects. (3.2)

fats. Type of nutrient largely made up of fatty acids, which provide a valuable source of energy. (7.1)

Español

endorfinas. Sustancias químicas del cerebro que mejoran el estado de ánimo; se liberan durante la actividad física. (8.1)

resistencia. Capacidad de continuar realizando una actividad física a lo largo del tiempo. (8.2)

entorno. Circunstancias, objetos, o condiciones que rodean una persona en la vida diaria. (1.2)

epidermis. Capa más externa de la piel. (2.1)

plan de evacuación. Estrategia que resume las rutas y los procedimientos seguros para salir de una casa en caso de que ocurra un incendio. (13.1)

estrógeno. Hormona que provoque el crecimiento y desarrollo de los órganos sexuales femeninas. (17.3)

eustress. Estrés positivo que fomenta el crecimiento y la motivación. (5.3)

exclusivo. Comprometido a ser involucrada románticamente con solamente uno pareja de citas. (15.4)

ejercicio. Actividad física estructurada y planificada que tiene el propósito de aumentar el estado físico. (8.1)

familia extensa. Parientes lejanos, incluidos tíos, primos y abuelos. (15.2)

condón externo. Objeto que se usa sobre un pene erecto durante la actividad sexual. (20.1)

extinguir. Apagar. (13.1)

dietas de moda. Planes modernos para perder peso que prometen una pérdida de peso significativa en cortos períodos de tiempo, a menudo mediante la eliminación de grupos de alimentos o la compra de comidas preparadas. (7.3)

terapia familiar. Tipo de terapia en que todos los miembros de la familia se reúnen juntos con una terapeuta para construir relaciones positivas y sanas. (6.2)

vista cansada. Condición en que objetos alejados se los ven con más claridad que objetos cercas. (3.2)

grasas. Tipo de nutrientes compuesto en gran parte de ácidos grasos, que provee una fuente de energía. (7.1)

English

feedback. Constructive response to a message to communicate that it was received and understood. (15.1)

fentanyl. Prescription opioid more powerful than morphine; sometimes cut with heroin. (11.2)

fertilization. Process by which the sperm and egg combine to create a zygote. (17.1)

fetus. Term that describes a developing baby during the fetal stage of prenatal development. (17.1)

fight-or-flight response. Body's impulse to either fight off or flee from threatening situations. (5.3)

financial abuse. Use of money to show power in a relationship and make others act in certain ways. (16.2)

fire triangle. Model to help you remember the elements that are needed for a fire to occur; elements include fuel, heat, and oxygen. (13.1)

first aid. Treatment given in the first moments of an accident or injury—usually before medical professionals arrive on the scene. (13.3)

first-aid kit. Container that includes the supplies needed to treat most types of minor injuries. (13.3)

FITT. Acronym used to focus on the key fitness factors of frequency, intensity, time, and type. (8.4)

flammable. Easily set on fire. (13.1)

food sanitation. Food safety practices that maintain the safety of food you handle and eat; includes refrigerating and freezing certain foods, cooking meat thoroughly, and washing vegetables and fruits. (12.3)

fossil fuels. Natural forms of energy, such as oil, natural gas, and gas, that were formed a very long time ago, when dinosaurs lived on Earth. (14.2)

fracture. Broken bone. (8.3)

friendship. Relationship between two or more people who share common interests, values, and goals and support each other. (15.3)

frostbite. Injury caused by the freezing of skin and body tissues. (8.3)

Español

retroalimentación. Respuesta constructiva a un mensaje para comunicar que fue recibido y entendido. (15.1)

fentanilo. Opioide recetado que es más potente que la morfina; a veces se corta con heroína. (11.2)

fertilización. Proceso por el cual el espermatozoide y el óvulo combinan para crear un cigoto. (17.1)

feto. Término que describe un bebé en desarrollo durante la etapa fetal del desarrollo prenatal. (17.1)

respuesta de lucha o huida. Impulso del cuerpo, ya sea de luchar o de huir de situaciones amenazantes. (5.3)

abuso financier. Uso del dinero para demostrar poder en una relación y hacer que otras personas actúen de determinada manera. (16.2)

triangulo del fuego. Modelo para ayudarle a recordar los elementos necesarios para que ocurra un fuego; los elementos incluyen combustible, calor, y oxígeno. (13.1)

botiquín de primeros auxilios. Tratamiento dado en los primeros momentos de un accidente o lesión—a menudo antes de que los profesionales médicos lleguen a la escena. (13.3)

botiquín. Recipiente que incluye las provisiones necesarias para tratar la mayoría de tipos de lesiones menores. (13.3)

FITT. Acrónimo usado para concentrarse en los factores claves de buena forma de frecuencia, intensidad, tiempo, y tipo. (8.4)

inflamable. Incendiado fácilmente. (13.1)

saneamiento de alimentos. Prácticas de seguridad de alimentos que mantienen la seguridad de la comida se maneja y se come; incluye refrigerar y congelar algas comidas, cocinar bien la carne, y lavar verduras y frutas. (12.3)

combustibles fósiles. Formas naturales de energía, tal como petróleo, gas natural, y gas, que fueran formados hace mucho tiempo, cuando los dinosaurios vivían en la Tierra. (14.2)

fractura. Rotura de un hueso. (8.3)

amistad. Relación entre dos o más personas que comparten intereses, valores y metas comunes y se apoyan mutuamente. (15.3)

congelación. Lesión resultada de la congelación de la piel y el tejido del cuerpo. (8.3)

English

G

gallbladder. Organ in which bile is stored until needed to digest food. (2.3)

gangs. Groups of people who carry out violent and illegal acts. (16.3)

gender. Characteristics a society associates with a particular biological sex. (19.1)

gender identity. Internal, deeply held thoughts and feelings about gender. (19.1)

gender roles. Behaviors society considers "appropriate" for a certain gender. (19.1)

genes. Segments of DNA that determine the structure and function of a person's cells and affect his or her development, personality, and health. (1.2)

genital herpes. Viral infection that results in sores on the genitals, mouth, or rectum. (18.1)

gingivitis. Inflammation of the gums. (3.2)

goal. Desired result of something you plan to do. (1.3)

gonorrhea. Bacterial infection that primarily affects the genitals, rectum, and throat. (18.1)

gratitude. Emotion that means being thankful or grateful. (5.2)

green products. Goods that have a less harmful impact on the environment than traditional products. (14.2)

group dating. Going out with a group that includes the person one is interested in rather than dating as a couple. (15.4)

growth spurt. Period of rapid physical growth that occurs during puberty. (19.2)

H

hackers. People who illegally access data on digital devices. (13.2)

hallucinogens. Drugs that alter the way people view, think, and feel about things, causing hallucinations. (11.2)

hangover. Negative symptoms caused by drinking large amounts of alcohol on one occasion. (10.1)

Español

G

vesícula. Órgano en que la bilis se almacena hasta que necesitan para digerir los alimentos. (2.3)

pandillas. Grupos de personas que llevar a cabo acciones violentos e ilegales. (16.3)

género. Características una sociedad asocial con un sexo biológico particular. (19.1)

identidad de género. Pensamientos y sentimientos internos profundos sobre el género. (19.1)

roles de género. Conductas que la sociedad considera "adecuadas" para cierto género. (19.1)

genes. Segmentos de ADN que determinan la estructura y la función de las células de una persona y afectan su desarrollo, la personalidad, y la salud. (1.2)

herpes genital. Infección vírica que produce úlceras en los genitales, la boca o el recto. (18.1)

gingivitis. Inflamación de las encías. (3.2)

meta. Resultado deseado de algo que planeas hacer. (1.3)

gonorrea. Infección bacteriana que afecta principalmente los genitales, el recto, y la garganta. (18.1)

gratitud. Emoción que significa ser agradecido. (5.2)

productos ecológicos. Bienes que tienen un impacto menos dañino por el ambiente que productos tradicionales. (14.2)

citas grupales. Salir con un grupo que incluye la persona uno está interesado en vez de salir en citas como pareja. (15.4)

estirón. Período de crecimiento físico rápido que ocurre durante la pubertad. (19.2)

H

piratas informáticos. Personas que acceden ilegalmente a los datos de los dispositivos digitales. (13.2)

alucinógenos. Drogas que alteran la manera en que personas ven, piensan, y sienten sobre cosas, causando alucinaciones. (11.2)

resaca. Síntomas negativos causados por beber grandes cantidades de alcohol de una sola ocasión. (10.1)

English

harassment. Type of bullying that targets a particular part of a person's identity, such as race, religion, or sex. (16.1)

hate crimes. Threats or violence against someone because of his or her race, ethnic origin, disability, sex, or religion. (16.3)

hazing. Use of pressure by a group to make someone do something embarrassing or even dangerous to be accepted by a group. (16.1)

health. State of complete physical, mental and emotional, and social well-being. (1.1)

healthcare. Treatment and prevention of illnesses, injuries, or diseases to improve wellness. (1.1)

health literacy. Person's ability to locate, evaluate, apply, and communicate information as it relates to health. (1.3)

health-related fitness. Type of physical fitness a person needs to perform daily activities with ease and energy. (8.2)

heart. Hollow, muscular organ located in the center of the chest; pumps blood into the circulatory system. (2.2)

heart attack. Medical emergency in which flow of blood to the heart is restricted, causing the heart to beat irregularly and inefficiently. (12.2)

heavy drinking. Consuming eight or more drinks for females and 15 or more drinks for males in one week; can lead to alcohol dependence. (10.1)

heroin. Illegal opioid that has dangerous side effects and is very addictive. (11.2)

homicide. Crime of killing another person. (16.3)

homophobia. Hostility, anger, exclusion, and violence directed at people who are LGBT+. (19.1)

hospice care. Type of care given to people who are dying that provides comfort and support to them and their families. (17.4)

Español

acoso. Tipo de intimidación dirigida a una parte particular de la identidad de una persona, como la raza, la religión o el sexo. (16.1)

crímenes de odio. Amenazas o violencia contra alguien debido a su raza, origen étnico, discapacidad, sexo o religión. (16.3)

novatadas. Uso de presión por un grupo a hacer que alguien haga algo embarazoso o hasta peligroso para ser aceptado por un grupo. (16.1)

salud. Estado de completa plenitud física, mental, emocional y social. (1.1)

cuidado de la salud. Tratamiento y la prevención de los padecimientos, heridas, o enfermedades a mejorar el bienestar. (1.1)

educación sobre salud. Capacidad de una persona para encontrar, evaluar, aplicar y comunicar información relacionada con la salud. (1.3)

estado físico relacionado con la salud. Tipo de estado físico que una persona necesita para realizar actividades diarias con facilidad y energía. (8.2)

corazón. Órgano hueco, muscular localizado en el centro del pecho; bombea la sangre en el sistema circulatorio. (2.2)

ataque cardíaco. Emergencia médica en que el flujo de la sangre al corazón se restringe, causando el corazón a batir irregularmente y de forma ineficiente. (12.2)

consumo excesivo de alcohol. Consumir ocho o más bebidas, en el caso de hembras, y 15 o más bebidas, en el caso de varones, durante una semana; puede conducir a una dependencia del alcohol. (10.1)

heroína. Opioide ilegal que tiene efectos secundarios peligrosos y es muy adictivo. (11.2)

homicidio. Crimen de matar otra persona. (16.3)

homophobia. Hostilidad, ira, exclusión y violencia dirigida a personas LGBT+. (19.1)

cuidado de enfermos terminales. Tipo de asistencia dado a las personas que están muriendo que provee comodidad y apoyo a ellos y sus familias. (17.4)

English

human immunodeficiency virus (HIV). Bloodborne virus that infects and kills white blood cells, weakening the immune system. (18.2)

human life cycle. Sequence of developmental stages a person experiences from birth through adulthood. (17.2)

human papillomavirus (HPV). Most commonly contracted STI that causes genital infections and sometimes cancer. (18.1)

human trafficking. Form of modern slavery in which people are forced or pressured to perform some type of job or service against their will. (16.3)

hyperthermia. Serious condition that results when the heat-regulating mechanisms of the body are unable to deal with the heat from the environment, which results in a very high body temperature. (8.3)

hypodermis. Innermost layer of the skin, which contains fat, blood vessels, and nerve endings; attaches to underlying bone and muscle. (2.1)

hypothermia. Serious condition that results when a person's body loses heat faster than it can produce it. (8.3)

I

identity. Who you are, which includes your physical traits, social connections, and internal thoughts and feelings. (5.1)

identity theft. Act of using people's personal information to pretend to be them. (13.2)

immediate family. Person's parents or guardians and siblings. (15.2)

individual therapy. Type of therapy that involves a one-on-one meeting with a therapist to discuss feelings and behaviors. (6.2)

infatuation. Intense romantic feelings for another person that develop suddenly and are usually based on physical attraction. (15.4)

Español

virus de inmunodeficiencia humana (VIH). Virus transmitido por la sangre que infecta y mata los glóbulos blancos, debilitando el sistema inmunológico. (18.2)

ciclo de vida humana. Secuencia de las etapas de desarrollo una persona experimenta desde el nacimiento hasta la adultez. (17.2)

virus del papiloma humano (VPH). ITS más comúnmente contratado que causa infecciones genitales y a veces cáncer. (18.1)

trata de personas. Forma moderna de esclavitud en la que se obliga o presiona a las personas a realizar algún tipo de trabajo o servicio contra su voluntad. (16.3)

hipertermia. Condición grave que resulta cuando los mecanismos del cuerpo por la regulación del calor no pueden resolver el calor del ambiente, que resulta en una temperatura corporal muy alta. (8.3)

hipodermis. Capa más interna de la piel, que contiene grasa, vasos sanguíneos, y terminaciones nerviosas; se une al hueso subyacente y al músculo. (2.1)

hipotermia. Condición grave que resulta cuando el cuerpo de una persona pierde el calor más rápido que puede producirlo. (8.3)

identidad. Quién eres, lo que incluye tus características físicas, conexiones sociales, así como sentimientos y pensamientos internos. (5.1)

robo de identidad. Acto de usar la información personal de las personas para pretender ser ellas. (13.2)

familia inmediata. Los padres o guardianes y hermanos de una persona. (15.2)

terapia individual. Tipo de terapia que consiste en una reunión uno a uno con una terapeuta para discutir los sentimientos y comportamientos. (6.2)

enamoramiento. Sentimientos intensos románticos por otra persona que desarrollan bruscamente y son por lo general basado en atracción física. (15.4)

English

influenza. Viral infection of the respiratory system; also known as the *flu*. (12.1)

inhalants. Chemicals that people breathe in to experience some type of high. (11.2)

inhibition. Self-control that keeps people from taking dangerous risks. (10.1)

inpatient treatment. Type of treatment that involves staying in a healthcare facility for a period of time. (6.2)

insomnia. Trouble falling or staying asleep. (4.2)

integumentary system. Body system that covers and protects the entire body. (2.1)

intensity. Amount of energy the body uses per minute during an activity. (8.4)

internal condom. Device similar to a pouch, which is placed inside the vagina or rectum. (20.1)

Internet predators. People who use personal information to find and harm people or violate their privacy. (13.2)

interpersonal skills. Skills that help people communicate and relate in positive ways with others. (15.1)

intimacy. Closeness. (15.4)

intimate partner violence. Abuse that involves couples who are or were in a romantic relationship. (16.2)

J

jet lag. Fatigue that people feel after changing time zones when they travel. (4.1)

joint. Location in the body where two or more bones meet and are held together. (2.1)

K

kidneys. Two bean-shaped organs that filter blood and make urine. (2.3)

Español

influenza. Infección vírica del sistema respiratorio; también conocido como *la gripe*. (12.1)

inhalantes. Productos químicos que las personas inhalan para experimentar algún tipo de colocón. (11.2)

inhibición. Autocontrol que prevenir personas a tomando riesgos peligrosos. (10.1)

tratamiento hospitalario. Tipo de tratamiento que consiste en quedarse en un centro de servicios médicos para un periodo de tiempo. (6.2)

insomnio. Dificultad de quedarse o permanecer dormido. (4.2)

sistema integumentario. Sistema corporal que cubre y protege todo el cuerpo. (2.1)

intensidad. Cantidad de energía que el cuerpo usa por minuto durante una actividad. (8.4)

condón interno. Dispositivo similar a una bolsa que se coloca dentro de la vagina o el recto. (20.1)

depredadores de internet. Personas que usan información personal para encontrar y dañar a personas o violar su privacidad. (13.2)

habilidades interpersonales. Habilidades que ayudan a personas comunicar y relacionar en maneras positivas con otros. (15.1)

intimidad. Cercanía. (15.4)

violencia de pareja. Abuso que involucra a parejas que están o estaban en una relación romántica. (16.2)

jet lag. Fatiga que las personas experimentan después de cambiar zonas de tiempo durante un viaje. (4.1)

articulación. Localización en el cuerpo donde dos o más huesos se unen y se mantienen juntos. (2.1)

riñones. Dos órganos con forma de frijol que filtran la sangre y hacen la orina. (2.3)

English

L

lice. Tiny insects that attach to hair and feed on human blood. (3.1)

life expectancy. Estimate of how long a person in a particular society is likely to live. (17.2)

life span. Actual number of years a person lives. (17.2)

ligaments. Strong bands of tissue that hold together bones at joints to allow movement. (2.1)

liver. Large brown organ to the right of the stomach that has many jobs, including making bile. (2.3)

long-term non-progressors. People living with HIV whose infection progresses to AIDS very slowly. (18.2)

lymphatic system. Body system of organs and tissues that help fight infections. (2.3)

M

major depressive disorder. Condition characterized by intense negative feelings that do not go away and negatively affect daily life; also known as *clinical depression*. (6.1)

malnutrition. Condition that results from people not eating the right amounts of nutrients. (7.2)

marijuana. Drug made up of dried parts of the cannabis plant. (11.2)

masturbation. Self-stimulation of the sex organ. (19.2)

maximum heart rate. Number of beats per minute a person's heart can achieve when working its hardest; varies by age. (8.4)

medical emergency. Urgent, life-threatening situation. (13.3)

medication abuse. Intentionally using a medication in an unintended way. (11.1)

Español

piojos. Minúsculos insectos que se adhieren al pelo y se alimentan de la sangre humana. (3.1)

esperanza de vida. Estimación de cuánto tiempo una persona en una sociedad particular es probable a vivir. (17.2)

período de vida. Número real de años una persona vive. (17.2)

ligamentos. Bandas fuertes de tejido que mantienen juntos los huesos a las articulaciones para permitir el movimiento. (2.1)

hígado. Órgano marrón grande al derecho del estómago que tiene muchos trabajos, incluyendo hacer la bilis. (2.3)

progresores lentos. Personas que viven con VIH y cuya infección avanza al SIDA muy lentamente. (18.2)

sistema linfático. Sistema corporal de órganos y tejidos que ayudan combatir las infecciones. (2.3)

trastorno depresivo mayor. Afección caracterizada por sentimientos negativos intensos que no desaparecen y que afectan de manera negativa la vida diaria; también se conoce como *depresión clínica*. (6.1)

desnutrición. Afección que se produce cuando una persona no consume la cantidad adecuada de nutrientes. (7.2)

marihuana. Droga hecha de partes secos de la planta cannabis. (11.2)

masturbación. Auto-estimulación del órgano del sexo. (19.2)

frecuencia cardiaca máxima. Número de latidos por minuto el corazón de una persona puede lograr cuando trabajando más duro; varía en edad. (8.4)

emergencia médica. Situación urgente, mortal. (13.3)

abuso de medicamentos. Usar intencionadamente un medicamento de una manera diferente al uso previsto. (11.1)

English

medication-assisted treatment (MAT). Use of medicinal and behavioral treatment together. (11.3)

medication misuse. Taking medication in a way that does not follow the medication's instructions; often unintentional. (11.1)

medications. Substances used to treat symptoms of an illness or to cure, manage, or prevent a disease. (11.1)

melatonin. Hormone that increases feelings of relaxation and sleepiness and signals that it is time to go to sleep. (4.1)

menstruation. Discharge of some blood and tissues from the uterus. (17.1)

mental and emotional health. Aspect of health that has to do with a person's thoughts and feelings. (1.1)

mental distress. Mental and emotional state in which negative thoughts interfere with daily function for a short amount of time. (5.1)

mental health conditions. Patterns of thoughts and feelings that decrease mental and emotional health. (5.1)

mental health medication. Substance that causes changes in the brain to reduce symptoms of a mental illness. (6.2)

mental illness. Mental or emotional condition so severe that it interferes with daily functioning; also known as a *mental disorder*. (6.1)

methamphetamine. Stimulant that speeds up brain functions. (11.2)

method of transmission. Way a disease gets from one organism or object to another; may be direct or indirect. (12.1)

middle adulthood. Stage of human development that occurs from 40 to 65 years of age. (17.4)

middle childhood. Period of time when children are between five and 12 years of age; also called the *school-age years*. (17.2)

milestones. Important events that occur in each of the developmental stages of the human life cycle. (17.2)

minerals. Inorganic elements found in soil and water that the body needs in small quantities. (7.1)

Español

tratamiento asistido con medicamentos (MAT). Uso de tratamiento medicinal y conductual al mismo tiempo. (11.3)

mal uso de medicinas. Tomando medicina en una manera que no siga las instrucciones de la medicina; a menudo accidental. (11.1)

medicamentos. Sustancias que se utilizan para tratar los síntomas de una afección o curar, controlar o prevenir una enfermedad. (11.1)

melatonina. Hormona que aumenta las sensaciones de relajación y cansancio y hace señales que es tiempo a dormir. (4.1)

menstruación. Emisión de algún sangre y tejidos del útero. (17.1)

salud mental o emocional. Aspecto de salud que refiere a los pensamientos y sentimientos de una persona. (1.1)

angustia mental. Estado mental y emocional en el que los pensamientos negativos interfieren en las funciones diarias por un período breve. (5.1)

afecciones de salud mental. Patrones de pensamientos y sentimientos que disminuyen la salud mental y emocional. (5.1)

medicamento para salud mental. Sustancia que causa cambios en el cerebro para reducir los síntomas de una enfermedad mental. (6.2)

enfermedad mental. Condición mental o emocional tan grave que interfiere con el funcionamiento diario; también llamado *trastorno mental*. (6.1)

metanfetamina. Estimulante que acelera las funciones cerebrales. (11.2)

método de transmisión. Manera en que una enfermedad se transfiere de un organismo u objeto a otro; puede ser directo o indirecto. (12.1)

edad adulta. Etapa de desarrollo humano que ocurre desde 40 hasta 65 años de edad. (17.4)

infancia media. Período de tiempo cuando niños tienen entre cinco y doce años; también llamado los *años de la edad escolar*. (17.2)

hitos. Eventos importantes que ocurren en cada de las etapas de desarrollo del ciclo de la vida humana. (17.2)

minerales. Elementos inorgánicos que se encuentran en el suelo y el agua que el cuerpo necesita en cantidades pequeños. (7.1)

English

miscarriage. Spontaneous loss of the fetus. (20.2)

moderate drinking. Consuming no more than one drink per day for females and no more than two drinks per day for males; also called *social drinking*. (10.1)

mononucleosis. Common viral infection that spreads through kissing or by sharing certain objects; also known as *mono* and the *kissing disease*. (12.1)

muscular system. Body system that helps the body move and aids other body systems. (2.1)

MyPlate food guidance system. United States government system that helps people put the *Dietary Guidelines* into practice. (7.2)

N

narcolepsy. Disorder that affects the brain's ability to control the sleep-wake cycle. (4.2)

natural disasters. Events or forces of nature that usually cause great damage. (13.1)

nearsightedness. Condition in which objects close to the eye appear clear, while objects farther away appear blurry. (3.2)

neglect. Type of child abuse in which a child's basic physical, emotional, medical, or educational needs are not met by parents or guardians. (16.2)

nervous system. Body system that allows people to think, use the senses, move, and maintain important body processes. (2.4)

neuron. Cell that is specialized to receive and send signals. (2.4)

nicotine. Toxic substance that gives tobacco products their addictive quality. (9.1)

nicotine replacement. Smoking cessation technique that involves the use of nicotine gum or the nicotine patch to lessen withdrawal symptoms. (9.3)

night-light. Small lamp, often attached directly to an electrical outlet, that provides dim light during the night. (4.3)

Español

aborto espontáneo. Pérdida espontánea del feto. (20.2)

consumo moderado de alcohol. Consumiendo no más de una bebida por día para hembras y no más de dos bebidas por día para varones; también llamado *consumo social de alcohol*. (10.1)

mononucleosis. Infección vírica común que propague mientras besando o compartiendo ciertos objetos; también conocido como *mono* y *enfermedad del beso*. (12.1)

sistema muscular. Sistema corporal que ayuda al cuerpo a mover y ayuda otros sistemas corporales. (2.1)

sistema de guía de comida MyPlate. Sistema del gobierno de los Estados Unidos que ayuda personas a poner en práctica las *Pautas Alimentarias*. (7.2)

narcolepsia. Trastorno que afecta la capacidad del cerebro a controlar el ciclo sueño-vigilia. (4.2)

desastres naturales. Eventos o fuerzas de la naturaleza que por lo general causan grandes daños. (13.1)

miopía. Condición en que los objetos cercas del ojo aparecen claros, mientras objetos más alejados aparecen nublados. (3.2)

negligencia. Tipo de abuso infantil en que los necesidades físicos, emocionales, médicos, o educativos básicos de un niño no se cumplen por los padres o guardianes. (16.2)

sistema nervioso. Sistema corporal que permite a las personas pensar, usar los sentidos, mover, y mantener procesos corporales importantes. (2.4)

neurona. Célula que está especializada por recibir y enviar señales. (2.4)

nicotina. Sustancia tóxica que le da a los productos de tabaco su cualidad adictiva. (9.1)

reemplazo de la nicotina. Técnica de dejar de fumar que consiste en el uso del chicle de nicotina o el parche de nicotina para disminuye los síntomas de abstinencia. (9.3)

luz de noche. Lamparilla, a menudo unido directamente a una toma de corriente, que provee luz débil durante la noche. (4.3)

English

noncommunicable diseases. Conditions that cannot be spread among living things and objects, but develop as a result of heredity, environment, and lifestyle factors; also known as *noninfectious diseases*. (12.2)

nonverbal communication. Communicating through facial expressions, body language, gestures, tone and volume of voice, and other signals that do not involve the use of words. (15.1)

nutrient-dense foods. Foods that are rich in needed nutrients and have little or no solid fats, added sugars, refined starches, and sodium. (7.2)

nutrients. Chemical substances that give your body what it needs to grow and function properly. (7.1)

O

obesity. Condition of excess body fat or excessive overweight. (7.3)

obstetrician/gynecologist (OB/GYN). Type of doctor who specializes in pregnancy, labor, and delivery. (17.1)

older adulthood. Stage of human development that begins at 65 years of age. (17.4)

online friends. People you met through social media, websites, chat rooms, or gaming. (15.3)

opportunistic infections. Conditions that occur when pathogens take advantage of a weakened immune system; the cause of death in HIV/AIDS cases. (18.2)

optimism. Ability to keep a positive outlook and focus on the good aspects of stressful situations. (5.2)

optometrist. Eye care specialist who examines and treats eyes for vision conditions. (3.2)

oral contraceptives. Pills that contain hormones to reduce the likelihood of pregnancy. (20.1)

Español

enfermedades no transmisibles. Afecciones que no pueden contagiarse entre seres vivientes u objetos, pero que se desarrollan como resultado de la herencia, el ambiente y los factores del estilo de vida; también se conocen como *enfermedades no infecciosas*. (12.2)

comunicación no verbal. Comunicarse a través de expresiones faciales, lenguaje corporal, gestos, tono y volumen de voz, así como otras señales que no involucran el uso de palabras. (15.1)

alimentos ricos en nutrientes. Alimentos que son ricos en nutrientes necesarias y tienen pequeño o no grasas sólidas, azucares agregadas, almidones refinados, y sodio. (7.2)

nutrientes. Sustancias químicas que le dan al cuerpo lo que necesita para crecer y funcionar correctamente. (7.1)

obesidad. Condición de exceso de grasa corporal o sobrepeso excesivo. (7.3)

obstetra/ginecólogo (obstetrician/gynecologist, OB/GYN). Tipo de médico que se especializa en el embarazo, el parto, y el alumbramiento. (17.1)

edad adulta mayor. Etapa de desarrollo humano que comienza a 65 años de edad. (17.4)

amigos por internet. Personas que conoce mientras la media social, sitios web, salas de chat, o los videojuegos. (15.3)

infecciones oportunistas. Afecciones que ocurren cuando los patógenos se aprovechan de un sistema inmunológico debilitado; causa de muerte en casos de VIH/SIDA. (18.2)

optimismo. Capacidad de mantener una actitud positiva y concentrarse en los aspectos buenos de situaciones estresantes. (5.2)

optometrista. Especialista en atención de la vista que examina y trata los ojos por las afecciones de visión. (3.2)

anticonceptivos orales. Pastillas que contienen las hormonas para reducir la probabilidad de embarazo. (20.1)

English

orthodontist. Dental specialist who prevents and corrects teeth misalignments. (3.2)

outpatient treatment program. Provides drug education or counseling without requiring a hospital stay. (11.3)

overdose. Taking more of a medication or drug than the body can process at one time. (11.1)

overnutrition. Condition that results from people eating too many foods that contain high amounts of added sugar, solid fat, sodium, refined carbohydrates, or too many calories. (7.2)

over-the-counter (OTC) medications. Medicines people can purchase without a doctor's prescription to treat the symptoms of many minor health conditions. (11.1)

overweight. Condition of excess body weight from fat, bone, muscle, water, or a combination of these factors. (7.3)

ovulation. Release of an egg from one of the follicles into the uterus. (17.1)

ozone. Gas made up of oxygen that naturally exists high above Earth's atmosphere. (14.1)

P

pancreas. Fish-shaped organ behind the stomach that makes many kinds of enzymes needed for digestion. (2.3)

parasomnia. Term for sleep disorders that occur when people are partially, but not completely, awoken from sleep. (4.2)

passion. Powerful feeling based on physical attraction. (15.4)

pathogens. Microorganisms that cause communicable diseases. (12.1)

pedestrians. People on foot or using methods of transportation with small wheels (for example, bicycles, skateboards, or wheelchairs). (13.2)

peer abuse. Violent mistreatment of one peer by another. (16.1)

peer mediation. Process in which specially trained students work with other students to resolve conflicts. (15.1)

Español

ortodoncista. Especialista dental quien previene y corrige las desalineaciones de los dientes. (3.2)

programa de tratamiento ambulatorio. Provee educación o terapia sobre las drogas sin requiere una estancia hospitalaria. (11.3)

sobredosis. Tomando demasiado mucho de una droga que el cuerpo puede procesar a un tiempo. (11.1)

sobrenutrición. Condición que resulta de personas comer demasiados alimentos que contienen cantidades altas de azúcar agregada, grasa sólida, sodio, carbohidratos refinados, o demasiado calorías. (7.2)

medicinas de venta libre. Medicamentos que se pueden comprar sin una receta del médico para tratar los síntomas de muchas afecciones menores de salud. (11.1)

sobrepeso. Condición de exceso de peso corporal por grasa, hueso, músculo, agua o una combinación de estos factores. (7.3)

ovulación. Liberación de un óvulo de uno de los folículos en el útero. (17.1)

ozono. Gas hecho de oxígeno que naturalmente existe alto sobre la atmosfera de la Tierra. (14.1)

páncreas. Órgano con forma de pescado detrás del estómago que hace muchos tipos de enzimas necesarias para la digestión. (2.3)

parasomnia. Término para trastornos del sueño que ocurren cuando la gente está parcialmente, pero no completamente, despierto del sueño. (4.2)

pasión. Sentimiento fuerte basado en atracción física. (15.4)

patógenos. Microorganismos que causan enfermedades transmisibles. (12.1)

peatones. Personas a pie o que utilizan medios de transporte con ruedas pequeñas (por ejemplo: bicicletas, patinetas o sillas de ruedas). (13.2)

abuso de pares. Maltrato violento de un par por un otro. (16.1)

mediación entre pares. Proceso en que estudiantes especialmente entrenados trabajan con otros estudiantes a resolver los conflictos. (15.1)

English

peer pressure. Influence that people your age or status have on your actions. (9.2)

peers. People who are similar in age to one another. (1.2)

periodontitis. Infection caused by bacteria getting under the gum tissue and destroying the gums and bone. (3.2)

physical abuse. Behaviors that cause physical harm to a person; may involve hitting, kicking, choking, slapping, or burning. (16.2)

physical activity. Any action in which the body uses energy. (8.1)

Physical Activity Guidelines for Americans. Resource health professionals use to provide guidance on how people can improve their health through physical activities. (8.1)

physical health. Aspect of health that refers to how well a person's body functions. (1.1)

pituitary gland. Master gland of the body, which releases hormones to control other endocrine organs. (2.4)

plaque. Sticky, colorless film that coats the teeth and dissolves their protective enamel surface. (3.2)

plasma. Liquid part of the blood. (2.2)

poisonous. Able to cause illness or death upon entering the body. (13.1)

pollutants. Substances that contaminate the environment and can harm people. (14.1)

post-exposure prophylaxis (PEP). Emergency course of ART that a person can take after potential exposure to HIV to reduce risk of transmission. (18.2)

precautions. Actions you take to prevent something bad from happening. (13.1)

pre-exposure prophylaxis (PrEP). Course of ART that helps prevent HIV transmission; comes in a pill taken daily. (18.2)

prenatal care. Medical care during pregnancy. (20.2)

prenatal development. Period of growth that occurs from conception to birth. (17.1)

Español

presión de pares. Influencia que tienen las personas de tu edad o estatus en tus acciones. (9.2)

pares. Personas quienes son similares en edad al otro. (1.2)

periodontitis. Infección debido a bacterias metiendo debajo del tejido de las encías y destruyendo las encías y el hueso. (3.2)

abuso físico. Conductas que causan daño físico a una persona; pueden implicar golpear, patear, ahogar, abofetear o quemar. (16.2)

actividad física. Cualquier acción en la cual el cuerpo usa energía. (8.1)

Pautas de Actividad Física para Estadounidenses. Recurso que profesionales de salud utilizan para proveer guía en como personas pueden mejorar sus saludes mientras actividades físicas. (8.1)

salud física. Aspecto de salud que refiere a como bien el cuerpo de una persona funciona. (1.1)

glándula pituitaria. Glándula maestra del cuerpo, que emite hormonas para controlar otros órganos endocrinos. (2.4)

placa. Capa pegajosa, incolora que cubre los dientes y disuelve su superficie de esmalte. (3.2)

plasma. Parte líquida de la sangre. (2.2)

venenoso. Capaz de causar una dolencia o la muerte al entrar en el cuerpo. (13.1)

contaminantes. Sustancias que contaminan el ambiente y puede dañarse a las personas. (14.1)

profilaxis posterior a la exposición (PEP). Curso de emergencia de la terapia antirretroviral que puede realizar una persona tras una exposición potencial al VIH para reducir el riesgo de transmisión. (18.2)

precauciones. Acciones se toma para prevenir algo malo suceda. (13.1)

profilaxis previa a la exposición (PrEP). Curso de TARV que ayuda a prevenir el transmisión de VIH; viene en una píldora que se toma todos los días. (18.2)

atención prenatal. Cuidado médico durante el embarazo. (20.2)

desarrollo prenatal. Período de crecimiento que ocurre desde la concepción hasta el nacimiento. (17.1)

English

prescription medications. Medicines that people can only purchase with a doctor's order for the treatment of a specific illness or condition. (11.1)

preventive healthcare. Going to the doctor when you are well to help you stay healthy; involves getting an annual physical exam, regular checkups, and screenings for conditions like hearing or vision loss. (1.1)

primary care physician. Regular doctor who provides checkups, screenings, treatments, and prescriptions. (1.1)

primary sexual characteristics. Changes to the sex organs during puberty. (17.3)

protective factors. Aspects of people's lives that reduce risk and increase the likelihood of optimal health. (1.2)

protein. Nutrient the body uses to build and maintain all of its cells and tissues. (7.1)

puberty. Stage of life when the body reaches sexual maturity. (17.3)

public service announcement (PSA). Media message that supports public health. (9.3)

pulse. Person's heart rate. (8.4)

purging. Attempts to rid the body of food. (7.4)

R

rape. Sexual intercourse that occurs without consent. (19.3)

recycling. Process in which used materials are turned into new products. (14.2)

refusal skills. Set of skills designed to help someone avoid participating in unhealthy behaviors. (1.3)

rehabilitation program. Treatment for substance use disorder that may involve detoxification, medications, or time spent in a rehabilitation facility. (11.3)

Español

medicamentos con receta. Medicamentos que se pueden comprar solo con una orden del médico para el tratamiento de una enfermedad o afección especifica. (11.1)

atención médica preventiva. Ir al médico cuando está bien para ayudarse mantiene la salud; consiste en recibiendo un examen físico anual, chequeos regulares, y proyecciones para condiciones como la pérdida de audición o visión. (1.1)

médico de atención primaria. Médico de cabecera que ofrece chequeos, proyecciones, tratamientos, y recetas. (1.1)

características sexuales primarias. Cambios en los órganos sexuales durante la pubertad. (17.3)

factores protectors. Aspectos de la vida de las personas que reducen el riesgo y aumentan la probabilidad de una salud óptima. (1.2)

proteína. Un nutriente que el cuerpo utiliza para construir y mantener todo tipo de células y tejidos. (7.1)

pubertad. Etapa de la vida cuando el cuerpo alcanza la madurez sexual. (17.3)

anuncio de servicio público (PSA). Mensaje que respalda la salud pública. (9.3)

pulso. Latido del corazón de una persona. (8.4)

purga. Intentos de limpiar al cuerpo de alimentos. (7.4)

violación. Relaciones sexuales que ocurren sin consentimiento. (19.3)

reciclaje. Proceso en que materiales usados se conviertan en productos nuevos. (14.2)

habilidades de rechazo. Conjunto de habilidades diseñadas para ayudar a alguien a evitar participar en comportamientos poco saludables. (1.3)

programa de rehabilitación. Tratamiento del trastorno por consumo de sustancias que puede involucrar la desintoxicación, el uso de medicamentos o pasar tiempo en un centro de rehabilitación. (11.3)

English

relapse. Occurrence when a person takes a medication or drug again after deciding to stop. (11.3)

relationships. Connections that people form and maintain with others. (15.1)

relaxation response. Reaction in which the body returns to its resting state after a stressful event. (5.3)

REM sleep. Active stage of sleep during which your breathing changes, your heart rate and blood pressure rise, and your eyes dart around rapidly. (4.1)

renewable energy. Type of energy that cannot be used up, such as wind, water, or solar power. (14.2)

reproductive system. Body system that consists of a group of organs working together to make the creation of new life possible. (17.1)

residential treatment program. Helps people get through the early stages of breaking an addiction in an inpatient environment with lots of support and few distractions. (11.3)

resilience. Ability to bounce back from traumatic or stressful events. (5.2)

resistance. Opposition. (8.2)

respiration. Exchange of oxygen and carbon dioxide between the body and the air around it. (2.2)

respiratory etiquette. Practice of covering your mouth and nose with a tissue while coughing or sneezing, or sneezing into your sleeve. (12.3)

respiratory system. Body system of organs that obtain vitally important oxygen from the outside world. (2.2)

response substitution. Smoking cessation technique that involves responding to difficult feelings and situations with behaviors other than smoking. (9.3)

risk factors. Aspects of people's lives that increase the chance of a disease, injury, or decline in health. (1.2)

rituals. Series of actions performed as part of a ceremony. (15.2)

Español

recaída. Incidencia cuando una persona toma un medicamento o droga nuevamente después de decidirse a abandonarlo. (11.3)

relaciones. Conexiones que las personas forman y mantienen con los demás. (15.1)

respuesta de relajación. Reacción en la que el cuerpo vuelve a su estado de reposo después de un evento estresante. (5.3)

sueño REM. Etapa activa de sueño mientras que su respiración cambie, su ritmo cardiaco y presión sanguínea suben, y sus ojos lanzan rápidamente por todo. (4.1)

energía renovable. Tipo de energía que no puede ser agotado, como tal la energía eólica, del agua, y solar. (14.2)

sistema reproductivo. Sistema corporal que consiste en un grupo de órganos trabajando juntos para hacer posible la creación de una vida nueva. (17.1)

programa de tratamiento residencial. Ayuda a las personas a superar las primeras etapas de romper una adicción en un ambiente hospitalario que ofrece mucho apoyo y pocas distracciones. (11.3)

resiliencia. Capacidad de recuperarse de eventos traumáticos o estresantes. (5.2)

resistencia. Oposición. (8.2)

respiración. Intercambio del oxígeno y el dióxido de carbono entre el cuerpo y el aire alrededor de ello. (2.2)

etiqueta respiratoria. Práctica de cubrir su boca y nariz con un pañuelo mientras tose o estornuda, o estornuda en su manga. (12.3)

sistema respiratorio. Sistema corporal de órganos que obtienen oxígeno de la vital importancia del mundo exterior. (2.2)

sustitución de respuesta. Técnica de dejar de fumar que consiste en contestando a sentimientos y situaciones difíciles con comportamientos aparte de fumar. (9.3)

factores de riesgo. Aspectos de las vidas de las personas que aumentan las probabilidades de una enfermedad, una lesión o el deterioro de la salud. (1.2)

rituales. Serie de acciones realizan como parte de una ceremonia. (15.2)

English

S

sandwich generation. Adults who care for their parents as well as their own children. (17.4)

saturated fats. Type of fat found mainly in animal-based foods, such as meat and dairy products. (7.1)

schizophrenia spectrum disorder. Condition characterized by having irregular thoughts and delusions, hearing voices, and seeing things that are not there. (6.1)

school violence. Any violent behavior that occurs on school property, at school-sponsored events, or on the way to or from school or school events. (16.3)

secondary sexual characteristics. Features that appear during puberty, but do not directly affect the sex organs. (17.3)

secondhand aerosol. Aerosol released into the environment by people who vape; other people nearby inhale secondhand aerosol. (9.1)

secondhand smoke. Tobacco smoke released into the environment by people who smoke; other people nearby inhale secondhand smoke. (9.1)

sedentary behaviors. Activities that consist of sitting or lying down and using very little energy. (8.1)

self-care. Practice of taking an active role in protecting your own health; involves eating healthy and getting plenty of sleep and physical activity. (5.3)

self-compassion. Treating oneself with kindness and understanding, even when experiencing setbacks and disappointments. (5.2)

self-esteem. How you feel about yourself. (5.1)

self-image. Your mental picture of yourself, which includes how you look, how you act, your skills and abilities, and your weaknesses; also called *self-concept*. (5.1)

self-talk. Thoughts and feelings about oneself. (5.1)

Español

generación sándwich. Adultos que cuidan a sus padres además de sus propios hijos. (17.4)

grasas saturadas. Tipo de grasa se encuentra principalmente en alimentos de origen animal, tal como carne y productos lácteos. (7.1)

trastorno del espectro esquizofrénico. Afección caracterizada por tener delirios y pensamientos irregulares, escuchar voces y ver cosas que no existen. (6.1)

violencia escolar. Cualquier comportamiento violento que ocurre en la propiedad escolar, en eventos patrocinados por la escuela o en el recorrido a la escuela o a los eventos escolares o desde estos. (16.3)

características sexuales secundarias. Características que aparecen durante la pubertad, pero que no afectan directamente los órganos sexuales. (17.3)

aerosol de segunda mano. Aerosol liberado en el ambiente por personas que vapean; otras personas que se encuentran cerca inhalan el aerosol de segunda mano. (9.1)

humo de segunda mano. Humo de tabaco liberado en el ambiente por personas que fuman; otras personas que se encuentran cerca inhalan el humo de segunda mano. (9.1)

comportamientos sedentarios. Actividades que consisten en sentarse o acostarse y consumen muy poca energía. (8.1)

autocuidado. Práctica de asumir un papel activo en la protección de tu propia salud; implica alimentarse de forma saludable y dormir y realizar actividad física lo suficiente. (5.3)

autocompasión. Tratarse uno mismo con amabilidad y comprensión, aun cuando se experimentan obstáculos y decepciones. (5.2)

autoestima. Como se siente sobre sí mismo. (5.1)

autoimagen. Su imagen mental de usted mismo, que incluye como se ve, como se comporta, sus habilidades y capacidades, y sus debilidades; también llamado *concepto de sí mismo*. (5.1)

diálogo interno. Pensamientos y sentimientos sobre uno mismo. (5.1)

English

sets. Anaerobic activities done in groups of repetitions followed by rest. (8.4)

sext. To send sexual content as digital text, a picture, or a video. (13.2)

sexual abuse. Sexual activity to which one person does not or cannot consent. (16.2)

sexual assault. Act of threatening, pressuring, or forcing someone into sexual activity. (19.3)

sexual harassment. Verbal or nonverbal sexual attention that occurs without consent. (19.3)

sexual intercourse. Any sexual activity that involves penetration. (19.2)

sexuality. Includes factors such as a person's biological sex, sexual expression and feelings, orientation, and gender identity. (19.1)

sexually transmitted infections (STIs). Communicable diseases spread from one person to another during sexual activity. (18.1)

sexual orientation. Continuing pattern of romantic and sexual attraction. (19.1)

short sleepers. People who can function well on less sleep than other people. (4.1)

sibling abuse. Violent behaviors that one sibling inflicts on another sibling. (16.2)

sibling rivalry. Competitive feelings between siblings; siblings may compete for material or nonmaterial items. (15.2)

side effect. Unpleasant and unwanted symptom that occurs from taking a medication. (11.1)

skeletal system. Body system made up of 206 bones that provides structure, shape, and protection to the body. (2.1)

skill-related fitness. Type of physical fitness that improves a person's performance in a particular sport or leisure activity. (8.2)

skills-training program. Teaches people skills for dealing with peer pressure and for handling stressful events without relying on medications or drugs. (11.3)

Español

series. Actividades anaeróbicas que se realizan en grupos de repeticiones seguidas de un descanso. (8.4)

sext. Enviar contenido sexual en forma de texto digital, una imagen o un video. (13.2)

abuso sexual. Actividad sexual para la cual una persona no da su consentimiento o no puede dar su consentimiento. (16.2)

agresión sexual. Acto de amenazar, presionar u obligar a alguien a tener actividad sexual. (19.3)

acoso sexual. Atención sexual verbal o no verbal que ocurre sin consentimiento. (19.3)

relaciones sexuales. Cualquier actividad sexual que implica penetración. (19.2)

sexualidad. Incluye factores como el sexo biológico, la expresión y los sentimientos sexuales, la orientación y la identidad de género de una persona. (19.1)

infecciones de transmisión sexual (ITS). Enfermedades transmisibles propagada de una persona a otro durante la actividad sexual. (18.1)

orientación sexual. Patrón continuo de atracción romántica y sexual. (19.1)

personas que duermen poco. Personas quienes pueden funcionar bien con dormir menos que otros. (4.1)

abuso de hermanos. Comportamientos violentos que un hermano dirige hacia otro hermano. (16.2)

rivalidad entre hermanos. Sentimientos competitivos entre hermanos; los hermanos pueden competir por temas materiales o no materiales. (15.2)

efecto secundario. Síntoma desagradable y no deseado que resulta de tomar medicina. (11.1)

sistema esquelético. Sistema corporal hecho de 206 huesos que proviene estructura, forma, y protección al cuerpo. (2.1)

estado físico relacionado con la habilidad. Tipo de estado físico que mejora el desempeño de una persona en un deporte o una actividad recreativa en particular. (8.2)

programa de entrenamiento de habilidades. Enseña a las personas habilidades para lidiar con la presión de pares y para manejar eventos estresantes sin depender de los medicamentos o drogas. (11.3)

English

sleep apnea. Potentially serious disorder in which a person stops breathing for short periods of time during sleep. (4.2)

sleep deficit. Condition that occurs when people frequently get less sleep than they should. (4.1)

sleep deprived. Term used to describe a person who gets inadequate amounts of sleep. (4.1)

sleep-wake cycle. Pattern of sleeping in a 24-hour period. (4.1)

sleep-wake schedule. Routine for going to bed at about the same time each night and getting up at about the same time each morning. (4.3)

SMART. Acronym used to guide goal setting; stands for specific, measurable, achievable, relevant, and timely. (1.3)

smog. Fog that has mixed with smoke and chemical fumes. (14.1)

sober living communities. Alcohol- and drug-free living environments that reduce some of the temptation and pressure people may feel to use alcohol and drugs. (11.3)

social health. Aspect of health that involves interacting and getting along with others in positive, healthy ways. (1.1)

socialize. Teaching children to behave in socially acceptable ways. (15.2)

spinal cord. Part of the nervous system that carries nerve signals between the brain and the body. (2.4)

spleen. Organ filled with white blood cells; filters blood. (2.3)

sprain. Injury to a ligament. (8.3)

stalking. Following and repeatedly contacting someone in a way that causes the person to feel scared, nervous, or threatened. (16.1)

standard precautions. Infection control practices that apply when giving first aid to any person under any circumstances. (13.3)

Español

apnea del sueño. Trastorno potencialmente grave en que una persona deja de respirar por periodos breves durante el sueño. (4.2)

déficit de sueño. Condición que ocurre cuando la gente frecuentemente recibe menos sueño que deben. (4.1)

con falta de sueño. Término usado por describir una persona que recibe cantidades deficientes del sueño. (4.1)

ciclo sueño-vigilia. Patrón de sueño en un periodo de 24 horas. (4.1)

plan de sueño-vigilia. Rutina para dormirse casi al mismo tiempo cada noche y despertarse casi al mismo tiempo cada mañana. (4.3)

SMART. Acrónimo en inglés utilizado para guiar el establecimiento de metas; significa específico (specific), mensurable (measurable), alcanzable (achievable), relevante (relevant) y oportuno (timely). (1.3)

smog. Niebla que se ha mezclado con humo y vapores químicos. (14.1)

comunidades de vida sobria. Ambientes libres de alcohol y drogas que reduzcan un poco de la tentación y presión personas pueden sentir a utilizar alcohol y drogas. (11.3)

salud social. Aspecto de salud que consiste en interactuando y llevando bien con otras personas en maneras positivas y sanas. (1.1)

socializar. Enseñar a los niños comportarse en maneras socialmente aceptables. (15.2)

médula espinal. Parte del sistema nervioso que lleva señales nerviosas entre el cerebro y el cuerpo. (2.4)

bazo. Órgano lleno de glóbulos blancos; filtra sangre. (2.3)

esguince. Lesión de un ligamento. (8.3)

acecho. Seguimiento y contacto reiterado con alguien a través de maneras que provocan que la persona se sienta atemorizada, nerviosa o amenazada. (16.1)

precauciones estándares. Prácticas de control de infecciones que aplican cuando se dé primeros auxilios a cualquier persona bajo cualquier circunstancia. (13.3)

English

statutory rape. Crime that takes place when someone over the age of consent engages in sexual intercourse with someone under the age of consent. (19.3)

stereotypes. Oversimplified ideas about a group of people. (15.3)

sterilization. Permanent birth control method in which a medical doctor performs a procedure on either male or female to prevent sperm and egg from uniting. (20.1)

stigma. Mark of shame or embarrassment that is usually unfair. (6.2)

stimulus control. Smoking cessation technique that involves avoiding tempting situations and managing feelings that lead to tobacco use. (9.3)

strangers. People whom you do not know. (13.2)

stress. Physical, mental, and emotional reactions of your body to the challenges you face. (5.3)

stress management. Process of using strategies to reduce the impact of the stress response and handle threatening situations in positive ways. (5.3)

stressor. Any factor that causes stress. (5.3)

stroke. Medical emergency in which blood flow to part of the brain is interrupted, injuring or killing brain cells. (12.2)

substance use disorder. Mental illness in which a person continues using a substance despite negative effects on health and life. (9.2)

suicide. Act of taking one's own life. (6.3)

suicide clusters. Series of suicides in a community that occur in a relatively short period of time. (6.3)

suicide contagion. Term that describes the copying of suicide attempts after exposure to another person's suicide. (6.3)

support groups. Gatherings in which a therapist meets with a group of people who share a common experience. (6.2)

survivors. People who lose a loved one to suicide. (6.3)

Español

estupro. Crimen que ocurre cuando alguien sobre la edad de consentimiento participa en relaciones sexuales con alguien bajo la edad de consentimiento. (19.3)

estereotipos. Ideas demasiadas simplificadas sobre un grupo de personas. (15.3)

esterilización. Método permanente de control de natalidad en el que un médico realiza un procedimiento en un varón o una hembra para prevenir que el esperma y el óvulo se unan. (20.1)

estigma. Marca de desgracia o vergüenza que es generalmente injusto. (6.2)

control de estímulos. Técnica para dejar de fumar que consiste en evitar las situaciones tentadoras y manejar los sentimientos que conducen al consumo de tabaco. (9.3)

desconocidos. Personas a las que no conoce. (13.2)

estrés. Reacciones físicas, mentales, y emocionales de su cuerpo a los retos que se enfrenta. (5.3)

manejo del estrés. Proceso de usar estrategias para reducir el impacto de la respuesta al estrés y manejar situaciones amenazantes de manera positiva. (5.3)

estresor. Cualquier factor que causa el estrés. (5.3)

accidente cerebrovascular. Emergencia medical en que el flujo sanguíneo a parte del cerebro se interrumpe, hiriendo o matando las células cerebrales. (12.2)

trastorno por consumo de sustancias. Enfermedad mental en la cual una persona continúa usando una sustancia a pesar de los efectos negativos sobre la salud y la vida. (9.2)

suicidio. La acción de quitarse la vida a sí mismo. (6.3)

grupos de suicidios. Series de suicidios en una comunidad particular que ocurren en un periodo de tiempo relativamente corto. (6.3)

contagio de suicidio. Termino que describe la copia de intentos de suicidio después de exposición al suicidio de otra persona. (6.3)

grupos de apoyo. Encuentros en los que un terapeuta se reúne con un grupo de personas que comparten una experiencia en común. (6.2)

sobrevivientes. Personas que pierden un ser querido por suicidio. (6.3)

English

sustainability. Actions that maintain the natural resources in the environment. (14.2)

syphilis. Bacterial infection divided into stages that causes extremely serious health conditions and disability. (18.1)

T

tar. Residue produced by burning tobacco; consists of small, thick, sticky particles. (9.1)

target heart rate. Number of heartbeats per minute that is safe and effective for a given intensity. (8.4)

teen parenthood. Act or process of an adolescent parent or parents raising a child. (20.2)

teen pregnancy. Pregnancy that occurs during the adolescent years when a teen's body is still developing and maturing. (20.2)

temper tantrum. Toddler's episode of emotional upset that often includes yelling, crying, hitting, kicking, or even biting. (17.2)

tendons. Structures made of tough tissue that connect muscle to bone. (2.1)

terrorism. Use of violence and threats to frighten and control groups of people to further an ideological aim. (16.3)

testosterone. Hormone that triggers growth and development of the male sex organs. (17.3)

therapist. Professional who diagnoses and treats people with mental health conditions. (6.2)

therapy. Treatment method that focuses on the psychological aspect of mental health. (6.2)

thirdhand aerosol. Particles and gases left over after someone vapes. (9.1)

thirdhand smoke. Particles and gases left over after someone smokes a cigarette; remains on surfaces nearby. (9.1)

thyroid hormone. Substance produced in the thyroid that increases the rate at which the body uses energy. (2.4)

Español

sostenibilidad. Acciones que mantienen los recursos naturales en el ambiente. (14.2)

sífilis. Infección bacteriana que se divide en etapas; causa condiciones de salud extremadamente graves y discapacidad. (18.1)

alquitrán. Residuo producido por la combustión del tabaco; consiste en partículas pequeñas, espesas, y pegajosas. (9.1)

frecuencia cardíaca objetivo. Número de latidos por minuto que es seguro y efectivo para una intensidad dada. (8.4)

paternidad adolescente. Acto o proceso de un padre adolescente o padres adolescentes criar a un niño. (20.2)

embarazo adolescente. Embarazo que ocurre durante los años de la adolescencia cuando el cuerpo de un adolescente aún se está desarrollando y madurando. (20.2)

rabieta. Episodio de un niño pequeño de trastorno emocional que a menudo incluye gritar, llorar, golpear, patear, o aún morder. (17.2)

tendones. Estructuras hechas de tejido duro que conectan musculo al hueso. (2.1)

terrorismo. Uso de violencia y amenazas para asustar y controlar grupas de personas para promover un objetivo ideológico. (16.3)

testosterona. Hormona que provoque el crecimiento y desarrollo de los órganos sexuales masculinos. (17.3)

terapeuta. Profesional que diagnostica y trata las personas con condiciones de salud mental. (6.2)

terapia. Método de tratamiento que se centra en el aspecto psicológico de la salud mental. (6.2)

aerosol de tercera mano. Partículas y gases que quedan después de que una persona vapea. (9.1)

humo de tercera mano. Partículas y gases que quedan después de que alguien fuma un cigarrillo; permanece en superficies cercanas. (9.1)

hormona tiroidea. Sustancia producida en la glándula tiroidea que aumenta la tasa a la que el cuerpo usa la energía. (2.4)

English

tinnitus. Pain or ringing in the ears after exposure to excessively loud sounds. (3.2)

tobacco. Plant with leaves that contain the chemical nicotine. (9.1)

tolerance. Body's need for an increased amount of a substance to experience the effects once felt with smaller amounts. (9.2)

tonsillitis. Bacterial or viral infection that affects the tonsils. (12.1)

toxic. Poisonous. (9.1)

toxic stress. Stress caused by repeated, long-lasting exposure to severe stressors, such as neglect and abuse, violence, or loss of a loved one. (5.3)

traditions. Specific patterns of behavior passed down in a culture. (15.2)

trans fats. Type of fat found in foods from animals, such as cows and goats; used to be found in many processed foods, such as packaged cookies and chips. (7.1)

transgender. Having a gender identity opposite of one's assigned, biological sex. (19.1)

trauma. Extreme stress due to deeply disturbing events, such as disasters, sexual assault, or violence. (5.3)

trichomoniasis. Curable infection caused by protozoa. (18.1)

triggers. Reminders that cause people to feel a strong desire for a substance. (9.2)

tryptophan. Amino acid that can help boost serotonin levels, which aid in sleep. (4.3)

tumor. Mass of abnormal cells. (12.2)

U

undernutrition. Condition that results from people not taking in enough nutrients for health and growth. (7.2)

Español

tinnitus. Dolor o acúfeno en las orejas después de exposición a sonidos excesivamente ruidosos. (3.2)

tabaco. Planta con hojas que contienen el químico nicotina. (9.1)

tolerancia. La necesidad del cuerpo de una cantidad mayor de una sustancia para experimentar los efectos que alguna vez se sintieron con cantidades más pequeñas. (9.2)

amigdalitis. Infección bacteriana o vírica que afecta las amígdalas. (12.1)

tóxico. Venenoso. (9.1)

estrés tóxico. Estrés causado por la exposición repetida y duradera a estresores severos, como negligencia y abuso, violencia o pérdida de un ser querido. (5.3)

tradiciones. Patrones específicos de comportamiento transmitido en una cultura. (15.2)

grasas trans. Tipo de grasa se encuentra en alimentos de origen animal, tal como vacas y cabras; solía ser encuentra en muchas comidas precocinadas, tal como galletas y papas fritas empacados. (7.1)

transgénero. Tener una identidad de género opuesta al sexo biológico asignado a una persona. (19.1)

trauma. Estrés extremo debido a eventos profundamente perturbadores, como desastres, agresión sexual o violencia. (5.3)

tricomoniasis. Infección curable causada por protozoos. (18.1)

desencadenantes. Recuerdos que causan a personas sentirse un deseo fuerte para una sustancia. (9.2)

triptófano. Aminoácido que puede ayudar a aumentar los niveles de serotonina, que ayudan a dormirse. (4.3)

tumor. Masa de células anormales. (12.2)

hiponutrición. Afección que se produce cuando una persona no consume una cantidad suficiente de nutrientes para la salud y el crecimiento. (7.2)

English

underweight. Condition of a body weight that is too low compared with others of the same sex and age. (7.3)

unsaturated fats. Type of fat found in plant-based foods, such as vegetable oils, some peanut butters and margarines, olives, salad dressing, nuts, and seeds. (7.1)

upstander. Person who recognizes when a behavior is wrong, takes steps to intervene and stop the behavior, and promotes positive change; also called an *ally*. (16.1)

urinary system. Body system that removes liquid waste from the body. (2.3)

V

vaccine. Substance that contains a dead or nontoxic part of a pathogen that is injected into a person to train his or her immune system to eliminate the live pathogen. (12.3)

vaginal ring. Small, flexible ring that releases hormones to stop ovulation. (20.1)

vaping device. Tobacco product that heats tobacco or synthetic nicotine without burning it, producing an aerosol. (9.1)

veins. Blood vessels that carry oxygen-poor blood. (2.2)

verbal communication. Use of words to send a spoken or written message. (15.1)

vitamins. Organic substances that come from plants or animals that are necessary for normal growth and development. (7.1)

W

weight stigma. Flawed belief that having a thinner body or lower weight is always better. (7.4)

well-being. Person's overall satisfaction that life's present conditions are good. (1.1)

wellness. Active process that involves becoming aware of and making choices toward improving aspects of health. (1.1)

Español

bajo peso. Condición de un peso corporal demasiado bajo en comparación con otras personas del mismo sexo y edad. (7.3)

grasas no saturadas. Tipo de grasa se encuentra en alimentos de origen vegetal, tal como aceite vegetal, algunas mantequillas de maní y margarina, olivas, arreglos de ensalada, nueces, y pepitas. (7.1)

espectador active. Persona que reconoce cuando un comportamiento es incorrecto, toma medidas para intervenir y detener el comportamiento, y promueve un cambio positivo; también denominado un *aliado*. (16.1)

sistema urinario. Sistema corporal que quita los residuos líquidos del cuerpo. (2.3)

vacuna. Sustancia que contiene un parte muerte o no tóxico de un agente patógeno en una persona para entrenar su sistema inmunológico a eliminar el agente patógeno vivo. (12.3)

anillo vaginal. Anillo pequeño y flexible que emite hormonas para parar la ovulación. (20.1)

dispositivo de vapeo. Producto de tabaco que calienta el tabaco o la nicotina sintética sin quemarlos, lo que produce un aerosol. (9.1)

venas. Vasos sanguíneos que llevan la sangre pobre en oxígeno. (2.2)

comunicación verbal. Uso de las palabras para enviar un mensaje hablado o escrito. (15.1)

vitaminas. Sustancias orgánicas derivadas de plantas o animales que son necesarias para el crecimiento y desarrollo normales. (7.1)

estigma de peso. Creencia errónea de que tener un cuerpo más delgado o un peso más bajo siempre es mejor. (7.4)

plenitude. Satisfacción general de una persona de que las condiciones presentes de la vida son buenas. (1.1)

bienestar. Proceso activo que implica tomar consciencia y hacer elecciones tendientes a mejorar los aspectos de la salud. (1.1)

English

wet dreams. Ejaculations that occur during sleep in males. (19.2)

withdrawal. Unpleasant symptoms that occur when someone with an addiction to a substance tries to stop using that substance. (9.2)

withdrawal. Natural birth control method based on the male pulling out of the female's vagina before ejaculation. (20.1)

Y

young adulthood. Stage of human development that occurs from 20 to 40 years of age. (17.4)

Z

zero-tolerance policy. Rule that results in punishment of young people caught driving with any level of alcohol in their system. (10.1)

zygote. Egg that has been fertilized by a sperm. (17.1)

Español

emisión nocturna. Eyaculaciones que ocurren durante el sueño de varones. (19.2)

abstinencia. Síntomas desagradables que ocurren cuando alguien adicto a una sustancia trata de dejar de consumir esa sustancia. (9.2)

retiro. Método natural de control de la natalidad basado en el varón retirándose de la vagina de la hembra antes de la eyaculación. (20.1)

adulto joven. Etapa de desarrollo humano que ocurre desde 20 hasta 40 años de edad. (17.4)

política de tolerancia cero. Regla que resulta en el castigo de jóvenes pillado manejando con cualquier nivel de alcohol en sus sistemas. (10.1)

cigoto. Ovulo que ha sido fecundado por un espermatozoide; también llamada *zigoto*. (17.1)

Index

A

AA. *See* Alcoholics Anonymous (AA)
abdominal muscles, 44
abdominal thrusts, 436
abortion, 640, 651–652
Above the Influence campaign, 360
abstinence. *See* sexual abstinence
abuse
    bullying, 518–526
    child abuse, 530–531
    defined, 527
    elder abuse, 532
    help and treatment, 535
    intimate partner violence, 529–530
    preventing and responding, 533–535
    reporting, 533–534
    sibling abuse, 531–532
    types of, 528–529
abuse hotlines, 533
ACA. *See Patient Protection and Affordable Care Act (ACA)*
Academy of Nutrition and Dietetics, 28
accidents
    alcohol and, 316–317
    falls, 407
    fire, 409–411
    marijuana and, 348
    medical emergencies, 425, 434–438
    motor vehicle accidents, 316–317, 423–425
    poisoning, 407–408
    providing first aid, 430–434
    water, 425–426
    weapons, 408
acetaminophen, 336, 429
acetylsalicylic acid. *See* aspirin
acid rain, 444, 447
acne, 76, 78–79, 566
acquaintance rape, 631. *See* rape; sexual assault

acquaintances, 496–497. *See also* friendships
acquired immunodeficiency syndrome (AIDS)
    defined, 594–595
    opportunistic infections, 597
    signs and symptoms, 596–597
    treatment, 599
acrophobia, 168
action plan, 22, 24–25. *See also* goal setting
active listening, 474, 480
acute stress, 151
addiction
    alcohol, 318–319
    defined, 287, 294
    drugs, 344
    medications, 341
    tobacco, 279–280
    treating, 300–302, 326–327, 360–361
    stages of substance use, 292–294
    support groups, 327, 361
    withdrawal, 287, 294, 318
    See also substance use disorder
ADHD. *See* attention-deficit hyperactivity disorder (ADHD)
adolescence, 557
    defined, 563–564
    emotional development, 568
    intellectual development, 567–568
    physical development and puberty, 557, 564–568, 619–622
    social development, 568
adoption, 651–652
adrenal glands, 69
adrenaline, 69
adulthood
    defined, 573
    health changes, 576
    signs of maturity, 573
    stages of, 573–575
advertisements. *See also* media
    alcohol, 324

    analyzing, 27–29, 80, 234–235, 298–299
    effect on body image, 229–231
    food, 215
    tobacco, 291, 298–299
advocacy
    community health, 31
    defined, 22, 29
    environment, 461, 466
    mental health, 185
    personal health, 29–30
    positive body image, 236
    substance abuse, 358–360
AED. *See* automated external defibrillator (AED)
aerobic activity, 248–251, 266–267
aerosol, 276, 281, 285–286
affirmative consent
    defined, 474, 477
    myths and facts, 629
    qualities of, 628–629
agender, 613
age of consent, 627–628
age spots, 576
aggressive behavior. *See* bullying; violence
aggressive communication, 481–482, 485
agility, 248, 253
aging, 573–578
agoraphobia, 168
AHA. *See* American Heart Association (AHA)
AIDS. *See* acquired immunodeficiency syndrome (AIDS)
air pollution, 446–448
Air Quality Index (AQI), 455, 457
Al-Anon Family Groups, 320, 328
Alateen, 320, 328
alcohol
    accidents, 316–317
    addiction, 318–319
    binge drinking, 310
    defined, 308–309
    factors affecting use, 321–324
    hangover, 312
    health effects, 311–313

heavy drinking, 310
legal consequences, 316
mental consequences, 314
moderate drinking, 310
pregnancy and, 313, 654
preventing use, 325–326
sexual activity, 311, 590, 633
social consequences, 314
support groups, 327
treating addiction, 326–327
violence, 318, 517
Alcoholics Anonymous (AA), 320, 327
alcohol poisoning, 312
alcohol use disorder, 308, 318–319, 327–328. *See also* alcohol
allergen, 385
allergic rhinitis, 385–386
allergies
bites and stings, 433
drug allergy, 337
first aid for, 433
respiratory, 385
ally. *See* upstanders
alveoli, 52
American Academy of Pediatrics, 28
American Cancer Society, 28
American Heart Association (AHA), 28, 428, 437
American Red Cross, 28, 50, 426, 428, 436–437
Americans with Disabilities Act (ADA) of 1990, 599
amino acids, 198–199
ammunition. *See* weapons
anabolic steroids, 342
anaerobic activity, 248–250, 267–268
anaphylaxis, 427, 433
anemia, 233, 571
anesthetics, 336
anger, 144–145. *See also* emotions
animal bites, 433
anorexia nervosa, 233
anti-anxiety medication, 177
antibiotic resistance, 376
antibiotics, 336, 370, 376, 586–587, 591, 593
antibodies, 61, 595, 598
antidepressants, 177
antihistamines, 429
antiperspirant, 76–77
antipsychotics, 177

antiretroviral therapy (ART), 594, 599–600
antisocial behavior, 165, 172
anus, 55, 57
anvil, ear, 67–68
anxiety. *See* anxiety disorders; stress
anxiety disorders
as a risk factor, 232
defined, 164, 166
generalized anxiety disorder (GAD), 166
panic attacks, 168
panic disorder, 168
phobias, 168
social anxiety disorder, 166–167
social media anxiety, 166–167
treatment, 176–177
aorta, 47, 49
appearance. *See* body image; hygiene
appendicitis, 58
appendix, 54–55, 58
appetite suppressants, 225
arachnophobia, 168
ARFID. *See* avoidant-restrictive food intake disorder (ARFID)
arousal, sexual, 618, 621
arsenic, 277, 451–452
arteriosclerosis, 380–381
artery, 46–47, 49
arthritis, 377–378, 388–389
asexual, 614
aspirin, 336, 451
assault, 529. *See also* sexual assault; violence
assertive communication, 480–483, 521
assisted living, 577
asthma, 281, 286, 384–385, 400
astigmatism, 87, 94
astraphobia, 168
atherosclerosis, 380–381
athlete's foot, 372
athletics. *See* physical activity
atrium, 47–48
attention-deficit hyperactivity disorder (ADHD), 164, 168–169, 177
attitude, 130, 133–134, 154. *See also* mental and emotional health

attraction, 506
atypical anorexia nervosa, 233
auditory canal, 67–68
autoimmune diseases, 377, 386, 388–389, 400
automated external defibrillator (AED), 427, 437–438
avoidant-restrictive food intake disorder (ARFID), 233
AWARxE Prescription Drug Safety Program, 359

B

BAC. *See* blood alcohol concentration (BAC)
back blows, 436
backbone. 42
bacteria, 371–372, 391, 450, 585
bad breath, 89, 91
balance, 506–507
barrier methods of contraception, 643–647
basal cell carcinoma, 81
batteries, 282, 450–451, 460
bed-wetting, 112
behavioral disorders, 171–172
behavioral factors. *See* lifestyle factors
behavioral treatment, 360
beliefs, 19, 130, 133–134
benign tumor, 381
best friends. *See* friendships
bias
evaluating information for, 29
weight-based, 231
biceps brachii, 44–45
bicycle. *See* biking
bifocals, 577
bigender, 613
biking, 257, 264, 317, 423–424
bile, 56
biological sex, 608–613, 615–616
binge drinking, 308, 310, 313. *See also* alcohol
binge-eating disorder, 231, 233
biodegradable, 455, 463
biotin, 84, 201
bipolar disorder, 164, 169–171, 177
birth control methods
birth control implant, 648–649

cartilage, 43–44
casual dating, 505–506
C.A.U.T.I.O.N. system for cancer detection, 382–383
cavities, 87, 89
CBD, 348
CDC. *See* Centers for Disease Control and Prevention (CDC)
cells, 16, 39
Centers for Disease Control and Prevention (CDC), 28, 220, 359, 431, 586, 598
central nervous system. *See* brain; spinal cord
central sleep apnea, 113
cerebellum, 62–64, 66, 311
cerebral cortex, 64, 311
cerebrum, 62, 64, 311
cervical cancer, 588–589
cervical cap, 644, 647
cervix, 552
chemicals
    pollution, 444, 446–457
    safe use, 453–454
    symbols, 453
    types of, 451–453
chemotherapy, 383
chewing tobacco, 279, 282
chicken pox, 372
child abuse, 527, 530–531
childcare, 655–657
child development, 559–562
Childhelp National Child Abuse Hotline, 533
child welfare agency, 534–535
chlamydia, 584–586, 590, 593
chloride, 202
choking, 428, 434–436
cholesterol, 197, 200, 221
chromium, 202
chromosomes, 16, 608–610. *See also* genetics
chronic diseases, 313, 378–389
chronic obstructive pulmonary disease (COPD), 384–385, 400
chronic stress, 151
cigarettes, 277–278, 280–281. *See also* tobacco
circadian rhythm, 102, 105–106, 245
circulatory system
    anatomy, 47–51

changes during adulthood, 576
defined, 46–47
diseases of, 380–381
effects of nicotine, 280
cirrhosis, 313
Civil Rights Act of 1991, 617
Civil Service Reform Act of 1978, 617
claustrophobia, 168
clavicle, 42
Clean Air Act, 456–457
clean energy, 455, 459
climate change, 448, 459–460
clinical depression, 164, 170. *See also* major depressive disorder
clique, 496, 501
clitoris, 552–553
closed adoption, 652
club drugs, 343, 352
cocaine, 343, 349, 351
cochlea, 68
codeine, 341
cold sores, 91
collaborative decision-making, 23–24
collagen, 41–43
collarbone. *See* clavicle
colon cancer, 381–382, 398
color blindness, 94–95
colorectal cancer. *See* colon cancer
combination pill, 647
combustible tobacco products, 277–278, 280–281
commercials. *See* advertisements; media
commitment, 477, 507
common cold, 372
communicable diseases
    conjunctivitis, 375
    defined, 370–371, 378
    influenza, 374
    mononucleosis, 374–375
    preventing, 391–396
    tonsillitis, 375
    transmission, 370, 373–374
    types of pathogens, 371–373
communication
    active listening, 480
    assertiveness, 480–483
    communication process, 474, 478
    communication skills, 479–483

feedback, 478
health promotion, 29–32
I-statements, 482–483
online communication, 420–423, 483
refusal skills, 25, 299–300, 325, 358–359, 590–591, 625-626
types of, 478–479, 483
community health, 31–32
community relationships, 475, 491, 518
community resources, 31–32, 327, 592, 656
community service, 17, 31
complex carbohydrates, 196–197
complications, of disease, 379, 386
composting, 455, 465–466
compromise, 485–486, 494
compulsion, 168–169
computers. *See* technology
concussion, 255, 260
condoms
    defined, 584, 590
    effectiveness, 591, 599, 644, 646
    how to use, 646
    pregnancy prevention, 644, 646
    STI prevention, 590–591, 599
    types of, 590–591, 644, 646
conduct disorder, 172
conflict management. *See* conflict resolution
conflict resolution
    compromise, 485–486, 494
    defined, 22, 26, 484
    importance of, 484
    mediation, 26, 486–487
    negotiation, 485–486
    peer mediation, 487
    sources of conflict, 25, 484
    steps of, 26, 485–486
conjunctivitis, 370, 375
connective tissue, 39
consent. *See* affirmative consent
conservation. *See* environmental health
constipation, 197, 233
Consumer Products Safety Commission, 28
contact lenses, 94

continuous positive airway pressure (CPAP) therapy, 113

contraception. *See* condoms; birth control methods; sexual abstinence

contraceptive sponge, 644, 646–647

co-occurring disorders, 233, 287, 291, 356

cooldowns, 268

coordination, 253–254

COPD. *See* chronic obstructive pulmonary disease (COPD)

copper, 202

copper intrauterine device (IUD), 649–650

cornea, 67

cortisol, 69

counselor, 30, 111, 158, 174, 176, 234, 300, 324, 328, 360–362, 419, 493, 504, 521, 535, 591, 614–615, 624, 630, 634

coxal bone, 42

CPAP therapy. *See* continuous positive airway pressure (CPAP) therapy

CPR. *See* cardiopulmonary resuscitation (CPR)

crack cocaine, 349, 351

cramps, menstrual, 553

cranium, 42

crimes, 518, 529, 538–541, 617, 630–631. *See also* violence

Crisis Text Line, 183

crush, 506

crystal meth, 350

culture, 14, 19–21, 133, 231, 490–491, 497–498

customs, 19

cuts, first aid for, 431–432

cyanocobalamin, 201

cyberbullying
    consequences of, 522, 524
    defined, 516, 522–523
    preventing, 420–423, 525–526, 538
    responding to, 420–423, 521, 524–525
    school violence, 537–538

cycle of abuse, 534

cynophobia, 168

D

dairy, 207

dandruff, 76, 85

date rape, 631. *See* rape; sexual assault

date rape drugs, 352

dating
    affirmative consent, 477, 628–629
    breakups, 509–510
    casual, 505–506
    exclusive, 505, 507
    group dating, 505, 508
    healthy versus unhealthy, 476–477, 506–507
    infatuation, 505–506
    passion, 505–506
    physical intimacy, 505, 507–508
    sexual abstinence, 507–508
    strategies for forming, 508–509
    violence, 529–530, 629–634

death and dying
    causes of, 309, 317, 336–337, 339, 341–342, 345, 349–353, 577
    grief, 185–186, 578
    hospice care, 577
    premature, 15
    suicide, 181–186

death of the tooth, 90

decibels, 96

decision-making
    about peer pressure, 569–570
    about sexual activity, 623–624, 656–658
    effect on health, 19–21, 559
    influences on, 137, 568–570
    process, 22–24, 324

deep breathing, 157

deforestation, 445

dehydration, 203, 233, 258

delayed sleep phase syndrome (DSPS), 109–111

deltoid, 44

dementia, 313, 587

dental caries. *See* cavities

dental health, 55–56, 88–93

dentin, 90

dentist, 88, 90–93

deodorant, 76–77

Department of Agriculture (USDA), 28, 205, 312

Department of Health and Human Services (HHS), 28, 205, 246

dependence, substance, 287, 293, 318, 341, 344

depressants, 308–309, 336, 341

depression. *See* major depressive disorder

dermatitis. *See* eczema

dermatologist, 12, 76, 79

dermis, 38, 40–41

detoxification, 320, 326, 360

development. *See* human development

developmental stages. *See* human life cycle

diabetes mellitus
    defined, 70, 377, 386
    family history, 16, 397
    preventing, 396, 400
    signs of, 388
    type 1, 386, 388
    type 2, 11, 387–388

diacetyl, 281–282

diaphragm, 46, 53

diaphragm, birth control, 644, 647

diet. *See* eating disorders; fad diets; nutrition

dietary fiber, 84, 194, 197

Dietary Guidelines for Americans, 204–206

diet pills, 223, 225, 342

difference of sex development (DSD), 610

digestion, 55–58

digestive system
    anatomy, 55–58
    changes during adulthood, 576
    defined, 54–55
    effects of nicotine, 280

digital citizenship, 417, 420

digital footprint, 417, 420

diphtheria, 396

direct transmission, 374

discrimination
    harassment, 518, 629–630
    HIV, 598–599
    LGBT+, 614, 616–617
    violence and, 517, 539–540
    weight-based, 231

diseases
    communicable, 59, 370–376

noncommunicable diseases, 379–380, 382, 396, 398

physical environment, 17

school environment, 30, 525

sexual orientation, 614

social environment, 18–19, 215, 229, 289, 321–324, 355

substance use, 289, 321–324, 355

environmental health

chemicals, 451–454

deforestation, 445

greener living, 461–466

greenhouse gases, 445

human impact, 445

laws affecting, 456–458

pollution, 446–450, 454

population, 445

protecting, 456–458

waste management, 445, 459–460

Environmental Protection Agency (EPA), 456–458

environmental protection hierarchy, 458–460

enzymes, 56, 61

EPA. *See* Environmental Protection Agency (EPA)

epidermis, 38, 40–41

epididymis, 551–552

e-pipe, 278

EpiPen, 433

equipment, sports and fitness, 256–257

erection, 552, 566, 620

escape plan, 406, 410–411

esophagus, 55–57

essential amino acid, 198–199

estrogen, 70, 552, 563, 567, 620

ethnicity. *See* race and ethnicity

eustress, 149, 151

executive function disorder (EFD), 168

exercise, 242, 244. *See also* physical activity

exhalation, 53

experimentation, substance use, 292, 318, 344

exploitation. *See* violence

explosives. *See* fire prevention and safety; weapons

extended-cycle birth control, 648

extended family, 488–489

external condom, 590, 640, 644, 646

external urethral sphincter, 59

eye contact, 478–480. *See also* nonverbal communication

eyelid, 67

eye protection, 257

eyes

anatomy, 67

bifocals, 577

common conditions, 94, 370, 375, 386

eyestrain, 93

protecting, 93

F

facial bones. *See* cranium

fad diets, 217, 223, 225

fallopian tube, 552–553

falls, 317, 407

FAM. *See* fertility awareness method (FAM)

families

coping with changes, 495

defined, 489

functions of, 489–491

parents and guardians, 491–493

sibling relationships, 488, 493–494

substance use, 289, 321–324, 355

types of, 489

violence, 517, 529–532

family history, 16, 165, 379–380, 386, 396–397. *See also* genetics

family therapy, 173, 176

farsightedness, 87, 94

FASD. *See* fetal alcohol spectrum disorder (FASD)

fats, 194, 199–200

fat-soluble vitamins, 201

FDA. *See* Food and Drug Administration (FDA)

feces, 57

feedback, 474, 478, 480

feelings. *See* emotions; mental and emotional health

female condom. *See* internal condom

female reproductive system, 552–553, 567–568

female sterilization, 651

feminine, 611. *See* gender

femur, 42–43

fentanyl, 341, 343, 351

fertility awareness method (FAM), 649

fertilization, 550, 553–554, 623

fertilizer, 449–450

fetal alcohol spectrum disorder (FASD), 313

fetal stage, 555

fetus, 550, 555, 641

fever blister. *See* cold sores

fiber. *See* dietary fiber

fibula, 42

fight-or-flight response, 149, 152

fights. *See* conflict resolution; violence

financial abuse, 527–528, 532

fine-motor skills, 561

firearms. *See* weapons

fire prevention and safety, 409–411

fire triangle, 406, 409

first aid

bites and stings, 433

burns, 434

cardiopulmonary resuscitation (CPR), 437–438

choking, 435–436

cuts, scrapes, puncture wounds, 431–432

defined, 427–428

electrical shock, 434

first-aid kits, 427–429

severe bleeding, 432

shock, 432

standard precautions, 431

fitness. *See* physical activity

fitness equipment, 256–257

fitness tracker, 262

FITT. *See* frequency, intensity, time, and type (FITT)

five-and-five method, 436

flashbacks, 169

flexibility, 251, 253, 262

floods, 412–413, 450

flu. *See* influenza

fluorescent light bulb, 462

fluoride, 88, 202

flu shot, 15, 396

folic acid, 201

follicle, 552–553

follicle-stimulating hormone, 620

food. *See also* nutrition
    choices, 214–215
        food safety, 216, 390, 394–395
        influence on health, 9, 77, 88, 119, 210–211
        preparing, 215
        reducing waste, 463
Food and Drug Administration (FDA), 28, 200, 213, 277
foodborne illness, 216
food diary, 226
food groups, 206–208
food poisoning, 216, 371–372
food preferences, 215
food safety and sanitation, 216, 390, 394–395
football, 257
fossil fuels, 445, 455, 459–460
foster care, 534, 577
foster family, 489
fracture, 255, 260
frequency, intensity, time, and type (FITT), 261, 264–265
friendships
    changes affecting, 502–503
    cliques, 496, 501
    defined, 496–497
    effect on health, 134, 297, 475–476, 498, 518
    face-to-face communication, 499
    gossip and rumors, 500
    healthy, 297, 476–477
    jealousy, 501–502
    online, 420–421, 483, 496, 498–499
    peer pressure, 289, 503–504, 569–570
    social health, 9
    strategies for building, 498–500
    toxic, 297, 477
    types of, 497–498
frontal lobe, 63–64, 311
frostbite, 255, 259
fruit, 206
fungi, 372–373

G

GAD. *See* generalized anxiety disorder (GAD)
gallbladder, 54–56
gangs, 518, 536, 538–539

gastrocnemius, 44
gastroenterologist, 12
gastroesophageal reflux disease, 280
gay. *See* homosexuality; LGBT+
gender
    defined, 608, 611
    expectations, 611
    identity, 613–614
    roles, 608, 611
gender binary, 611
gender expression, 613
gender identity, 608–609, 613–614, 616–617
gender stereotypes, 611
generalized anxiety disorder (GAD), 166
genes, 14, 16, 614
genetics
    body composition, 219
    development, 558–559
    genetic makeup, 16–17
    influence on health, 15–17, 165, 288, 379–380, 382, 398
    reproduction, 553
genetically modified organisms (GMOs), 213
genital herpes, 584–585, 588, 590, 593
genital warts, 588
germinal stage, 554
germs. *See* pathogens
GHB (gamma hydroxybutyrate), 352
gingivitis, 87, 90
glands, 39, 56, 68–70
global warming. *See* climate change
glucagon, 69–70
glucose, 196–197
gluteus maximus, 45
gluteus medius, 45
GMOs. *See* genetically modified organisms (GMOs)
goal setting
    defined, 22–23
    physical activity, 263–265
    setting and achieving, 24–25
    SMART goals, 22, 24–25, 263
    weight management, 222
gonadotropin-releasing hormone, 619–620
gonorrhea, 584–586, 590, 593

gossip, 500, 518–519
grains, 206–207
grandparents, 489
gratitude, 139, 146–147
gray matter. *See* cerebral cortex
greater vestibular gland, 552
greenhouse gases, 445, 448
green products, 455, 463
grief, 186, 578
grooming, human trafficking, 539
grooming, personal. *See* hygiene
gross-motor skills, 561
group dating, 505, 508
growth hormone, 619
growth spurt, 618, 620
gum disease, 89
gums, 88
guns. *See* weapons

H

hacking, 417, 420
hair, 40–41, 83–85
hair follicle, 40–41
halitosis, 91
hallucinogens, 343, 350, 352
hammer, ear, 67–68
hamstring, 45
Hands-Only CPR, 437
hand washing, 392–394
hangnail, 86
hangover, 312
harassment, 516, 518, 629–630
hate crime, 536, 539–540, 617
hay fever, 385–386
hazards. *See* safety
hazing, 516, 518–519
health
    aspects of, 7–10
    defined, 6–7
    effect on life expectancy, 15, 558
    factors affecting, 15–21
    healthcare, 10–13
    interrelatedness, 10
healthcare
    access to, 13
    defined, 6, 10
    insurance, 12–13
    preventive, 10
    services, 11–12
    settings, 12

incus. *See* anvil
indirect transmission, 374, 394
individuality, 506
individual therapy, 173, 176
infancy, 560
infatuation, 505–506
infection control. *See*
    communicable diseases;
    standard precautions
infectious disease. *See*
    communicable diseases
infertility, 586
influences on health. *See*
    protective factors; risk factors
influenza, 370, 372, 374, 396
ingrown toenail, 86
inhalants, 343, 352–353
inhalation, 53
inhibition, 308, 311
injuries
    medical emergencies, 434–438
    responding to, 430
    treatment, 259–260, 431–434
inner conflict, 150
inpatient treatment, 12, 173, 177,
    360
insect bites and stings, 433
insomnia, 109, 111, 629
insulin, 69–70. *See also* diabetes
    mellitus
insurance, health, 12–13
integumentary system
    anatomy, 40–41
    defined, 38, 49
    diseases of, 78–81, 83–85
intellectual development
    adolescence, 567–568
    defined, 558
    early childhood, 559–561
    middle childhood, 561–562
intensity, 261, 263
internal condom, 590, 640, 644,
    646
internal urethral sphincter, 59
Internet predator, 417, 420
Internet safety
    cyberbullying, 522–526
    online behavior, 420
    online communication, 483
    online relationships, 421, 498
    privacy, 420–421
    sexting, 421, 423, 622

thinking before posting, 421,
    423
interneuron, 63
interpersonal communication.
    See communication
interpersonal skills, 474, 477. *See
    also* communication; conflict
    resolution
intersex, 610
intestine, 55–58
intimacy, 505, 507–508
intimate partner violence, 527,
    529–530
intrauterine device (IUD), 649
iodine, 202
iris, 67
iron, 84, 202–203, 208
iron deficiency, 210
I-statements, 144, 482–483
IUD. *See* intrauterine device (IUD)

J

James, Josh, 113
jealousy, 501–502, 623
jet lag, 102, 106
jock itch, 372
joints, 38, 43–44, 388–389
jumping rope, 264
juvenile diabetes. *See* type 1
    diabetes mellitus

K

Kaposi's sarcoma, 597
keratin, 41, 85
kidneys, 54, 58, 386
kissing. *See* dating
kissing disease. *See*
    mononucleosis
kneecap. *See* patella; sesamoid
    bone

L

labium majus, 552–553
labium minus, 552–553
lacto-ovo vegetarian, 199
lactose, 207
lactose intolerance, 207
lacto-vegetarian, 199
lambskin condom, 591, 644
Land Revitalization Program, 458

landfills, 445, 450, 460, 463
large intestine, 55, 57–58
larynx, 51–52
LASIK (laser in-situ
    keratomileusis), 94
lead, 277, 451
LED light bulb, 462
lens, of eye, 67
lesbian. *See* homosexuality;
    LGBT+
leukoplakia, 282
LGBT+
    defined, 615
    discrimination, 616–617
    gender identity, 613–614
    homophobia, 616–617
    sexual orientation, 614–615
    support for, 617
lice, 76, 85
life expectancy, 556–558
life span, 556–557
lifestyle factors
    influence on health, 19–21
    noncommunicable diseases,
        379–380, 382, 396
    nutrition, 210–211
    physical activity, 244
    sleep, 103–104
ligaments, 38, 43–44, 259
liquor. *See* alcohol
liver, 54–56, 313, 576
long-term goal, 24
long-term non-progressors, 594,
    597
loss. *See* death and dying; grief
love, 506. *See* dating; romantic
    relationships
lower respiratory system, 52
lung cancer, 281, 381–382, 398
lung diseases, 378–379, 384–386
lungs, 51–53
luteinizing hormone, 620
lymph, 60
lymph nodes, 59–60
lymphatic system, 54, 59, 280

M

magazines. *See* media
magnesium, 202, 208
major depressive disorder
    defined, 164, 170
    drug abuse, 347

schizophrenia spectrum
disorder, 172
substance use disorders, 288,
290–294, 318–319, 341, 345
therapy, 173, 176
treatment options, 176–177
mercury, 451
metabolic syndrome, 221
metacarpals, 42
metatarsals, 42
methadone, 342
methamphetamine, 343, 349
methane, 445
methanol, 277
meth mouth, 350
microorganisms, 371, 391. *See
also* communicable diseases;
pathogens
middle adulthood, 572–575
middle childhood, 556–557,
561–562
milestones, 556–557
mindfulness, 158, 167, 225
mindfulness-based stress
reduction (MBSR), 158
minerals, 184, 202–203
miscarriage, 653–654
moderate drinking, 308, 310
Molly. *See* MDMA
molybdenum, 202
mono. *See* mononucleosis
mononucleosis, 370, 374–375, 585
mood disorders
bipolar disorder, 170–171
major depressive disorder,
169–170
seasonal affective disorder
(SAD), 170
treating, 176–177
mood stabilizer, 177
morphine, 342
motor neuron, 63
motor vehicles
energy-efficient, 466
pollutants, 456, 459
motor vehicle accidents
alcohol and, 316–317
marijuana and, 348
preventing, 423–425
mouth and teeth
care, 88–89
common conditions, 89–93
digestive system, 55–57

respiratory system, 51, 53
mouth guard, 257
mucus, 51–52
mumps, 372
muscle endurance, 250–251, 262
muscle flexibility, 250–251
muscle pairs, 45
muscle strength, 250, 253, 262,
399, 576–577
muscle tissue, 39, 45
muscular system, 38, 40, 44–45
mutual consent. *See* affirmative
consent
mutual respect, 477
mycoses, 373
MyPlate food guidance system,
204, 206–209

N

nails, 40–41, 85–86
naphthalene, 277
napping, 114, 116–118
narcolepsy, 109, 114
Narcotics Anonymous, 361
National Domestic Violence
Hotline, 533
National Eating Disorders
Association Helpline, 234, 236
National Emergency Number,
182
National Highway Traffic Safety
Administration, 28
National Institute of Mental
Health, 28
National Institute on Drug Abuse
(NIDA), 28, 348, 359
National Sexual Assault Hotline,
633
National Suicide Prevention
Lifeline, 179, 183
National Teen Dating Abuse
Hotline, 533
natural disasters, 406, 412–414,
450
nearsightedness, 87, 94
neglect, 527, 530–532
negotiation, 485–486
nerve tissue, 39
nervous system
anatomy, 62–68
changes during adulthood, 576
defined, 62–63

diseases of, 386
effects of substances on, 280,
311, 313, 341, 344
neurologist, 12
neuron, 62–63
niacin, 201, 208
nicotine
addiction, 291–294
defined, 276–277
effect on mental health, 166,
284
health effects, 279–280, 380
mental, social, and legal
consequences, 284–285
tobacco products, 277–279
treating addiction, 300–302
nicotine gum, 301
nicotine lozenges, 301
nicotine patch, 301
nicotine replacement, 295, 301
NIDA. *See* National Institute on
Drug Abuse (NIDA)
night eating syndrome, 233
night-light, 115, 122
nightmares, 112
night owl syndrome, 110. *See also*
delayed sleep phase syndrome
(DSPS)
nitrogen dioxide, 457
noise pollution, 454
noncombustible tobacco
products, 278–279, 281–282
noncommunicable diseases
arthritis, 388–389
cancer, 381–383
chronic respiratory diseases,
384–385
defined, 377–378
diabetes mellitus, 386–388
factors affecting, 379–380
heart disease, 380–381
preventing, 396–400
nonessential amino acids, 198–199
non-GMO foods, 213
noninfectious diseases. *See*
noncommunicable diseases
nonverbal communication
awareness of, 483
defined, 474, 478
eye contact, 479–481
online communication, 479,
483
using, 478–479

nucleus, 16
nurse practitioner, 11
nursing home, 577
nutrient-dense foods, 204–205, 212
nutrients
  carbohydrates, 196–197
  defined, 194–195
  digestion, 56–57
  fats, 199–200
  minerals, 202–203
  proteins, 198–199
  vitamins, 200–201
  water, 203
nutrition
  facts and food labels, 213
  guidelines, 205–208
  hair and, 83
  influence on health, 8, 19–21, 210–211, 559
  nutrients, 195–203
  pregnancy, 209
  skills for good nutrition, 211–216
Nutrition Facts label, 213

O

oatmeal, 197
obesity
  defined, 217, 220
  diabetes and, 387
  during childhood, 561
  health effects, 221
  physical activity, 243–244
OBGYN. *See* obstetrician/gynecologist (OBGYN)
obsession, 168–169
obsessive-compulsive disorder (OCD), 168–169, 177
obstetrician/gynecologist (OBGYN), 550, 553, 655
obstructive sleep apnea, 113
occipital lobe, 63–64, 66–67, 311
occupational post-exposure prophylaxis (oPEP), 600
OCD. *See* obsessive-compulsive disorder (OCD)
ODD. *See* oppositional defiant disorder (ODD)
Office of the Surgeon General, 28, 279–280
oil gland, 41

older adulthood, 572, 574–577
omega-3, 84
oncologist, 12, 383
online communication, 421, 423, 479, 483, 499, 526
online relationships, 421, 496, 498
online safety
  cyberbullying, 522–526
  hacking, 420
  identity theft, 420
  Internet predators, 420–421
  positive behavior, 420
  privacy, 420–421
  sexting, 421, 423, 622
  thinking before you post, 421, 423, 526
open adoption, 652
oPEP. *See* occupational post-exposure prophylaxis (oPEP)
ophidiophobia, 168
opioids
  abuse and addiction, 342, 358
  defined, 341–342
  effects on the brain, 341
  overdose, 351
  purpose of, 336
  symptoms of abuse, 341
  types of, 341
opportunistic infections, 594, 597
oppositional defiant disorder (ODD), 172
optimism, 139, 145, 148
optometrist, 87, 93
oral contraceptives, 640, 647–648
oral health, 88–93. *See also* mouth and teeth
oral thermometer, 429
organ, body, 39–40, 551
organic foods, 213
orthodontist, 87, 90
orthopedist, 12
orthorexia, 232
OSFED. *See* otherwise specified feeding or eating disorder (OSFED)
ossicles, 68
osteoarthritis, 389
osteoporosis, 280
OTC. *See* over-the-counter (OTC) medications
otherwise specified feeding or eating disorder (OSFED), 233
outer ear. *See* pinna

outpatient treatment, 12, 354, 360
ova. *See* egg, human
ovarian cyst, 567
ovaries, 69–70, 552–553
overbite, 90
over-the-counter (OTC)
  medications, 334, 336–339, 341, 429
overdose
  alcohol poisoning, 312
  defined, 334, 341
  drug abuse, 345
  medication abuse, 341
  opioids, 351
  symptoms of, 312, 341
overnutrition, 204, 210–211
overweight
  body-fat distribution, 221
  defined, 217, 220
  diabetes mellitus, 387
  physical activity, 243–244
ovo-vegetarian, 199
ovulation, 550, 553
ozone, 444, 448, 457

P

padding, 257
pancreas, 55–56, 69–70
panic attack, 168
panic disorder, 168
pantothenic acid, 201
parasites, 450
parasomnia, 109, 111–112
parathyroid gland, 69
parathyroid hormone (PTH), 69
parenthood, 570–571, 651–652
parents and guardians, 491–493. *See also* families
parietal lobe, 63–64, 311
particulate matter, 447. *See also* air pollution
passion, 505–506
passive communication, 480, 482–483
patella, 42–43
pathogens, 370–373, 391, 585. *See also* communicable diseases
Patient Protection and Affordable Care Act (ACA), 12
pectoralis major, 44
pedestrian safety, 417, 423–424
pediatrician, 12

protective factors
  body image, 229–232
  defined, 14, 17
  eating disorders, 232–233
  environmental, 17–19
  food choices, 214–215
  genetic, 16–17
  lifestyle, 19–21
  noncommunicable diseases,
    379–380
  substance use, 288–291,
    321–324, 355–356
  suicide, 181–183
protein, 84, 194, 198–199, 208
protozoa, 373, 376, 584–585, 587.
  See also communicable diseases;
  pathogens
PSA. *See* public service
  announcement (PSA)
psychiatrist, 12
psychological abuse, 528
psychological dependence, 293,
  310
psychologist, 158, 176
PTH. *See* parathyroid hormone
  (PTH)
PTSD. *See* post-traumatic stress
  disorder (PTSD)
puberty, 551, 563–567, 619–622
public health department, 592
public service announcement
  (PSA), 295, 297, 359
public transportation, 423–425
pulmonologist, 12
pulp cavity, 90
pulse, 261–262
puncture wound, 431–432
pupil, 67
purging, 228, 233
pyridoxine, 201

Q

quadriceps, 44

R

race and ethnicity
  identity, 133
  influence on BAC, 311
  influence on body image,
    231, 235

valuing diversity, 497–498,
  525, 533, 540, 616
radiation therapy, 383
radius, 42
rape, 352, 529, 627, 630. *See also*
  sexual assault
reaction time, 253–254
rectum, 55, 57
recycling, 455, 458–460
red blood cells, 49, 51
refined grains, 206–207
reflective gear, 257
reflex, 66
refusal skills
  defined, 22, 25
  sexual activity and
    abstinence, 590–591, 625
  sexting, 423
  substance use, 299–300, 325,
    358–360, 590
Rehabilitation Act of 1973, 599
rehabilitation program, 354,
  360–361
rejuvenate, 104
relapse, disease, 379
relapse, substance use, 354, 361
relationships
  dating, 505–510
  defined, 474–475
  family, 182, 475, 488–493, 495
  friendships, 496–504
  healthy versus unhealthy,
    476–477, 506–507
  influence on health, 17, 148,
    150, 245, 297, 475–476
  influence on human
    development, 559
  online, 421, 498
  skills for relationships, 478–487
  types of, 475
relaxation response, 149, 152
relaxation techniques, 120, 153,
  157–158
religious practices, 19–20
REM (rapid eye movement)
  sleep, 102, 106–107
remission, 378
renewable energy, 455, 459
reproductive system
  caring for, 566–567, 589–593,
    655
  changes during adulthood,
    576, 654

defined, 550–551
  female, 552–553, 567–568, 576
  male, 551–552, 576
rescue breaths, 437
residential treatment program,
  354, 360
resilience, 139, 148
resistance, 152, 248, 250
*Resource Conservation and
  Recovery Act*, 457
respect, 506
respiration, 46, 53, 279
respiratory diseases
  allergies, 385–386
  asthma, 384–385
  chronic obstructive
    pulmonary disease
    (COPD), 385
  preventing, 396, 400
respiratory etiquette, 390, 394
respiratory system, 40
  anatomy, 51–53
  changes during adulthood, 576
  defined, 46, 51, 384
  diseases of, 384–386
  effects of nicotine, 280–281
response substitution, 295, 302
responsibility, 492
restless leg syndrome (RLS), 112
restricted eating, 233
retina, 67
retirement, 575
retirement community, 577
reusing, 458–460
rheumatoid arthritis, 389
rheumatologist, 12
riboflavin, 201, 208
ribs, 42
R.I.C.E. treatment, 259
ringworm, 372
risk factors
  body image, 229–232
  defined, 14, 17
  eating disorders, 232–233
  environmental, 17–19
  food choices, 214–215
  genetic, 16–17
  lifestyle, 19–21
  noncommunicable diseases,
    379–380
  substance use, 288–291,
    321–324, 355–356
  suicide, 181–183

Special Supplemental Nutrition Program for Women, Infants, and Children (WIC), 657
speedballing, 351
sperm, 551, 553–554, 641
spermicide, 644, 646–647
SPF. *See* sun protection factor (SPF)
sphincter, 56, 59
spinal cord, 62–63, 66
spine, 42
spiritual practices, 19–20
spleen, 54, 58–59, 61
split nail, 86
sports. *See* physical activity
sports equipment, 256–257
sportsmanship, 256
spousal violence, 529
sprain, 255
squamous cell carcinoma, 81
stalking, 516, 518
standard precautions, 427, 431
stapes. *See* stirrup, ear
staph infection, 372
starches. *See* complex carbohydrates
statutory rape, 627, 630. *See also* rape; sexual assault
stent, 381
stepfamily, 489
stereotypes, 231, 496, 498
sterilization, 640, 650–651
sternocleidomastoid, 44
sternum, 42–43
STI. *See* sexually transmitted infections (STI)
stigma, 173, 177
stimulants, 177, 336, 342
stimulus control, 295, 302
stirrup, ear, 67–68
stomach, 55–57
strain, 259
stranger, 417, 419
stress
    bodily response, 151–152
    defined, 149–150
    influence on health, 17, 20, 132, 142, 182, 185, 356
    post-traumatic stress disorder (PTSD), 169, 531, 632
    sources of, 150–151, 454, 495
    strategies for managing, 143, 152–158, 245

substance use, 297, 356
    types of, 150
stressor, 149–150
stretching, muscle, 250–251, 264
stroke, 378–379, 381
Substance Abuse and Mental Health Services Administration (SAMHSA), 361
substance use
    addiction, 294
    alcohol, 309–319
    drug abuse, 344–353
    factors affecting, 288–291, 321–324, 355–356
    medication abuse, 339–342
    overdose, 312, 341
    preventing, 296–300, 325–326, 356–360
    substance use disorder, 291–294
    tobacco products, 277–286
substance use disorders
    alcohol use disorder, 318–319
    co-occurring disorders, 166, 291
    defined, 287, 291
    drugs, 344
    helping someone get treatment, 327–328, 361–362
    medications, 341
    nicotine, 291–294
    stages of, 291–294, 344
    treatment, 300–302, 326–327, 360–361
sugar, 196, 205–206, 211–212, 399
suicide
    defined, 180
    factors affecting, 181–182, 233
    helping someone get treatment, 178–179
    helping survivors, 180, 185–186
    hospital supervision, 177
    preventing, 183, 185
    substance use, 317, 341
    warning signs of, 184
suicide cluster, 180, 182
suicide contagion, 180, 182
sulfur, 202
sulfur dioxide, 457
sunburn, 78, 80–81
sunlight
    energy source, 459

seasonal affective disorder (SAD), 170
    skin cancer, 80–81, 382, 398
    sleep and, 122
sun protection factor (SPF), 81
sun safety, 78–81, 382, 398
Supplemental Nutrition Assistance Program (SNAP), 215
support groups, 173, 176, 327, 354, 361, 656
surgeon, 12
surgery, 383
sustainability, 455, 461
sweat gland, 40–41
swimming
    accidental death, 317
    calories burned, 264
    eye protection, 257
    safety, 425–426
synergism, 336
synthetic cannabinoids, 348
synthetic marijuana, 348
syphilis, 584–585, 587, 590, 593

T

tablets. *See* technology
tar, 276–277, 280–281
target heart rate, 261, 267
tarsals, 42
taste. *See* sensory organs
tattoo, 78, 83
Tdap vaccine, 396
tears, 67
teasing, 232
technology
    analyzing media, 27–29, 80, 234–235, 298–299
    blue light, 102, 106, 122
    cyberbullying, 523–526
    evaluating health information, 27–29
    heart rate monitors and fitness trackers, 262
    limiting screen time, 223, 499
    media influence, 215, 229–232, 234, 236, 290–291, 324, 355
    online communication, 421, 423, 479, 483, 499, 526
    online safety, 420–422
    stressor, 150

teen pregnancy and parenthood
　　challenges of, 655–657
　　factors affecting, 654
　　resources for, 657
teeth. *See* mouth and teeth
teeth grinding, 91, 112
television. *See* media
temper tantrum, 556, 560
temperature, 66. *See also* sensory
　　organs
temporal lobe, 63–64, 311
tendon, 38, 44
terminal illness, 379
terrorism, 536, 541
testes, 69–70, 551–552, 564
testosterone, 50, 551, 563–564, 620
tetanus, 396, 431
texting
　　online communication, 421,
　　　423, 479, 483, 499, 526
　　sexting, 421, 423, 622
　　while driving, 15, 425
　　while walking, 423–424
thalamus, 66
THC, 348
therapist, 138, 158, 173–174, 176,
　　234, 535, 615
therapy, mental health, 173, 176
thiamin, 201, 208
thirdhand aerosol, 276, 285–286
thirdhand smoke, 276, 285–286
throat. *See* pharynx
thrush, 597
thymus, 59, 61, 69
thyroid gland, 69
thyroid hormone, 62, 69
tibia, 42–43
tibialis anterior, 44
tidal wave, 450
time management, 153, 155–156
tinnitus, 87, 96
tissue, 39
tobacco
　　cigarettes, 277–278, 280–281
　　defined, 276–277
　　factors affecting use, 288–291,
　　　517
　　health effects on others, 285
　　health effects on self, 77,
　　　279–283, 399–400
　　legal consequences, 284–285
　　mental consequences, 284
　　oral health, 88

preventing use, 296–300
smokeless tobacco, 279, 282
social consequences, 284
tobacco products, 277–279
treating addiction and
　　quitting, 300–302
vaping, 278–279, 281–282
toddler, 560
tolerance, substance use, 287,
　　292–293, 318–319, 337, 344
tongue, 56
tonsillitis, 370, 375
tonsils, 59, 61
tooth decay, 89–90
tornado, 412–413
touch. *See* sensory organs
toxic substances. *See* carcinogens;
　　poisoning
toxic shock syndrome (TSS), 567
toxic stress, 149, 151
trachea, 51–52
traditions, 488, 490
tranquilizers. *See* depressants
trans fats, 194, 199–200
transfusion, 50
transgender, 608, 613–614
trapezius, 44
trauma, 149, 151, 232
trees, planting, 465
triceps brachii, 44
trichomoniasis, 584–585, 587,
　　589–590, 593
triggers, 287, 293
trust, 477, 623
tryptophan, 115, 119
TSS. *See* toxic shock syndrome
　　(TSS)
tsunamis, 450
tubal ligation, 651
tuberculosis, 597
Tufts University Health &
　　Nutrition Letter, 28
tumors, 377, 381. *See also* cancer
TV. *See* media
type 1 diabetes mellitus, 386, 388,
　　400
type 2 diabetes mellitus
　　defined, 388
　　factors affecting, 210, 212,
　　　221, 400
　　physical activity, 243–244
　　signs of, 388
typhoon, 450

U

ulcer, 280
ulna, 42
ultrafine particles, 281
ultraviolet (UV) light, 78, 81
umbilical cord, 554–555
underage drinking, 315. *See also*
　　alcohol
underbite, 90
undernutrition, 204, 210
understanding, 477
underweight, 217, 220–221
unemployment, 17, 518
unhealthy relationships, 476–477.
　　See also violence
universal donor, 50
unsaturated fats, 194, 199–200
upstanders, 516, 521, 524–526
ureter, 59
urethra, 59, 551
urinary bladder, 551
urinary system, 54, 58–59, 576
urinary tract, 576
urine, 58–59. *See also* bladder;
　　kidneys
urologist, 12
USDA. *See* Department of
　　Agriculture (USDA)
uterus, 552–554

V

vaccines
　　common, 396
　　defined, 390, 395
　　how they work, 395
　　human papillomavirus
　　　(HPV), 589
vagina, 59, 552–554
vaginal ring, 640, 648–649
values, 19, 23, 133–134
valves, heart, 47–48
vaping
　　factors affecting, 288–291
　　health effects, 281–282, 345
　　marijuana, 348
　　mental, social, and legal
　　　consequences, 284–285
　　myths and facts, 283
　　nicotine, 279–280, 291–294
　　preventing, 296–300
　　quitting, 300–302